*Fourth Edition*

# UNDERSTANDING PHARMACOLOGY
## for Health Professionals

## Susan M. Turley
*MA(Educ), BSN, RN, RHIT, CMT*

## Pearson

Boston   Columbus   Indianapolis   New York   San Francisco   Upper Saddle River
Amsterdam   Cape Town   Dubai   London   Madrid   Milan   Munich   Paris   Montreal   Toronto
Delhi   Mexico City   Sao Paulo   Sydney   Hong Kong   Seoul   Singapore   Taipei   Tokyo

**Library of Congress Cataloging-in-Publication Data**

Turley, Susan M.
  Understanding pharmacology for health professionals / Susan M. Turley—4th ed.
    p. ; cm.
  Includes bibliographical references and index.
  ISBN-13: 978-0-13-514570-8
  ISBN-10: 0-13-514570-8
  1. Pharmacology. 2. Allied health personnel. I. Title.
  [DNLM: 1. Pharmaceutical Preparations. 2. Drug Therapy.
QV 55 T941ua 2010]
  RM300.T85 2010
  615'.1—dc22

                                                        2009000027

Notice: The author and the publisher of this volume have taken care that the information and technical recommendations contained herein are based on research and expert consultation, and are accurate and compatible with the standards generally accepted at the time of publication. Nevertheless, as new information becomes available, changes in clinical and technical practices become necessary. The reader is advised to carefully consult manufacturers' instructions and information material for all supplies and equipment before use, and to consult with a healthcare professional as necessary. This advice is especially important when using new supplies or equipment for clinical purposes. The author and publisher disclaim all responsibility for any liability, loss, injury, or damage incurred as a consequence, directly or indirectly, of the use and application of any of the contents of this volume.

**Publisher:** Julie Levin Alexander
**Publisher's Assistant:** Regina Bruno
**Editor-in-Chief:** Mark Cohen
**Development Editor:** Melissa Kerian
**Assistant Editor:** Nicole Ragonese
**Director of Marketing:** Karen Allman
**Executive Marketing Manager:** Katrin Beacom
**Marketing Specialist:** Michael Sirinides
**Marketing Assistant:** Judy Noh
**Managing Production Editor:** Patrick Walsh
**Production Liaison:** Christina Zingone
**Production Editor:** Kate Boilard, Laserwords Maine
**Senior Media Editor:** Amy Peltier
**Media Project Manager:** Lorena Cerisano

**Manufacturing Manager:** Ilene Sanford
**Manufacturing Buyer:** Pat Brown
**Senior Art Director:** Maria Guglielmo
**Interior Designer:** Nesbitt Graphics Inc.
**Cover Designer:** Anthony Gemmellaro
**Manager, Rights and Permissions:** Zina Arabia
**Manager, Visual Research:** Beth Brenzel
**Manager, Cover Visual Research
  and Permissions:** Karen Sanatar
**Image Permission Coordinator:** Angelique Sharps
**Composition:** Laserwords India
**Printing and Binding:** Courier/Kendallville
**Cover Printer:** Lehigh Phoenix
**Cover Image:** Istockphoto/Curt Pickens

All drug names/brands are owned and trademarked by their respective companies.

10  9  8  7  6  5  4  3  2  1

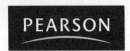

www.pearsonhighered.com

ISBN-13: 978-0-13-514570-8
ISBN-10: 0-13-514570-8

## Dedication

*To my husband Al for his support and love*

*To our children Daniel, Minh, and Lien*

# Contents

## Unit One — The Past History, Present Uses, and Future of Drugs   1

## Unit Two — Drugs by Body Systems   97

# *Foreword*

The classical Greek word *pharmakon*, on which the word *pharmacology* is based, has three related meanings: *charm*, *poison*, and *remedy*. These variant senses of the word spotlight important aspects of the history of pharmacology.

In the prescientific age, issues of cause and effect were frequently assumed without experimental proof. What we now call superstition and magic took the place of more rational modes of thought and action. Primitive healers used natural substances of animal, vegetable, and mineral origin with boundless confidence in their power to cure, even though objective evidence of their efficacy was lacking. And we can be sure that many cures took place through the power of suggestion, a potent force still recognized today as the "placebo effect."

But if some patients recovered after dosing with crude, prehistoric remedies, others were killed outright. It cannot have escaped the early medicine men—or their patients—that some "medicines" were more useful for getting rid of enemies (or inconvenient friends) than for treating the sick. Hence, the second meaning of the word *pharmakon*. Even today, the toxicity of drugs is a major problem, for some of our most effective drugs also have the narrowest margins of safety.

Only after centuries of observation and experimentation has medical science achieved an understanding of the way drugs work and a sound basis for their safe and effective use. The third sense of *pharmakon*, a sense hedged about with a great deal of wishful thinking in primitive times, has thus largely been realized today. And yet, in many ways, we have only scratched the surface.

Many medicines achieve their effects not by neatly eliminating or neutralizing the source of symptoms but by inducing abnormalities in body chemistry or function that tend to offset the abnormalities caused by the disease. Except for a few naturally occurring enzymes, hormones, vitamins, and minerals, most substances administered as medicines are foreign to the body and are therefore capable of causing annoying side effects and allergic reactions. Clearly, this state of affairs leaves much to be desired and presents a continuing challenge to pharmacologic chemists and clinical researchers.

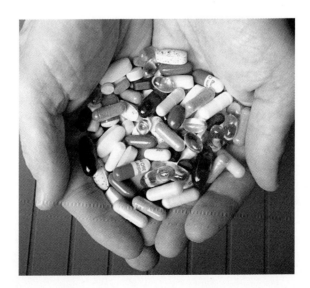

> The fact that we don't have a single perfect drug, much less a panacea or cure-all, accounts for the staggering multitude and diversity of imperfect drugs in current use.
>
> —John H. Dirckx, M.D.

The great number and variety of drugs are apt to prove daunting at first sight to the student or health professional who undertakes the study of pharmacology. I, as a physician, am sometimes asked, "How can you possibly remember all those drugs?" The answer is simple: I can't, and neither can anyone else. The typical practicing physician has a working knowledge of just one or two drugs in each pharmacologic category—perhaps more in categories pertaining to his or her specialty, perhaps none in categories he or she never has occasion to prescribe. Once a physician is fully familiar with the characteristics, indications, side effects, and doses of one drug in a pharmacologic category, similar information about all the others in the same category would be excess baggage.

Just as the range of useful information for the practicing physician doesn't include the whole field of pharmacology, students in health care don't need to memorize huge masses of information or endless lists of drugs. What they need is a good general understanding of how various kinds of drugs work, their potentials and limitations, some of the reasons for their number and diversity, and the rationale behind their bewildering and often tongue-twisting names.

This is exactly the kind of mental database that *Understanding Pharmacology for Health Professionals* will give you. The author, drawing from her diversified background in nursing, medical transcription, health information management, and healthcare education at the college level, has produced a clear, well-organized, stimulating textbook that takes the student step by step through the whole subject of pharmacology without going into needless complexities or irrelevant details. The facts are accurate and up to date, and their logical connections are presented with clarity. Historical sidelights and pertinent illustrations keep the interest level high. A comprehensive drug reference (Appendix D) at the end of the textbook gives capsule information about all current prescription drugs and many over-the-counter drugs, as well as their pronounciations.

*Understanding Pharmacology for Health Professions* is not only a superb introductory textbook but is a reference work that you will consult often and with profit.

—*John H. Dirckx, M.D.*

# *Preface*

This textbook serves as your guide as you study pharmacology. The road of pharmacology is paved with extensive and often unrecognized research on the part of thousands of doctors and scientists around the world. Pharmacology is built layer by layer upon previous discoveries and consists of equal parts of hard work, astute observation, sudden insights, and divinely appointed coincidences. Indeed, the road of pharmacology is constantly being built anew with each new drug discovery. This is the interesting road you will be following as you study this textbook!

The purpose of this textbook is to provide a framework of knowledge to help you (whether you are a student or a health professional) to do the following:

1. Recognize drug categories and generic and trade name drugs
2. Understand therapeutic drug effects and the rationale for using drugs to prevent, diagnose, and treat disease
3. Understand why side effects, allergic effects, and other effects of drugs occur
4. Distinguish between sound-alike drugs
5. Explore clinical applications and current healthcare issues relating to pharmacology and drugs.

By providing this foundation of knowledge, *Understanding Pharmacology for Health Professionals* will help you be prepared to deal with drugs currently on the market and also with the myriad new drugs that are approved each year.

With the help of *Understanding Pharmacology for Health Professionals*, the road of pharmacology that stretches ahead of you will become both familiar and nonthreatening, one that you will travel frequently and confidently in the future!

## A Guide to the Fourth Edition

Thanks to valuable input from students, instructors, and reviewers, the fourth edition includes an abundance of new features. In the pages that follow, please explore what makes this fourth edition an ideal teaching and learning tool.

### Organization Refinements

The organization of chapters by body systems or drug categories has proven very effective in the past editions. This format was retained, but a new overarching structure was created to organize the chapters into three broad units for clarity and ease of instruction.

**Unit One: The Past History, Present Uses, and Future of Drugs**
This unit consists of six chapters that introduce the field of pharmacology. These chapters build a strong foundation of basic knowledge that facilitates learning specific drugs introduced in later chapters.

**Unit Two: Drugs by Body Systems**
This unit consists of 13 chapters of drugs related to specific body systems. The body system approach is the most efficient way to learn anatomy and physiology, human disease, and pharmacology.

**Unit Three: Other Drug Categories**
This unit consists of five chapters of drug categories that are not directly related to any specific body system.

Other organizational changes included combining some shorter chapters, so that all chapters in the fourth edition are now of relatively the same length. This makes it easier for both students and instructors to cover approximately the same amount of material during each week or class session. Although there are now a total of 24 chapters, no material from the previous edition has been deleted.

## Richer Features than Ever Before

**Drugs Updates.** Each chapter has been updated to include the most current drug names and drug information available—right up to the day of publication. Also, references to reliable and continuously updated Websites have been included in the *Instructor's Resource Manual* as sources of information about new drugs as they come on the market.

**Visual Enhancements.** The quantity and quality of images throughout the textbook have been greatly increased to include full-color photographs of prescriptions, drug name labels, and drugs being administered to patients.

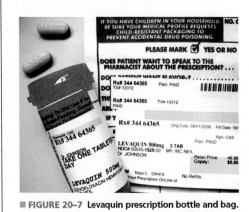

■ FIGURE 20–7 **Levaquin prescription bottle and bag.**
Levaquin is the trade name for the generic drug levofloxacin, an antibiotic drug that belongs to the fluoroquinolone category. This prescription is for a 3-day supply to treat a mild urinary tract infection prior to a surgical procedure. Although most antibiotic drugs have plain and unlabeled tablets, the Levaquin tablet is not only labeled with the drug name on one side of the tablet, but the reverse side of the tablet has the tablet strength of 500 (for 500 mg). Notice the red warning label on the prescription bottle that says "Do not use if you are breastfeeding." Notice the blue notice on the prescription bag that requests child-resistant packaging.

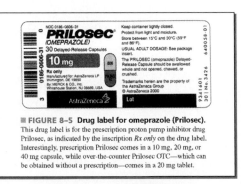

■ FIGURE 8–5 **Drug label for omeprazole (Prilosec).**
This drug label is for the prescription proton pump inhibitor drug Prilosec, as indicated by the inscription *Rx only* on the drug label. Interestingly, prescription Prilosec comes in a 10 mg, 20 mg, or 40 mg capsule, while over-the-counter Prilosec OTC—which can be obtained without a prescription—comes in a 20 mg tablet.

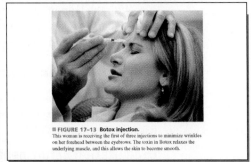

■ FIGURE 17–13 **Botox injection.**
This woman is receiving the first of three injections to minimize wrinkles on her forehead between the eyebrows. The toxin in Botox relaxes the underlying muscle, and this allows the skin to become smooth.

**Drug Alert!** This special box appears in most chapters and calls attention to

■ unusual and harmful drug effects
■ sound-alike drug names that could result in taking or administering the wrong drug
■ drug-drug and drug-food interactions
■ other areas of special interest that are currently in the news.

### Drug Alert!

Well-known chemotherapy protocols CHOP and MOPP include the chemotherapy drug vincristine, which is represented by the "O" in the protocol abbreviations. The "O" stands for Oncovin, a former trade name of vincristine. Even though Oncovin has been discontinued and is no longer available, these chemotherapy protocols have kept their original abbreviation that includes the "O." Healthcare professionals are expected to know that the "O" stands for "Oncovin" (even though that trade name drug is no longer on the market) and that the generic drug vincristine is part of the chemotherapy protocol.

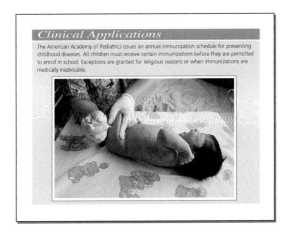

*Clinical Applications*

The American Academy of Pediatrics issues an annual immunization schedule for preventing childhood diseases. All children must receive certain immunizations before they are permitted to enroll in school. Exceptions are granted for religious reasons or when immunizations are medically inadvisable.

**Clinical Applications**

1. Look at this handwritten prescription and answer the following questions.
   a. What drug has been prescribed?
   b. To what drug category does this drug belong?
   c. What is the therapeutic effect of this drug?
   d. What is the strength of this drug?
   e. In what drug form does it come?
   f. Translate the rest of the prescription into plain English.

PAT SMITH, M.D.
27 Oak Leaf Lane
Baltimore, MD 12121
Phone: 322–7890
Name_____
Address_____
Age_____

Rx  Timoptic 0.25%
     Ophthalmic drops
     #1
     S. gtts ī o.u. BID

**Clinical Applications.** This new feature helps students take what they have learned and relate it to actual patient and clinical situations. Some examples include

■ how pediatric immunizations are given
■ how the genetic makeup of a person influences drug effects
■ polypharmacy and challenges that the elderly face in taking drugs
■ how to avoid theft of prescription pads in the physician's office
■ how drug advertising affects consumers.

A Clinical Applications section also appears at the end of nearly all chapters, featuring the following types of job-skill exercises:

■ Handwritten and electronic prescriptions. Challenge students' ability to read, decipher, and interpret written drug information on a prescription form.
■ Drug forms. Quiz students on identifying the pictured drug form.
■ Drug labels. Pose questions about the specific information on the label.
■ Patient photographs. Prompt students to link the pictured disease to a particular drug category from that chapter.
■ Clinical scenarios. Display excerpts from medical case histories with accompanying questions.

The answers to the Clinical Applications questions can be found in the *Instructors Resource Manual.*

## New Appendices Provide Added Value

There are all new and comprehensive appendices at the conclusion of the textbook. They include the following:

**Appendix A    Sound-Alike Drug Names**
Extensive list of sound-alike drugs that often cause drug errors.

**Appendix B    Glossary of Key Words with Definitions**
Bolded drug words/phrases and their definitions that appear in the chapters as well as from Chapter 8 of the previous edition.

**Appendix C    Glossary of Abbreviations, Symbols, and Their Meanings**
A comprehensive list of drug abbreviations and symbols often seen in medical documents and drug articles. This list includes dangerous abbreviations of drugs as identified by JCAHO (Joint Commission on Accreditation of Healthcare Organizations) and ISMP (Institute for Safe Medication Practices).

**Appendix D    Glossary of Generic and Trade Name Drugs, Categories, Indications, Doses, and Drug Pronunciations**
Comprehensive, quick-reference list for verifying generic and trade name drugs, their indications for use, their drug forms, available strengths/doses, and see-and-say pronunciations that are easy to follow and ensure accurate pronunciation of every drug name.

## A Consistent Format in Every Chapter

**Learning Objectives.**  Set of goals that should be previewed before reading the chapter and then reread upon completing the chapter to verify that key concepts have been mastered.

**Drug Categories.**  Drugs are grouped into categories according to their therapeutic effects or by the disease they are used treat. Each drug category includes a description of how those drugs work in the body and their therapeutic effects.

**Drug Terminology.**  Key words and phrases are highlighted in bold throughout the text.

**Generic and Trade Name Drugs.**  Comprehensive coverage includes prescription as well as over-the-counter drugs. Generic drugs currently on the market are listed for each drug category. After each generic drug, one or two of the most common trade name drugs for that generic drug are listed in parentheses.

**Special Features.**  The special features "Did You Know?," "Historical Notes," and "In Depth," so popular with students, instructors, and practitioners, have been retained and expanded. Touches of humor throughout this textbook—one of its best-known and most-appreciated features—have been retained.

---

### *Did You Know?*

Sometimes, an alcoholic patient will drink methanol instead of ethanol (liquor). In the body, methanol is metabolized into formaldehyde, a toxic chemical that is used by pathologists to preserve biopsied tissue specimens.

Methylene blue is a dye that is used to stain tissue samples (Gram's stain, Wright's stain). It is used during surgery to stain tissue that is abnormal so that it can be excised. It is also an antiseptic drug that is included in many combination drugs to treat urinary tract infections (hence its trade name Urolene Blue).

---

### *Historical Notes*

Dr. John Eng, an endocrinologist in New York in the early 1980s noticed that persons bitten by venous animals often developed pancreatitis because the venom overstimulated the pancreas. Dr. Eng remembers, "So we ordered up a whole variety of venoms—from snakes and other animals, including the Gila monster—and started looking for the compound that stimulated the pancreas." Dr. Eng worked on this research for 20 years until he discovered a compound in Gila monster saliva that stimulates the pancreas to secrete insulin. "The Gila monster is a beautiful reptile. All I can say is, without the Gila monster, this would never have happened and, to me, that is kind of humbling."

Carla McClain, "Gila monster spit aids diabetics," *Arizona Daily Star,* May 9, 2005.

---

### *In Depth*

Prostaglandin is a naturally occurring body substance that was first isolated from the prostate gland, from which it derives its name. Prostaglandins are present in many different tissues in the body and, when used as drugs, they have several different actions. Prostaglandin $E_1$ drugs cause vasodilation, which is useful in treating erectile dysfunction. Prostaglandin $E_1$ drugs are also used to keep open a patent ductus arteriosus to sustain life in a newborn with a congenital heart defect such as tetralogy of Fallot. Prostaglandin $E_2$ drugs stimulate smooth muscle in the wall of the uterus and are used to induce premature labor and terminate a pregnancy.

**Quiz Yourself.** Detailed and thought-provoking questions are included at the end of each chapter. The answers to the Quiz Yourself questions can be found in the *Instructor's Resource Manual.*

## Quiz Yourself

1. Name six things that support the normal balance between new bone deposition and bone resorption.
2. Which bone cells are inhibited by bone resorption inhibitor drugs?
3. Describe the various routes of administration and timing of doses for the different bone resorption inhibitor drugs.
4. Why are hormone (estrogen) replacement drugs not used as often for the long-term treatment of osteoporosis as they once were?
5. Give the meaning of the abbreviations *ASA, COX,* and *NSAID.*
6. Name the categories of drugs used to treat osteoarthritis and give examples of drugs from each category.
7. Contrast the therapeutic action of aspirin with that of acetaminophen.
8. How does enteric-coated aspirin help prevent gastric ulcers in patients with osteoarthritis?
9. Indocin is an NSAID that is used to treat osteoarthritis in the elderly and patent ductus arteriosus in premature infants. True or false?
10. Why are gold compound drugs useful in treating rheumatoid arthritis but not osteoarthritis?
11. List the medical conditions for which a muscle relaxant drug might be prescribed.
12. To what category of drugs does each of these drugs belong?
    a. abatacept (Orencia)
    b. alendronate (Fosamax)
    c. allopurinol (Zyloprim)

**Spelling Tips.** Provides tips to help students watch out for unusual spellings of drug names and correctly use internal capitalization.

## Spelling Tips

| | |
|---|---|
| **BuSpar** | Unusual internal capitalization. |
| **ClimaraPro** | Unusual internal capitalization. |
| **CombiPatch** | Unusual internal capitalization. |
| **Femhrt** | Unusual word ending that actually is the abbreviation *hrt* (for *hormone replacement therapy*). |
| **MetroGel-Vaginal** | Unusual internal capitalization. |
| **MICRhoGAM** | Unusual internal capitalization. |
| **NuvaRing** | Unusual internal capitalization. |
| **RhoGAM** | Unusual internal capitalization. |
| **YAZ** | All capital letters. |

**Multimedia Extension Exercises.** Link to the Companion Website created for this textbook. Features include links to find out about new drugs and additional chapter-specific exercises for further practice.

## Multimedia Extension Activities

- Go to www.pearsonhighered.com/turley and click on the photo of the cover of *Understanding Pharmacology for Health Professionals* to access the interactive Companion Website created for this textbook.

## A Note About Drug Doses and Calculations

It is not the purpose of this textbook to instruct in the actual prescribing or administration of drugs. Calculation of drug doses and administration of drugs are entirely different topics of study. For those students seeking resources dedicated to this aspect of pharmacology, *Medical Dosage Calculations* by Olsen, Giangrasso, Shrimpton, and Dillon (Pearson, 2008) and *Ratio & Proportion Dosage Calculations* by Giangrasso and Shrimpton (Pearson, 2010) are ideal companion textbooks. Instructors and bookstores may wish to contact their Pearson representative to arrange a value-priced bundle package of these two textbooks.

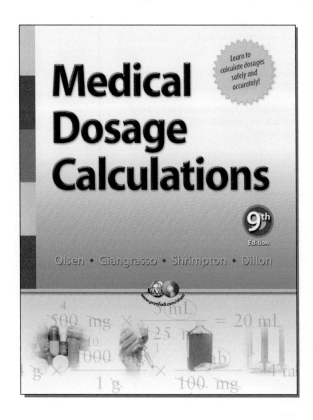

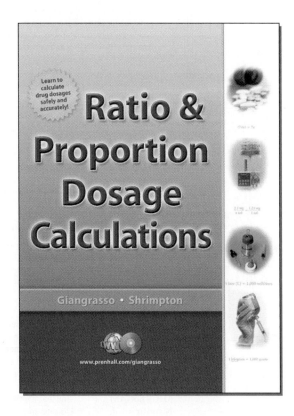

# Acknowledgments

I wish to acknowledge Mark Cohen, Editor-in-Chief for Health Professions at Pearson Health Science, for his expertise, creative insights, support, professionalism, and enthusiasm for Understanding Pharmacology for Health Professionals through the years. I also wish to thank Melissa Kerian, Development Editor, for expertly overseeing the details for the textbook and its ancillary products.

I wish to thank the many instructors who have used the various editions of this textbook since it was first published in 1991. I also wish to acknowledge the many students who have studied from this textbook and the healthcare professionals who use this textbook as a day-to-day drug reference on the job. The insightful comments of all of these individuals have helped to continuously improve this textbook from edition to edition.

I wish to acknowledge Sally C. Pitman and Health Professions Institute for publishing the first edition of this textbook.

Finally, I wish to thank John H. Dirckx, M.D., for being an expert reviewer of the textbook and as the author of the Foreword.

# Reviewers

**Dale Brewer, BS, MEd, CMA (AAMA)**
Program Director/Professor of Medical Assisting
Pensacola Junior College
Pensacola, Florida

**Carol Hendrickson, MS Ed.**
Instructor, Medical Coding/ Pharmacology
Pasco Hernando Community College
New Port Richey, Florida

**Maria Teresa Lopez-Hill, MS**
Associate Faculty
Collin County Community College, Central Park Campus
McKinney, Texas

**Michele G. Miller, CMA, M.Ed**
Program Director, Medical Assisting
Lakeland Community College
Kirtland, Ohio

**Linda Parks, MA, RHIT**
Program Director, Health Information Technology
Darton College
Albany, Georgia

# About the Author

**Susan M. Turley**, MA (Educ), BSN, RN, RHIT, CMT, is an experienced educator and practitioner in many areas of health care. She has worked in acute care, managed care, long-term care, and physician offices, and held positions in nursing, quality management, risk management, infection control, medical assisting, medical transcription, and health information management.

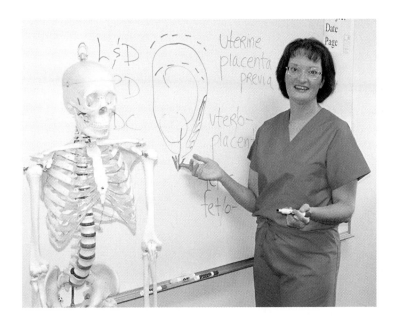

As an educator, she has taught college and community college courses in medical terminology, pathophysiology, pharmacology, and medical transcription. She has presented numerous staff inservices in acute care, managed care, and long-term care settings, and co-presented numerous all-day seminars for instructors throughout the country.

She is the author of *Medical Language* (Pearson, 2007) and co-author of *Medical Language STAT!* (Pearson, 2009), as well as numerous medical and educational articles for national journals. She is also the co-author of two funded national healthcare grants, and co-author (with physicians) of a peer-reviewed physician journal article and chapters in two reference textbooks for physicians.

She has a Master of Arts degree in adult education, a Bachelor of Science degree in nursing, and national certification in the fields of both health information management and medical transcription.

Her writing is well known for its clarity in presenting technically difficult material and for a special blend of in-depth coverage that includes humor and interesting anecdotes to stimulate learning and keep interest high.

# A Note to Students

## The Beginnings of this Textbook

A number of years ago, I began to teach a course in pharmacology (lecture and clinical lab) at a local community college. By the third semester of teaching, I had selected, used, and subsequently discarded three different pharmacology textbooks from three different publishers. Some of my objections to these textbooks were that they were

- dry and uninteresting
- inconsistent in the depth of content presented
- unclear in their explanation of drug effects
- visually uninviting
- lacking in humor and anecdotal information.

By the fourth semester of teaching pharmacology, I made the decision to begin writing student handouts for each drug category studied to supplement my weekly lecture. I tried to make the explanations of drug effects and other in-depth topics as clear and straightforward as possible. This often necessitated prolonged research on certain topics until I was certain I could convey a complicated concept in a concise and understandable way.

After many revisions, additions, and much research, this material became the basis for the first edition of *Understanding Pharmacology for Health Professionals*.

Just prior to completing the manuscript for the first edition, I received a Master's degree in adult education. Having thoroughly studied the techniques of the best educators, I was more convinced than ever that these techniques could be applied to the teaching of pharmacology, and that pharmacology could be presented in an interesting, stimulating, challenging, and even humorous way to enhance the total learning experience. So I searched for interesting anecdotal material as well as humorous material/cartoons/quotes to enliven the text.

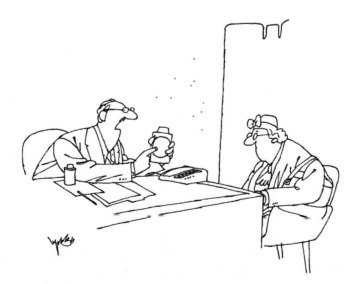

*"This drug was tested on 2000 white mice, and they had a ball."*

Abundant positive feedback from instructors, students, and practitioners from across the country overwhelmingly validated this combination of clear explanations and attention-holding techniques as a successful educational and professional tool.

## How to Use This Textbook

As you begin each chapter, do these things first before reading the chapter text.

- ■ **Review the Chapter Contents list.** This will alert you to all of the topics that will be presented in the chapter.
- ■ **Review the Learning Objectives.** This will give you key concepts from the chapter and a general idea of what types of information you will be expected to know when you finish the chapter.
- ■ Browse through the pages of the chapter. This will give you an idea of the length of the chapter and more specific information about its contents.
- ■ Look at some of the illustrations and cartoons in the chapter and feature boxes entitled *Did You Know?* and *Historical Notes.* These will entice you to begin reading the chapter material!

When you are ready to read, break the chapter into manageable sections and read those pages. Do not attempt to read too much material at once. After you have finished reading the chapter, answer the Quiz Yourself and Clinical Applications questions at the end of the chapter. This will help you assess your level of learning and apply what you have learned.

## Practical Applications of Knowledge

It is important that you be able to relate the information you are learning to your own life experiences, whether personal or professional. Everyone has at least some familiarity with drugs. In addition, most people have a family member or friend who is taking one or more drugs. As you begin to study a particular chapter, your instructor may ask you to document (in writing) conversations with family members or friends about drugs they are taking, the symptoms that prompted the prescription of those drugs, and whether or not their symptoms improved (while keeping the person's identity confidential, of course!). You may also include drugs you are taking and why, but this is optional (to preserve your privacy).

In this way, you become an active participant in the information-gathering process and begin to see yourself as a researcher. The facts you gather will form a mental framework upon which to place the information you learn in the textbook. You will remember that your sister takes Flovent for her asthma, that you use Claritin for your seasonal allergies, and that your elderly aunt takes Celebrex for her arthritis and hydrochlorothiazide for her blood pressure.

Besides having a knowledge of drug uses and effects, it is important for you to know how to communicate your knowledge through speaking and writing. This means mastering the pronunciation and spelling of drug names and recognizing common generic drugs and their trade name equivalents.

While I was teaching pharmacology at the community college, a student in the Emergency Medical Technician (EMT) Program approached me and asked for assistance in learning to pronounce drug names. This student stated that he was being ridiculed when he called ahead to the hospital from the ambulance and couldn't correctly pronounce drug names during the conversation. I made a tape of the pronunciation of the most common generic and trade name drugs for him. He studied it and later reported that he was successfully pronouncing the drug names and that the healthcare professionals he dealt with had noticed his improvement in this area.

The pronunciation of drug names should be practiced during the study of each chapter. Many drug names, particularly the generic names, have multiple syllables, and correct pronunciation requires some practice. Hearing your instructor pronounce the drug name is just the first step. You need to practice pronouncing drug names for yourself. An easy-to-use, see-and-say pronunciation guide for each of the generic and trade name drugs in the textbook can be found in Appendix D at the end of the textbook.

While studying pharmacology, it is easy to become buried by the sheer volume of drug names, drug facts, and other details. It is important to recognize common generic and trade name drugs for each category of drugs, and recognize the suffixes that are common to generic drug names that relate to specific categories of drugs.

However, long after you have forgotten some of the specific drug facts, it is critical that you retain the ability to research and find information about new drugs as they come on the market. You need to know how to locate new drugs on the Internet, how to interpret printed drug information, how to formulate questions to obtain additional information, and how to contact appropriate individuals (pharmacists, doctors, etc.) to obtain information.

On a personal note, I would encourage you to constantly increase your knowledge of pharmacology during your study of this textbook and in the future. I hope this textbook will make your study of pharmacology relevant and interesting! Blessings to you as you study and learn about pharmacology!

—*Susan M. Turley*

# Unit One

# THE PAST HISTORY, PRESENT USES, AND FUTURE OF DRUGS

# 1

# Introduction to Pharmacology and the History of Drugs

**CHAPTER CONTENTS**

## Learning Objectives

After you study this chapter, you should be able to

1. Describe the origin of the words *pharmacology, drug, medicine,* and other words related to specialty fields within pharmacology.

2. Describe the three general medical uses for drugs.

3. Give the origin and meaning of the symbol *Rx*.

4. Name at least five drugs historically derived from plant, animal, or mineral sources that are still in use today.

5. Describe the process of the preparation of drugs in the 1800s to early 1900s.

6. Name 10 major pharmaceutical milestones that have occurred since the 1800s.

7. Describe the use of mislabeled and dangerous drugs and the problem they presented in the past for consumer safety.

8. Describe the origin and content of the various drug laws.

9. Describe the function of the Food and Drug Administration (FDA) with respect to approving or removing drugs from the market.

10. Differentiate between prescription and over-the-counter (OTC) drugs.

11. Define *schedule drugs* and describe the five categories of controlled substances.

12. Define *orphan drugs.*

Pharmacology is a fascinating and multifaceted discipline that impacts not only our chosen career in health care, but also our personal lives. From our role as members of the healthcare team to that of consumers, pharmacology plays a part in our lives.

The study of pharmacology covers a broad spectrum of diverse, yet interrelated, topics: botany, molecular chemistry, research, toxicology, legislation, and patient education.

There is an excitement inherent in the study of pharmacology. The field of pharmacology is amazing in its scope, ranging from the historical and present day uses of herbs and plant extracts to day-to-day painstaking research that produces unusable products as well as life-saving drugs to the future with genetic manipulation, molecular pharmacology, adult stem cell therapy, and a seemingly limitless potential for discovery.

## Origins of Pharmacology Words

### Pharmacology

Pharmacology is the study of drugs and their interactions with living organisms. The word *pharmacology* comes from the Greek word *pharmakon,* which means *medicine* or *drug,* and the suffix *-logy,* which means *the study of.* Pharmacology is concerned with the nature of drugs, their effects in the body, drug doses, side effects, and so forth.

*Pharmacology* is a general word. Other more specific words related to specialty fields within the field of pharmacology include the following:

**molecular pharmacology** the study of the chemical structures of drugs and the effects of drugs at the molecular level within cells

**pharmacodynamics** the mechanisms of action by which drugs produce their effects (desired or undesired) based on time and dose

**pharmacogenetics** how the genetic makeup of different people affects their responses to certain drugs

**pharmacogenomics** using genome technology to discover new drugs

**pharmacokinetics** how drugs move through the body in the processes of absorption, distribution, metabolism, and excretion

**pharmacotherapy** using drugs to affect the body therapeutically.

### Drugs and Medicines

The word *drug* is derived from the Dutch word *droog,* which means *dry,* and refers to the use of dried herbs and plants as the first medicines. The Latin word for *drug* is *medicina,* from which we derive the words *medicine* and *medication.* A drug or a medicine can be thought of as any nonfood chemical substance that affects the mind or the body. The word *medicine* refers to a drug that is deliberately administered for its medicinal value as a preventive, diagnostic, or therapeutic agent (see ■ **FIGURE 1–1**). The word *drug* can be used interchangeably with the word *medicine,* but *drug* can also refer specifically to chemical substances that do not have a preventive, diagnostic, or therapeutic use (e.g., illicit or street drugs).

## Medical Uses for Drugs

Drugs have three medical uses. They are used to prevent disease, to diagnose disease, and to treat symptoms, signs, conditions, and diseases. The study of these uses is known as ***pharmacotherapy.***

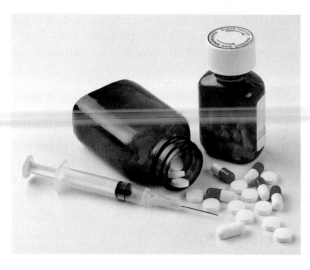

■ **FIGURE 1–1  Medications.**
Medications or medicines are drugs that are used to prevent, diagnose, or treat symptoms, signs, conditions, and diseases.

1. **Preventive use.**   Drugs are used to prevent the occurrence of diseases or conditions. The administration of a preventive drug is known as ***prophylaxis***. *Prophylaxis* is from a Greek word meaning *to keep guard before.* Examples of the preventive uses of drugs include the following:
   - ■ Drugs taken prior to traveling to prevent motion sickness (see ■ **FIGURE 1–2**)
   - ■ Contraceptive drugs taken to prevent pregnancy
   - ■ Vaccinations given to immunize children or adults against certain diseases, such as polio, diphtheria, or influenza.
2. **Diagnostic use.**   Drugs are used by themselves or in conjunction with radiologic procedures and other types of medical tests to provide evidence of a disease process. Examples of the diagnostic uses of drugs include the following:
   - ■ Radiopaque contrast dyes used during x-ray procedures
   - ■ Drugs that mimic the cardiac effect of exercise in patients who cannot undergo regular cardiac exercise stress testing.

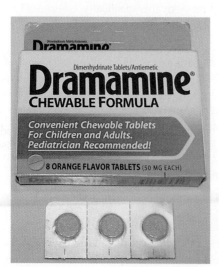

■ **FIGURE 1–2  Preventive use of drugs.**
Dramamine is an over-the-counter drug that is taken to prevent motion sickness and vomiting. The word *vomiting* does not appear on the drug package, but the word *antiemetic,* which means *pertaining to against vomiting,* appears at the top right.

## Clinical Applications

The American Academy of Pediatrics issues an annual immunization schedule for preventing childhood diseases. All children must receive certain immunizations before they are permitted to enroll in school. Exceptions are granted for religious reasons or when immunizations are medically inadvisable.

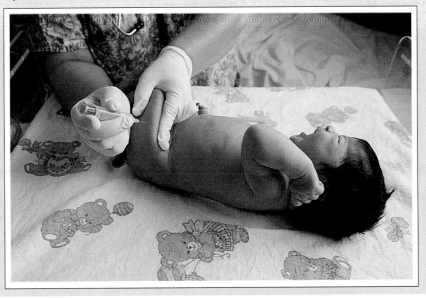

3. **Therapeutic use.** The majority of drugs are used to control, improve, or cure symptoms, signs, conditions, or diseases of a physiologic or psychological nature. Examples of the therapeutic uses of drugs include the following:
   - Antibiotic drugs to kill bacteria and cure an infection
   - Analgesic drugs to control the pain and inflammation of arthritis
   - Insulin to treat diabetes mellitus.

## Drugs in Ancient Times

Pharmacology is one of the oldest branches of medicine. Ancient peoples such as the Sumerians and Egyptians recorded the use of drugs on clay tablets, on wall paintings in tombs, and on papyrus as early as 2000 B.C. The Egyptians treated diseases with substances such as frogs' bile, sour milk, lizards' blood, pigs' teeth, sugar cakes, dirt, spiders' webs, hippopotamus' oil, and toads' eyelids. The Egyptians applied moldy bread to abrasions, a practice that actually had some therapeutic basis as, many centuries later, penicillin was extracted from a mold. An Egyptian medicinal scroll, the Ebers Papyrus from 1500 B.C. (discovered in the early 1800s), contained the names of 800 different herbal formulations and prescriptions. The Egyptians also extracted the oil from various plants known for their healing properties. In 1922 when King Tutankhamun's tomb was opened, archeologists discovered 350 alabaster jars of plant oils in it.

The ancient Chinese practiced healing arts that emphasized the use of herbs and some minerals, but few animal products (see ■ **FIGURE 1–3**). Herbal preparations were used in conjunction with acupuncture, massage, and exercise. Shen Nong completed the first Chinese book on herbal medicine in 3494 B.C. It included 365 different herbal remedies.

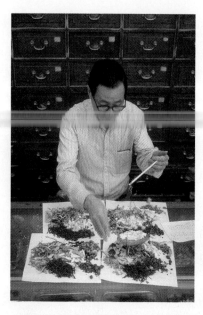

■ **FIGURE 1–3  Chinese herbal medicines.**
This Chinese pharmacist prepares herbal medicines in much the
same way that his ancestors did, by using dried herbs which are
then crushed into powder. He is making four batches of the same
medicine, each of which contains the same mixture of herbs. The
wall behind him holds drawers of many different types of dried
herbs. In 1970, the Chinese Academy of Medical Science compiled
a collection of traditional herbal remedies. American pharmacists
evaluated those remedies and found that 45 percent of them were
therapeutic, according to Western standards of medicine.

Many other cultures around the world furthered the use of drugs within their own cultures,
including the Native Americans of North America. The Aztec Indians of Mexico grew many
herbs with medicinal properties. Aztec King Montezuma maintained royal gardens of medicinal plants.

The Greeks and Romans furthered the study of medicine through an understanding of anatomy
and physiology, which was an important first step toward understanding how drugs exert their
effects in the body.

Ancient drugs were prepared according to standard recipes that involved drying, crushing, and
combining a variety of plants, substances from animals, or minerals. The symbol **Rx**, which comes
from the Latin word *recipe,* meaning *take,* indicates a prescription, the combining of ingredients to
form a drug. The use of some ingredients was based on medical lore and superstition. Some ingredients had therapeutic value, but others were worthless or actually harmful.

Medieval physicians prescribed a broad range of drugs from herbs to metals (e.g., powdered
gold) to addictive substances (e.g., opium). In the 1600s, patients were advised to eat soap to cure
blood in the urine and put mercury in beer to cure intestinal worms. Because little was known about
even the most fundamental physical and chemical processes of the body, the therapeutic use of
drugs was not an exact science.

## Modern Drugs Derived from Natural Sources

Amazingly, there are a number of drugs, based on old prescriptions, that are still in use today. These
include drugs derived from plants, animals, and minerals.

### Drugs Derived from Plants

The medicinal use of the foxglove plant was noted in 13th-century writings (see ■ **FIGURE 1–4**).
A derivative of this plant is used to make the drug digoxin (Lanoxin), which is still used today to
treat congestive heart failure.

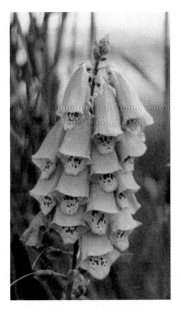

**■ FIGURE 1–4  Foxglove plant.**
This beautiful wild flowering plant is commonly known as foxglove, but its scientific name is *Digitalis lanata.* The drug digitalis (which is no longer in use) came from this plant, as does the modern drug digoxin (Lanoxin), which is used to treat congestive heart failure.

The belladonna plant was the original source of two drugs that are still in use today—atropine and scopolamine. Belladonna means *beautiful lady* in Italian. "Sixteenth century Italian women … squeezed the juice of the berries of these plants into their eyes to widen and brighten them." (Michael C. Gerald, *Pharmacology: An Introduction to Drugs,* 2nd ed. Englewood Cliffs, NJ: Prentice Hall, 1981, p. 149, out of print.) Atropine is still used to dilate the pupil in patients with inflammatory conditions of the iris. Scopolamine is used to treat motion sickness.

The opium poppy has been used for centuries as a painkiller and also as a recreational drug to induce euphoria and a trance-like state. The sap from the seedheads of the poppy flower *Papaver somniferum* contain opium, a substance that is the source of the illegal street drug heroin, which has no medical use, as well as the prescription drug morphine, which is a potent analgesic drug used to treat severe pain.

Colchicine, a drug still used to treat gout, was used for that same purpose in the sixth century. It was originally derived from the autumn crocus known as *Colchicum autumnale.*

Ephedrine is present in the leaves of a bushy shrub (species name, *Ephedra*). The leaves were burned and used by the ancient Chinese to treat respiratory ailments. Today, ephedrine is present in over-the-counter bronchodilator drugs.

## *Did You Know?*

Herbs have been a part of all cultures for centuries and have been mentioned frequently in literature. Henbane, a very toxic herb, was supposed to have been the poison that Claudius used to kill his brother, Hamlet's father. "Henbane should not be confused with wolfsbane. Students of literature know wolfsbane to be useful as a vampire repellant (Dracula, 1897); however, we should point out that double-blind studies demonstrating the effectiveness of this plant have not as yet been conducted." (Michael C. Gerald, *Pharmacology: An Introduction to Drugs,* 2nd ed. Englewood Cliffs, NJ: Prentice Hall, 1981, p. 149, out of print.)

Some estrogen hormone replacement therapy drugs are derived from yams. The drug galanta-mine (Razadyne), which is used to treat Alzheimer's disease, is derived from daffodil bulbs. In addition, many of the gums, oils, and bases in which drugs are dissolved come from plant sources. Many drugs contain soybean oil, sesame seed oil, or olive oil.

Other plants have also become the sources of some modern drugs (see ▪ TABLE 1–1).

▪ TABLE 1–1  **Other plant sources of some modern drugs**

| Plant Sources | Modern Drug |
|---|---|
| black cohosh | Remifemin (used to treat menopause hot flashes) |
| cinchona bark | quinine (used to treat malaria) |
| cocoa butter | binder or filler ingredient |
| hot pepper plant | capsaicin (topical pain relief) |
| mold | penicillin (antibiotic drug) |
| | statin drugs (used to treat high cholesterol) |
| periwinkle (vinca) | vincristine (used to treat cancer) |
| rose hips | vitamin C (see ▪ FIGURE 1–5) |
| snakeroot | reserpine (used to treat hypertension) |
| willow bark | aspirin (used to treat pain) |

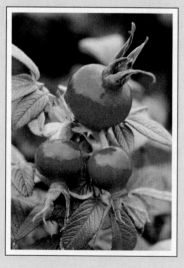

▪ FIGURE 1–5  **Rose hips.**
Hips are the botanical name for the rounded fruit of a rose. Powdered rose hips are still the source of natural vitamin C in some over-the-counter vitamin C dietary supplements. Other products use synthetic vitamin C.

## Drugs Derived from Animals

Thyroid supplement drugs are composed of dried (desiccated) thyroid gland tissue taken from animals. Thyroid supplement drugs are used to treat patients with hypothyroidism.

The drug Premarin, a female hormone replacement drug used to relieve the symptoms of menopause, is derived from **pre**gnant **mar**es' ur**in**e, and the trade name is formed from selected letters taken from that phrase.

Lanolin, a common ingredient of topical skin drugs, is obtained from the purified fat of processed sheeps' wool.

In the past, the only source of insulin used to treat diabetes mellitus was from ground-up animal pancreas (see ▨ **FIGURE 1–6**). This type of insulin is still available.

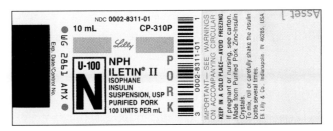

▨ **FIGURE 1–6   NPH Iletin II insulin.**
The drug label clearly shows that the source of this insulin is from pork (in vertical capital letters).

## Drugs Derived from Minerals

Minerals, such as calcium and iron, are available as individual dietary supplements, and trace minerals, such as copper, magnesium, selenium, and zinc, are included in many multivitamin supplements. Centrum multivitamins use the advertising slogan "From A to Zinc," to show that they contain vitamins and minerals alphabetically from vitamin A through zinc.

Potassium, in the form of potassium chloride, is given in conjunction with diuretic drugs because diuretic drugs cause increased excretion of potassium (and water).

The cardiac drug quinapril (Accupril) contains red iron oxide as an inert ingredient in its brown tablets.

# Drugs in the 1800s and 1900s

It was not until the 1800s that chemists developed techniques to extract and isolate pure substances from crude drug preparations. The isolation of morphine in 1803 by a German pharmacist marked the beginning of modern drug therapy using chemically pure ingredients.

In the early 1900s, the extraction and preparation of drugs was still a time-consuming process that utilized test tubes, filters, and Bunsen burners. Pharmacists at that time actually prepared the drugs they dispensed. Daily, they made milk of magnesia, paregoric, and syrup bases for liquid medicines. In addition, they hand-rolled cocoa butter suppositories. They measured out drugs in minims, drams, ounces, grains, and scruples (the apothecary system of measurement).

Much has changed since then. Many drugs are now completely synthetic rather than derived from natural sources. Other natural drugs have undergone chemical modification and molecular restructuring to create new drugs that possess superior pharmacologic action. In addition, the pharmacist no longer prepares drugs, but dispenses them and provides patient information and education.

## Pharmaceutical Timeline

The following list briefly notes some major pharmaceutical milestones dating from the 1800s to the present time (see ▣ TABLE 1–2).

▣ TABLE 1–2  **Major pharmaceutical milestones of the 1800s to the present**

| Year | Major Pharmaceutical Milestone |
|------|-------------------------------|
| 1803 | Morphine isolated from crude opium |
| 1827 | Merck & Company, a German drug company, begins the first commercial production of morphine |
| 1843 | Dr. Alexander Wood of Scotland creates the syringe and injects patients with morphine |
| 1899 | Aspirin introduced |
| 1908 | Sulfanilamide introduced (first anti-infective drug) |
| 1912 | Phenobarbital introduced for epilepsy (first antiepileptic drug) |
| 1913 | Vitamins A and B discovered |
| 1922 | Insulin introduced (first drug for diabetes mellitus) |
| 1938 | Dilantin introduced for epilepsy |
| 1941 | Penicillin introduced (first antibiotic drug) |
| 1945 | Benadryl introduced (first antihistamine drug) |
| 1948 | Cortisone introduced (first corticosteroid drug) |
| 1952 | Thorazine introduced for psychosis (first antipsychotic drug) |
| 1952 | Hydrocortisone introduced (first topical corticosteroid drug) |
| 1957 | Librium introduced for neurosis (first antianxiety drug) |
| 1958 | Haldol introduced for psychosis |
| 1966 | Clotting factors introduced for hemophilia |
| 1967 | Inderal introduced for hypertension (first beta-blocker drug) |
| 1970 | Levodopa introduced for Parkinson's disease |
| 1972 | Researchers discover a receptor in the brain that responds to drugs derived from opium |
| 1977 | Tagamet introduced for peptic ulcers (first $H_2$ blocker drug) |
| 1978 | First portable insulin pump introduced |
| 1981 | Verapamil introduced for heart arrhythmia (first calcium channel blocker drug) |
| 1982 | Humulin (human insulin) introduced (first drug made by recombinant DNA technology) |

*(continued)*

**▪ TABLE 1–2** *(continued)*

| Year | Major Pharmaceutical Milestone |
|------|-------------------------------|
| 1983 | Topical prescription drug hydrocortisone approved for over-the-counter sales |
| 1985 | ACE inhibitor drugs introduced for hypertension |
| 1986 | Orthoclone OKT3 introduced (first monoclonal antibody drug) |
| 1987 | Mevacor introduced (first statin drug for high cholesterol) |
| 1987 | Alteplase (Activase) introduced for dissolving blood clots (first tissue plasminogen activator drug) |
| 1987 | AZT (zidovudine, Retrovir) introduced (first drug for HIV) |
| 1992 | Proscar introduced for benign prostatic hypertrophy (first nonsurgical treatment) |
| 1993 | Cognex introduced (first drug for Alzheimer's disease) |
| 1994 | Combination drug therapy introduced for peptic ulcers caused by *Helicobacter pylori* |
| 1995 | Cozaar introduced for hypertension (first angiotensin II receptor blocker drug) |
| 1996 | Invirase introduced for HIV (first protease inhibitor drug) |
| 1996 | Fosamax introduced for osteoporosis (first nonhormonal drug treatment) |
| 1996 | Nicoderm introduced (first prescription-strength, over-the-counter drug for stopping smoking) |
| 1997 | Plavix introduced for the treatment of acute coronary syndrome |
| 1998 | Viagra introduced (first oral drug for erectile dysfunction in men) |
| 1999 | Celebrex introduced for arthritis (first COX-2 inhibitor drug) |
| 2000 | Deciphering of the human genome opens the field of gene therapy in pharmacology |
| 2001 | Anthrax attack on the United States creates high demand for the antibiotic drugs ciprofloxin and doxycycline |
| 2002 | Botox introduced for the treatment of facial wrinkles |
| 2003 | Fuzeon introduced (first fusion inhibitor drug for HIV) |
| 2004 | Lunesta introduced for the long-term treatment of chronic insomnia |
| 2005 | Requip introduced (first drug for restless legs syndrome) |
| 2006 | Gardasil introduced (first vaccine against cervical cancer caused by HPV) |
| 2007 | Exelon introduced (first transdermal drug patch for Alzheimer's disease) |
| 2007 | Zyrtek is the first drug to have the same dose strength for both its prescription and over-the-counter forms |
| 2007 | Isentress introduced (first integrase inhibitor drug for HIV) |
| 2008 | Xenazine introduced (first FDA-approved drug for Huntington's disease) |

## Mislabeled and Dangerous Drugs

From the early history of pharmacology, most physicians attempted to treat patients based on what little scientific knowledge was available to them. As early as 2100 B.C., the Code of Hammurabi gave severe penalties for malpractice.

However, throughout medical history many ineffective, mislabeled, and even dangerous drugs have been manufactured, advertised, and prescribed. In 1680, English apothecary (pharmacist) Thomas Sydenham created the drug *Sydenham's Laudanum*, which contained powdered opium, wine, and herbs. During the 1700s and 1800s, drugs with names such as *Warner's Safe Cure for Diabetes, Dr. Shreve's Anti-Gallstone Remedy,* and *Anti-Morbific Great Liver and Kidney Medicine* were commonly sold without regulation and were accompanied by extravagant claims of cures. Drugs often contained one of the addicting ingredients of opium, morphine, or cocaine without its presence being listed on the label. *Ayer's Cherry Pectoral,* advertised for respiratory ailments, contained cherry flavoring and heroin. Even when a drug included the name of the addictive ingredient in its title or on its label (see ■ FIGURE 1–7), consumers were often not aware of its addictive qualities. One drug prescribed for respiratory ailments, hydrocyanic acid, caused many deaths. (This poison, which as a gas contains cyanide, is used for legal executions.)

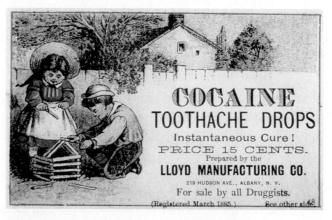

■ **FIGURE 1–7  Cocaine in a common drug.**
This 1885 advertisement was for the drug *Cocaine Toothache Drops*.
It was not known at that time that cocaine was a highly addictive drug.
Children as well as adults became addicted to this drug.

It is estimated that in the early 1900s one out of every 200 Americans was addicted, most of them middle-class women who used these drugs for themselves and their children.

Consumer warnings against the misuse of drugs, the possibility of addiction, or dangerous drug side effects did not exist. At that time, the prevailing dictum was "Let the buyer beware."

## Drug Legislation and Drug Agencies

Laws were passed in the 1900s to protect the public from unscrupulous drug sellers, as well as from worthless, mislabeled, and dangerous drugs that were then on the market. The drug manufacturers strongly opposed drug laws, but public outrage resulted in the passage of **The Food and Drugs Act** of 1906, the first federal drug law. A 1912 amendment to this act required the accurate labeling of drugs to prevent substitution or mislabeling of ingredients. It also stated that only drugs listed in the

*United States Pharmacopeia* or *National Formulary* could be prescribed. Nevertheless, many worthless drugs remained on the market because the burden of proof lay with the government to show fraud on the part of the seller.

It took a national tragedy to force a much-needed update of The Food and Drugs Act of 1906. Sulfonamide, an early anti-infective drug, was widely used in the United States in 1937. After an extensive advertising campaign aimed at physicians, a Tennessee company marketed this drug in a raspberry-flavored base and called it "Elixir of Sulfonamide." This base had been tested by the manufacturer for flavor and fragrance but not for safety. Elixirs are made from a sweetened alcohol base, but this drug base was an industrial-strength liquid solvent. A number of children died after taking less than one ounce of this drug, and over 350 individuals were poisoned. At that time, a drug manufacturer did not need FDA approval before marketing a drug. Because of this tragedy, Congress passed **The Food, Drug, and Cosmetic Act** of 1938 that previously had lacked the support it needed to pass. As a result, the government no longer needed proof of fraud to stop the sale of a drug. It could seize any drug suspected of being toxic. Secondly, the burden of proof was shifted to the drug manufacturers, who were required to provide data based on scientific experiments to show that their product was safe before they were allowed to market it. It became the job of the **Food and Drug Administration (FDA)** to review these data and evaluate the safety of drugs.

In 1951, the **Durham-Humphrey Amendment** to The Food, Drug, and Cosmetic Act defined prescription drugs as those drugs that could only be given to patients under the care of a physician.

In the late 1950s, the drug thalidomide was developed in West Germany and was used extensively during early pregnancy to treat morning sickness in women. The FDA refused to approve its use in the United States without further studies. Before these additional studies could be completed by the manufacturer, evidence against the safety of the drug began to accumulate. Over 8,000 babies in Europe were born with deformed limbs ("seal limbs," or phocomelia). This tragedy resulted in the passage of the 1962 **Kefauver-Harris Amendment** to The Food, Drug, and Cosmetic Act, which tightened control on existing prescription drugs and new drugs. It required that drugs be shown to be both safe and effective before being marketed. It also required manufacturers to report adverse side effects from new drugs. Since that time, many drugs have been kept from the market or have been removed from the market because of a lack of safety.

## *Historical Notes*

Because of its devastating adverse effects in unborn children, thalidomide would have been relegated to an obscure footnote in medical history, but in 1997 it was discovered to be a useful drug in treating cancer, AIDS, and leprosy. The potential adverse effects of this drug are so great that it is only considered as a viable treatment option for these life-threatening diseases. The FDA regulates the use of thalidomide in two ways: (1) by limiting the number of physicians who can prescribe it and (2) by requiring women taking the drug not to have sexual intercourse or to use two forms of birth control (so that there is virtually no risk of them giving birth to a child with phocomelia). Thalidomide is now an official prescription drug used to treat multiple myeloma, leprosy, graft-versus-host disease, and several types of cancers. It is also officially recognized as an orphan drug that is used to treat wasting syndrome from HIV, as well as Crohn's disease.

For each new drug, the FDA must weigh the inherent risks of the drug against its potential benefits. To do this thoroughly, the FDA must take the time to complete its review process before it issues a final approval (or rejection) of a new drug. In 1988, the Food and Drug Administration was moved under the federal Department of Health and Human Services.

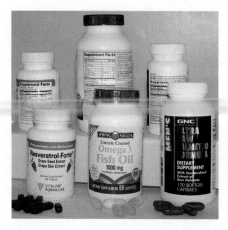

**■ FIGURE 1–8  Dietary supplements.**
Dietary supplements, such as vitamins, minerals, and herbs, are manufactured in tablets and capsules that resemble prescription and over-the-counter drugs. However, the bottle label clearly states "Dietary Supplement," and the reverse side of the bottle provides information under the heading of "Supplement Facts."

In 1994, the **Dietary Supplements and Health and Education Act** was passed. This legislation allowed the FDA to set up guidelines for the manufacturers of herbal products and dietary supplements (see ■ **FIGURE 1–8**). Although the FDA could not regulate these products and the products were still available without a prescription, the drug manufacturers were now liable for any claims against their products in accordance with the FDA guidelines.

In the early 1990s, FDA approval of a new drug took an average of 34 months. However, for certain critical drugs the process could be much shorter. The first drug effective against HIV was approved by the FDA in 1987 in just 107 days. Despite the rapid handling of many critical drugs, critics still pointed to a time lag in the approval of other new drugs. They argued that some drugs were available in other countries for quite some time before they received approval by the FDA for use in the United States. For example, Inderal, a widely used drug for hypertension and arrhythmias, was available in Europe for nearly 10 years before it was finally approved for use in the United States in 1967. In response to this criticism, the FDA made a concerted effort to streamline the approval process, particularly with respect to drugs used to treat life-threatening diseases. In 1996, indinavir (Crixivan), a protease inhibitor drug used to treat HIV, was approved by the FDA in record time, just 42 days after the new drug application was submitted. In 1997, then-President Clinton signed the **Food and Drug Administration (FDA) Modernization Act**. It gave the FDA the authority to accelerate the approval process for certain types of drugs. By 2000, the average review time for new drugs had fallen to less than 15 months. Critically needed drugs (as well as those for whom the drug manufacturer pays a special fee) can be approved in as little as 6 months.

In addition, the FDA allows physicians to prescribe some investigational drugs even before they are officially approved for marketing. These drugs are for life-threatening diseases for which no other alternative therapy exists. In order to prescribe such a drug, the FDA requires an **Emergency Treatment Investigational New Drug (IND)** application to be filed. This is also known as a **Compassionate Use IND** application. In the 1970s, long before the cardiac drug amiodarone (Cordarone) was on the market (final approval, 1985), cardiologists prescribed it as an investigational new drug to treat patients with life-threatening cardiac arrhythmias that did not respond to other antiarrhythmic drugs. Similarly, the first drug for HIV was prescribed for patients before its approval in 1987. This was done under a Compassionate Use IND application.

Under the federal regulations of HIPAA (pronounced "hip-ah"), the **Health Insurance Portability and Accountability Act** of 1996, all healthcare settings must provide patients with a statement that verifies that their health record information, including all drug information, is kept secure and is only released to authorized inquiries from other healthcare providers, insurance companies, or healthcare quality monitoring organizations.

## Prescription and Over-the-Counter Drugs

The Food and Drug Administration (FDA) regulates prescription drugs and over-the-counter drugs. **Prescription drugs** are defined as those drugs that are not safe to use except under professional medical supervision. Prescription drugs can only be obtained with a written prescription or verbal order from a physician, dentist, nurse practitioner, or other healthcare provider whose license permits this. Prescription drugs are also known as *legend drugs* because the drug manufacturer and pharmacist add one of these two legends (inscriptions) to the drug package and to the filled prescription bottle: "Caution: Federal law prohibits dispensing without a prescription" or "Rx only."

In addition to prescription drugs, the FDA also regulates **over-the-counter (OTC) drugs**. An OTC drug is defined as one that can be purchased without a prescription and is generally considered safe for consumers to use if the label's directions and warnings are followed carefully. OTC drugs comprise more than half of all the drugs used in the United States.

For many years, there was a clear distinction between prescription drugs and OTC drugs. Then, in 1983, the topical prescription drug hydrocortisone was approved for over-the-counter sales and many other drugs followed. The OTC drug is the same as the original prescription drug, but the recommended dose is usually just a fraction (often half) of the dose of the prescription drug. An exception to this is cetirizine (Zyrtec), a prescription antihistamine drug whose over-the-counter dose, as approved by the FDA, is the same as its prescription dose.

In 1992, the OTC Drugs Advisory Committee was created to assist the FDA in reviewing drugs and determining which ones were safe and appropriate for over-the-counter use (see ■ TABLE 1–3).

■ TABLE 1–3  **Some prescription drugs that are also OTC drugs**

| Generic Name | Prescription Trade Name | OTC Trade Name | Therapeutic Use |
|---|---|---|---|
| butenafine | Mentax | Lotrimin Ultra | skin fungal infection |
| butoconazole | Gynazole-1 | Mycelex-3 | vaginal yeast infection |
| cetirizine | Zyrtec | Zyrtec | nasal allergies |
| cimetidine | Tagamet | Tagamet HB 200 | heartburn/ulcer |
| cromolyn | Intal | Nasalcrom | nasal allergies |
| famotidine | Pepcid | Pepcid AC | heartburn/ulcer |
| hydrocortisone | Hycort | Cortizone-5 | skin inflammation |
| ibuprofen | Motrin | Advil, Motrin IB | pain |
| naproxen | Naprosyn | Aleve | pain |
| nicotine | Nicotrol Inhaler | Nicoderm CQ | quit smoking |
| nizatidine | Axid | Axid AR | heartburn/ulcer |
| omeprazole | Prilosec | Prilosec OTC | heartburn/ulcer |
| ranitidine | Zantac | Zantac 75 | heartburn/ulcer |

This committee consists of physicians and pharmacists, as well as one nonvoting member from the drug/cosmetics industry. The FDA approves a prescription drug being reclassified as an OTC drug if the following criteria are met: (1) the indication for the drug's OTC use is similar to its use as a prescription drug, (2) the patient can easily diagnose and monitor his or her own condition when using the OTC drug, (3) the OTC drug has a low rate of side effects/toxicity and a low potential for abuse, and (4) use of the OTC drug does not require the patient to have any special monitoring or testing.

## Focus on Healthcare Issues

Supporters of the reclassification of some prescription drugs to an OTC status claim that this will lower drug prices and allow better access to treatment and fewer visits to the doctor. Opponents to reclassification have these arguments: (1) consumers may actually pay more because health insurance plans will not reimburse for OTC drug purchases, (2) excessive use of OTC drugs may increase the number of adverse drug–drug interactions, and (3) consumers may try to self-medicate serious illnesses instead of visiting their physicians for appropriate treatment.

## Schedule Drugs

Drugs with the potential for abuse and dependence were first regulated by **The Harrison Narcotics Act** of 1914. This act established the legal framework for controlling these drugs and introduced the word *narcotic*. This act was replaced in 1970 by **The Comprehensive Drug Abuse Prevention and Control Act**. Title II of this act, **The Controlled Substances Act**, established the **Drug Enforcement Administration (DEA)** in 1973 to regulate the manufacturing and dispensing of these drugs. The act also divided potentially addictive drugs into five categories or schedules based on their potential for physical or psychological dependence. These drugs are known as *schedule drugs* or *controlled substances.* The labeling and packaging for a controlled substance and all of its advertisements must clearly show the drug's assigned schedule (see ▪ **FIGURE 1–9**). The manufacturing, storage, dispensing, and disposal of controlled substances are strictly regulated by both federal and state laws.

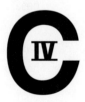

▪ **FIGURE 1–9  Controlled substance symbol.**
The capital *C* stands for *controlled substance.* The number written inside (always a Roman numeral) indicates the assigned schedule. It is important to remember that a *C* with the Roman numeral IV inside it does *not* mean that the drug is to be given by the intravenous (I.V.) route; it means that the drug is a Schedule IV controlled substance.

**Schedule I**

Extremely high potential for abuse and addiction

No currently accepted medical use

Not available under any circumstances, even with a prescription

Examples: heroin, LSD, marijuana, methaqualone, peyote, psilocybin

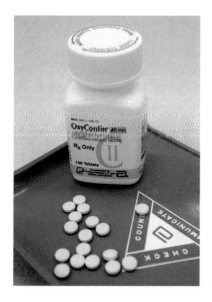

**■ FIGURE 1–10  Schedule II drug.**
OxyContin is a prescription drug that is used to treat severe pain.
It is also a popular drug of abuse. Because it is a Schedule II
drug—see the symbol on the label—it has a high potential for
addiction. The drug bottle is sitting on a blue pill-counting tray in
the pharmacy. This tray helps the pharmacist accurately count out
the exact number of tablets specified in the patient's prescription.
The logo in the center of the tray reminds the pharmacist to
"Check, Counsel, Communicate."

**Schedule II**    (see ■ **FIGURE 1–10**)

High potential for abuse and addiction

Currently accepted medical uses

Requires an official prescription form

Severe physical and psychological dependence may result

Examples: cocaine, codeine, Demerol, Dilaudid, methadone, morphine, OxyContin, Percodan, Ritalin

**Schedule III**

Less potential for abuse and addiction than Schedule II drugs

Currently accepted medical uses

Moderate physical and psychological dependence may result

Examples: anabolic steroid drugs, dronabinol (Marinol), Hycodan, paregoric, phenobarbital, testosterone, Tylenol w/ Codeine, Vicodin

**Schedule IV**

Less potential for abuse and addiction than Schedule III drugs

Currently accepted medical uses

Limited-to-moderate physical and psychological dependence may result

Examples: Ambien, Darvon, Librium, Meridia, Sonata, Valium, Xanax

**Schedule V**

Limited potential for abuse

Currently accepted medical uses

Some physical and psychological dependence may result

Examples: cough syrups with codeine, Lomotil

## Focus on Healthcare Issues

There has been a longstanding debate over whether marijuana (a Schedule I drug) should be legally available to treat patients with certain medical conditions. In 1996, voters in California passed Proposition 215 to allow seriously ill patients to use marijuana if approved by their primary care physician. Eight other states passed similar laws.

However, the federal law that prohibits the manufacturing and distribution of marijuana supersedes individual state laws. In November 2000, the U.S. Supreme Court agreed to hear a case that sought an exemption from the federal law for cases of medical necessity. The American Medical Association (AMA) advised that marijuana did provide medical benefit to patients with certain conditions, and many other groups supported the legalization of marijuana to varying degrees. In May 2001, however, the Supreme Court issued a decision that federal drug laws that ban the manufacture and distribution of marijuana allow for no exceptions, even for medical necessity.

   Despite this ruling, many patients do use the marijuana plant to treat themselves. Of note is that the main active ingredient in marijuana is available as the prescription drug dronabinol (Marinol). It is a Schedule III drug and is used to treat nausea and vomiting caused by chemotherapy and to stimulate the appetite in patients with HIV.

Physicians, dentists, podiatrists, nurse practitioners, and other healthcare providers whose state licenses allow them to may prescribe controlled substances. First, however, they must register with the federal Drug Enforcement Agency and be issued a DEA certificate and number to prescribe or dispense a schedule drug (controlled substance). The provider's DEA number must be clearly written on any prescription for a schedule drug. In addition, some states require the healthcare provider to register with the state agency that controls schedule drugs and be issued a state certificate and number in order to prescribe or dispense schedule drugs in that state.

## Orphan Drugs

In 1983, **The Orphan Drug Act** was passed. Its purpose was to facilitate the development of new drugs to treat rare diseases. Normally, drug companies are reluctant to spend large amounts of time and money to research and test a drug if it will have a limited market. In the past that meant that drugs for rare diseases that only affected a few patients were not being developed. The Orphan Drug Act provided special incentives to a drug company, including grants to offset drug development costs, a tax credit that allowed the drug company to deduct up to 75 percent of the cost of clinical trials, a streamlined process for obtaining FDA approval, and exclusive marketing rights for seven years. This encouraged the development of orphan drugs to treat rare diseases, and now there are more than 1,000 orphan drugs.

# Chapter Review

## Quiz Yourself

   1. Describe the linguistic origin/etiology of the following words.
      **a.** pharmacology
      **b.** medicine
      **c.** drug

2. How are the definitions of *drug* and *medicine* the same? How are they different?
3. Describe the three medical uses for drugs and give examples.
4. Give the meaning of and describe the linguistic origin of the symbol *Rx*.
5. Give the name of a drug in current usage that originated from the natural sources listed below.

   | Natural Source | Drug |
   |---|---|
   | **a.** foxglove plant | _____ |
   | **b.** sheeps' wool | _____ |
   | **c.** rose hips | _____ |
   | **d.** poppy | _____ |
   | **e.** mold | _____ |
   | **f.** periwinkle | _____ |

6. In what decade was each of the following drugs first introduced? Circle the correct answer.

   | | | | | | | |
   |---|---|---|---|---|---|---|
   | **a.** insulin | 1890s | 1900s | 1910s | 1920s | 1930s | 1940s |
   | **b.** penicillin | 1890s | 1900s | 1910s | 1920s | 1930s | 1940s |
   | **c.** aspirin | 1890s | 1900s | 1910s | 1920s | 1930s | 1940s |
   | **d.** cortisone | 1890s | 1900s | 1910s | 1920s | 1930s | 1940s |
   | **e.** vitamin A | 1890s | 1900s | 1910s | 1920s | 1930s | 1940s |
   | **f.** phenobarbital | 1890s | 1900s | 1910s | 1920s | 1930s | 1940s |
   | **g.** Viagra | 1950s | 1960s | 1970s | 1980s | 1990s | 2000s |
   | **h.** Tagamet | 1950s | 1960s | 1970s | 1980s | 1990s | 2000s |
   | **i.** Librium | 1950s | 1960s | 1970s | 1980s | 1990s | 2000s |
   | **j.** 1st recombinant DNA drug | 1950s | 1960s | 1970s | 1980s | 1990s | 2000s |
   | **k.** Thorazine | 1950s | 1960s | 1970s | 1980s | 1990s | 2000s |
   | **l.** Gardisil | 1950s | 1960s | 1970s | 1980s | 1990s | 2000s |
   | **m.** Inderal | 1950s | 1960s | 1970s | 1980s | 1990s | 2000s |
   | **n.** $H_2$ blocker drugs | 1950s | 1960s | 1970s | 1980s | 1990s | 2000s |
   | **o.** Nicoderm | 1950s | 1960s | 1970s | 1980s | 1990s | 2000s |
   | **p.** First drug for HIV | 1950s | 1960s | 1970s | 1980s | 1990s | 2000s |
   | **q.** Botox | 1950s | 1960s | 1970s | 1980s | 1990s | 2000s |

7. Name three ancient "medicines" that seem silly or outrageous to us today.
8. Is it possible that some of the "medicines" you named for Question 7 could be found to have some therapeutic value in the future? State the reason for your answer.
9. In the 1700s and 1800s, drugs frequently contained addictive ingredients not listed on the label. Name two such ingredients.
10. Describe the social and consumer safety circumstances that led to the passage of each of these drug laws.
    **a.** The Food and Drugs Act of 1906
    **b.** The Food, Drug, and Cosmetic Act of 1938
    **c.** Kefauver-Harris Amendment of 1962
    **d.** FDA Modernization Act of 1987
11. What federal agency is empowered to review data on a drug's safety and clinical effectiveness and approve drugs for marketing?
12. What is a Compassionate Use IND application?
13. Define the following phrases: *prescription drug, over-the-counter drug.*
14. Describe how The Controlled Substances Act categorized drugs of potential abuse.
15. What is the purpose of the 1983 Orphan Drug Act? What three incentives does it offer to drug companies to develop orphan drugs?
16. What part of the wording of a drug label tells you that it is a prescription drug?

**17.** Why was the drug thalidomide, which caused severe birth defects in thousands of babies, allowed on the market again?

**18.** What is the meaning of this symbol?

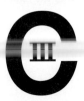

## Clinical Applications

**1.** In 2001, the manufacturer of lovastatin (Mevacor) asked the FDA to allow this prescription drug to switch from being a prescription drug to being an OTC drug. The FDA did not approve this change. Describe the four criteria mentioned in this chapter for prescription-to-OTC approval. Explain why you think the FDA OTC Drugs Advisory Committee ruled against this request? If you had been on the committee, would you have voted for or against approving this drug for OTC use? (*Hint:* Look up lovastatin in Appendix D of this textbook and see what category of drugs it belongs to; then look up that category of drugs in Chapter 11 and read about it.)

**2.** You are caring for a patient who is extremely ill but might be able to be helped if he could get access to a drug that is already approved in Europe. Write a paragraph criticizing the time lag in the United States for the approval of new drugs that are already in clinical use in other countries. Give a drug example to support your position.

**3.** You read in the newspaper about an FDA-approved drug that has now suddenly been withdrawn from the market because of causing serious adverse reactions and several deaths. Write a paragraph defending the time needed to investigate drugs before approving them. Give a drug example to support your position.

**4.** Look at this drug label and answer the following questions.
   **a.** What is the name of this drug?
   **b.** To what schedule does this drug belong?
   **c.** Is this a prescription drug or an over-the-counter drug? How can you tell?

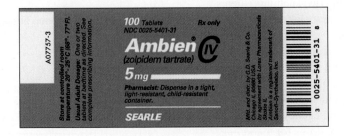

## Multimedia Extension Exercises

■ Go to www.pearsonhighered.com/turley and click on the photo of the cover of *Understanding Pharmacology for Health Professionals* to access the interactive Companion Website created for this textbook.

# Drug Design, Testing, Manufacturing, and Marketing

## CHAPTER CONTENTS

## Learning Objectives

After you study this chapter, you should be able to

1. Name several ways in which drugs are discovered or created.

2. Describe how computers facilitate drug design.

3. Differentiate between the chemical, generic, and trade/brand names of a drug.

4. List at least five things that the trade names of drugs might tell you about those drugs.

5. Describe the three phases of the human testing of new drugs.

6. Define the phrases *in vitro, in vivo, clinical trials, control group, drug patent, isomer,* and *placebo.*

7. Describe how inert ingredients might affect the bioavailability of a drug.

8. Describe how direct marketing of prescription drugs has affected consumers and drug costs.

9. Give four reasons why a drug might be withdrawn from the market or recalled.

The development, testing, manufacturing, and eventual marketing of any drug is a time-consuming and expensive process. A drug company may evaluate thousands of different chemicals before finding one that moves successfully through all phases of testing and is finally approved by the FDA for release and marketing. This chapter traces the steps from a newly discovered or designed chemical to final FDA approval and clinical use of a drug.

## Drug Discovery and Creation

Drugs are discovered or created in several ways.

1. **Ancient sources.** Many drugs still in use today were originally derived from plant, animal, or mineral sources hundreds or even thousands of years ago. Many of these were described in Chapter 1.

2. **A totally new chemical can be discovered in the environment, from plants, from animals, from the ocean, or from the soil.**

   Example: The chemotherapy drug Taxol was originally derived from the needles of the Pacific yew tree.

   Examples: The antituberculosis drug streptomycin was first isolated from the stomach of a sick chicken. Most recently, the drug Byetta for diabetes mellitus was created from a protein found in the saliva of the Gila monster, a lizard found in desert areas.

   Examples: Over the years, thousands of soil samples have been evaluated for evidence of antibiotic activity because many new antibiotic drugs have been discovered in this way. The fungus from which cephalosporin antibiotic drugs were derived was first isolated near a sewer outlet in Sardinia. Coal tar drugs used to treat psoriasis, a skin condition, are a by-product of coal mining.

3. **A totally new chemical can be derived from molecular manipulation of a drug that is already in use.** An **isomer** is a drug that has the same chemical formula (same types and numbers of atoms in its molecule) as another drug, but has those atoms arranged in a different way—either with different chemical bonds or in a different structural relationship to each other (such as a mirror image). Dextrorotary drugs (such as dextromethorphan) and levorotary drugs (such as levothyroxine) are examples of isomers that are rotated and are the right-facing (or left-facing) mirror image compared to a related isomer (*dextr/o-* means *right* and *lev/o-* means *left*). Other types of molecular manipulation create drugs that are similar in structure but are not isomers, although these drugs often have a similar therapeutic effect (see ■ **FIGURE 2–1**). Other examples of molecular manipulation to create new drugs include the following.

   Example: Penicillin G is derived from the mold *Penicillium chrysogenum*. One of the drug's major drawbacks is that it is destroyed by stomach acid and cannot be administered orally. When the penicillin structure was changed by adding certain chemicals to the vats where the penicillin was fermenting, a semisynthetic penicillin was obtained that was not destroyed by stomach acid. This penicillin derivative was named *ampicillin.*

   Example: In 1991, when reports of a severe cardiac adverse reaction were linked to the then-popular antihistamine drug terfenadine (Seldane) and it was taken off the market, researchers were able to manipulate its molecular structure and derive the new drug fexofenadine (Allegra), which did not cause that adverse reaction.

   Example: When the drug erythropoietin was used to treat anemia in patients undergoing kidney dialysis, enzymes in the blood broke it down too rapidly to maintain an effective blood level over time. When researchers added two more sugar molecules to its molecular structure, they created the new drug Aranesp, which keeps an effective blood level and requires fewer doses.

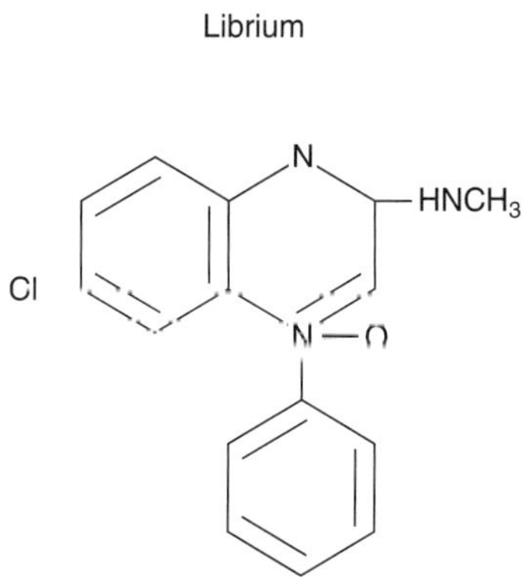

Librium                               Valium

**■ FIGURE 2–1  Derivative chemical structure.**
In 1957, the first benzodiazepine antianxiety drug was synthesized:
chlordiazepoxide (Librium). Its chemical structure is shown on the left.
Working with that molecule, the same researcher then derived
diazepam (Valium). Its chemical structure is shown on the right. Both
drugs are still in use today to treat anxiety and neurosis.

In the distant past, designing a new drug by changing the molecular structure of an existing drug was a slow process of trial and error, using intuition and molecular models made
from wood and wire.

Now, a computer can display the molecular structure of any drug from a listing of thousands contained in its database (see **■ FIGURE 2–2**). With only very slight molecular

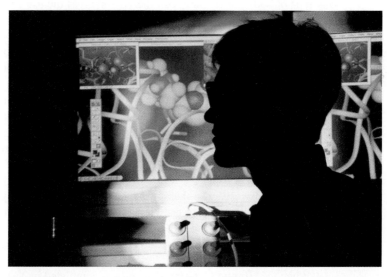

**■ FIGURE 2–2  Creating new drugs with computer-aided design
(CAD).**
With computers, researchers can study any molecule, rotating it in three
dimensions on the computer screen. By analyzing the molecules, researchers
can tell if that particular arrangement of atoms is the "key" that will open the
"lock"—that is, activate a particular receptor on the cell membrane. When a
researcher wants to know why different-looking drugs seem to produce a similar
effect on the same receptor, he/she can have the computer superimpose all of the
drugs on the screen to see how their atoms match up.

changes, the original drug may be significantly changed in a variety of ways that influence absorption, metabolism, half-life, therapeutic effect, or side effects. The computer can also identify those chemicals that would probably not be successful in treating a particular disease before time and money are invested in extensive testing. Using computers to manipulate chemicals at the molecular level and design new drugs is based on **molecular pharmacology**, the study of the chemical structures of drugs and their actions at the molecular level within a cell and even within DNA in the nucleus.

4. **A totally new chemical can be created through genetic manipulation.    Recombinant DNA (rDNA) technology**, (also known as *gene splicing* or *genetic engineering*), involves using enzymes in a test tube (*in vitro*) to cut apart a segment of a DNA molecule from a human cell. This segment specifically directs the production of a particular substance in the body. The technique of gene cloning allows the production of a large supply of this DNA segment. The DNA segments are then spliced together (recombined) with the DNA in a bacterial cell. As the bacterium multiplies, it carries the new DNA within it as part of its genetic makeup. All subsequent generations of bacteria are now preprogrammed to make supplies of that particular substance that can be used as a drug. In huge vats, these bacteria can produce unlimited quantities of the drug.

   In 1982, human insulin (Humulin) became the first recombinant DNA technology drug approved by the FDA. Drugs created through recombinant DNA technology include recombinant human erythropoietin, recombinant human growth factor, recombinant clotting factors, and others. The **Recombinant DNA Advisory Committee** is a group of physicians and pharmacists who review the clinical trials of these genetically engineered new drugs and make recommendations to the FDA.

5. **Stem cell therapy.**    Stem cells are immature cells that are capable of differentiating into any type of body tissue. Stem cell therapy involves the use of stem cells to repair or replace damaged cells in the body. In 2001, the first embryonic stem cell was manipulated to become a mature red blood cell. This breakthrough ignited a controversy over the use of human embryonic cells in stem cell research. Umbilical cord blood can also be used for stem cell therapy, but only if the umbilical cord is saved and preserved after birth. Now, it is known that stem cells can be harvested from the patient's own bone marrow or blood. This approach has no ethical concerns; it also involves no chance of tissue rejection because the stems cells are harvested from the patient. Stem cell therapy has been used since 1988 to replenish cells in the bone marrow after they have been destroyed by chemotherapy drugs used to treat cancer, but researchers are eager to treat a wider range of diseases with stem cell therapy.

6. **Gene therapy.**    In patients who are missing a specific gene or have an abnormal gene that is the cause of a disease, gene therapy can be used. In gene therapy, a normal version of the gene is linked to a harmless virus. The virus (known as a *vector*) then carries the gene into body cells affected by the disease. The world's first gene therapy occurred in 2007, in which the normal version of a gene was used to correct an inherited disorder of the retina of the eye in a 23-year-old patient in England.

   When the **Human Genome Project** was completed in 2000, the map of all 3.2 billion parts of the human genome had been deciphered. This opened up an entirely new area of opportunity to drug researchers—gene therapy that replaces defective genes in the body at the molecular level. Now through a computer database known as The Connectivity Map, researchers are able to do an online match between the genetic profile of a disease and the genetic profile of a drug that could be used to treat that disease.

   Information from the human genome has led to the development of the subspecialty areas of pharmacogenetics and pharmacogenomics in research and drug design.

**pharmacogenetics**   how the genetic makeup of different people affects their response to certain drugs

**pharmacogenomics**   using genome technology to discover new drugs

## Drug Names

From the moment of its discovery or design, every drug has a **chemical name** that is assigned by the International Union of Pure and Applied Chemistry (IUPAC). The chemical name accurately describes its molecular structure and distinguishes it from all other chemicals. The chemical name is commonly used by drug companies and researchers, but is too lengthy and complicated for everyday use by healthcare professionals (see ■ **FIGURE 2–3**). So the drug company, together with an organization known as the **United States Adopted Names (USAN) Council,** determines a second name for the drug—its **generic name**. There is only one generic drug name related to a specific chemical name. When the FDA gives final approval for marketing, the drug company creates a third name for the drug known as the *trade name* or *brand name*. The trade name is specifically designed to be easy for physicians and patients to remember and, if possible, to suggest how the drug is used.

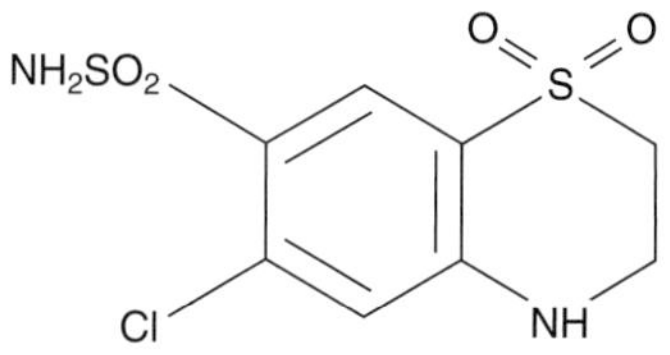

■ **FIGURE 2–3  Molecular structure and chemical name.** The chemical name of this drug actually describes its molecular structure: 6-chloro-3,4-dihydro-2H-1,2,4-benzothiadiazine-7-sulfonamide 1,1-dioxide. The generic name of this drug is hydrochlorothiazide, a diuretic drug. It is also available as the trade names HydroDIURIL (from the Merck drug company) and Microzide (from the Watson drug company), among others.

## *Clinical Applications*

The accurate spelling of drug names is critical. Some trade name drugs are difficult to spell because drug manufacturers are not held to any linguistic standards. For example, the trade name drug Rythmol is used to normalize the rhythm of the heart, and yet the *h* found in *rhythm* is not in the drug name. The trade name drug Levothroid is a thyroid hormone replacement, and yet the *y* found in *thyroid* is not in the drug name. Throughout this textbook, there are tips to assist you in the accurate spelling of generic and trade name drugs.

**Tip 1:**   The spellings of generic drugs that belong to the same drug category often reflect their similar chemical structure.

Example: All of the following generic drugs belong to the beta-blocker class of drugs and are used to treat hypertension and some types of heart arrhythmias. They all have the suffix *-olol.*

acebutolol, atenolol, betaxolol, metoprolol, nadolol, pindolol, propranolol

Example: All of the following generic drugs belong to the benzodiazepine class of tranquilizer drugs and are used to treat anxiety and neurosis. They all have the suffix *-azepam.*

clonazepam, diazepam, lorazepam, oxazepam

*(continued)*

## *Clinical Applications* *(continued)*

Example: All of the following generic drugs belong to the penicillin class of drugs and are used to treat infections. They all have the suffix -*cillin*.

ampicillin, amoxicillin, nafcillin, oxacillin, penicillin

**Tip 2:**   The drug manufacturer selects a trade name that indicates what disease condition or symptom the drug is being used to treat. However, the spelling of the drug is often slightly different from the spelling of the disease.

Azmacort    treats asthma
Nicorette    decreases the craving for nicotine in smokers
Mucinex     removes mucus from the lungs
Pepcid       treats peptic ulcers
Rythmol      treats an irregularity of the heart rhythm

**Tip 3:**   The drug manufacturer selects a trade name that indicates what part of the body is being treated.

Boniva        strengthens the bones
Bronkaid     aids in dilating the bronchi in the lungs
Dermatop    a lotion for the skin
Nasalcrom    treats nasal allergies

**Tip 4:**   The drug manufacturer selects a trade name that simplifies the generic name while retaining parts of its phonetic sound.

Cipro          ciprofloxacin
Haldol         haloperidol
Humulin       human recombinant DNA insulin
Levothroid    thyroid hormone replacement
Sudafed       pseudoephedrine

**Tip 5:**   The drug manufacturer selects a trade name that indicates the ingredients or source of the drug.

Fer-In-Sol    iron (**Fe**) **in sol**ution
Kay Ciel      composed of potassium (**K**) chloride (**Cl**)
Premarin      obtained from **pre**gnant **mar**es' ur**in**e
cetuximab    a **m**onoclonal **a**nti**b**ody

**Tip 6:**   The drug manufacturer selects a trade name that indicates the therapeutic effect of the drug.

Elimite        eliminates mites (scabies)
Glucotrol     controls the level of glucose (blood sugar)
Lipitor         decreases the level of blood lipids
Restoril        restores rest/sleep to treat insomnia

**Tip 7:**   The drug manufacturer selects a trade name that indicates how often the drug is to be taken.

Lithobid     lithium drug given twice a day to treat bipolar disorder
                 (*b.i.d.* is a Latin abbreviation that means *twice a day*)
Nitro-Bid    nitroglycerin drug given twice a day to treat angina

**Tip 8:** The drug manufacturer selects a trade name that indicates the duration of the drug's therapeutic effect.

Cardizem LA **l**ong-**a**cting drug for hypertension
Pronestyl-SR **s**ustained-**r**elease drug for heart arrhythmia
Zyflo CR **c**ontrolled-**r**elease tablet for asthma

**Tip 9:** The drug manufacturer selects a trade name that indicates the strength of the drug.

Bactrim DS **d**ouble-**s**trength dose of antibiotic drug
Cortizone-5 0.**5**% hydrocortisone anti-inflammatory ointment

**Tip 10:** The drug manufacturer selects a trade name that indicates the route of administration.

Bactrim IV          intravenous (**IV**) antibiotic drug
Transderm-Scōp **transderm**al skin patch for motion sickness

**Tip 11:** The drug manufacturer selects a trade name that indicates the amount of a particular active ingredient.

Tylenol w/ Codeine No. 2  contains 15 mg of codeine
Tylenol w/ Codeine No. 3  contains 30 mg of codeine

**Tip 12:** The drug manufacturer selects a trade name that reflects the manufacturer's identity.

ED Tuss HC cough syrup          manufactured by **Ed**wards drug company
Wytensin for hypertension          manufactured by **Wy**eth-Ayerst drug company

## Testing of New Drugs

No matter how a drug was originally discovered or designed, it must be thoroughly tested by the drug company before it can be marketed. It is tested to determine the drug's effectiveness and safety according to certain guidelines specified by the FDA.

Chemical analysis of a drug done in a laboratory in test tubes is known as ***in vitro* testing** (*in vitro* is Latin for *in glass*). Testing carried out in animals or humans is known as ***in vivo* testing** (*in vivo* is Latin for *in living*).

The animal phase of drug testing precedes testing on humans. During animal testing, any side effects, toxic effects, addictions, cancerous tumors, or fetal deformities are noted and evaluated. Also during this phase, the **pharmacodynamics** of the drug are explored. This involves using mathematics to describe the mechanism of action by which the drug produces its effects (desired or undesired), based on time and dose. It includes calculating the following.

**frequency distribution curve**   the number of animals that respond or do not respond to the drug and at what dose

**half-life**   the time required for the drug level in the serum to decrease from 100 percent to 50 percent. The half-life of a drug can be prolonged significantly when liver or kidney diseases decrease metabolism or excretion of a drug. The shorter a drug's half-life, the more frequently it must be given.

**median effective dose ($ED_{50}$)**   the dose at which 50 percent of animals tested show a therapeutic response to the drug

**median toxicity dose ($TD_{50}$)**   the dose at which 50 percent of animals tested had toxic levels of the drug

**therapeutic index (TI)**   the relative margin of safety between the dose that produces a therapeutic effect and the dose that produces a lethal effect in animals. Animal studies, however, are limited in their application as they are not always a reliable indicator of how well a drug will perform in humans. For example, penicillin is toxic to some animals, even in small doses, but causes few side effects in humans even at fairly high doses. If animal studies alone had been used to evaluate the potential of penicillin, it might not even be marketed for human use.

The higher the therapeutic index, the more desirable it is, because it indicates that the drug has a wide margin of safety. For example, penicillin has a therapeutic index of greater than 100. The therapeutic index of digoxin (Lanoxin) is less than 2, and it is not uncommon for patients being given a therapeutic dose of digoxin to begin to exhibit symptoms of toxicity.

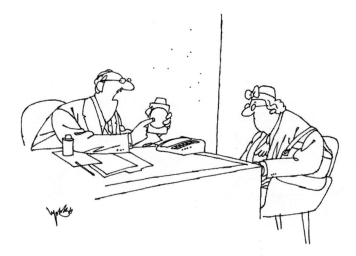

*"This drug was tested on 2000 white mice, and they had a ball."*

When animal studies are complete, the drug company submits an **Investigational New Drug (IND)** application to the FDA to request permission to test the drug in humans. The IND contains information from the animal studies to show that the drug will not pose an undue risk to humans. It also includes information about the chemistry and manufacturing process for the drug. If the IND application is approved, then the drug company can ship the drug to clinical investigators at a number of clinical sites and begin human testing.

There are three phases of human testing, which are known as *clinical trials.* During phase I, about 10 to 100 healthy volunteers are used to study a safe dose range, evaluate side effects, and establish a final, correct dose. The pharmacokinetics of the drug (movement of the drug through the body via the processes of absorption, distribution, metabolism, and excretion) are also studied. It is not uncommon to see "want ads" in the classified section of newspapers of large cities for volunteers for phase I clinical drug trials (see ■ **FIGURE 2–4**). Informed consent is mandatory, and, during the testing, volunteers are monitored and given medical examinations. Phase I testing of a new drug generally takes 1 1/2 years.

In phase II, the drug is given on an experimental basis to about 50 to 500 patients who actually have the disease that the drug is intended to treat. This is done to determine the extent of its therapeutic effect. Phase II testing of a new drug usually takes two years.

During phase III, the drug is administered to several hundred or several thousand ill patients in exactly the way (dose, route of administration, frequency, etc.) in which it will be used once it is on

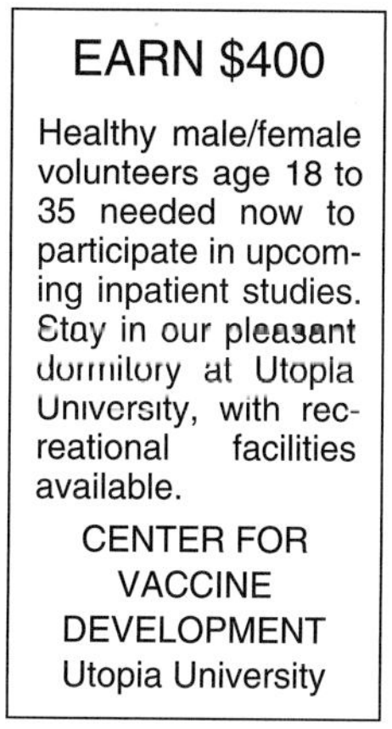

EARN $400

Healthy male/female volunteers age 18 to 35 needed now to participate in upcoming inpatient studies. Stay in our pleasant dormitory at Utopia University, with recreational facilities available.

CENTER FOR VACCINE DEVELOPMENT
Utopia University

■ **FIGURE 2–4  Newpaper advertisement.**
A typical newspaper ad seeking volunteers to participate in clinical trials to test a new drug.

the market. The performance of the drug is compared with that of other drugs currently being used to treat the same disease in order to evaluate its relative effectiveness. In addition, double-blind studies with the drug and a **placebo** are performed, in which neither the patients nor the physician-investigators know which patients are receiving the drug and which patients (the **control group**) are receiving the placebo. In 1993, the FDA issued guidelines that clinical trials should also address the issue of gender: how a drug acts in both men and women. In addition, drug manufacturers who agree to test their new drugs on children so that pediatric doses can be standardized, receive a six-month extension on the standard 17-year patent on new drugs. Phase III testing of a new drug usually lasts three years.

## Drug Alert!

A placebo is a drug form that exerts no pharmacologic effect, no therapeutic effect, and has no side effects when administered. The word *placebo* means *I will please* in Latin. Placebos are used in double-blind research studies in which neither the researcher nor the patient knows whether the drug given was the drug being tested or was a placebo. Placebos are commonly sugar pills or injections of sterile normal saline solution. Interestingly, while it is physiologically impossible for a placebo to exert any pharmacologic effect, patients often report a decrease in certain types of symptoms and can even experience "side effects" when given a placebo. These effects are quite real and demonstrate that, in some situations, the power of suggestion can produce changes within the body that closely mimic the pharmacologic effect of an actual drug.

Once phase III is completed, the drug company submits all of its documentation on the drug to the FDA in a **New Drug Application (NDA)** and waits for a final FDA decision for approval or denial. It is the responsibility of the FDA to evaluate a new drug based on the drug company's documentation and an examination of the relative risks and benefits of the drug. Only about 20 percent of the NDA applications that are filed with the FDA ever receive final FDA approval for marketing.

*Did You Know?*

The data collected for just one patient in just one clinical drug trial can exceed 100 pages of documentation, and the total documentation for all aspects of the drug testing can exceed 100,000 pages.

The ulcer drug cimetidine (Tagamet) is a case in point. After four years of testing, the SmithKline company had accumulated a stack of documents 17 feet high that had to be taken to the FDA in a truck. Denise Grady, "Bottleneck at the FDA," *Discover* (November 1981), p. 56.

Once a drug has received its final approval from the FDA, its ingredients, doses, manufacturing process, labeling, and packaging cannot be changed. With further clinical trials, however, a drug's indicated uses can be expanded. Although new clinical indications for a drug often seem far removed from a drug's original use, they are based on the drug's therapeutic effects or even its side effects.

Example: Propranolol (Inderal) was originally approved by the FDA in 1967 for heart arrhythmias. In 1973, it was approved for hypertension. In 1979, it was approved for migraine headaches.

Example: Indomethacin (Indocin) was originally approved for arthritis and gout. In 1985, it was approved for use in premature infants to close a patent ductus arteriosus (a heart defect).

## Drug Manufacturing

The FDA carefully monitors the quality of both generic and trade name drugs manufactured by all drug companies. Unlike in years past when pharmacists hand-mixed drug ingredients and molded drugs into tablets, today's manufacturing processes are strictly regulated for drug quality, as well as for sanitation and packaging.

Generic drugs, as well as trade name drugs that are in the same drug form and have the same dose strength—even if they are from different drug companies—must all contain exactly the same active drug ingredient and must be able to be administered in exactly the same way. That does not mean, however, that the **bioavailability** will be identical for each of those drugs. Drug companies use different types of **inert ingredients** (binders, fillers), as well as different preservatives, antioxidants, and buffers in a drug. In most cases, these differences only minimally affect the disintegration, absorption, metabolism, and excretion of the drug. However, in some cases, the inert ingredients do seem to affect the therapeutic effect of the drug.

The bioavailability of the active drug ingredient can be particularly crucial in drugs with a low therapeutic index (a low margin of safety between the therapeutic dose and the toxic dose). The inert ingredients can affect the bioavailability of certain drugs. A study in *The New England Journal of Medicine* compared four preparations of digoxin. All met FDA standards, but the bioavailability of the active drug was much higher for one preparation than for the others. This resulted in blood levels of the drug that ranged from toxic for that one drug to subtherapeutic for some of the other drugs.

The manufacturing process also includes securing the drug in an appropriate container. This could require adding a packet of a desiccant (a moisture-absorbing silica gel), if necessary, tightly sealing the top of the container with foil to prevent tampering, or placing the drug in individually sealed blister paks (see ■ FIGURE 2–5).

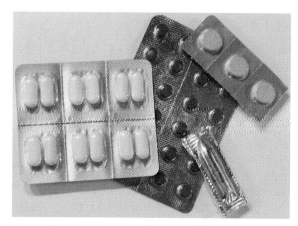

**■ FIGURE 2–5 Protective packaging.**
Blister paks protect the integrity of the drug while allowing
the drug form to be seen through a protective plastic
window. Access is through a peel-off backing.

## Drug Marketing

The advertising of over-the-counter drugs is regulated by the **Federal Trade Commission**. The advertising of prescription drugs is regulated by the FDA based on the federal Food, Drug, and Cosmetic Act.

For many years, drug companies only promoted their prescription drugs by advertising to physicians in the form of visits from a drug sales representative, free samples, promotional literature and videos, and advertising in medical journals. This is still the most prevalent form of prescription drug advertising.

Now, however, direct-to-consumer (DTC) marketing has become common, beginning with magazine ads and moving to television (see ■ TABLE 2–1). Sports magazines contain ads for prescription drugs for men (for erectile dysfunction or an enlarged prostate gland), while drugs for women (for birth control, infertility, menopause, and osteoporosis) are featured in women's magazines.

Consumers are watching these television prescription drug ads and then following the suggestion to "Ask your doctor if [this drug] is right for you." Many critics of television advertising of prescription drugs feel that the final direct appeal to consumers, the phrase "Ask your doctor if [this drug] is right for you," has created a consumer-driven shift in which consumers proactively ask for certain prescription drugs by name that they might not even need and pressure physicians to prescribe the more expensive advertised prescription drugs.

■ TABLE 2–1  **Direct-to-consumer drug marketing timeline**

| Year | DTC Marketing Milestones |
| --- | --- |
| 1981 | The first direct-to-consumers (DTC) print advertisement appears for an analgesic drug. |
| 1985 | FDA rules that drug ads marketed to consumers must include risk information. |
| 1997 | FDA allows drug manufacturers to direct market their ads to consumers via TV. |
| 2001 | More than 100 prescription drugs are regularly marketed directly to consumers. Advertising slogans like "the little purple pill" (for Nexium) become well known. |
| 2004 | Cialis, a drug for erectile dysfunction in men, advertised during TV broadcasts of the 2004 Super Bowl. |

## Drug Patents

The trade name of a drug is registered with the U.S. Patent Office as a registered trademark. While the drug remains under patent, only the original drug company has the right to advertise and market the drug under that trade name.

A drug company is protected by a 17-year patent on any new drug that is approved by the FDA. This means that, during those 17 years, no other company can manufacture or market an identical drug. However, part of the 17-year patent period is used up during the testing process before the drug is even approved. In 1984, a law was passed that allows the drug company to get back up to 5 years of patent protection that were used up during the approval process.

When the patent expires at the end of the 17 years, the original drug company hopes that its drug has been so successful and that its trade name is so firmly entrenched in the mind of the prescribing physician that it will maintain its market share. However, when the patent expires, any other drug company can manufacture that drug under its original generic name or under a new trade name and compete for a place in the market.

The drug's original trade name can only be used by the original drug company. If a generic drug is manufactured by several different drug companies, it will be listed under several different trade names (see ▥ TABLE 2–2).

▥ TABLE 2–2 **Example of generic name and related trade names**

| Type of Name | Drug Name and Drug Company |
|---|---|
| Generic name | mesalamine (approved by the FDA in 1992 to treat ulcerative colitis) |
| Original trade name | Rowasa (manufactured by Solvay) |
| Subsequent trade names | Asacol (manufactured by Procter & Gamble) |
| | Canasa (manufactured by Axcan Scandipharm) |
| | Lialda (manufactured by Shire US) |
| | Pentasa (manufactured by Shire US) |

Some drug companies begin to seek FDA approval for their own version of another drug company's popular trade name drug even before the 17-year patent expires. As early as 2001, three different drug companies had begun production of their version of the popular antidepressant fluoxetine (Prozac), even though the original drug company's patent did not expire until 2003. Today, the generic drug fluoxetine is manufactured by many different drug companies: The drug company Warner Chilcott manufactures it as the trade name drug Sarafem, while the original drug company Eli Lilly still markets it as Prozac.

All drug companies must provide the FDA with a complete list of all of the prescription drugs they currently have on the market. Each of those drugs has a unique identifier number known as the *National Drug Code (NDC)* (see ▥ FIGURE 2–6). The NDC is a multi-digit number, given in

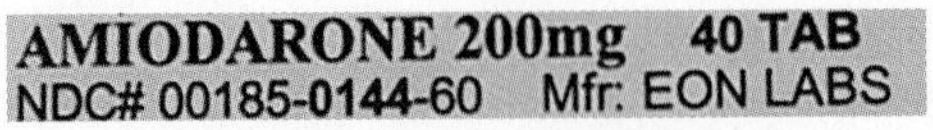

▥ FIGURE 2–6 **National Drug Code.**
Each prescription drug has a National Drug Code or NDC. The NDC identifies the drug manufacturer (Eon Labs), drug strength/dose (amiodarone 200 mg), and package size and type. The NDC may also appear on the label on the prescription bottle or on other printed labels generated by the pharmacy.

**AMIODARONE 200mg    40 TAB**
NDC# 00185-0144-60    Mfr: EON LABS

three segments. The first segment identifies the drug company (this part of the number is assigned by the FDA); the next segment identifies the drug's specific strength/dose; and the last segment is a package code that identifies the package size and type.

## Drug Withdrawals and Recalls

Just because a drug has been approved by the FDA and is on the market does not guarantee that it will remain on the market indefinitely. The drug companies and the FDA continue to monitor the effectiveness and safety of approved drugs. This is known as ***post-marketing surveillance.*** Certain adverse drug effects only become apparent over time, after a drug has been taken by thousands of patients, rather than by the hundred or so tested during the clinical trials. Healthcare professionals and consumers can report adverse events concerning drugs through MedWatch, the FDA's safety information and adverse event reporting system on the Internet. The FDA continually evaluates current reports of adverse effects of drugs, especially those that involve death, and will remove a drug from the market, if warranted.

If a drug is associated with an adverse event, the FDA may elect to have the drug company expand its existing warning label to include that new information, rather than withdrawing the drug from the market.

> Example: In 2007, the FDA suggested that the labeling for all antidepressant drugs include additional information that their use could lead to an increased risk of suicide in young adults between ages 18 and 24.

In addition to concerns about the adverse effects of drugs, the FDA also removes (recalls) certain batches of drugs from the market because of various types of manufacturing defects. A recall can be done for several different reasons.

1. The drug does not contain the correct amount of active ingredient.
2. The drug does not remain stable until its expiration date.
3. The drug is contaminated with particulate matter from the manufacturing process.

> Example: In 2000, the manufacturer of a drug used to treat arthritis, recalled the drug because the capsules were contaminated with acebutolol, a cardiac drug.

> Example: In 2007, certain drug lots of an injectable pediatric vaccine were recalled because the fluid was not sterile.

> Example: In 2008, many batches of heparin whose active ingredient had been manufactured in an uninspected drug manufacturing plant in China were withdrawn from the market when they were linked to many allergic reactions and even some deaths.

It is the responsibility of the drug manufacturer to notify physicians, hospitals, and pharmacies of a drug recall. Once notified, it is the responsibility of the physician, hospital, or pharmacy to dispose of the recalled lots of drugs.

# *Chapter Review*

## Quiz Yourself

1. What are the three names that can be associated with a drug?
2. The spellings of the suffixes of generic drugs may be similar if they belong to the same drug classification. True or false?
3. Describe six ways in which drug companies select a trade name for a drug.
4. Describe four ways in which a new drug can be discovered or created.
5. Describe recombinant DNA technology and how it helps drug companies to produce certain drugs.

6. What is meant by tests that are performed *in vitro? In vivo?*
7. What types of drug characteristics/effects are studied during each of the three phases of human testing of a drug prior to FDA approval?
8. How do computers assist in the designing of new drugs?
9. How can inert ingredients affect the bioavailability of a drug?
10. According to consumer groups and insurance companies, what are the disadvantages of direct-to-consumer advertising of prescription drugs?
11. Name four reasons why a drug can be withdrawn from the market or recalled.

## Clinical Applications

1. This label appeared on the patient's pharmacy prescription drug bottle. Answer the following questions.
   a. What is the name of this drug?
   b. What is the strength of this drug?
   c. Who is the manufacturer of this drug?
   d. Which numbers in the NDC correspond to the code for the drug company?
   e. Which numbers in the NDC correspond to the code for the drug's strength?
   f. What is the total number of tablets to be dispensed for this prescription?

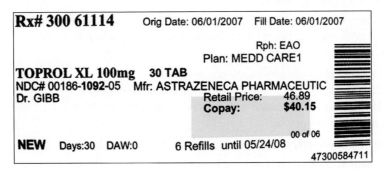

2. What is unique about the technology used to create the drug whose label is pictured below? Where is this technology named in the information on the drug label?

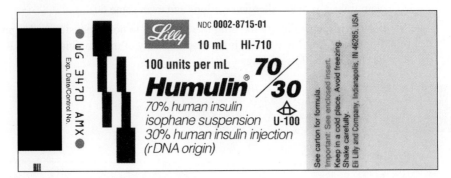

## Multimedia Extension Exercises

■ Go to www.pearsonhighered.com/turley and click on the photo of the cover of *Understanding Pharmacology for Health Professionals* to access the interactive Companion Website created for this textbook.

# Drug Forms

## Learning Objectives

After you study this chapter, you should be able to

1. Name eleven forms in which drugs are manufactured.

2. Describe seven different types of tablets.

3. Describe the difference between a solution and a suspension.

4. Name eight different types of drugs that come in a solution form.

5. Describe how pellets, beads, and wafers are used as drug forms.

6. Define these words and phrases: *ampule, elixir, lozenge, transdermal patch,* and *vial.*

Before a drug can receive final approval by the FDA, the drug company must clearly state in what form or forms the drug will be manufactured. Different forms of a drug are appropriate for different routes of administration. Some drugs are ineffective when administered in a certain form; other drugs can seriously injure the patient if administered in the wrong drug form.

## Drug Forms

Drugs are manufactured in the following different forms.

1. **Tablet.**   A tablet is a solid drug form that contains an active drug (as a dried powder) plus inert ingredients (binders and fillers) to provide bulk and ensure a standardized tablet size. In written prescriptions, *tablet* is sometimes abbreviated as *tab* or *tabs*. Tablets come in many colors, many standard shapes (round, oval, square, oblong), and some unusual shapes (triangle, baseball-diamond shape [see ■ **FIGURE 3–1**], pentagon, hexagon, and others).

   Example: Tablets of Cialis, a drug used to treat erectile dysfunction, are mustard colored and manufactured in the shape of a teardrop.

   Example: Tablets of Valium, a drug used to treat anxiety, have a tiny, V-shaped opening cut in the center of each tablet.

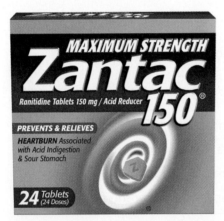

■ **FIGURE 3-1  Drug label for over-the-counter Zantac.**
Over-the-counter Zantac also comes in a 75 mg strength. Zantac is a nonprescription acid reducer available for prevention and relief of heartburn associated with acid indigestion and sour stomach.

## *Clinical Applications*

A 2006 survey of pharmacists found that a tablet with a unique color and shape, one that had the drug name and dose imprinted on it, and one that had a distinctive aroma was the best combination to help positively identify the drug and decrease drug errors. Nearly 70 percent of pharmacists report that patients ask them weekly to identify tablets or capsules that have been taken out of the original packaging.

The Food and Drug Administration (FDA) advises patients who take more than one drug to be able to tell them apart by size, shape, color, imprint, or drug form.

Tablets are also manufactured in several specialized types: scored tablet, effervescent tablet, enteric-coated tablet, slow-release tablet, caplet, lozenge, and troche.

A **scored tablet** has an indented line running across it, from one side to the other, so that it can be easily broken into equal pieces to produce an accurate, but reduced, dose (see ■ **FIGURE 3–2**).

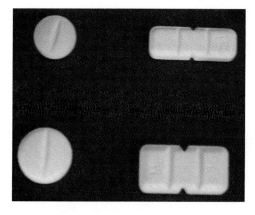

**■ FIGURE 3–2 Scored tablets.**
A scored tablet can be divided easily and
accurately. These scored tablets can be divided into
two or three equal doses, depending on the number
of score marks on the tablet.

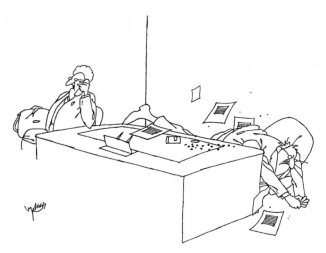

*"While the doctor's trying to split one of the tablets he prescribed, I
thought I'd give you a call."*

An **effervescent tablet** is one that is dissolved in a glass of water before being swallowed
(e.g., Alka-Seltzer for a head cold). An **enteric-coated tablet** is covered with a special coating that resists stomach acid, but dissolves in the alkaline environment of the small intestine to
avoid irritating the stomach (e.g., Ecotrin for pain). The *ec* in the trade name Ecotrin reminds
that it is enteric coated). A **slow-release tablet** is manufactured to provide a continuous, sustained release of the drug. The drug's trade name often includes the abbreviation **CR** (controlled release), **LA** (long acting), **SR** (slow  release), or **XL** (extended length). **Caplets** are
coated tablets in the form of an elongated capsule.

Some over-the-counter drugs come in the form of **lozenges**. These tablets are formed
from a hardened base of sugar and water containing the drug and other flavorings. Lozenges
are never swallowed whole, but are allowed to disintegrate slowly into a liquid form that
releases the drug topically in the mouth and throat (e.g., Cepacol lozenge for a sore throat).
A **troche** is an oblong tablet that has a base of sugar and disintegrates into a paste to release
the drug topically in the mouth (e.g., Mycostatin Pastilles for a yeast infection in the mouth.
A *pastille*, a French word that means *little lump of bread,* is another name for a *troche*).

2. **Capsule.**   A capsule comes in two varieties. The first is a soft, one-piece gelatin shell with the liquid drug inside (e.g., fat-soluble vitamins such as A and E). The second type of capsule is a hard shell manufactured in two pieces that fit together and hold the powdered or granular drug inside (see ■ **FIGURE 3–3**). In written prescriptions, the word *capsule* is sometimes abbreviated as *cap* or *caps.* Hard shell capsules come in a variety of colors.

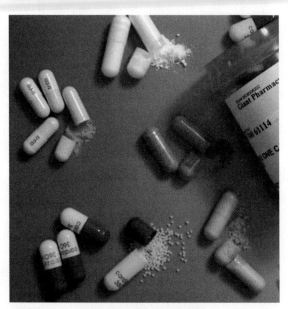

■ **FIGURE 3–3  Hard shell capsules.**
The trade name drug Cardizem is used to treat hypertension. It comes in a blue and white, hard shell capsule that contains the drug in a granular form.

Example: Nexium, a drug used to treat heartburn and ulcers, is a distinctive deep purple–colored capsule with three gold bands around one end and the drug name in large letters. Its marketing campaign is built around the phrase "the little purple pill." Even its Website www.purplepill .com is done in purple!

## *Historical Notes*

Many over-the-counter cold remedies and drugs to treat pain were manufactured as capsules until some Tylenol capsules were purposely contaminated with cyanide in the early 1980s. Now, most drug companies manufacture their over-the-counter drugs for pain in a tablet or caplet form that prevents tampering with the contents. Many prescription drugs, however, are still manufactured as two-piece, hard shell capsules.

3. **Ointment.**   An ointment is a semisolid emulsion of oil (lanolin or petroleum) and water, the main ingredient being oil (see ■ **FIGURE 3–4** and ■ **TABLE 3–1**). Many topical drugs are manufactured in an ointment base (e.g., Kenalog ointment for skin inflammation). Specially formulated ophthalmic ointments can be applied topically to the eye without causing irritation. Ointments are absorbed into the area to which they are applied; most exert a local, not systemic, drug effect.

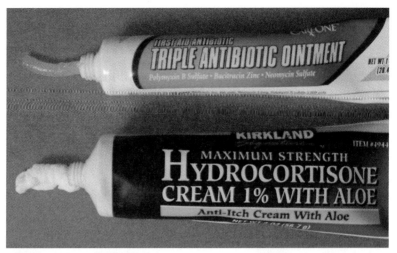

**■ FIGURE 3–4** **Ointment and cream drug forms.**
These over-the-counter drugs are triple antibiotic ointment and hydrocortisone
cream. The feel, appearance, and consistency of the two drug forms are different.

4. **Cream.**    A cream is a semisolid emulsion of oil (lanolin or petroleum) and water, the main
ingredient being water (see **■ FIGURE 3–4**). Emulsifying agents are added to keep the oil and
water mixed together. Many topical drugs are manufactured in a cream base (e.g., hydrocortisone cream for skin inflammation). Creams are absorbed into the skin and exert a local, not
systemic, drug effect.

5. **Lotion.**    A lotion is a suspension of a drug in a water base (e.g., Keri lotion or Calamine
lotion for skin dryness and irritation). Lotions are absorbed into the skin and exert a local, not
systemic, drug effect.

**■ TABLE 3–1** **Comparison of ointment, cream, and lotion drug forms**

| Drug Form | Feel | Appearance | Consistency | Dispensed from |
|---|---|---|---|---|
| Ointment | Greasy | Clear | Firm | Tube |
| Cream | Nongreasy | Opaque/milky | Semiliquid | Tube or bottle |
| Lotion | Nongreasy | Opaque/milky | Liquid | Bottle |

6. **Powder.**    A powder is a finely ground form of a drug. Powdered drugs can be found within
capsules; they are also placed in glass vials where they must be reconstituted with sterile
water before they can be injected (e.g., powdered ampicillin, an antibiotic drug in a vial).
Powders come in individual packets. The powder is reconstituted with water for oral use (e.g.,
Metamucil, a laxative). Powders can also be sprinkled topically or sprayed onto the skin (e.g.,
Tinactin, an antifungal drug for the skin). Powders also come in a canister that is activated and
the powder is inhaled into the lungs with the help of a special inhalation device (e.g., Serevent
Diskus, a bronchodilator drug).

7. **Liquid.**    A liquid drug comes in the form of a solution or a suspension. Two general words
used to describe liquid drugs are *aqueous* (from the Latin word *aqua,* water), meaning *of a
watery consistency,* and *viscous,* meaning *nonwatery* or *thick.*

**Solutions** contain the drug in a base of sterile water, saline, or water and alcohol. Solutions never need to be mixed, as the drug concentration is always the same in every part of the solution, even after prolonged standing. Solutions come in three forms.

A. Solutions in which the drug is dissolved in sterile water or saline for injection into body tissue or the blood. These drugs are packaged in **ampules** (see ■ FIGURE 3–5) or **vials** (see ■ FIGURE 3–6).

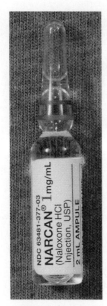

■ **FIGURE 3–5  Ampule.**
An ampule is a small, slender glass container with a main body and a narrow, extended top. An alcohol swab is placed around the neck (narrowed indentation) of the ampule, and the ampule is quickly snapped into two pieces. A syringe is used to withdraw the drug solution from the body of the broken ampule. An ampule can be used only once and the remaining, unused drug must be discarded because it contains no preservative. This ampule contains the liquid drug Narcan, which is used to treat an overdose of narcotic drugs.

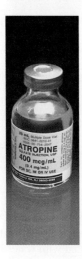

■ **FIGURE 3–6  Vial.**
A vial is a small glass bottle. The top has an aluminum cap that protects a rubber stopper beneath until the vial is opened. To withdraw the liquid drug from a vial, the vial is turned upside down, the needle of a syringe is inserted through the rubber stopper, air is injected into the vial, and the drug dose is withdrawn. A vial can be used multiple times. The rubber stopper is cleansed with alcohol before each dose is withdrawn. This vial contains the liquid drug atropine, which is used to treat an abnormally slow heart rate. Some vials contain a powdered drug that must be reconstituted to a liquid before it can be drawn up into the syringe.

B. Solutions in which the drug is dissolved in a liquid base (elixirs, syrups, tinctures, liquid sprays, foams, mousse) are for topical or oral administration.

**Elixirs** are solutions that contain the drug in a water and alcohol base with added sugar and flavoring (e.g., Tylenol elixir for fever and pain). Elixirs are commonly used for pediatric or elderly patients who cannot swallow the tablet or capsule form of a drug (see ■ FIGURE 3–7).

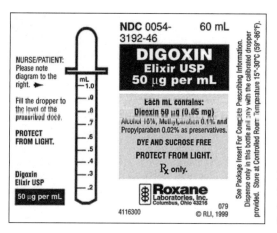

■ **FIGURE 3–7  Elixir.**
Digoxin elixir is used to treat congestive heart failure in children. Notice the illustration of the calibrated dropper on the label. The dropper allows a very precise, small dose of the elixir to be given.

**Syrups** are solutions that contain the drug in a thickened water base with added sugar and flavorings, but no alcohol. Syrups are sweeter and more viscous (thicker) than elixirs. Most over-the-counter cough drugs are syrups that coat the mucous membranes for a soothing effect in addition to the drug effect (e.g., Robitussin for coughs).

**Tinctures** are solutions that contain the drug in a water and alcohol base (e.g., topical iodine tincture to disinfect the skin). Tinctures are never taken internally.

**Liquid sprays** are solutions that contain the drug in a water or alcohol base. They are sprayed manually by a pump or by squeezing a bottle or they are forced from a can by an aerosol propellant. Spray liquid drugs are commonly used for topical application (example: Afrin nasal spray, a decongestant drug).

**Foams** are solutions that contain the drug in a water base that is expanded by tiny aerosol bubbles when expelled from the container (e.g., over-the-counter contraceptive foams; Rogaine foam for male baldness).

**Mousse** is a solution that contains the drug in a thickened alcohol base. It is expanded by tiny aerosol bubbles when expelled from the container (e.g., RID mousse to kill lice on the body).

C. Solutions in which the drug form remains separate from the base (emulsions, gels) but is still evenly distributed throughout the solution. Even though the drug particles never dissolve in the base, they never settle to the bottom over time, so they do not need to be shaken prior to administration.

**Emulsions** are solutions that contain  fat globules dispersed uniformly throughout a water base (e.g., Intralipid intravenous fat solution).

**Gels** are solutions that contain fine, undissolved drug particles dispersed uniformly throughout a thickened water base (e.g., MetroGel for acne rosacea).

## *Did You Know?*

Liquid drugs that are given orally come in a variety of flavors to please everyone and "help the medicine go down": grape, cherry, bubblegum, pineapple, maple, wine, raspberry, mocha, butterscotch, strawberry, mint, orange, honey lemon, root beer, watermelon, coconut, licorice, banana, etc.

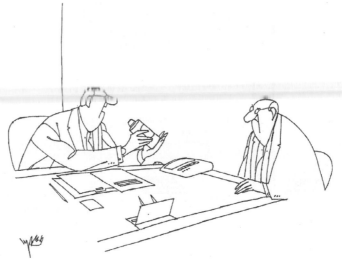

*"I think you'll like this new medication, . . . it's a little spritzy, sweet and spicy with some bite, but not abrupt . . . and it has a rich, toasted almond-peach aftertaste with lots of character."*

**Suspensions** contain fine, undissolved particles of a drug suspended in a water or oil base (see ■ **FIGURE 3–8**). After prolonged standing, these fine particles gradually settle to the bottom of the container (due to the action of gravity). It is always important to shake suspensions well before using them, a fact that is noted on the label of the drugs (e.g., Maalox, an antacid drug).

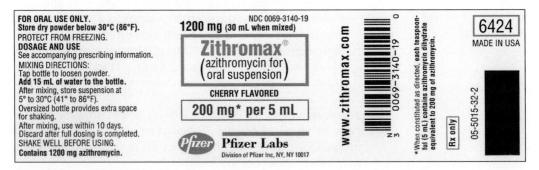

■ **FIGURE 3–8 Suspension form of a drug.**
This drug label is for the antibiotic drug azithromycin (Zithromax). It is in the form of a powder that is reconstituted with water to make an oral suspension. Notice the fine print (bottom left) that says "Shake Well Before Using," because the fine drug particles of a suspension will settle to the bottom of the container over time.

8.  **Suppository.**   A suppository is composed of a solid base of glycerin or cocoa butter that contains the drug. Suppositories are manufactured in appropriate sizes for vaginal or rectal insertion and also come in adult and pediatric sizes. Vaginal suppositories are used to treat vaginal yeast infections, but can also be inserted into the mouth to treat oral yeast infections. Rectal suppositories can be used to administer drugs to patients who are vomiting and cannot take oral drugs.

9.  **Transdermal patch.**   Transdermal patches contain drugs and are applied to the skin (see ■ **FIGURE 3–9** and ■ **FIGURE 3–10**). The patch releases a small amount of drug over a long period of time, usually for one to two days. The drugs in transdermal patches are designed to exert a systemic effect in the body, not a topical effect on the skin.

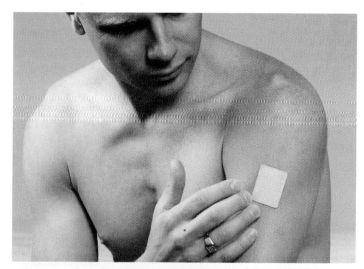

■ **FIGURE 3–9 Transdermal patch.**
Transdermal patches release drugs slowly over a long period of time.
They are used to treat chronic conditions, such as severe pain, to relieve
the urge to smoke, and to prevent angina attacks in patients with heart disease.

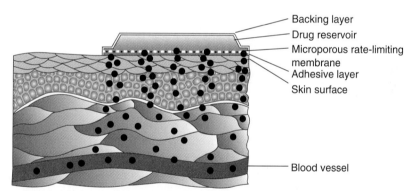

■ **FIGURE 3–10 Cross section of a transdermal patch.**
A transdermal patch consists of a multilayered disk containing a drug reservoir, a
porous membrane, and an adhesive layer to hold it to the skin. The porous membrane
regulates the amount of drug entering the skin, releasing small amounts over time.

10. **Pellet, bead, wafer, insert, and device.** A drug in the form of a pellet, bead, wafer, or insert
    can be placed within a body space or body cavity, where it slowly releases drug to the sur-
    rounding tissues (e.g., a Muse pellet inserted into the urethra to treat erectile dysfunction;
    Septopal beads on a wire implanted in bone to treat chronic infection; a Gliadel wafer, a
    chemotherapy drug, implanted near a cancerous tumor; Lacrisert inserts placed in the lower
    eyelid sac to treat dry eye syndrome; Mirena, a T-shaped device, inserted into the uterus to
    prevent pregnancy).
11. **Gas.** A drug can be inhaled in the form of a gas (e.g., a general anesthetic gas used during
    surgery).

## Focus on Healthcare Issues

Studies have shown that patients usually take their prescribed drugs accurately only 50 percent of the time. Researchers want to improve that percentage by inventing new drug forms. Development is nearly completed on an artificial tooth that contains a tiny mechanism that is preprogrammed to dispense a drug at specific times. Another drug researcher wants to make drugs in the form of a tasteless powder that can be sprinkled on food. A Massachusetts company has created a computer chip that contains up to 100 doses of a drug; the chip is implanted in the body and receives wireless signals that tell it when to release a drug dose. In the future, drug researchers will work closely with biomedical engineers to create drug forms and drug-delivery technology so small that they are measured in nanometers (billionths of a meter).

# Chapter Review

## Quiz Yourself

1. What is the reason for manufacturing a drug as an enteric-coated tablet?
2. What are caplets?
3. Besides tablets and capsules, list five other forms in which drugs are manufactured.
4. Describe the difference between an elixir and a syrup.
5. Which drug form contains a built-in drug reservoir?
6. What is the difference between an ampule and a vial?
7. What can be done with a scored tablet that cannot be done with other tablets?
8. What phrase is written on the drug label of a suspension that would not be on the drug label of a solution?
9. A suppository can only be given rectally: true or false?
10. Differentiate between the feel, appearance, and consistency of an ointment versus a cream versus a lotion.
11. What do the abbreviations CR, LA, SR, and XL have in common?

## Spelling Tips

**lozenge**    no final *r*, although it is often mispronounced as "lozenger."

## Clinical Applications

1. Carefully examine this photograph and identify what drug forms are represented by each of the four pictured over-the-counter drugs.

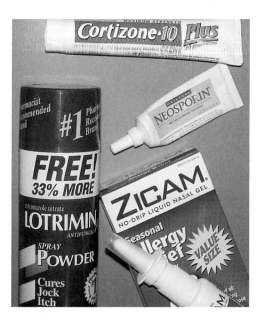

2. This nurse is preparing a drug dose. What two pieces of drug-related equipment are shown here? What form of drug would be in the container?

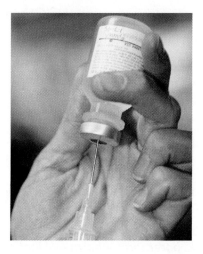

## Multimedia Extension Exercises

■ Go to www.pearsonhighered.com/turley and click on the photo of the cover of *Understanding Pharmacology for Health Professionals* to access the interactive Companion Website created for this textbook.

# 4

# Routes of Administration and the Drug Cycle

## CHAPTER CONTENTS

Routes of Administration

The Drug Cycle

Quiz Yourself

Spelling Tips

Clinical Applications

Multimedia Extension Exercises

## Learning Objectives

After you study this chapter, you should be able to

1. Name 11 routes of drug administration.

2. Describe the advantages and disadvantages of oral administration of a drug.

3. Describe the differences between an intradermal, subcutaneous, and intramuscular injection.

4. Recognize and define Latin abbreviations for topical administration.

5. Define the role of plasma proteins and the blood–brain barrier in the distribution of a drug.

6. Describe how the liver metabolizes drugs.

7. Describe how the kidneys excrete drugs.

8. Describe how drug doses are adjusted for patients with liver or kidney disease, elderly patients, or premature infants.

9. Define the words and phrases *buccal route, intracardiac route, intrathecal route, intravesical route, I.V. piggyback, parenteral, pharmacokinetics, receptor,* and *sublingual route.*

Before a drug can receive final approval by the FDA, the drug company must clearly state what routes of administration have been found to be safe and effective for that drug. Different forms of a drug are appropriate for different routes of administration. Some drugs are ineffective when administered by a certain route; other drugs may seriously injure the patient if administered by the wrong route.

Once a drug is administered, it goes through the steps of the drug cycle. These steps include absorption, distribution, metabolism, and excretion.

## Routes of Administration

There are various routes by which drugs can be administered. Some drugs are approved for use via more than one route and are manufactured in different drug forms appropriate for those different routes. Each route of administration has distinct advantages and disadvantages. A drug given by the recommended route of administration will be therapeutic; if given by another route, it may be ineffective, harmful, or even fatal.

1. **Topical.**    When a drug is applied directly to the skin or the eyes or ears, it is administered via the topical route (see ■ **FIGURE 4–1**). The therapeutic effect of the drug only extends to the local area (e.g., antibiotic ointment for a skin injury, Timoptic eye drops for glaucoma, or antibiotic drops for an ear infection). The word *topical* contains the combining form *topic/o-* (a specific area) and the suffix *-al* (pertaining to); the word means *pertaining to a specific area.*

   Sites of topical administration are abbreviated as follows (see ■ TABLE 4–1).

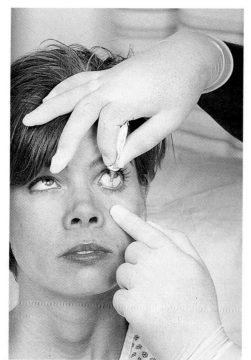

■ **FIGURE 4–1  Topical route of administration.**
The nurse is administering a topical ophthalmic antibiotic ointment to the patient's eye by pulling down the lower eyelid so that a ribbon of ointment can be laid in the sac between the eye and the lower eyelid. As the patient blinks, the ointment is distributed across the eye. Topical ophthalmic ointment is specially formulated to be nonirritating to the eye; it is not interchangeable with other topical ointments that are used on the skin.

■ **TABLE 4–1 Abbreviations for topical administration**

| Abbreviation | Latin Meaning | Medical Meaning |
|---|---|---|
| A.D. | *auris dextra* | right ear |
| A.S. | *auris sinistra* | left ear |
| A.U. | *auris unitas* | both ears |
| | *auris uterque* | each ear |
| O.D. | *oculus dexter* | right eye |
| O.S. | *oculus sinister* | left eye |
| O.U. | *oculus unitas* | both eyes |
| | *oculus uterque* | each eye |

## *Clinical Applications*

When you are administering a topical drug to a patient, remember that, as you face the patient, your right-hand side corresponds to the patient's left-hand side. If the physician's order is for ointment in the right eye, you have to consciously think about correctly identifying the patient's right side.

2. **Transdermal.** This route of administration differs from the topical route in that the drug is applied to the skin, but the therapeutic effect is felt systemically, not just at the site of administration. Drugs delivered by the transdermal route are manufactured in the form of a transdermal patch (see Chapter 3). A transdermal patch is worn on the skin and releases the drug slowly over one or more days, providing a sustained therapeutic blood level (e.g., Nicoderm CQ patch to stop smoking). The word *transdermal* contains the prefix *trans-* (across; through), the combining form *derm/o-* (skin), and the suffix *-al* (pertaining to); the word means *pertaining to through the skin*.

3. **Oral.** The oral route is the most convenient route of administration and the one most commonly used. The oral route involves placing the drug in the mouth and swallowing it (see ■ **FIGURE 4–2**). Tablets, capsules, and liquids are all given orally. The drug is then absorbed from the stomach or small intestine into the blood. The oral route is routinely abbreviated as PO or p.o. (Latin for *per os*, meaning *through the mouth*).

   Disadvantages of the oral route include the following.

   ■ It is difficult for some patients to swallow the largest tablets and capsules (see ■ **FIGURE 4–3**).

   ■ The oral route cannot be used for patients who are unconscious or vomiting.

   ■ Some drugs (e.g., penicillin, an antibiotic drug) are inactivated by stomach acid and cannot be given orally. After oral administration, some drugs (e.g., lidocaine for cardiac arrhythmias) are metabolized so quickly by the liver as they pass through the portal circulation that a therapeutic blood level cannot be achieved.

   ■ Some drugs (e.g., tetracycline, an antibiotic drug) cannot be taken with certain foods and beverages because they combine chemically to form an insoluble complex.

   ■ Some drugs (e.g., MAO inhibitor drugs for depression) cannot be taken with certain foods because they produce severe adverse effects.

4. **Sublingual and buccal.** Sublingual administration involves placing the drug (usually in a tablet form) under the tongue and allowing it slowly to disintegrate. Buccal administration involves placing the drug (usually in a tablet form) in the pocket between the cheek and the lower teeth on one side of the mouth and allowing it slowly to disintegrate. The tablet is not swallowed (as this would be oral administration). The dissolved drug is absorbed quickly through the oral mucous membranes and absorbed into the large blood vessels under the tongue and oral mucosa. Drugs

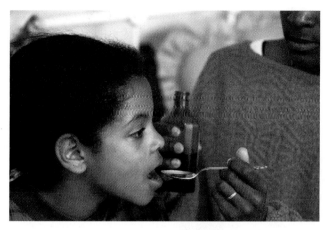

**■ FIGURE 4–2  Oral route of administration.**
This is the most common route of drug administration. Drugs can be given as tablets, capsules, or liquids. Many pediatric drugs are in a liquid form. For oral administration of a drug to an infant, the liquid drug is mixed with a small amount of formula and given orally through the nipple which has been removed from the bottle of formula.

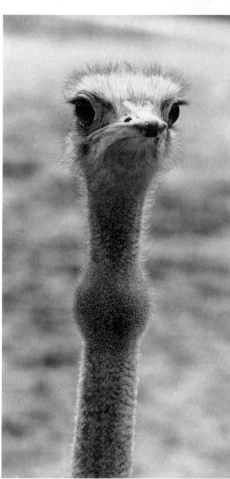

**■ FIGURE 4–3  Oral route of administration.**
Some patients have difficulty swallowing very large tablets or capsules. Their physicians can prescribe an alternate drug form, such as a liquid.

given by the sublingual route provide a faster therapeutic effect than those given by the oral route (e.g., nitroglycerin tablets and spray for treating angina attacks). At the present time, few drugs are administered by the buccal route. The word *sublingual* contains the prefix *sub-* (below; underneath), the combining form *lingu/o-* (tongue), and the suffix *-al* (pertaining to); the word means *pertaining to underneath the tongue.* The word *buccal* contains the combining form *bucc/o-* (cheek) and the suffix *-al* (pertaining to); the word means *pertaining to the cheek.*

5. **Nasal.** Nasal administration involves spraying a drug into the nasal cavity. This is usually done topically to treat allergy symptoms of nasal stuffiness (e.g., Nasonex, a topical corticosteroid drug for inflammation), but some nasal spray drugs act systemically throughout the body (e.g., Miacalcin nasal spray for Paget's disease of the bones).

6. **Inhalation.** This route of administration involves the inhaling of a drug that is in a gas, liquid, or powder form (see ■ FIGURE 4–4). The drug is absorbed through the alveoli of the lungs (e.g., an anesthetic gas). The word *inhalation* contains the prefix *in-* (in; within), the combining form *hal/o-* (breathe), and the suffix *-ation* (a process); the word means *a process of breathing in.*

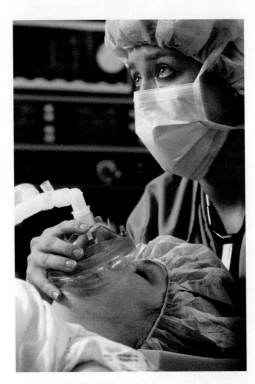

■ FIGURE 4–4 **Inhalation route of administration.**
This patient is receiving a drug in the form of an anesthetic gas to produce unconsciousness prior to having surgery.

7. **Nasogastric.** This route is used to administer drugs to patients who cannot take oral drugs. Nasogastric administration is accomplished with a nasogastric tube that is passed from the nose through the esophagus and into the stomach. Any liquid drug that can be given by the oral route can be given by this route. *Nasogastric* is abbreviated as *NG*. The word *nasogastric* contains the combining form *nas/o-* (nose), the combining form *gastr/o-* (stomach), and the suffix *-ic* (pertaining to); the word means *pertaining to the nose and stomach.*

## Did You Know?

The first nasogastric tube, developed in the late 1700s, was constructed from eel skin. It was used for several weeks to feed a patient who could not eat.

8. **Gastrostomy and jejunostomy.** These routes are used to administer drugs to patients who cannot take oral drugs. These routes use a surgically implanted feeding tube to deliver liquid drugs directly into the stomach (gastrostomy) or jejunum (jejunostomy). Any liquid drug that

can be given orally can be given by these routes. The word *gastrostomy* contains the combining form *gastr/o-* (stomach) and the suffix *-stomy* (surgically created opening); the word means *a surgically created opening in the stomach.* The word *jejunostomy* contains the combining form *jejun/o-* (jejunum) and the suffix *-stomy* (surgically created opening); the word means *a surgically created opening in the jejunum.*

9. **Vaginal.** The vaginal route is used to treat vaginal infections by means of creams, ointments, and suppositories (e.g., Monistat vaginal cream or suppositories for a yeast infection). Contraceptive foams are inserted vaginally as well.

10. **Rectal.** This route is reserved for certain situations, such as when the patient is vomiting, is unconscious, or the drug cannot be given by injection (e.g., Tylenol suppository for a fever). Systemic absorption of a drug via the rectal route of administration is slow and often unpredictable, so this route is not used often. However, the rectal route is the preferred route when drugs are administered topically to relieve constipation (e.g., Fleet enema) or to treat hemorrhoids (e.g., Anusol cream or suppositories) or ulcerative colitis (e.g., Proctofoam-HC aerosol foam).

11. **Parenteral.** Parenteral administration theoretically includes all routes of administration other than the oral route; but in clinical usage, parenteral administration commonly includes these routes: intradermal, subcutaneous, intramuscular, and intravenous. The word *parenteral* contains the prefix *par-* (beside; apart from), the combining form *enter/o-* (intestine), and the suffix *-al* (pertaining to); the word means *pertaining to apart from the intestine*, i.e., a route other than through the mouth.

   **Intradermal** administration involves using a syringe to inject a liquid drug into the dermis, the layer of skin just below the epidermis or skin surface (see ▩ **FIGURE 4–5** and ▩ **FIGURE 4–6**). Intradermal administration is used for allergy scratch tests and for the Mantoux test that screens for tuberculosis. The word *intradermal* contains the prefix *intra-* (within), the combining form *derm/o-* (skin), and the suffix *-al* (pertaining to); the word means *pertaining to within the skin.*

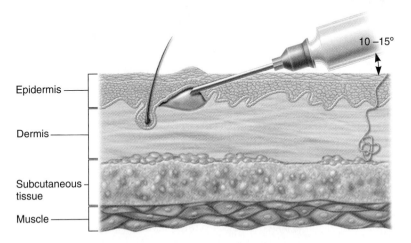

Epidermis

Dermis

Subcutaneous tissue

Muscle

10–15°

▩ **FIGURE 4–5 Intradermal route of administration.**
The needle is inserted at a 10- to 15-degree angle so that it does not penetrate too deeply. The epidermis itself is less than 1/20 inch thick; therefore, when an intradermal injection is positioned correctly, the tip of the needle is still visible through the epidermis.

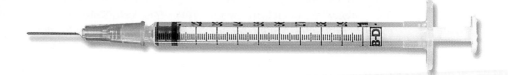

**■ FIGURE 4–6  Syringe.**
A syringe is used to withdraw a liquid drug from an ampule or vial. This tuberculin syringe is
calibrated to measure liquid drug doses to the hundredth of a milliliter (mL). The needle on the
syringe is used to penetrate the skin to the correct depth to administer the liquid drug. This type
of syringe is used to give either intradermal or subcutaneous injections. A longer needle and a
larger syringe are used to administer liquid drug doses via the intramuscular route.

**Subcutaneous** administration involves using a syringe to inject a liquid drug into the subcutaneous tissue (the fatty layer of tissue just beneath the dermis of the skin but above the
muscle layer) (see **■ FIGURE 4–7**). There are only a few blood vessels in this fatty layer,
so drugs are absorbed more slowly than by the intramuscular route. Examples of drugs given
via the subcutaneous route include insulin for diabetes mellitus, allergy shots, and heparin.
This route is abbreviated as *subQ*, *SQ*, or *subcu*; there is no one official abbreviation. The word
*subcutaneous* contains the prefix *sub-* (below; underneath), the combining form *cutane/o-*
(skin), and the suffix *-al* (pertaining to); the word means *pertaining to below the skin*.

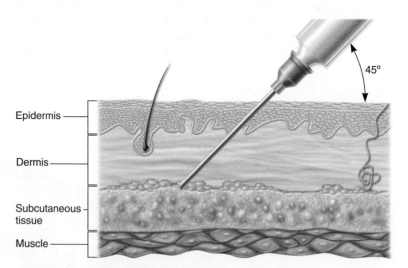

**■ FIGURE 4–7  Subcutaneous route of administration.**
The needle is inserted at a 45-degree angle to reach the fatty subcutaneous tissue,
but not penetrate into the muscle layer. Diabetic patients who inject insulin daily
use the subcutaneous route. A subcutaneous injection can also be classified as a
**hypodermic** injection (*hypo-* means *below* and *derm/o-* means *skin*).

**Intramuscular** administration involves the injection of a liquid drug into the belly (area of
greatest mass) of a muscle (see **■ FIGURE 4–8** and **■ FIGURE 4–9**). The muscles of the
body are well supplied with blood vessels, and drugs injected intramuscularly are absorbed
more quickly than with subcutaneous administration. Also, a muscle is able to absorb a
larger amount of a liquid drug (up to 5 mL). An intramuscular injection must be given into

a muscle that is large enough that the needle will not accidentally injure a nearby nerve. Examples of drugs given intramuscularly include meperidine (Demerol) for severe pain and penicillin for bacterial infection. Some liquid drugs, such as Valium (an antianxiety drug), can never be given by intramuscular injection because they are not water soluble and, if injected, would form precipitate particles in the muscle tissue. The word *intramuscular* is abbreviated as either *IM* or *I.M.* The word *intramuscular* contains the prefix *intra-* (within), the combining form *muscul/o* (muscle), and the suffix *-ar* (pertaining to); this word means *pertaining to within the muscle.*

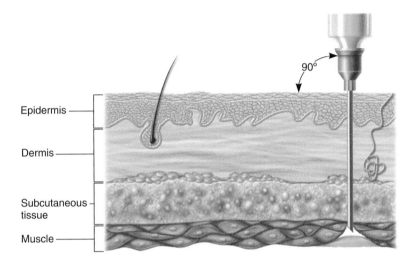

■ **FIGURE 4–8 Intramuscular route of administration.**
The needle is inserted at a 90-degree angle to reach the muscle layer. An intramuscular injection can also be classified as a **hypodermic** injection.

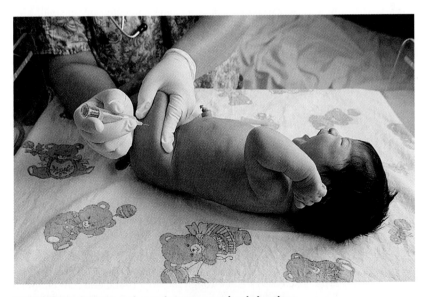

■ **FIGURE 4–9 Newborn intramuscular injection.**
The vastus lateralis muscle is the preferred site for giving injections such as infant immunizations, as this is the muscle that has the greatest bulk.

In adults, there are only four large muscle sites that are recommended for intramuscular injection of drugs: ventrogluteal, deltoid, dorsogluteal, and vastus lateralis.

## Did You Know?

Fans of the Star Trek television series and movies have long been familiar with this futuristic drug delivery system: the imaginary hypospray! The injection requires no needle and causes no pain.

**Intravenous** administration involves the injection of a liquid drug into a vein. A bag of intravenous fluid is hung from an I.V. pole that is elevated above the patient. The effect of gravity moves the fluid through the I.V. tubing, and into the patient's vein, with the drug flowing in drip by drip through the needle. Alternatively, an I.V. pump can be used to precisely regulate the amount of I.V. fluid given. The therapeutic effect of a drug given intravenously is often seen immediately. The intravenous route entirely bypassses the step of absorption because the drug is not absorbed from the tissues or stomach. Examples of drugs given intravenously include thiopental (Pentothal) for induction of general anesthesia, diazepam (Valium) to control continuous epileptic seizures, and most chemotherapy drugs. The word *intravenous* is abbreviated as either *IV* or *I.V.* The word *intravenous* contains the prefix *intra-* (within), the combining form *ven/o-* (vein), and the suffix *-ous* (pertaining to); the word means *pertaining to within the vein.*
Intravenous administration can be done in one of three ways.

- **Bolus.**   The whole amount of a drug can be injected in a short period of time through a **port** (rubber stopper) in the I.V. tubing by gently pushing on the plunger of the syringe. This is often referred to as *I.V. push.*
- **I.V. infusion.**   The drug can be injected into the fluid of a large I.V. bag and administered continuously over several hours. This is known as *I.V. drip.*
- **I.V. piggyback.**   The drug can be injected into a small I.V. bag of fluid that is then attached (or piggybacked) onto an existing primary I.V. line. For some drugs, the small I.V. bag already comes premixed (see ▪ **FIGURE 4–10**).

12. **Other routes of administration.**   The following routes of administration are used less frequently and only in special situations. They include the central venous line, endotracheal tube, implantable port, intra-arterial route, intra-articular route, intracardiac route, intrathecal route, intraperitoneal route, intravesical route, and the umbilical artery or vein.

- **Central venous line.**   This route is used to continuously administer intravenous fluids or drugs to critically ill patients or to administer chemotherapy drugs to patients with cancer. A special catheter (Broviac, Hickman, or Groshong) is tunneled through the subcutaneous tissue of the upper chest, inserted into a large vein, and advanced until its tip is positioned in the superior vena cava. For administration of chemotherapy drugs, the external end of the catheter is sealed, and is only uncapped when the chemotherapy drug is administered. This allows the patient to be ambulatory because there is no attached I.V. line.
- **Endotracheal tube.**   This route is used to administer drugs through an endotracheal tube inserted through the mouth into the trachea (see ▪ **FIGURE 4–11**). This route is especially useful if there is no established intravenous access. With endotracheal administration, the drug dose is absorbed through the lung tissue and into the blood. Emergency drugs administered through the endotracheal route are identified by the memory aid NAVEL (naloxone, atropine, Valium, epinephrine, or lidocaine). The endotracheal route is also used to administer synthetic lung surfactant drug to treat respiratory distress syndrome in premature

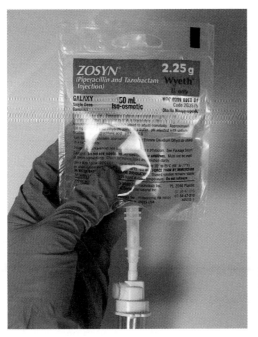

**■ FIGURE 4–10  I.V. piggyback route of administration.**
Because I.V. antibiotic drugs are frequently ordered in the hospital, small I.V. bags often come premixed with the antibiotic drug already in them; they can be attached quickly to the patient's existing I.V. line. This I.V. bag contains the trade name antibiotic drug Zosyn, a combination drug that contains the generic antibiotic drugs piperacillin and tazobactam; it is used to treat severe infections.

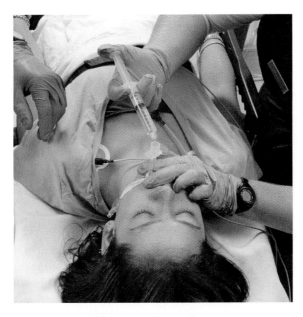

**■ FIGURE 4–11  Endotracheal tube route of administration.**
The paramedic is injecting a liquid drug in a syringe into the open end of the clear plastic endotracheal tube. After the drug is injected, it will be absorbed by the lungs and go into the blood. The patient also will receive oxygen and manual ventilation to assist her breathing until she can be evaluated in the emergency room.

infants. The word *endotracheal* contains the prefix *endo-* (within), the combining form *trache/o-* (trachea), and the suffix *-al* (pertaining to); the word means *pertaining to within the trachea.*

■ **Implantable port.**    This is a special intravenous access device that is used to administer a chemotherapy drug to treat cancer. The port is a thin metal or plastic reservoir that is placed in a subcutaneous pocket of tissue. The reservoir is attached to a catheter that is threaded into the patient's superior vena cava. The chemotherapy drug is administered by inserting a needle through the skin overlying the reservoir and injecting the drug into the reservoir. The reservoir then releases the drug slowly into the blood. Another type is an Ommaya reservoir that is placed beneath the scalp with the catheter placed in the ventricle of the brain. In the same way, this reservoir is filled with a chemotherapy drug that then circulates throughout the brain via the cerebrospinal fluid.

■ **Intra-arterial route.**    This route is used for administration of a chemotherapy drug directly into the area of a cancerous tumor. A catheter is inserted into the main artery that brings blood to the organ where the cancerous tumor is located. The catheter is connected to an infusion pump that is implanted under the skin or worn externally. This pump administers doses of chemotherapy drug through the intra-arterial catheter at preprogrammed intervals. The word *intra-arterial* contains the prefix *intra-* (within), the combining form *arteri/o-* (artery), and the suffix *-al* (pertaining to); the word means *pertaining to within the artery.*

■ **Intra-articular route.**    This route is used to administer a drug into a joint (e.g., corticosteroid drugs to decrease pain and inflammation). These drugs are injected once every few weeks or months. The word *intra-articular* contains the prefix *intra-* (within), the combining form *articul/o-* (joint), and the suffix *-ar* (pertaining to); the word means *pertaining to within the joint.*

■ **Intracardiac route.**    This route is only used during emergency resuscitation associated with cardiac arrest. If external compressions do not cause the heart to begin to beat again, then the intracardiac route is used with a needle inserted through the chest wall, between the ribs, and into one of the heart chambers. Then the drug epinephrine (Adrenalin) is injected to stimulate the heart muscle to begin to contract. The word *intracardiac* contains the prefix *intra-* (within), the combining form *cardi/o-* (heart), and the suffix *-ac* (pertaining to); the word means *pertaining to within the heart.*

■ **Intrathecal route.**    This route is used to administer drugs within the meninges around the spinal cord and into the cerebrospinal fluid (e.g., spinal anesthesia). The word *intrathecal* contains the prefix *intra-* (within), the combining form *thec/o-* (layers of membranes), and the suffix *-al* (pertaining to); the word means *pertaining to within the layers of membranes (meninges).*

■ **Intraperitoneal route.**    This route is used to administer drugs or fluids into the peritoneal cavity. A catheter is surgically implanted through the abdominal wall into the peritoneal cavity. Sometimes the intraperitoneal route is used to administer chemotherapy drugs. As the chemotherapy drug is dispersed throughout the peritoneal fluid, it comes in contact with the surfaces of all of the organs in the abdominopelvic cavity where there might be cancerous tumors present. In other cases, the intraperitoneal route is used to administer dialysis fluids for peritoneal dialysis in patients with kidney failure. The fluid draws waste products out of the blood of the abdominal organs and, after a period of time, the dialysis fluid is removed and discarded. The word *intraperitoneal* contains the prefix *intra-* (within), the combining form *peritone/o-* (peritoneum), and the suffix *-al* (pertaining to); the word means *pertaining to within the peritoneum.*

■ **Intravesical route.**    This route is used for the administration of chemotherapy drugs into the bladder to treat bladder cancer. A catheter inserted into the urethra carries the chemotherapy drug into the bladder, where it remains for a predetermined period of time. The word *intravesical* contains the prefix *intra-* (within), the combining form *vesic/o-* (bladder), and the suffix *-al* (pertaining to); the word means *pertaining to within the bladder.*

■ **Umbilical artery or vein.**    This route is accessible only in newborn infants before the umbilical cord has dried. It is used to administer intravenous fluids and draw blood. It is generally not used to give drugs. Instead, an I.V. line is inserted peripherally in the hand, foot, or scalp for drug administration.

# The Drug Cycle

Following administration, most drugs go through a well-defined sequence of four steps before being excreted from the body. These steps are known as the ***drug cycle***.

**1.** Absorption from the site of administration

**2.** Distribution via the circulatory system

**3.** Metabolism

**4.** Excretion from the body

**Pharmacokinetics** is the study of how drugs move through the body in the processes of absorption, distribution, metabolism, and excretion.

## Absorption

Absorption involves the movement of a drug from the site of administration through tissues and into the blood. For most drug forms, absorption involves three steps.

- **Disintegrate.** Tablets, capsules, suppositories, and so on, are drug forms that must first disintegrate before they can be absorbed; this step is omitted for drugs that are already in a liquid form or those that are effervescent tablets that disintegrate outside the body in a glass of water before being swallowed (see ■ **FIGURE 4–12**).

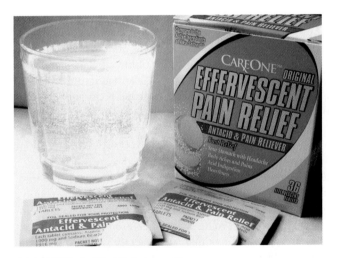

■ **FIGURE 4–12 Disintegration.**
These two tablets are disintegrating in a glass of water before they can be taken by the oral route.

- **Dissolve.** Once the drug is in a liquid form, it dissolves in the surrounding body fluids (saliva, gastric juice, or tissue fluid).
- **Absorb.** From the body fluids, the drug passes through the walls of nearby capillaries and is absorbed into the blood.

**Absorption after topical administration.** Following topical administration of a drug, the drug form does not need to undergo disintegration; it quickly dissolves in the tissue fluids of the skin. However, topical drugs do not complete the final step of absorption and do not go into the blood. Their therapeutic effect is only exerted locally at the site of administration.

**Absorption after transdermal administration.** Following application of a transdermal patch, the drug in the patch reservoir begins to be released. Because the drug is in a liquid form, it does not need to undergo disintegration; it quickly dissolves in the tissue fluids of the skin, passes through the walls of nearby capillaries, and is absorbed into the blood.

**Absorption after oral administration.** Following oral administration of a drug, the drug form disintegrates, if necessary. It then dissolves in stomach or intestinal fluids, passes through the mucous membrane lining of the stomach or intestine into nearby capillaries, and then is absorbed into the blood.

The presence or absence of food (particularly a large or fatty meal) can influence the rate of drug absorption. The presence of food in the GI tract can reduce absorption of a drug from 30 percent to as much as 80 percent.

Some drugs are not absorbed at all following oral administration (e.g., neomycin, an antibiotic drug). This drawback can be overcome by administering the drug via a different route. However, nonabsorption of a drug via the oral route can also be turned into a therapeutic advantage. For example, neomycin can be given orally to exert its antibiotic effect solely in the intestinal tract to kill intestinal bacteria prior to abdominal surgery. Carafate, an antiulcer drug, is not absorbed following oral administration, but that is acceptable because its therapeutic effect is to bind directly to a stomach ulcer and form a protective coating so that the ulcer can heal. Another drug, Metamucil, also is not absorbed, but passes through the intestine, where it binds with water to increase stool bulk and exert its therapeutic effect to relieve constipation.

**Absorption after inhalation administration.** Following administration of a drug by inhalation, the vaporized liquid or gas does not need to undergo disintegration. The drug immediately dissolves in the tissue fluids of the mucous membranes lining the lungs, passes through the walls of nearby capillaries, and is absorbed into the blood. Some drugs given by inhalation exert a topical effect (e.g., Maxair, an inhaled bronchodilator drug for asthma), while other drugs produce a systemic effect throughout the whole body (e.g., general anesthetic gas administered prior to surgery).

**Absorption after vaginal or rectal administration.** Following vaginal administration, the drug form disintegrates and releases the drug topically into the vagina. Drugs administered vaginally are always intended to have only a topical therapeutic effect, and there is minimal absorption into the blood. The rate of absorption following rectal administration is rather slow and variable; therefore, the rectal route is not often used for drugs that act systemically. The rectal route is usually reserved for drugs that act topically within the rectum (e.g., Anusol to treat hemorrhoids). However, in a situation in which the patient is vomiting and the drug (e.g., Tylenol for fever) cannot be given orally and is not manufactured for I.M. or I.V. administration, it can be given rectally as a suppository.

**Absorption after parenteral administration.** Following intradermal, subcutaneous, and intramuscular injections, the drug is already in a liquid form and so it quickly dissolves in the tissue fluids of the skin, passes through the walls of nearby capillaries, and is absorbed into the blood.

Only intravenous injections entirely bypass the step of absorption because the drug is administered directly into a vein and immediately enters the blood.

## Distribution

Once a drug has been absorbed into the blood, it is distributed throughout the body via the circulatory system (see ■ **FIGURE 4–13**).

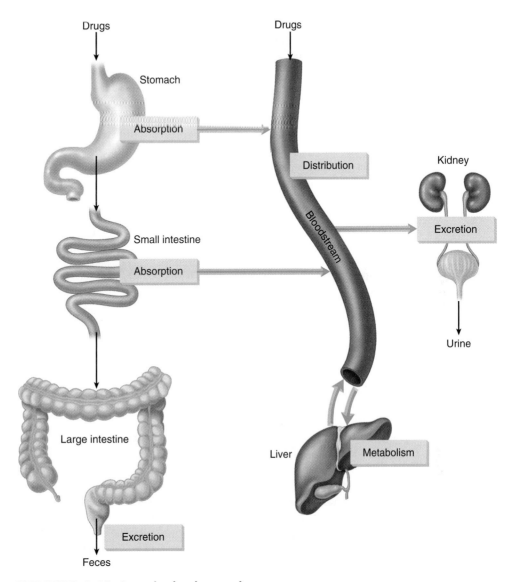

■ **FIGURE 4–13  Steps in the drug cycle.**
Drugs pass through the four steps in the drug cycle: absorption, distribution, metabolism, and excretion.

As a drug enters the blood, some of the drug binds to circulating **plasma proteins**, such as **albumin**. These large molecules have indentations in their molecular surfaces that permit drug molecules to bind to them. Drug molecules that are bound to plasma proteins are essentially pharmacologically inactive as they are carried through the blood.

The other portion of the drug that did not bind to plasma proteins moves through the circulatory system, passing through the walls of capillaries, and into body tissues. As this portion of the drug leaves the blood, some of the bound drug is released by the plasma proteins so as to maintain an equilibrium of unbound drug in the blood.

When a drug moves into body tissues, it comes in contact with a cell membrane and exerts an effect by interacting with one or more **receptors**. This process will be discussed in the next chapter.

There is one area of the body where some drugs are not readily distributed. The brain is protected by the **blood–brain barrier** that exists between the capillary walls of blood vessels in the brain and the surrounding brain tissues. Some drugs are able to pass through the blood–brain barrier and exert a therapeutic effect (e.g., Ritalin for attention deficit–hyperactivity disorder; a general anesthetic drug given prior to surgery to produce unconsciousness). Other drugs are able to pass through the blood–brain barrier and cause side effects such as drowsiness (e.g., antihistamine drugs) or euphoria (e.g., drugs for pain or addictive drugs). However, some classes of drugs are, for the most part, unable to cross the blood–brain barrier. Unfortunately, sometimes the blood–brain barrier actually blocks drugs that are needed to treat diseases of the brain. Some chemotherapy drugs for brain cancer cannot penetrate the blood–brain barrier. Instead, a wafer form of the drug must be implanted directly in the brain (e.g., Gliadel wafer for brain tumors). Another example is Parkinson's disease, which is due to a deficiency of the neurotransmitter dopamine in the brain. Dopamine as a drug cannot cross the blood–brain barrier. Fortunately, levodopa, which has a slightly different molecular structure, can cross the blood–brain barrier; once in the brain, it is converted to dopamine to correct the deficiency and treat Parkinson's disease. Researchers have found a way to use genetic engineering to link a drug that cannot penetrate the blood–brain barrier to an antibody that can, and so the drug-antibody combination easily passes through to the brain.

At one time, it was thought that the placenta formed a barrier to protect the developing fetus from harmful substances. It is now known that the placenta allows nearly all drugs to pass from the maternal circulation to the fetus. Each year, many infants are born addicted to drugs that their mothers took, or they are born with birth defects due to the effect of drugs taken by their mothers. Therefore, pregnant women are advised not to take any drugs, even over-the-counter drugs, except those prescribed by a healthcare provider who knows that the woman is pregnant.

## Metabolism

The process of metabolism is also known as *biotransformation* because the drug is gradually transformed or metabolized from its original active form to a less active, or even inactive, form. This process is accomplished in the liver, the principal organ of metabolism, by the action of liver enzymes.

Drugs given orally are absorbed through the mucous membranes of the stomach or intestines and enter the blood of the portal vein. Before this vein empties into the inferior vena cava, it passes through the liver. Therefore, all drugs given by the oral route are absorbed into the blood of the portal vein and are immediately subjected to metabolism by liver enzymes. This initial metabolism by the liver is referred to as the *first-pass effect*, because the drug must first pass through the liver before it can enter the general circulation to exert a systemic effect. For some drugs, the first-pass effect is so extensive that most of the drug dose is immediately metabolized, and the drug must be given by a different route of administration in order to be therapeutic.

Lidocaine (Xylocaine) cannot be given orally because no active drug remains after the first-pass effect. Therefore, lidocaine is given intravenously to treat cardiac arrhythmias or via the topical or transdermal routes to produce local anesthesia.

If nitroglycerin is administered orally, 90 percent of the dose is metabolized by the liver in the first-pass effect. Therefore, the standard dose of nitroglycerin is set to take this into account and to make certain that sufficient amounts of the drug remain in the blood to be therapeutic in treating the symptoms of angina.

Some drugs are actually administered in an inactive form and remain inactive until they are metabolized by the liver. So it is the **metabolite** form of the drug that is active and actually exerts a therapeutic effect. This type of drug is classified as a **prodrug**. The prefix *pro-* means *before*. A prodrug is a form of the drug that comes before the active drug is produced. Some classes of drugs such as ACE inhibitor drugs used to treat hypertension are examples of prodrugs (e.g., Mavik, Vasotec).

## Clinical Applications

Because the liver is the principal organ for drug metabolism, a decreased rate of drug metabolism occurs in patients with chronic liver disease, such as hepatitis, or in elderly patients with decreased liver function due to degenerative changes associated with aging. In these patients, drug doses need to be reduced to compensate for the prolonged action of unmetabolized drug in the blood and to prevent toxicity from high levels of drug.

Premature infants have very immature livers that are unable to metabolize drugs efficiently. The doses of their drugs must be carefully calculated to avoid toxicity.

**Chronotherapy** is a method of drug therapy that attempts to coordinate the administration and metabolism of a drug to the body's own biological rhythms. Certain diseases, such as hypertension or asthma, tend to be worse at certain times of the day. If an antihypertensive drug is taken at bedtime, it is metabolized and reaches its highest therapeutic level in the early morning, just when the blood pressure rises dramatically and there is an increased incidence of heart attacks and strokes.

## Excretion

The excretion of drugs is a necessary step in ridding the body of waste products (inactive drug metabolites) and removing active drugs that are not metabolized by the liver. The principal organ of drug excretion is the kidney, although other organs are involved to a limited degree. The lungs excrete certain inhaled drugs each time the patient exhales. Also, trace amounts of drugs are excreted in saliva, tears, sweat, and breast milk.

A drug is not automatically excreted by the kidney just because it reaches the renal artery that leads to the kidney. A drug that remains bound to albumin does not pass through the glomerular membrane in the nephron of the kidney. Drug bound to albumin remains in the general circulation. However, unbound drug, which exists by itself as a small molecule, does pass through the glomerular membrane. Once through the glomerular membrane, a further distinction is made between water-soluble drugs and fat-soluble drugs. An unbound molecule of a water-soluble drug is excreted in the urine because of its affinity for the water content of urine. An unbound molecule of a fat-soluble drug is more attracted to the lipid (fat) structure of the renal tubule wall than to the urine. Its molecule passes through the wall of the renal tubule, into a nearby capillary, and returns to the blood. Eventually, molecules of the fat-soluble drug are metabolized by the liver into a more water-soluble form that can be excreted in the urine. Without the action of the liver, it would be difficult for any fat-soluble drug to be excreted by the kidneys. Indeed, it has been estimated that some fat-soluble barbiturate drugs could remain in the blood for years if the liver did not metabolize them to a water-soluble form.

Poor renal function can significantly prolong the effects of some drugs. Patients with renal disease and elderly patients with decreased levels of kidney function due to aging are prescribed lower doses of drugs to prevent toxic symptoms due to decreased rates of drug excretion.

# Chapter Review

## Quiz Yourself

1. List two disadvantages encountered when administering some drugs by the oral route.
2. The sublingual route of administration provides more rapid absorption of a drug than the oral route. True or false?

3. What is the meaning of the abbreviation A.S.? O.U.?
4. A diabetic patient would inject insulin via what route of administration?
5. Name three acceptable sites for an intramuscular injection in an adult.
6. Differentiate between the I.V. push, I.V. drip, and I.V. piggyback methods of administration.
7. A drug administered via the intravesical route would be administered into what organ?
8. Describe the steps of absorption, distribution, metabolism, and excretion of a drug that is administered orally.
9. What is meant by the phrase *first-pass effect*?
10. How do plasma proteins such as albumin regulate the amount of drug circulating in the blood?
11. What is the function of the blood–brain barrier?
12. Give two reasons why standard drug doses may need to be decreased for elderly patients.
13. Give two reasons why drugs reaching the kidney may not be immediately excreted in the urine.
14. What is chronotherapy and how is it useful in determining when to administer drugs?
15. Define the words *biotransformation*, *albumin*, *metabolite*, and *prodrug*.

## Spelling Tips

**intravenous**    not *inter*venous. Also with *intra-arterial*, *intracardiac*, *intradermal*, *intramuscular*, and *intrathecal.* The prefix *intra-* means *within.* The prefix *inter-* means *between.*

**parenteral**    not *parental.*

## Clinical Applications

1. What route of administration is shown here?

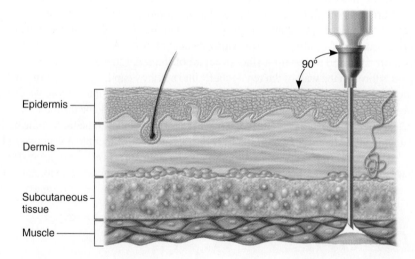

**2.** What route of administration is shown here? (*Hint:* You can look up the drug name in Appendix D for additional information.)

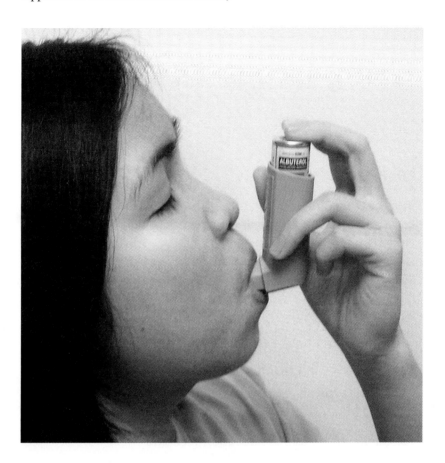

## Multimedia Extension Exercises

- Go to www.pearsonhighered.com/turley and click on the photo of the cover of *Understanding Pharmacology for Health Professionals* to access the interactive Companion Website created for this textbook.

# 5

# Using Drugs Therapeutically

## Learning Objectives

After you study this chapter, you should be able to

1. Describe the physiologic basis of all drug effects.

2. Differentiate between a local and a systemic drug effect.

3. Define the phrases *therapeutic effect, side effect, adverse effect*, and *target organ*.

4. Describe two actions the physician might take to reverse drug toxicity.

5. Describe the physiologic basis of an allergic drug reaction.

6. Describe the physiologic basis of drug-drug and drug-food interactions.

7. Define the words *receptor, agonist, antagonist, synergism*, and *antagonism*.

8. Describe the metric system of drug measurement.

9. Describe these drug measurements: units, inches, drops, milliequivalents, percentages, and ratios.

10. Recognize and define Latin abbreviations indicating frequency of doses.

11. Describe how dose calculations are made for adults, infants, and patients on chemotherapy.

12. Name the five rights of drug administration.

A drug is given to prevent, diagnose, or treat a disease or condition. The effect that a drug exerts is directed toward one of those three goals. Drugs can also exert other effects in the body, however, and these effects are often undesirable. A drug's effect can also be altered by an interaction with other drugs or foods taken at the same time.

## Basis of Drug Effects

Drug effects are initiated through **receptors**. Receptors are special protein molecules located on the cell membranes of every cell. They are specifically designed to interact with body chemicals (hormones, enzymes, neurotransmitters, etc.), but they can also interact with drugs. There are many different kinds of receptors located on the cells of organs and tissues throughout the body.

You can think of a receptor as a lock and a drug as a key (see ▪ **FIGURE 5–1**). A drug can unlock (or activate) a receptor. In fact, chemically similar drugs can unlock and activate the same receptor. A drug that is able to unlock and activate a receptor and produce an effect is known as an ***agonist drug***.

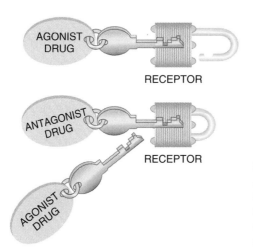

▪ **FIGURE 5–1  Agonist and antagonist drugs.** An agonist drug (key) unlocks and activates a receptor (lock). An antagonist drug (key) occupies and blocks a receptor (lock), but does not activate it. An antagonist drug also keeps an agonist drug from unlocking and activating the receptor.

Some drugs appear to fit into a receptor, but cannot actually unlock and activate the receptor to produce an effect. These drugs are known as ***antagonist or blocker drugs***. When an antagonist drug combines with a receptor, it is similar to inserting the wrong key into a lock. The key may fit, but it cannot be turned to unlock the lock. Instead, the antagonist drug's therapeutic effect is to occupy the receptor site and block body hormones, enzymes, neurotransmitters, or other drugs from activating the receptor.

It should also be noted that one drug can act as a master key to unlock several different receptors in different organs and tissues. This action accounts for the therapeutic effect plus various side effects that can be produced throughout the body by just one drug.

There are many types of receptors throughout the body. **Adrenergic receptors** respond to the neurotransmitters epinephrine and norepinephrine from the sympathetic division of the nervous system, as well as to certain drugs. Adrenergic receptors include alpha$_1$, alpha$_2$, as well as beta$_1$ and beta$_2$ receptors. Alpha$_1$ and alpha$_2$ receptors (also known as α–*adrenergic receptors*) respond to norepinephrine and drugs that act in a similar way. Beta$_1$ and beta$_2$ receptors (also known as β-*adrenergic receptors*) respond to epinephrine and drugs that act in a similar way. (The Greek letters α and β mean *alpha* and *beta*.) **Cholinergic receptors** respond to the neurotransmitter acetylcholine from the parasympathetic division of the nervous system, as well as to certain drugs. The adjective *cholinergic* is derived from the word *acetylcholine*. There are many other types of receptors, including those that respond to histamine, which are known as $H_1$ and $H_2$ *receptors*.

## Local and Systemic Effects of Drugs

Basically, drugs act in one of two ways, either locally or systemically. A **local effect** is limited to the site of administration and those tissues immediately surrounding it. Most drugs applied topically exert a local effect (e.g., nasal sprays in the nose, topical creams and ointments on the skin). A few drugs applied topically exert a systemic effect (e.g., Nicoderm CQ patch to stop smoking).

Except for some skin diseases, most medical conditions and diseases cannot be treated by a drug that acts only at the site of administration; they must be treated with a drug that acts systemically. A **systemic effect** is felt throughout the body. Drugs taken orally usually exert a systemic effect. (In a previous chapter, we discussed how some oral drugs are not absorbed and only exert a local effect in the gastrointestinal tract.) Inhaled drugs exert either a local effect or a systemic effect, depending on the type of drug. Drugs given subcutaneously, intramuscularly, or intravenously exert a systemic effect. Drugs given vaginally exert a local effect. Drugs given rectally exert either a local or a systemic effect, depending on the type of drug.

The same drug given by different routes can exert either a local or a systemic effect.

Example: The over-the-counter antihistamine drug diphenhydramine (Benadryl) can be purchased as a spray or cream that has a local effect to relieve itching of the skin. It can also be purchased as a tablet or capsule that, when swallowed, has a systemic effect to relieve allergy symptoms of itching and hives anywhere on the skin, as well as nasal stuffiness and red, watery eyes.

Example: The prescription drug lidocaine (Xylocaine) has a local effect when it is gargled for topical anesthesia in the mouth, applied to the skin as a cream or ointment for topical anesthesia, or injected subcutaneously for local anesthesia; however, when it is given intravenously to treat cardiac arrhythmias, it has a systemic effect.

## Other Drug Effects

### Therapeutic Effect

The **therapeutic effect** is the drug's main action for which it was prescribed by the physician or other healthcare provider. The therapeutic effect of a drug is intended to prevent a disease, to diagnose a disease, or to treat a disease by controlling, improving, or curing the symptoms of the disease.

The therapeutic effect of a drug can be directed toward the specific area of the body that has the disease—toward a **target organ** (e.g., the heart, in patients with congestive heart failure). However, the therapeutic effect is not always directed toward a target organ. For example, when a physician prescribes an antibiotic drug, the therapeutic effect is intended to destroy or inhibit the growth of disease-causing bacteria, wherever they are within the body.

Sometimes the therapeutic effect is actually one of the side effects of the drug. Many antihistamine drugs, when given orally to treat allergies, produce significant drowsiness. This side effect is undesirable, particularly in patients who must drive or operate machinery. However, this side effect of drowsiness can be utilized as a therapeutic effect when an antihistamine drug is incorporated into a drug that is used to treat insomnia. Antihistamine drugs are a common ingredient in over-the-counter sleep aids.

The perfect drug would have a complete therapeutic effect that is perfectly suited to its medical purpose and no other effects. Unfortunately, the perfect drug does not exist!

## Side Effects

Drug effects other than the therapeutic effect are known as *side effects.* **Side effects** can be mild and temporary, moderate and annoying, or severe enough that the patient must stop taking the drug.

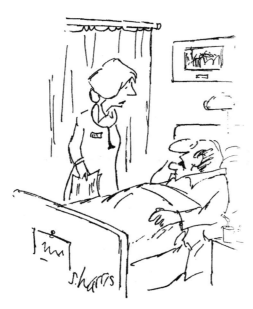

*"I stopped taking the medicine because I prefer the original disease to the side effects."*

A list of common side effects is developed as a new drug is tested. If the side effects are severe, the FDA may not approve the drug. It should be noted that no drug is entirely safe and without potential side effects and risks. Even one of the oldest and most widely used over-the-counter drugs—aspirin—can cause serious side effects, such as gastric bleeding and ulcers.

Examples of side effects vary widely with the type of drug. Some drugs produce few side effects, but most drugs are associated with at least one or two side effects that are frequently observed after administration of the drug. Common gastrointestinal side effects of many drugs include anorexia (lack of appetite), nausea, vomiting, or diarrhea. A common side effect of narcotic drugs is constipation. Common central nervous system side effects include drowsiness, excitement, or depression. Some antidepressant drugs cause significant side effects of blurred vision, dry mouth, and fatigue. Common side effects of chemotherapy drugs include nausea, vomiting, chills, fever, loss of hair, and depression of the bone marrow. Even though these side effects are more severe than those of other drugs, the FDA does not take these drugs off the market because chemotherapy drugs are used to treat cancer—a life-threatening condition.

Once a drug is approved by the FDA, its advertisements, informational literature, prescribing information, and package inserts must list the drug's side effects.

## Adverse Effects

Severe side effects are often referred to as *adverse effects.* **Adverse effects** are not as commonly observed as side effects. Some adverse effects become apparent only after a drug has been on the market for some time and has been prescribed for large numbers of patients. The FDA can remove a drug from the market, even after it has been approved, if there are reports of severe adverse effects.

Example: The drug tegaserod (Zelnorm) was approved by the FDA in 2002 for the treatment of irritable bowel syndrome and was also approved in 2004 for chronic constipation. This drug was heavily advertised on television. However, in 2007 it was taken off the market because of an increased risk of heart attack and stroke.

## Focus on Healthcare Issues

In 2000, the FDA proposed regulations to make the prescribing information provided with drugs easier for doctors to use. The FDA acknowledged that too few doctors read these lengthy, fine-print information sheets. The newly revised drug information begins with a section describing the most important warnings for not prescribing a drug for particular types of patients and ends with a patient-counseling checklist that the doctor can review with the patient. Seven of the eleven drugs taken off the market by the FDA from 1997 to 2000 were taken off because doctors kept prescribing those drugs to particular patients despite warnings to the contrary in the drug information.

## Historical Notes

In 1997, the FDA removed from the market one of the two drugs in the widely popular "fen-phen" combination drug for weight loss. Fenfluramine (Pondimin) was removed from the market; the other drug, phenteramine (Fastin), was allowed to remain on the market as an appetite suppressant. At the same time, the chemically related drug dexfenfluramine (Redux) was also taken off the market. Both fenfluramine (Pondimin) and dexfenfluramine (Redux) were linked to cases of patients developing primary pulmonary arterial hypertension and damage to the heart valves. Before it was taken off the market, Redux had already been prescribed for 2 million people.

Often an adverse effect is so unusual and seemingly unrelated to the drug's usual effect that it takes some time before a causal relationship is established.

## Clinical Applications

Isotretinoin (Accutane) is a vitamin A–type (retinoid) drug that was first approved by the FDA in 1982 for the treatment of severe cystic acne vulgaris of the skin. It was not until 2001 that the FDA required patients to sign a consent form prior to taking Accutane because of a possible link to suicide. See Chapter 17 for a feature on how the Accutane controversy affected one family.

Pramipexole (Mirapex) was approved by the FDA in 1997 to treat the symptoms of Parkinson's disease. More recently it was approved to treat restless legs syndrome. However, even the television advertisements warn of the adverse reactions of compulsive gambling and sexual activity.

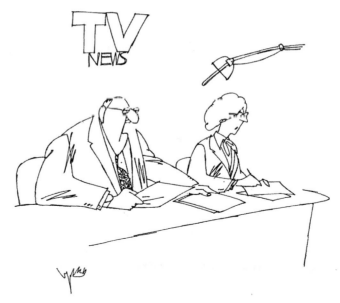

*"Six white mice were ordered to appear today before a Senate subcommittee concerning their alleged adverse reaction to a new drug."*

According to a study published in *Archives of Internal Medicine*, the incidence of death or adverse reactions to drugs more than doubled between 1998 and 2005. Adverse drug reactions account for 1.5 million hospitalizations each year, or about 4,000 every day. An additional 770,000 patients develop an adverse drug reaction after being admitted to the hospital and receiving more drugs. As many as 100,000 Americans die each year as a result of an adverse drug reaction. It has been estimated that for every dollar spent on prescription drugs, another dollar is spent to treat adverse reactions caused by those drugs.

Physicians and pharmacists can report adverse drug effects to the FDA (see ■ **FIGURE 5–2**). The FDA's phone number must be published in bold type on all drug information, effective as of 2000. The FDA also maintains the national Adverse Event Reporting System (AERS). Almost half of the reports of patients' deaths sent to the FDA were due to adverse drug reactions.

## Toxic Effects

Toxic effects result when the serum level of a drug rises above the therapeutic level to a higher level that is toxic. Before FDA approval, the drug company must show that a drug does not produce a toxic effect when administered in a therapeutic dose. However, when a drug with a low **therapeutic index** (a narrow margin of safety between the therapeutic dose and the toxic dose)—such as the heart drug digoxin (Lanoxin)—is administered, it is not uncommon to see toxic symptoms, particularly in elderly patients whose liver and kidneys are less able to metabolize and excrete the drug.

When toxic effects occur, the physician may elect to decrease the dose of the drug, lengthen the time between doses, or discontinue the drug altogether. Patients taking drugs that are known to frequently cause toxic effects are scheduled for blood tests to monitor the drug level and other laboratory tests to monitor the function of particular organs that might be affected.

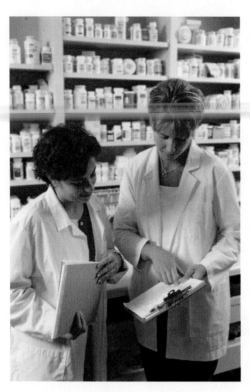

■ **FIGURE 5–2 Pharmacists.**
Pharmacists check each patient's list of prescribed drugs, watching for drugs that might cause an adverse effect or interact with other drugs. Pharmacists also consult with physicians. This collaborative communication is one way to avoid adverse drug effects.

Example: The antibiotic drugs gentamicin and kanamycin are known to exert toxic effects on the ears (**ototoxicity**) and kidneys (**nephrotoxicity**). Patients on these drugs have audiograms to monitor hearing acuity and their BUN and creatinine levels are also monitored by blood tests to assess kidney function. The word *ototoxicity* contains the combining form *ot/o-* which means *ear*; the word *nephrotoxicity* contains the combining form *nephr/o-* which means *nephron or kidney*.

Example: Liver function tests are done for patients on some cholesterol-lowering drugs (e.g., Lipitor, Mevacor, Zocor) because of their possible toxic effect on the liver.

## Allergic Reactions

An allergic reaction is a type of side effect that differs from other side effects because of its specific underlying cause: the release of **histamine** that occurs even when a drug is at a therapeutic level. The word *allergy* was introduced in the early 1900s. An allergy is a reaction that occurs when the body's immune system identifies a foreign substance (which is known as an ***antigen***) and initiates an antibody response against it. The antigen (pollen, dust, or a drug) does not provoke an allergic reaction in everyone, only in certain hypersensitive people. The presence of the antigen combined with an antibody stimulates the release of histamine.

Histamine produces mild-to-severe allergic symptoms, depending on the amount released. Mild allergic reactions are characterized by itching, swelling, redness, and sneezing. Severe or life-threatening allergic reactions involve bronchospasm, edema, shock, and death. The most severe symptoms of an allergic reaction are collectively known as ***anaphylaxis*** or ***anaphylactic shock***.

# Drug Alert!

Anaphylactic shock is not common, but is often associated with antibiotic drugs, although other drugs may also produce it. Interestingly, a patient may take several courses of an antibiotic drug over the years without any reaction, but then the next course of the drug will cause an allergic reaction. Once a patient is sensitized to a particular drug, even a small dose can trigger an allergic reaction. In addition, some drugs show cross allergies to other drug groups because of similarities in their molecular structures. For example, patients allergic to penicillin should avoid other drugs in the penicillin group, such as ampicillin, and may also exhibit hypersensitivity to cephalosporin antibiotic drugs (Keflex, Velosef, Ceclor) because of their similar chemical structure.

### Idiosyncratic Reactions

A **drug idiosyncrasy** is a type of drug reaction that is not a side effect and is not based on an allergic reaction. It is an individual's unique reaction to a drug, and it differs from side effects commonly associated with that drug. A drug idiosyncrasy has its basis in the genetic makeup of the individual, as certain genetic factors are responsible for variations in the metabolism and action of a drug. Certain ethnic groups, such as those of Asian, Jewish, and African descent, have well-studied idiosyncratic reactions to certain drugs. **Pharmacogenetics** is the study of how the genetic makeup of different people affects their response to certain drugs.

Example: Malignant hyperthermia (uncontrolled elevated body temperature) is a type of drug idiosyncrasy. It occurs in 1 out of every 20,000 patients who are given the inhaled general anesthetic drug halothane. It can also occur in some patients who are given the muscle relaxant drug succinylcholine prior to surgery. This idiosyncratic reaction is caused by a genetic variation in one known gene that controls a particular receptor, but the reaction may involve up to six different genes. The patient experiences severe, continued muscle contractions followed by malignant hyperthermia. Unless the symptoms are treated quickly, they can result in death.

## Drug–Drug and Drug–Food Interactions

### Drug–Drug Interactions

Drug–drug interactions occur because of polypharmacy, synergism, and antagonism.

**Polypharmacy.** Many patients take more than one drug on a daily basis. In particular, elderly patients with chronic medical problems may consume a number of drugs several times a day. The elderly make up 15 percent of the population in the United States, but they take 33 percent of the prescription drugs. The risk of an adverse reaction to a drug is one-third higher in people ages 50–59 than in those just 10 years younger. This is because there is a marked increase in the number of drugs prescribed to the average person after age 50. In addition, many patients take both prescription drugs and several over-the-counter drugs of their own choice. **Polypharmacy** increases the likelihood of a drug–drug interaction.

**Synergism.** When administered simultaneously, some drugs interact with each other in a particular way that either accentuates or diminishes the action of each. **Synergism** occurs when two drugs combine to produce an effect that is greater than the independent effect of each drug. In many cases, synergism is beneficial.

## Clinical Applications

The way to optimize the therapeutic effect of a drug and minimize the occurrence of adverse or toxic effects is to take the drug exactly as prescribed. For many elderly people, this is easier said than done. The multiple drugs they take are on varying schedules, given several times a day, or daily, or only weekly—and this can be confusing. Add to that the common problems of memory and vision loss, and this increases the possibility of noncompliance (missed drug doses) or toxicity (overdoses). A drug dose container purchased at a drug store (see ■ FIGURE 5–3) can be an inexpensive solution. A new FDA-approved computerized unit the size of a bread box and known as EMMA (Electronic Medication Management Assistant) holds individualized doses of a month's worth of drugs. EMMA plugs into a regular outlet and has a wireless connection to the Internet to access the patient's electronic medication administration record. When it is time for a drug dose, an audible alert sounds. The patient then pushes a button on the touch screen, and the drug dose is dispensed.

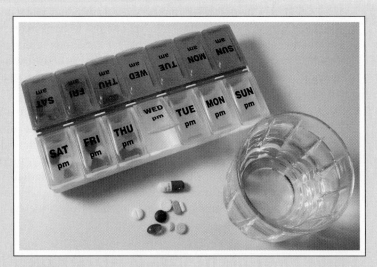

■ **FIGURE 5–3 Polypharmacy.**
Elderly patients often take multiple prescription and over-the-counter drugs each day. Drug dose containers help organize the patient's various drugs. This container has sections for each day of the week, for both A.M. and P.M. drug doses. The patient is getting ready to take his Wednesday P.M. drugs. The use of a drug dose container helps remind the patient to take all of the drugs at the correct time each day, but it does not prevent the occurrence of a drug-drug interaction. Polypharmacy increases the likelihood of a drug-drug interaction.

Example: Tylenol is combined with codeine to provide more complete pain relief than either drug alone can provide.

Example: A potassium-wasting diuretic drug is combined with a potassium-sparing diuretic drug to achieve effective water loss while conserving potassium.

However, an undesirable type of synergism can also occur. One well-publicized undesirable synergistic drug combination is that of tranquilizer drugs taken with alcohol or antihistamine drugs taken with alcohol. In both cases, the drug side effect of drowsiness is heightened by the sedative effect of alcohol, often with fatal results.

## Did You Know?

Although Elvis Presley officially died of a heart attack in 1977, the State Board of Medical Examiners found that he had been prescribed some 12,000 pills— tranquilizers, stimulants, sedatives, and painkillers—in the 18 months prior to his death.

According to the *Washington Post* newspaper, Prozac (an antidepressant drug) and alcohol taken by the chauffeur driving Princess Diana may have contributed to the car accident in which she was tragically killed in 1997.

## Historical Notes

In 1988, astemizole (Hismanal) and terfenadine (Seldane) antihistamine drugs were hailed as superior to older antihistamine drugs because they did not cause sedation. After they had been on the market for 10 years, the FDA required them to carry a warning label that they should not be used by patients taking the antibiotic drug erythromycin or the antifungal drugs ketoconazole or itraconazole. Taking just a little more than the prescribed dose of either of these antihistamine drugs in combination with the antibiotic or antifungal drug could cause a fatal cardiac arrhythmia. In 1999, the FDA removed both of these antihistamine drugs from the market.

**Antagonism.** Another type of drug–drug interaction is known as *antagonism*. **Antagonism** occurs when two drugs combine to produce an effect that is less than the intended effect for either drug (see ■ **FIGURE 5–4**).

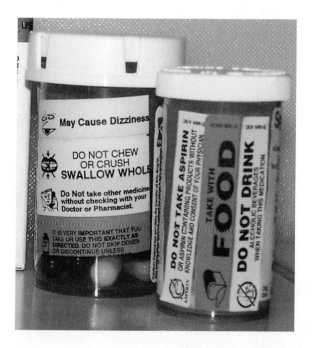

■ **FIGURE 5–4 Warning labels on prescription bottles.** The pharmacist applies labels to the prescription bottle to warn the patient of a possible drug-drug interaction, drug–food interaction, side effects, and so forth. These two prescription bottles have a total of seven warning labels on them. On the bottle on the left, the patient is warned (1) that it might cause dizziness (a side effect), (2) that it should not be chewed or crushed, (3) that it should not be taken with other drugs without checking first with the doctor or pharmacist (drug-drug interaction of antagonism), and (4) that it should be taken exactly as directed. On the bottle on the right, the patient is warned (1) not to take it with aspirin (drug-drug interaction of synergism), (2) to take it with food (to avoid the side effect of stomach irritation), and (3) not to drink alcoholic beverages with it (drug–drug interaction).

Example: When the antibiotic drug tetracycline is taken with an antacid, these two drugs combine in the stomach to form an insoluble compound that prevents either drug from exerting a therapeutic effect.

### Drug–Food Interactions

Synergistic and antagonistic drug–food interactions also occur (see ■ **FIGURE 5–5**).

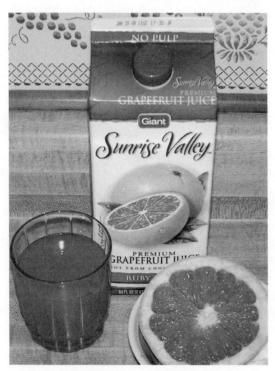

■ **FIGURE 5–5  Grapefruit and grapefruit juice.**
This delicious, nutritious, and healthful fruit and its juice can cause serious adverse effects and even toxic effects when taken together with certain drugs.

## *Drug Alert!*

The beneficial effects of drinking grapefruit juice may turn into toxic effects if you are taking certain drugs. This is because grapefruit juice blocks an enzyme in the intestine that normally breaks down part of a drug dose before it even enters the blood. With decreased levels of this enzyme, much more active drug enters the blood, and this can result in a toxic level of the drug.

Example: Tetracycline cannot be taken with milk because together they form an insoluble compound in the stomach.

Example: MAO inhibitors, a class of antidepressant drugs, cannot be taken with foods rich in the amino acid tyramine because that will cause hypertension, headache, and a possible stroke. Tyramine is present in aged cheeses, alcoholic beverages, bananas, liver, avocados, and chocolate, and patients taking MAO inhibitor drugs must avoid these foods.

Example: An antihistamine drug taken with grapefruit juice can cause the adverse effect of a heart arrhythmia.

Example: A cholesterol-lowering drug taken with grapefruit juice can result in toxicity with blood levels 15 times higher than normal.

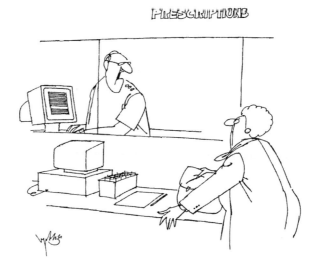

"*I'm not cruising the Internet ... I'm checking your prescription drug interactions.*"

## Systems of Drug Measurement

In the early history of pharmacology, the measurement of drug doses was crude and imprecise. The powdered, dried herbs in many prescriptions contained varying amounts of active drug that could not be measured accurately. There is one system of drug measurement (e.g., the apothecary system) that is of historic interest and other systems of drug measurement (e.g., the metric system and other types of drug measurements) that are currently in use.

### Apothecary System of Drug Measurement

In the 1700s, the apothecary system was introduced from England. The word *apothecary* comes from a Greek word that referred to a person who combined and dispensed drugs. Some apothecary measurements are still in use today. These include the liquid measurements of the pint, quart, and gallon that are used in the home. Apothecary measurements for drug doses included the minim, grain, scruple, and dram. (The standard of a grain of drug was originally based on the average weight of one grain of wheat.) The use of these apothecary drug measurements has been nearly discontinued. Phenobarbital, desiccated thyroid, and iron are just a few of the remaining drugs that have equivalent apothecary and metric doses printed on the drug label. The drug label for dessicated thyroid shows both systems of measurement (e.g., 1 grain and the metric equivalent of 60 mg). The abbreviation of the apothecary measurement *grain* (gr) was often confused with the abbreviation of the metric measurement *gram* (g).

Roman numerals were often used with the apothecary measurements. Today, Roman numerals are still used in handwritten prescriptions, at the discretion of the physician writing the prescription. The Roman numeral is not written in its standard form as I, II, III, or IV, but is written as a variation (see ■ FIGURE 5–6).

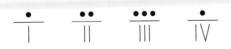

■ **FIGURE 5–6 Roman numerals for drug doses.**
Special Roman numerals are often used for drug doses in handwritten prescriptions. *Note:* These do not represent fractions, although they do resemble them to some extent.

## Metric System of Drug Measurement

The metric system was invented by the French in 1790. It is based on the length of a meter, which was originally calculated by dividing the earth's circumference by 10 million. The use of the metric system was made legal, but not mandatory, in the United States in 1866. In 1975, Congress passed the Metric Conversion Act, but with the exception of scientists, doctors, and other professionals in scientific fields, few laypersons in the United States use the metric system on a regular basis.

The metric system is officially known as the International System of Units (SI). This abbreviation is derived from the original French name, Système International d'Unites. The SI was officially adopted as the exclusive unit of measurement by the American Medical Association in 1988. The SI system is based on the meter (for length measurements), the kilogram (for weight measurements), and the liter (for volume measurements). The metric system is used for nearly all drug doses.

Metric length measurements include the meter and centimeter. A centimeter is equivalent to 1/100 of a meter. When a cube is formed that is 1 cm long on each side, it becomes a measurement of volume known as the *cubic centimeter* ($cm^3$ or cc). This volume measurement is equivalent to the volume contained in a milliliter (mL), and the two volume abbreviations *mL* and *cc* are used interchangeably to express the volume of liquid drug doses.

Metric weight measurements include the kilogram, gram, milligram, and microgram. Each of these differs by a factor of 1,000.

Drug measurements are not expressed in terms of kilograms. Kilograms are used to measure a person's weight, which can be important in calculating the correct drug dose (e,g., a 50-kilogram woman weighs 110 pounds). Extremely premature infants are measured in grams (e.g., a 900-gram premature infant weighs just about 2 pounds). Drug dose measurements are expressed in milligrams and occasionally in micrograms.

Metric volume measurements include the liter and milliliter with one liter equaling 1,000 milliliters. Drugs are not prescribed by the liter; however, the milliliter (mL) is used frequently as a measurement for liquid drugs. As mentioned previously, a milliliter (mL) and a cubic centimeter ($cm^3$ or cc) are equivalent and interchangeable.

Example: A common dose for the antacid drug Maalox is 30 mL or 30 cc. The Mantoux intradermal test for tuberculosis involves the injection of 0.1 mL (or 0.1 cc) of a liquid drug.

Drug measurements in the metric system are never expressed in fractions. Also, a drug dose with a metric number less than 1 is written as a decimal and always has a zero added to the left of the decimal point (e.g., 0.5 mg, not .5 mg). The decimal point must be placed carefully in a drug dose, as an error in placement can mean a 10-fold increase or decrease in the drug dose.

## Other Drug Measurements

Other types of drug measurements include the unit, inch, drop, milliequivalent, percentage, ratio, and household.

1. **Units.**   The doses of certain drugs are never measured by the metric system but instead by a special designation called a *unit*. Some penicillins, some vitamins, and all types of insulin are measured in units (see ■ **FIGURE 5–7**). The exact value of the unit varies from drug to drug. A unit of penicillin was standardized in 1944 as 0.6 mcg of penicillin G based on its ability to cause a ring of inhibition of a certain size on a bacterial culture. A unit of insulin is defined on the weight basis of pure insulin. Insulin is manufactured with 100 units per milliliter, which is abbreviated as U 100. A few drugs are measured in international units (IU).

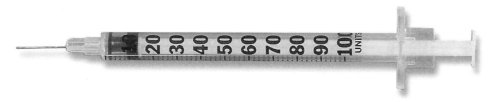

■ **FIGURE 5–7  Insulin syringe.**
An insulin syringe is used to administer liquid insulin, and its calibrations are in units, not in milliliters as are other syringes. This system of measurement (units) is clearly marked at the base of the syringe. This syringe can administer up to 100 units of liquid insulin. It cannot be used to administer liquid drugs that are measured in milliliters.

2. **Inches.**   Only one commonly prescribed drug is measured in inches, and that is nitroglycerin ointment (Nitro-Bid), a cardiac drug used to treat angina pectoris. A pad of specially marked papers is supplied with the tube of ointment so that the patient can accurately measure each dose. The ointment is squeezed onto the paper along a preprinted line that is marked off in ½-inch increments. The prescribed dose may range from 1/2 inch to 4 inches of ointment.
3. **Drops.**   The Latin word for *drops* is *guttae*, and the abbreviation is *gtt*. Eye and ear liquid drugs are often prescribed in the number of drops to be given.
4. **Milliequivalents.**   An equivalent is the molecular weight of an ion divided by the number of hydrogen ions it reacts with. A milliequivalent is 1/1000 of an equivalent and is abbreviated as *mEq*. The combining form *mill/i-* means *one thousand*. Doses of electrolyte drugs such as potassium are measured in milliequivalents, although the doses can also be given in milligrams.
5. **Percentage.**   A percentage is one part in relationship to the whole, based on a total of 100.

   Example: A 10 percent solution would be composed of 10 mL of drug in 100 mL of liquid, or 1 mL of drug in 10 mL of liquid.

   Example: A 0.25 percent ointment of the topical corticosteroid drug desoximetasone (Topicort) would contain 0.25 mg of drug in 100 mg of white petrolatum base.

6. **Ratio.**   A ratio expresses the relationship between the concentrations of two substances together in a solution. A ratio is expressed as two numbers with a colon mark between them.

   Example: Epinephrine for intracardiac injection during resuscitation is supplied in a ratio of 1:10,000 (1 part epinephrine to 10,000 parts of solution). Epinephrine used as a local anesthetic drug for subcutaneous injection is supplied in a less concentrated solution, with a ratio of 1:100,000 (1 part epinephrine to 100,000 parts of solution).

7. **Household measurement**.   The household system of measurement is an unofficial system for measuring drugs that is only used by people in their homes. It includes measuring spoons as well as silverware teaspoons and tablespoons. This is an inaccurate measurement system because there is no standard size for silverware teaspoons and tablespoons. In fact, a silverware

teaspoon can hold anywhere from 4 to 7 mL of liquid. Many over-the-counter liquid drugs (e.g., cough syrup) include in the package either a standardized plastic medicine cup or medicine spoon with teaspoon markings to ensure accurate measurement.

## The Five Rights of Drug Administration

Every year, about 1.5 million people are harmed by drug errors according to the Institute of Medicine (IOM). To reduce drug errors, the IOM recommends that all prescriptions be created electronically and drug information inserts be standardized and simplified.

In the hospital, the IOM found that each patient has approximately one drug error per day. A study published in *Archives of Internal Medicine* found that drug errors occur in one of every five doses of drugs administered in the hospital.

For drugs to be given correctly, healthcare professionals need to observe the five rights of drug administration. These include (1) the right patient, (2) the right drug, (3) the right dose, (4) the right route, and (5) the right time.

1. **The right patient.**   In a home situation, the patient is dispensing a drug to himself or to a family member, and it is not difficult to determine who should receive the drug. However, in a nursing home, hospital, or other healthcare facility where there are many patients receiving drugs, patient identification becomes crucial.

2. **The right drug.**   Generic drug names are often complex and trade name drugs can have similar-sounding names. Similar-sounding drug names can result in confusion and a drug error. For a complete list of sound-alike drugs, see Appendix A. The nurse or medication aide should check the drug name against the drug order three different times: when the drug is taken from the medication cart or shelf in the medication room, as it is being poured or placed in a paper cup, and before giving it to the patient. Also, a nurse or medication aide knows never to administer a drug prepared by another person.

3. **The right dose.**   Calculating a drug dose is an extremely important process. While it is not within the scope of this textbook to teach dose calculations, for those students who need to know how to calculate drug doses, we recommend *Medical Dosage Calculations* by Olsen, Giangrasso, Shrimpton, and Dillon (9th edition, 2008) and *Ratio-Proportion Dosage Calculations* by Giangrasso and Shrimpton (1st edition, 2010) published by Pearson/Prentice-Hall, as companion textbooks.

   The standard adult dose for a drug is appropriate for most adults. It is preset by the drug company during the drug's clinical trials to encompass the range of sizes and ages of most adult patients. However, patients who are elderly, extremely thin, or extremely obese fall outside this range and may need to have their drug dose adjusted by the physician.

   Pediatric doses, especially those for infants and premature babies, must be calculated with great accuracy. A pediatric drug dose is calculated based on the total body weight of the patient, not the age and, because the weight of a child increases regularly, the drug dose needs to be recalculated periodically when a child is on long-term drug therapy. Pediatric drug doses are expressed as mg/kg/day (milligrams of drug per kilogram of body weight per 24-hour period).

   Chemotherapy drug doses are calculated based on the patient's total body surface area. This method customizes the dose for each patient to maximize the effectiveness of the drug while minimizing its severe side effects. Chemotherapy drug doses are expressed as $mg/m^2$ (milligrams of drug per meter squared of body surface area).

4. **The right route.**   Because some drugs can be given therapeutically via several different routes of administration, it is always important to check the prescribed route of administration and also make sure that the drug form is compatible with that route.

5. **The right time.**   Drugs are measured not only in terms of the amount of the dose but also in terms of the frequency of the dose. There are a number of commonly used abbreviations that indicate the frequency of administration. These abbreviations are based on Latin phrases (see ▥ TABLE 5–1). See Appendix C for a more complete list of abbreviations, including those that are not recommended for use by the Joint Commission for Accreditation of Healthcare Organizations (JCAHO).

▥ **TABLE 5–1** **Common abbreviations for frequency of drug administration**

| Abbreviation | Latin Meaning | Medical Meaning |
|---|---|---|
| a.c. | *ante cibum* | before meals |
| ad lib. | *ad libitum* | as needed |
| b.i.d. | *bis in die* | twice a day |
| c̄ | *cum* | with |
| h.s. | *hora somni* | at bedtime (hour of sleep) |
| n.p.o., NPO | *nil per os* | nothing by mouth |
| p.c. | *post cibum* | after meals |
| p.r.n. | *pro re nata* | as needed |
| q.d. | *quaque die* | every day |
| q.h. | *quaque hora* | every hour |
| q.h.s. | *quaque hora somni* | at bedtime (hour of sleep) |
| q.i.d. | *quater in die* | four times a day |
| q.o.d. | (informal usage) | every other day |
| s̄ | *sine* | without |
| t.i.d. | *ter in die* | three times a day |

# Chapter Review

## Quiz Yourself

1. Describe the difference between local and systemic drug effects.
2. Give an example of a drug that can act either locally or systemically to produce a therapeutic effect, depending on the route of administration.
3. Differentiate between a drug's therapeutic effect and a side effect.
4. List several common side effects involving the GI tract and the central nervous system.
5. How does a toxic effect differ from a side effect?
6. Define the phrase *therapeutic index*.
7. What is the basis for all of the symptoms associated with an allergic reaction?
8. Describe the lock-and-key concept as it pertains to a drug and a receptor.
9. Give an example of a synergistic drug–drug interaction and of an antagonistic drug–drug interaction.

10. Define the word *polypharmacy*.
11. To what system of measurement do the words *cubic centimeter* and *milliliter* belong?
12. Name a drug that is measured in units. In inches. In milliequivalents.
13. A milliliter is equivalent in volume to a cubic centimeter. True or false?
14. Give the English definition of these common abbreviations that pertain to drug doses.

 **a.** a.c.
 **b.** b.i.d.
 **c.** g
 **d.** h.s.
 **e.** mcg
 **f.** mg
 **g.** mL
 **h.** mEq.
 **i.** p.r.n.
 **j.** t.i.d.

15. Pediatric drug doses are individually calculated on the basis of what criterion?
16. Chemotherapy drug doses are individually calculated on the basis of what criterion?

## Spelling Tips

**milliequivalent** often mispronounced as "millequivalent." Also, the abbreviation *mEq.* is unusual for its internal capitalization.

## Clinical Applications

1. Pharmacists place drug warning labels on prescription bottles before giving them to patients. Look at the warning labels on these prescription bottles. Write down the wording of each warning. Indicate whether it warns of a drug–drug interaction, a drug–food interaction, or is some other type of warning.

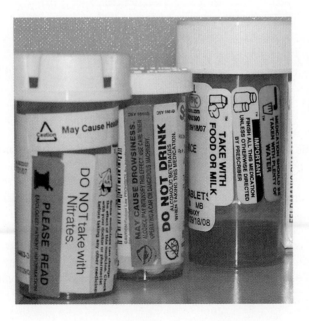

**2.** The excerpt below is from an actual medical report. Read it and then answer these questions.

**a.** Does this represent polypharmacy?

**b.** What two organs in this patient's body might be functioning at a decreased level and so prolong the effect of these drugs?

**c.** State what each of these drugs is used to treat. (*Hint*: Use Appendix D at the back of this textbook to look up the drug names.)

**d.** Is this patient at risk for drug-drug interactions?

### *Excerpt from a Medical Report*

This is a 76-year-old white female, who is currently taking Accupril 20 mg q.d., Actos 45 mg q.d., aspirin 81 mg q.d., Catapres-TTS-1 patch weekly, Lasix 40 mg q.d. (we will increase to 80 mg q.d. today), Glucotrol XL 10 mg q.d., Humulin N 12 units q.a.m. (we will decrease to 8 units q.a.m. today), K-Dur 10 mEq. q.d., Lanoxin 0.125 mg q.d., lorazepam 0.5 mg b.i.d., Metamucil p.r.n., Prozac 20 mg q.d., Zantac 150 mg b.i.d., Risperdal 0.5 mg q.h.s., Serevent inhaler 2 puffs q.12h., Synthroid 0.1 mg q.d., Celebrex 200 mg q.d., Zaroxolyn 10 mg q.d., and Ambien 5 mg q.h.s. p.r.n. She presents today with increasing fatigue, fever, and a productive cough. She is to begin Levaquin 250 mg q.d. for 10 days.

| Drug name | Used to treat |
|---|---|
| Accupril | _____ |
| Actos | _____ |
| aspirin | _____ |
| Catapres-TTS-1 | _____ |
| $B_{12}$ injections | _____ |
| Lasix | _____ |
| Glucotrol XL | _____ |
| Humulin N | _____ |
| K-Dur | _____ |
| Lanoxin | _____ |
| lorazepam | _____ |
| Metamucil | _____ |
| Prozac | _____ |
| Zantac | _____ |
| Risperdal | _____ |
| Serevent | _____ |
| Synthroid | _____ |
| Celebrex | _____ |
| Zaroxolyn | _____ |
| Ambien | _____ |
| Levaquin | _____ |

## Multimedia Extension Exercises

■ Go to www.pearsonhighered.com/turley and click on the photo of the cover of *Understanding Pharmacology for Health Professionals* to access the interactive Companion Website created for this textbook.

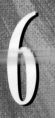

# The Prescription

## CHAPTER CONTENTS

## Learning Objectives

After you study this chapter, you should be able to

1. Give the definition of a prescription.

2. Name the types of prescriptions.

3. Describe medication orders and other types of orders

4. Describe the difference between the components of a prescription and a medication order.

5. Describe the role of the pharmacist in filling a prescription.

## Definition of a Prescription

The etiology or origin of the word *prescription* is from the Latin word *praescriptio*, meaning *a written order*. The word *prescription* is composed of the prefix *pre-* (before), the combining form *script/o-* (write), and the suffix *–ion* (action). The definition of *prescription* is *the action of writing [that takes place] before [a drug is dispensed]*.

A **prescription** is a written, computerized, electronic, or verbal order from a physician (or other qualified healthcare provider) to a pharmacist, giving instructions as to how to dispense a drug to a specific patient who requires drug therapy. A prescription is a medicolegal document; it conveys precise medical information, and it is a legal document that can be used as evidence in a court of law.

Nonprescription (over-the-counter) drugs do not require a prescription and can be purchased by any adult. Prescription drugs can only be ordered by a licensed physician or doctor of osteopathy (M.D. or D.O.), dentist (D.D.S), podiatrist (D.P.M.), or other appropriately licensed healthcare provider, such as a physician's assistant (PA), nurse practitioner (NP), or optometrist (O.D.).

## Types of Prescriptions

1. **Written prescription.** A written prescription is handwritten on a single preprinted form taken from a prescription pad (see ▦ **FIGURE 6–1**). All handwritten prescriptions must be written in ink, not pencil. The prescription must also be recorded in the patient's paper medical record on a drug list for future reference. The written prescription is the traditional way in which prescriptions have been done for centuries.

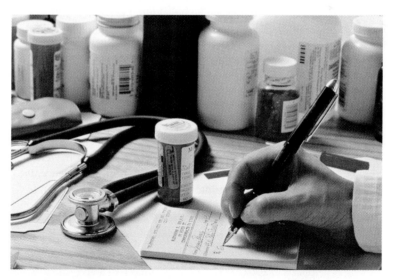

▦ **FIGURE 6–1 Prescription form.**
A prescription form is used to convey to a pharmacist a written record of a physician's order of a drug for a patient. This physician may be prescribing a new drug or ordering a refill of the drug that is in the prescription bottle.

## Drug Alert!

Handwritten prescriptions can be notoriously difficult to read. Various studies have found that 5 percent or 16 percent or even 25 percent of all handwritten prescriptions are illegible. Pharmacists often become familiar with a particular physician's handwriting and can decipher illegible handwriting. However, when in doubt, the pharmacist always calls the physician to confirm the drug and dose. Some states, such as Florida, have passed a law that all handwritten prescriptions must be legible!

## Clinical Applications

It is not uncommon for people to steal prescription pads and write prescriptions on them for drugs of abuse. To prevent theft of prescription pads, medical office personnel know that it is important to take these precautions.

1. Store extra prescription pads in a locked drawer or closet.
2. Have the physician carry just one prescription pad on his/her person from examining room to examining room.
3. Never leave a prescription pad on the counter or in an unlocked drawer in the examining room.
4. The physician should sign the prescription form only at the time he/she writes the prescription. The physician should never pre-sign blank prescription forms.

2. **Computerized prescription.**   More recently, with the advent of the electronic patient record, a prescription can be typed into the medical office's software system, a copy of the prescription printed out, signed by the physician, and given to the patient. A computerized prescription can be faxed directly to the pharmacist.
3. **Electronic prescription.**   An electronic prescription is also generated by a computer, but is not signed by the physician. Instead, the physician's digital electronic signature is automatically imprinted at the bottom of the prescription. An electronic prescription can be faxed directly to the pharmacist.
4. **Verbal prescription.**   A verbal prescription is not written but is given over the telephone. In cases in which the physician cannot see the patient in the medical office (e.g., on a weekend), the physician may verbally give a prescription over the telephone to a pharmacist. When the prescription is for a drug that is not a controlled substance, the pharmacist can fill the prescription without having a printed-out prescription and without having the physician's signature.

## Did You Know?

About 3.3 billion prescriptions were filled in the United States in 2006; this was up from 3 billion prescriptions in 2002, 2.5 billion prescriptions in 1998, and 1.5 billion prescriptions in 1989.

## Medication Orders and Other Types of Orders

### Medication Order

A **medication order** is the written record of a physician's order to the pharmacist to dispense a drug to a patient who is in a hospital or other healthcare facility. Medication orders are handwritten on a large preprinted form known as the *physician's order sheet* or *physician's order record* (see ▨ FIGURE 6–2). The physician's order sheet is located at the front of the patient's hospital or facility medical record. For facilities with an electronic patient record, medication orders are typed into the computer on a designated screen that serves as a physician's order sheet.

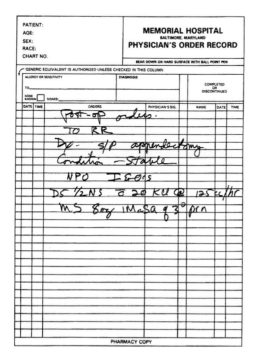

▨ **FIGURE 6–2** **Physician's order sheet.**
The physician's order sheet is used to write medication orders for a patient in the hospital. This patient has just come out of surgery, and all drug orders must be rewritten to reflect the patient's change in status. This is what the orders say:

Post-op orders (postoperative orders)
To RR (to the recovery room)
Dx—S/P appendectomy (diagnosis—status post appendectomy)
Condition—stable.
NPO (nothing by mouth). I&O's (measure intake and output of fluids)
D5 ½ NS with 20 KCl @ 125 cc/hr (intravenous fluids of dextrose 5% with half normal saline with potassium chloride at 125 cubic centimeters per hour)
MS 8 mg IM or SQ q3° p.r.n (morphine sulfate 8 milligrams, intramuscular or subcutaneous, every 3 hours, as needed)

## Verbal Order

When a patient has been admitted to the hospital, the patient's physician can give a verbal drug order over the telephone to a licensed nurse, who then writes the order on the physician's order sheet, marks it as a **verbal order** (V.O.), and then signs her name and the initials of her license. The order is then sent to the pharmacy. The physician must come to the facility to personally sign the order within a specific amount of time. Verbal orders are also known as *telephone orders*.

## Standing Orders

**Standing orders** are a group of specific orders that are preprinted on a facility's physician's order sheet. They often pertain to a protocol of treatment related to a specific disease or surgical procedure. They contain standard common orders that are the same for any patient who has that specific disease or is scheduled for that surgical procedure. For example, a patient admitted for bowel surgery would have preoperative standing orders for a clear liquid diet and enemas, for an antibiotic drug to kill bacteria in the bowel, and for no food (NPO) after midnight before the surgery. Some parts of the preoperative standing orders are often completed at home by the patient prior to admission to the facility. In addition to the standing orders, the physician would also write more specific medication orders to address a particular patient's other medical needs for drugs for ongoing disease processes (diabetes, hypertension, etc.).

### Automatic Stop Orders

**Automatic stop orders** are a type of medication order that originates not with the physician but with the hospital pharmacy. Medication orders for certain types of drugs (e.g., controlled substances) are only valid for a certain number of days while the patient is in the hospital. (The exact number of days is determined by the hospital's Pharmacy Committee.) After that time, the pharmacy automatically stops sending the drug to the patient's nursing unit, and the attending physician must write an entirely new order if the patient is to continue to receive that drug.

All drug orders carry an automatic stop order that is activated whenever a patient's situation changes in the hospital (e.g., the patient goes to surgery, is transferred to another nursing unit within the hospital, is discharged to another healthcare facility, or is discharged to home). If the patient is discharged to another healthcare facility, the physician lists all of the patient's drugs in the discharge summary. The discharge summary is faxed to the other healthcare facility, and the attending physician there must reorder the patient's drugs. If the patient is discharged to home, the attending physician at the hospital provides individual prescriptions that the patient can take to a local pharmacy to be filled.

## Components of Prescriptions and Medication Orders

Prescriptions that are written on prescription forms (see ■ FIGURE 6–3) or printed out electronically and medication orders that are written on a physician's order sheet (see Figure 6–2) or typed into the hospital computer system are composed of several components. Not every component is present in all types of forms.

**1. Identifying information about the prescriber.**

| | |
|---|---|
| Prescription form | The physician's name (and/or the name of the medical group), office address, and phone number are preprinted at the top of the prescription form to positively identify the prescriber. |
| Physician's order sheet | This information is not included on the physician's order sheet. The physician's signature after the written order provides his/her name; all other information about the physician is already on file with the hospital. |

**2. Identifying information about the patient.**

| | |
|---|---|
| Prescription form | The patient's first and last name and his/her address are handwritten on the prescription form by the physician in order to positively identify the patient. |
| Physician's order sheet. | This information is already preprinted on the physician's order sheet. It is preprogrammed to appear there if it is a computerized patient record. If a paper medical record is being used, the patient's hospital card (that was created at the time of the patient's admission) is used to imprint this information in the top corner of the physician's order sheet. |

### *Clinical Applications*

In a hospital or other healthcare facility, the physician's office address and phone number are not needed on the physician's order sheet because the physician is already a member of the facility's medical staff. Prior to joining the medical staff, each physician must provide his/her name, office address, home address, and phone numbers (as well as Social Security number, state medical license number, federal and state DEA number, educational background, and board certifications) in a written application that is kept on file in the facility's credentialing department. No physician is permitted to write orders, including medication orders, unless he/she is already an approved member of that facility's medical staff.

**KELVIN SELCHER, M.D.**
Chartwell Professional Group
398 Medical Way
Pittsburgh, PA  15228
Phone: 312-555-1000

Name_____Age_____Date_____
Address_____

R⨯

[  ] Do not substitute        Refills: 0  1  2  3 Other_____

Signature: _____M.D.
DEA #_____

■ **FIGURE 6–3  A prescription form.**
Prescription forms are used for handwritten prescriptions when
patients are seen in a medical office or when patients are discharged from the hospital. The blank prescription form has several
standard component parts, as described in the text.

### 3. Age and weight of the patient.

Prescription form   This information is not always included on a prescription form, but it can be
useful. The age is more important when the patient is a child.
Prescriptions for children less than five years of age should give an accurate
age in years and months. It is mandatory to include the age of the patient in
any prescription written for a Schedule II drug. The doses of some drugs may
need to be adjusted if the patient's weight is very low or very high.

Physician's order   The age of a patient in the hospital is already entered on the demographics
sheet   face sheet in the patient's medical record upon admission and is not included
in the medication order.

### 4. Date of the order.

Prescription form   The physician writes the full date (month/day/year) on the prescription form.
A prescription for a prescription drug is only valid for one year from the date on
the prescription form. A prescription for a Schedule III through Schedule V
drug is only valid for six months from the date. A prescription for a Schedule II
drug is only valid for seven days from the date.

Physician's order   The physician writes the full date next to each medication order. In addition, the
sheet   time of the order is written next to the date. This is because medication orders
in the hospital setting are time sensitive and must be filled by the pharmacy and
administered by the nurse in a timely manner.

5. **Rx.**    Prescriptions have been written since ancient times. The practice of medicine began with the Romans and Greeks, and so many medical words are Latin or Greek. This symbol stands for the Latin word *recipere*, meaning *to take*. Prescriptions were, at one time, actually recipes listing several ingredients to be crushed and mixed by the pharmacist before dispensing.

Prescription form    Most prescription forms come with a large preprinted *Rx* just to the left of the area where the prescription itself will be handwritten.

Physician's order sheet    The *Rx* symbol is not preprinted on a physician's order sheet because the page is large and is used to order other types of treatments and services (e.g., physical therapy, social services) in addition to drugs.

6. **Drug name.**

Prescription form    The physician writes either the drug's generic name or its trade name on the prescription form. The chemical name of a drug is not used in writing a prescription. Abbreviations of drug names are avoided because they may be misread and mistaken for a different drug.

Physician's order sheet    Same.

7. **Drug strength.**

Prescription form    A number appears right after the name of the drug. This number, which indicates the drug strength, is followed by an abbreviation of a unit of measurement. This number may be omitted if the drug is only available in a single strength. The physician must prescribe a drug strength that corresponds exactly to the strength in which the drug is manufactured.

> Example: If the drug is manufactured in 25 mg and 50 mg tablets, the physician cannot write a prescription for an 80 mg tablet. However, if the drug is manufactured as a scored tablet, the physician can write a prescription for exactly one-half of the amount in one tablet, knowing that the correct dose can easily be administered by dividing the scored tablet into two equal pieces.

Physician's order sheet    Same.

8. **Drug form.**

Prescription form    The specific drug form must be included. Some drugs come in several different forms (e.g., capsules, tablets, liquids, intravenous solutions).

Physician's order sheet    Same.

9. **Quantity to be dispensed.**

Prescription form    The symbol # is read as *number* and indicates to the pharmacist the total number of capsules, tablets, milliliters, ounces, etc., of drug to dispense to the patient. Sometimes the physician will preface the number sign with the abbreviation for the word *dispense* (e.g., Disp. #30). The total amount dispensed equals the length of treatment times the number of doses to be taken each day.

| | |
|---|---|
| Physician's order sheet | The physician does not need to indicate the total number of capsules, tablets, milliliters, or ounces of drug to dispense, as the medication order continues as long as the patient is in the hospital (with the exception of certain drugs such as controlled substances). The amount of drug needed for one day is dispensed to each nursing unit's medication room or cart by the hospital pharmacy, and this continues for as long as the patient is on that nursing unit. |

### 10. Directions for use.

| | |
|---|---|
| Prescription form | The abbreviation *Sig.* stands for the Latin word *signetur*, meaning *write on the label*. It indicates that the directions for how to use the drug will follow. The pharmacist is to type these directions on the label of the prescription bottle that is given to the patient. These directions include Latin abbreviations; however, when the prescription is filled, the pharmacist translates these directions into English so that the patient can understand them. These directions describe the amount of the dose (e.g., 1 tablet), the route of administration (e.g., P.O.), and frequency of the dose (e.g., b.i.d.). |
| | *Note:* Sometimes the abbreviation *Sig.* is written as just an *S* or may not be handwritten at all on the prescription form. |
| Physician's order sheet | The abbreviation *Sig.* is usually not included. The physician writes the directions using Latin abbreviations. These directions describe the amount of the dose, the route of administration, and the frequency of the dose. The hospital pharmacist does not need to translate the directions into English because the nurse on the unit understands these abbreviations. |

### 11. Signature.

| | |
|---|---|
| Prescription form | At the bottom of a prescription form, there is a preprinted line with *M.D.* at the far right-hand side (if the provider is an M.D.). The physician must sign his or her name on that line for the prescription to be valid. |
| Physician's order sheet | The physician signs his/her name and *M.D.* directly below the last medication order, not at the bottom of the page. This prevents anyone from illegally inserting additional medication orders at a later time in any blank space above the physician's signature. |

### 12. Refills.

| | |
|---|---|
| Prescription form | The physician indicates how many times the patient is permitted to refill the prescription before he/she must be re-evaluated medically. On prescription forms, there is a preprinted area that says *Refills* followed by the numbers 0 (if no refills are permitted), 1, 2, and 3. Instead of the *0*, some prescription forms have *NR*, which stands for *no refills*. The physician simply circles the appropriate number to indicate how many refills are allowed. The number of refills may also be written out (e.g., Refills × 2). Prescription drugs may be refilled for only one year. No refills are permitted for Schedule II drugs. |
| Physician's order sheet | The physician does not indicate the number of refills because the pharmacy continues to send the drug to the nursing unit as long as the patient is on that unit or until the physician orders that drug to be discontinued. |

### 13.  Generic substitution.

Prescription form    Some states mandate that the pharmacist must fill each prescription with a generic drug. If the physician wants the prescription filled with a trade name drug, he/she must specifically indicate this either by writing the trade name and checking a preprinted box that says "Dispense as written" ("DAW") or by writing the trade name and also writing "No substitution" or "Do not substitute." Other prescription forms include a preprinted message such as this: "A generically equivalent product will be dispensed unless the practitioner handwrites 'Brand Necessary' or 'Brand Medically Necessary' on the prescription form."

Physician's order sheet    Each hospital has its own formulary that contains all of the drugs that are stocked by the hospital pharmacy. The hospital pharmacist will dispense the generic equivalent of a drug unless the physician specifically requests a particular trade name.

## *Did You Know?*

In 2002, physicians wrote the equivalent of over 10 prescriptions for every person in America.

### 14.  DEA number.

Prescription form    Prescribing prescription drugs with a potential for abuse or physical/psychological dependence (e.g., schedule drugs or controlled substances) is restricted under the Controlled Substances Act of 1970. For schedule drugs, the physician's assigned federal DEA (Drug Enforcement Agency) number must be included for the prescription to be valid. Preprinted prescription forms provide a line on which to write this information. Prescriptions for drugs that are not controlled substances do not require the physician's DEA number. The DEA number consists of nine characters, the first two of which are A, B, or C for physicians and M for other practitioners.

Physician's order sheet    The physician does not need to provide his/her DEA number when writing a medication order for a controlled substance for a patient in the hospital or other healthcare facility. When the physician became a member of the medical staff of that hospital, his/her DEA certification was verified and is kept on file.

## *Clinical Applications*

Prescriptions for Schedule II drugs must be written on a special prescription form. This is known as an "official prescription form," and it is only printed by certain printing companies designated by that state. Official prescription forms contain security features (a control number, thermochromatic ink, and an imprinted seal) that are designed to prevent alterations and forgeries. This is a precaution to avoid the unauthorized use of drugs that have a high potential for drug abuse and addiction. In addition, these prescription forms may include background repetition of the word "void" that becomes visible if someone attempts to photocopy or fax these forms. Even with this precaution, thousands of prescriptions for Schedule II drugs are forged each year. A pharmacist may contact a physician's office to verify that a Schedule II prescription is indeed valid and not forged. Occasionally, unscrupulous physicians, dentists, and pharmacists prescribe or dispense Schedule II drugs to patients who have a drug habit in exchange for money. These individuals can be investigated by the state licensing board and the DEA and denied renewal of the federal DEA number needed to prescribe schedule drugs. Of interest is the fact that some states (e.g., New York in 2006) now require that an "official prescription form" be used to prescribe all prescription drugs, not just Schedule II drugs.

The use of generic rather than trade name drugs can result in considerable savings to consumers, but for certain critical drugs—such as digoxin (Lanoxin) for congestive heart failure, phenytoin (Dilantin) for seizures, and anticoagulant drugs—many physicians prefer to rely on the therapeutic effect of a trade name drug.

Prescriptions for generic drugs only accounted for 13 percent of all new prescriptions filled in 1995, but accounted for 45 percent of all new prescriptions filled in 2006.

## The Pharmacy and the Pharmacist

Once a prescription is submitted to the pharmacy, it becomes the property of the pharmacy, and the pharmacy is responsible for keeping it on file for several years (as specified by state law). After a prescription is received, the pharmacist verifies the drug and dose prescribed and then fills the prescription (see ▧ **FIGURE 6–4**). In a large facility, these tasks may be completed by a pharmacy technician and then checked for accuracy by a pharmacist. A label is placed on each prescription

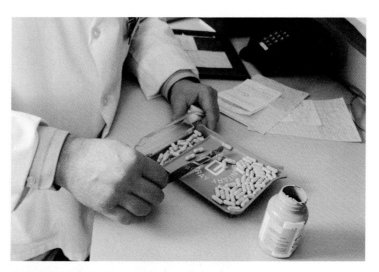

▧ **FIGURE 6–4  Filling a prescription.**
Tablets or capsules are removed from a larger stock bottle in the pharmacy and placed on a manual pill-counting tray. The number specified in the prescription is counted out, moved into the side section, and then poured into the plastic prescription bottle that is given to the patient.

bottle (see ▧ **FIGURE 6–5**). The pharmacist also assigns a prescription number (Rx #) that is printed on the label of the prescription bottle and is unique to that prescription. To obtain a refill, the patient must provide this unique prescription number to the pharmacy.

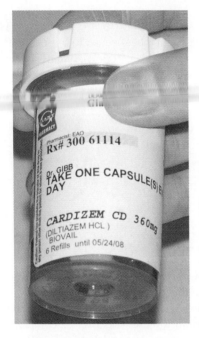

**■ FIGURE 6–5  Label on a prescription bottle.**
The label includes the name, address, and phone number of the
pharmacy, the patient's name, Rx #, and date. It includes the drug
name. This prescription is for Cardizem CD, a heart drug. Because
the physician requested a trade name drug, the generic name of the
drug (diltiazem HCl) is also written below in parentheses. The label
also includes the dose (360 mg), frequency, amount of drug
dispensed, and number of refills allowed (6), as well as the name of
the prescribing physician.

The childproof safety cap for prescription drug bottles was invented in 1984. It is the pharmacist, not the prescribing physician, who places a childproof cap on a prescription bottle
(see **■ FIGURE 6–6**).

As the number of prescriptions filled each year has increased, pharmacies have looked for ways
to more effectively serve their customers. Pharmacies that are part of a corporate chain are linked

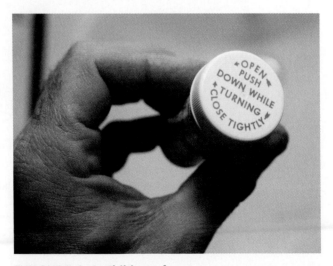

**■ FIGURE 6–6  Childproof cap.**
The pharmacist asks patients if they would like childproof caps on
their prescription bottles to keep children in their homes from
mistaking colored prescription drug capsules and tablets for candy.

through a common computer system. That means that patients can have their prescriptions refilled quickly at any one of the many pharmacies in that chain because the drug information is shared via computerized patient records. In addition, pharmacists offer personalized assistance to customers (see ■ **FIGURE 6–7** and ■ **FIGURE 6–8**).

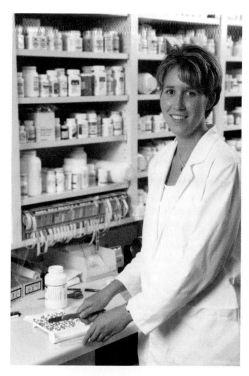

■ **FIGURE 6–7  The pharmacist.**
A pharmacist offers personalized services by answering questions and helping customers understand what drugs they are taking and when and how to take them.

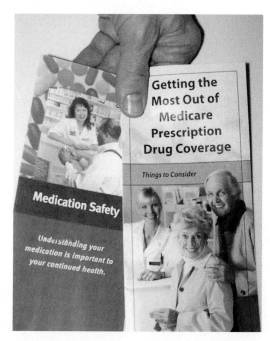

■ **FIGURE 6–8  Drug information.**
Pharmacists provide free pamphlets to customers to explain how to take drugs safely and, for senior customers, how to enroll and pay for drugs through the Medicare Part D Prescription Drug Program.

## *Clinical Applications*

The president of the National Association of Chain Drug Stores (which represents 94,000 pharmacists and 32,000 drug stores) reported that pharmacists "see firsthand the struggle of seniors having to choose between food and their drugs because they lack prescription drug coverage for what have become increasingly complex and effective, but expensive drugs." Many seniors rely on the kindness of their primary care physicians to supply them with enough drug samples to last until their next visit, they cut down on the frequency of doses, or they simply do without their drugs.

More recently, online pharmacies have provided a convenient service to patients who want to order their prescriptions over the Internet and have their drugs mailed to them. Legitimate Internet pharmacies have a seal on the home page of their Website that says "Verified Internet Pharmacy Provider Site." Patients mail in their actual prescriptions, and the Internet pharmacy calls the doctor to verify the validity of the prescription before filling it. However, some Internet pharmacies do not require a prescription form and do not check with the patient's physician. They advertise that they will provide "prescription drugs without a prescription." The patient fills out a medical question-naire online, and the company's doctor, without examining the patient, writes a prescription for the drug the patient wants. Internet pharmacies can be an easy source of drugs for an addict. Persons can forge a prescription for a prescription drug or even a schedule drug, fax it to several Internet pharmacies at the same time, and obtain multiple bottles of drugs. Another issue with Internet phar-macies is that some obtain their drugs from foreign countries where the quality and purity of the drugs can be compromised.

# *Chapter Review*

## Quiz Yourself

1. Define these abbreviations and symbols: *Rx*, *#*, *Sig.*, and *DEA*.
2. Name the 14 component parts of a prescription.
3. How does a prescription differ from a medication order?
4. Describe how verbal orders for drugs are handled by a nurse in the hospital.
5. What precautions should be taken to prevent the theft of prescription pads from the medical office?
6. What precaution is taken to prevent prescriptions for schedule drugs from being written by an unlicensed individual?
7. What precaution is taken to prevent additional medication orders from being illegally inserted at a later time after the physician signs the physician's order sheet?
8. How can a physician indicate on the prescription that the patient should receive a trade name drug and not a generic drug equivalent?

## Spelling Tips

**prescription**   not "perscription," although it is pronounced this way by some people.

## Clinical Applications

1. Demonstrate that you can identify the components of this sample prescription by answering the following questions.

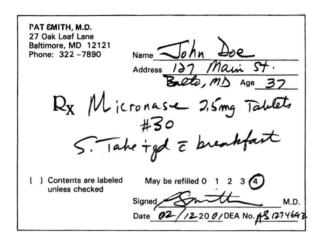

a. What is the name and address of the physician?

b. What is the name and address of the patient?

c. What is the name of the drug that was prescribed by the physician?

d. What disease is this drug prescribed to treat? (*Hint:* Look up this drug in Appendix D at the end of the textbook.)

e. What is the strength and unit of measurement of the dose?

f. What is the form in which this drug is manufactured?

g. How many did the physician prescribe to be given to the patient when this prescription is filled?

h. What does the abbreviation "S." mean?

i. How many is the patient to take and when? (*Hint:* Look up the two symbols and the abbreviation "q.d." in Appendix C at the end of the textbook to understand what the physician is saying.)

j. How many refills are allowed?

## Multimedia Extension Exercises

■ Go to www.pearsonhighered.com/turley and click on the photo of the cover of *Understanding Pharmacology for Health Professionals* to access the interactive Companion Website created for this textbook.

# Unit Two

## DRUGS BY BODY SYSTEMS

# CHAPTER

# 7

# Urinary Drugs

## CHAPTER CONTENTS

## Learning Objectives

After you study this chapter, you should be able to

1. Compare and contrast the sites of action and therapeutic effects of various diuretic drugs.

2. Explain why potassium supplements are given to patients taking diuretic drugs.

3. Describe the therapeutic effects of drugs used to treat urinary tract infections, urinary pain, urinary spasm, and overactive bladder.

4. Compare and contrast the therapeutic effects of drugs used to treat benign prostatic hypertrophy and erectile dysfunction.

5. Given the generic and trade names of a urinary drug, identify what drug category they belong to or what disease they are used to treat.

6. Given a urinary drug category, identify several generic and trade name drugs in that category.

Urinary drugs are used to treat diseases of the kidneys, bladder, urinary tract, and some parts of the male reproductive system. These diseases include urinary tract pain and spasms, urinary tract infections, prostatitis, overactive bladder, benign prostatic hypertrophy, and erectile dysfunction. Urinary drugs are also used to treat hypertension and edema in the body.

Urinary drugs include diuretic drugs, potassium supplements (taken concurrently with some diuretic drugs), drugs used to treat urinary tract infections, urinary analgesic drugs, urinary antispasmodic drugs, and drugs used to treat overactive bladder, benign prostatic hypertrophy, prostatitis, and erectile dysfunction.

# Diuretic Drugs

The kidneys continuously filter the circulating blood, extracting waste products of metabolism and nonwaste products such as water, sodium, potassium, other **electrolytes** (positively or negatively charged molecules), glucose, etc. The kidneys excrete all of the waste products and either excrete or reabsorb the nonwaste products, depending on the needs of the body. When blood levels of sodium or potassium are normal, anything in excess is excreted in the urine. As these electrolytes are excreted, they hold water to them with osmotic pressure, and this contributes to the amount of urine that is produced. When blood levels of sodium or potassium are low, these electrolytes are reabsorbed from the fluid in the kidney tubules back into the blood in a nearby capillary.

Diuretic drugs keep sodium and potassium from being reabsorbed from the tubules back into the blood (see ■ **FIGURE 7–1**). The extra sodium and potassium cause an increase in the volume of urine. By causing sodium, potassium, and water to be excreted, diuretic drugs are useful in the treatment of hypertension, the edema associated with congestive heart failure, renal failure, and cerebral edema.

Diuretic drugs are divided into several different categories based on the site of the drug's effect in the nephron of the kidney. Diuretic drugs include thiazide diuretic drugs, loop diuretic drugs, potassium-sparing diuretic drugs, osmotic diuretic drugs, and carbonic anhydrase inhibitor diuretic drugs.

## Thiazide Diuretic Drugs

Thiazide diuretic drugs act at the loop of Henle and the distal convoluted tubule in the nephron. There, they block sodium and potassium from being reabsorbed from the tubule back into the blood. More sodium and potassium than usual are excreted in the urine and therefore more water as well.

| | |
|---|---|
| bendroflumethiazide (Naturetin) | indapamide (Lozol) |
| chlorothiazide (Diuril) | methyclothiazide (Enduron) |
| chlorthalidone (Hygroton) | metolazone (Zaroxolyn) |
| hydrochlorothiazide (HCTZ, HydroDIURIL, Microzide) | |

*Note:* The suffix *-thiazide* is common to generic thiazide diuretic drugs.

## Loop Diuretic Drugs

Loop diuretic drugs act at the proximal convoluted tubule, the loop of Henle, and the distal convoluted tubule, but they derive their name from their action at the loop of Henle. These drugs block sodium and potassium from being reabsorbed from the tubule back into the blood. More sodium and potassium than usual are excreted in the urine and therefore more water as well.

| | |
|---|---|
| bumetanide (Bumex) | furosemide (Lasix) (see ■ **FIGURE 7–2**) |
| ethacrynic acid (Edecrin) | torsemide (Demadex) |

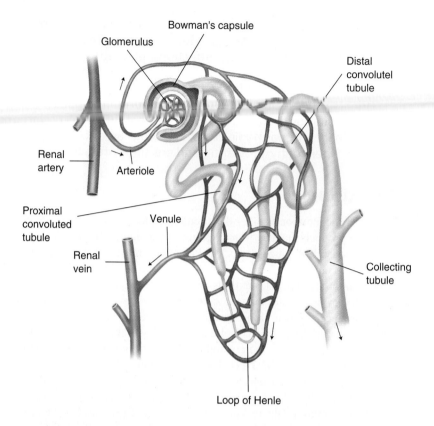

Bowman's capsule

Glomerulus

Distal convolutel tubule

Renal artery

Arteriole

Proximal convoluted tubule

Venule

Renal vein

Collecting tubule

Loop of Henle

Thiazide Diuretic Drugs

Act at the loop of Henle and the distal convoluted tubule.

Loop Diuretic Drugs

Act at the proximal convoluted tubule, the loop of Henle, and the distal convoluted tubule.

Potassium-Sparing Diuretic Drugs

Act at the proximal convoluted tubule and the loop of Henle.

Osmotic Diuretic Drugs

Act at Bowman's capsule, the proximal convoluted tubule, the loop of Henle, and the distal convoluted tubule.

Carbonic Anhydrase Inhibitor Diuretic Drugs

Act at the proximal convoluted tubule.

**▧ FIGURE 7–1  Diuretic drugs and the nephron of the kidney.**
Nephrons in the kidney are the site of urine production. Blood that contains waste products, electrolytes, other substances, and water enters the first part of the nephron, a spherical collecting structure known as *Bowman's capsule.* Inside it is a network of intertwining capillaries known as the *glomerulus.* In the glomerulus, the pressure of the blood pushes water and other substances from the blood out into Bowman's capsule, a process known as *filtration.* The resulting solution is known as *filtrate.* The filtrate then flows into the proximal convoluted tubule. There some of the water and nonwaste substances move out of the tubule and back into the blood, a process known as *reabsorption.* Reabsorption also occurs in the U-shaped loop of Henle and the distal convoluted tubule before the final product, urine, is excreted by the kidney. Diuretic drugs act at different areas of the nephron, as shown. Laypersons often refer to diuretic drugs as "water pills."

# Drug Alert!

The thiazide group of diuretic drugs causes adverse drug interactions with many different kinds of drugs. Thiazide diuretic drugs keep anticoagulant drugs from working effectively to prevent blood clots. They decrease the effect of some types of insulin used to treat diabetes mellitus. However, when taken in combination with other types of drugs, they have an opposite effect and actually prolong the effect of the other drug, causing severe side effects or toxicity. This is true when thiazide diuretic drugs are taken with chemotherapy drugs which are used to treat cancer, or with lithium which is used to treat the manic phase of bipolar disorder.

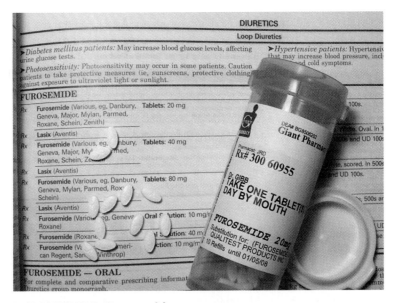

■ **FIGURE 7–2  Furosemide.**
This prescription bottle contains the generic drug furosemide, a loop diuretic drug. Each tablet contains a dose of 20 mg. If the trade name drug had been used to fill this prescription, the label would have read "Lasix 20 mg."

## Potassium-Sparing Diuretic Drugs

Potassium-sparing diuretic drugs act at the proximal convoluted tubule and the loop of Henle. They cause sodium and water to be excreted in the urine, but they spare (or conserve) potassium and allow it to be reabsorbed from the tubule back into the blood.

amiloride (Midamor)

spironolactone (Aldactone)

triamterene (Dyrenium)

## Osmotic Diuretic Drugs

Osmotic diuretic drugs are interesting because it is the presence of the drug itself (which always stays in an inactive form) that causes the diuretic effect. So many molecules of the inactive drug are present in the filtrate within Bowman's capsule that this causes an increase in the concentration (osmolarity) of the filtrate. As the filtrate moves through the tubules, its higher osmolarity continues to hold water and electrolytes to it and prevents water from being reabsorbed from the tubules back into the blood. This is because of the principle of osmosis, in which water will not flow from a region of greater concentration—in the tubules—to a region of lesser concentration—in the blood.

mannitol (Osmitrol)

### Carbonic Anhydrase Inhibitor Diuretic Drugs

Carbonic anhydrase is an enzyme that is normally present inside cells in the wall of the proximal convoluted tubule. Inside each tubule wall cell, carbonic anhydrase constantly reacts with carbon dioxide and water to produce bicarbonate and hydrogen. The negative bicarbonate ion then moves out of the tubule wall cell and into the blood in a nearby capillary. The positive hydrogen ion then moves out of the tubule wall cell and into the filtrate within the tubule, where it does a quick exchange with another positive ion—sodium. As the sodium ion moves into the tubule wall cell, it brings water from the filtrate with it (by osmotic pressure). This decreases the amount of filtrate within the tubule and is part of the normal process of concentrating the urine before it is excreted.

Carbonic anhydrase inhibitor diuretic drugs inhibit the enzyme carbonic anhydrase in the tubule wall cells. This means that bicarbonate and hydrogen ions are not formed. When no positive hydrogen ions are available to exchange places with positive sodium ions, the sodium ions stay in the filtrate and hold water to them, and this produces a greater volume of urine.

Carbonic anhydrase inhibitor diuretic drugs are used to treat the edema associated with congestive heart failure.

acetazolamide (Diamox)

### Combination Diuretic Drugs

These combination drugs contain a thiazide diuretic drug (hydrochlorothiazide) and a potassium-sparing diuretic drug (amiloride, spironolactone, triamterene)

Aldactazide (hydrochlorothiazide, spironolactone)

Dyazide (hydrochlorothiazide, triamterene)

Maxzide (hydrochlorothiazide, triamterene)

Moduretic (hydrochlorothiazide, amiloride)

## *Clinical Applications*

Both thiazide diuretic drugs and loop diuretic drugs cause sodium, potassium, and water to be excreted in the urine, but this extra loss of potassium can cause adverse effects in some patients, including cardiac arrhythmias. Patients who take a thiazide diuretic or loop diuretic drug also take a potassium-sparing diuretic drug to offset the loss of potassium from the other diuretic drug, or they can take an oral potassium supplement.

## Potassium Supplements

Potassium supplements are frequently prescribed for patients taking thiazide diuretic and loop diuretic drugs in order to avoid excessive loss of potassium. Potassium supplements are manufactured as liquids (patients often object to the taste), powders, effervescent tablets (to be dissolved in water), capsules, and tablets. Doses are measured in milliequivalents (mEq.) (see ■ FIGURE 7–3).

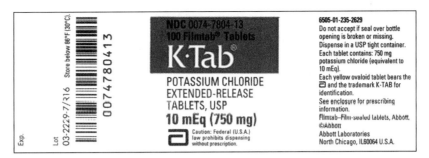

**■ FIGURE 7–3** **Potassium supplement.**
The *K* in the trade name K-Tab signifies that this is a potassium supplement because *K* is the chemical symbol for potassium. This drug is measured in milliequivalents (10 mEq.), but the equivalent metric measurement in milligrams (750 mg) is also given on the label. This drug is in the form of an extended-release tablet.

| | |
|---|---|
| Kay Ciel | Klotrix |
| K-Dur | K-Lyte |
| K-Lor | K-Tab |
| Klor-Con | Micro-K |
| Klorvess | |

*Note:* The presence of *K* in each trade name refers to $K^+$, the symbol for the chemical element *potassium.*

# Drug Alert!

Although foods such as bananas are rich in potassium, dietary sources alone are usually not sufficient to replenish the loss of potassium caused by taking a thiazide diuretic drug or a loop diuretic drug. If not given supplemental potassium, patients on these drugs can develop the adverse effect of hypokalemia, an extremely low level of potassium in the blood. This can lead to life-threatening cardiac arrhythmias because the electrolyte potassium is crucial to the normal contraction of the heart muscle.

## Drugs Used to Treat Urinary Tract Infections

Urinary tract infections (UTIs) are treated with drugs that are particularly effective against gram-negative bacteria (e.g., *Eschericia coli*) that are always present in the gastrointestinal tract and are a frequent cause of UTIs. Antibiotic drugs kill bacteria; anti-infective drugs inhibit their growth.

There are several categories of drugs that act systemically to treat UTIs: penicillin-type antibiotic drugs, cephalosporin antibiotic drugs, quinolone antibiotic drugs, fluoroquinolone antibiotic drugs, sulfonamide anti-infective drugs, folic acid antagonist drugs, and other antibiotic-type drugs.

### Penicillin-Type and Cephalosporin Antibiotic Drugs for UTIs

Penicillin-type antibiotic drugs, such as ampicillin, and the structurally related cephalosporin antibiotic drugs are used to treat UTIs as well as other types of infections in the body. These two categories of antibiotic drugs are discussed in more detail in Chapter 20.

### Quinolone Antibiotic Drugs for UTIs

Quinolone antibiotic drugs are only used to treat UTIs.

cinoxacin

nalidixic acid (NegGram)

*Note.* The trade name *NegGram* was selected by the drug company because the drug is effective against the gram-negative bacteria that cause urinary tract infections.

### Fluoroquinolone Antibiotic Drugs for UTIs

Fluoroquinolone antibiotic drugs are similar in chemical structure to the quinolones. Some drugs in this class are indicated for the treatment of UTIs and related types of infections, such as prostatitis and nongonoccocal urethritis.

ciprofloxacin (Cipro)          norfloxacin (Noroxin)

levofloxacin (Levaquin)     ofloxacin (Floxin)

lomefloxacin (Maxaquin)

*Note:* The suffix *-floxacin* is common to generic fluoroquinolone antibiotic drugs.

### Sulfonamide Anti-Infective Drugs for UTIs

These anti-infective drugs are not true antibiotic drugs because they only inhibit the growth of bacteria but do not kill them as antibiotic drugs do. Sulfonamide drugs inhibit one step in the formation of folic acid by certain bacteria. Bacteria that do not make folic acid are not susceptible to the effect of sulfonamide drugs. These drugs are used to treat UTIs as well as many other types of infections. Sulfonamide drugs are also known as *sulfa drugs*.

sulfadiazine

sulfisoxazole (Gantrisin Pediatric)

### Folic Acid Antagonist Drugs for UTIs

These anti-infective drugs block the formation of folic acid in bacterial cells. This interferes with the ability of some bacteria to grow and reproduce.

trimethoprim (Primsol, Proloprim)

### Other Antibiotic-Type Drugs for UTIs

These antibiotic-type drugs have a special affinity for the tissues of the urinary tract.

Acetohydroxamic acid inhibits an enzyme that is present in some bacteria that split urea in the urine and cause UTIs. Fosfomycin is metabolized to an acid that is excreted unchanged (and in a still-active form) in the urine, where it kills bacteria until it is excreted from the body. Once it is in the urine, methenamine is changed to ammonia and formaldehyde, chemicals that are lethal to bacteria and kill them. Nitrofurantoin is changed by the bacteria into a substance that alters bacterial RNA and therefore kills the bacteria.

acetohydroxamic acid (Lithostat)       methenamine (Hiprex, Urex)

fosfomycin (Monurol)                          nitrofurantoin (Macrobid, Macrodantin)

### Combination Antibiotic and Anti-Infective Drugs for UTIs

These combination drugs contain an antibiotic drug (trimethoprim) and an anti-infective sulfa drug (sulfamethoxazole). Trimethoprim blocks one step in the synthesis of folic acid by bacteria; sulfamethoxazole blocks the next step in the same process. Used in combination, these two drugs work synergistically. They are indicated for the treatment of UTIs and prostatitis, as well as other types of infections.

Bactrim (sulfamethoxazole, trimethoprim)

Septra (sulfamethoxazole, trimethoprim)

## *Did You Know?*

Cranberry juice is effective in preventing urinary tract infections. Cranberries are acidic, which is why eating the berries makes your mouth pucker! Cranberries temporarily increase the acidity of the urine; this suppresses the growth of bacteria because the bacteria prefer an alkaline environment. Also, cranberry juice contains the simple sugar fructose, which acts as an antiadhesion factor that keeps bacteria from adhering to the bladder wall. A cranberry dietary supplement for urinary tract health is available in softchew tablets or capsules.

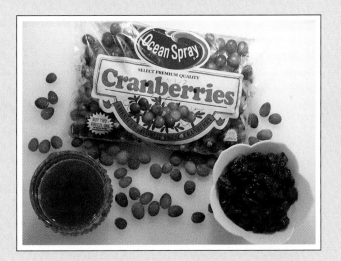

# Urinary Analgesic Drugs

Urinary tract infections, interstitial cystitis, other urinary tract diseases, and urinary tract surgery or endoscopic procedures produce symptoms of burning, urgency, and painful urination. Urinary analgesic drugs exert a local, pain-relieving effect on the mucous membranes of the urinary tract, even though these drugs are given orally.

dimethyl sulfoxide (DMSO, Rimso-50)

pentosan (Elmiron)

phenazopyridine (Pyridium, Urogesic)

## Urinary Antispasmodic Drugs

Irritation in the urinary tract from infection, catheterization, kidney stones, or urinary retention can result in ureteral spasms, renal colic, spasm of the bladder sphincter, and urinary retention or urinary incontinence. Antispasmodic drugs relax the smooth muscle in the walls of the ureters and bladder and promote normal bladder function.

| | |
|---|---|
| atropine (Sal-Tropine) | L-hyoscyamine (Anaspaz, Cystospaz) |
| bethanechol (Urecholine) | neostigmine (Prostigmin) |
| flavoxate (Urispas) | oxybutynin (Ditropan) |

## Combination Antibiotic, Analgesic, and Antispasmodic Drugs

These combination drugs contain a urinary antibiotic drug (methenamine), a urinary analgesic drug (phenazopyridine, phenyl salicylate), a urinary antispasmodic drug (atropine, hyoscyamine), a urinary antiseptic drug (methylene blue), and/or a sedative drug (butabarbital).

Dolsed (atropine, hyoscyamine, methenamine, methylene blue, phenyl salicylate)

Pyridium Plus (butabarbital, hyoscyamine, phenazopyridine)

Urised (atropine, hyoscyamine, methenamine, methylene blue, phenyl salicylate)

Urogesic Blue (hyoscyamine, methenamine, methylene blue, phenyl salicylate)

## *Drug Alert!*

Pyridium and Pyridium Plus turn the urine red-orange in color. Dolsed, Urised, and Urogesic Blue turn the urine a blue-green color because of the presence of methylene blue.

## Drugs Used to Treat Overactive Bladder

Overactive bladder is characterized by urinary urgency and frequency due to involuntary contractions of the bladder wall as the bladder fills with urine. There is also urinary incontinence at times. These drugs block the action of acetylcholine and reduce the smooth muscle tone of the bladder wall to decrease bladder contractions, bladder spasms, and incontinence (see ■ FIGURE 7–4).

| | |
|---|---|
| darifenacin (Enablex) | tolterodine (Detrol) |
| solifenacin (Vesicare) | trospium (Sanctura) |

## *Did You Know?*

The trade name Vesicare is an appropriate name for this drug because it implies caring for the bladder; the combining form *vesic/o-* means *bladder*.

## Drugs Used to Treat Benign Prostatic Hypertrophy

Benign prostatic hypertrophy (BPH) is common in men over age 50, with the incidence increasing with age. The prostate gland hypertrophies (enlarges) due to a chain reaction in which the male hormone

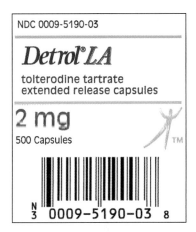

■ **FIGURE 7–4  Drug label for tolterodine (Detrol LA).**
The *LA* in the drug name stands for *long-acting*, because the drug is
manufactured as an extended-release capsule. Extensive magazine
and television advertising of this drug popularized the condition of
overactive bladder, and the catchy phrase "Gotta go, gotta go, gotta go
right now!" became well known. According to analysts, the number
of patients asking their physicians for Detrol increased by 45 percent
because of this direct-to-consumer advertising.

testosterone is acted on by an enzyme in prostatic cells and is converted to dihydrotestosterone. It is the
action of dihydrotestosterone that causes the prostate gland to enlarge or hypertrophy. This enlargement
is a benign, not cancerous, process. Symptoms of BPH include difficulty initiating urination, hesitancy,
and decreased urinary stream. Androgen inhibitor drugs and alpha$_1$-receptor blocker drugs are used to
treat BPH, and decrease the size of an enlarged prostate gland.

## Androgen Inhibitor Drugs for BPH

The word *androgen* refers to all of the various male hormones. Androgen inhibitor drugs inhibit the
male hormone dihydrotestosterone and reduce its effect on the prostate gland. The drug needs to be
taken for 6 to 12 months to see if it will be effective in decreasing the size of the prostate gland. If it
is effective, treatment must continue indefinitely. Finasteride has also been found to decrease the
incidence of cancer of the prostate gland (see ■ **FIGURE 7–5**).

dutasteride (Avodart)          finasteride (Proscar)

*Note:* The suffix *-asteride* is common to androgen inhibitor drugs.

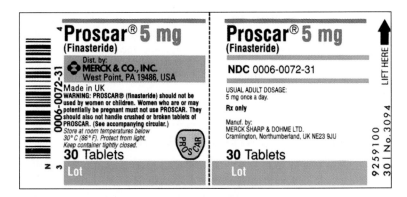

■ **FIGURE 7–5  Drug label for finasteride (Proscar).**
This drug was approved in 1992 as the first nonsurgical treatment for benign
prostatic hypertrophy (BPH). Finasteride, under the trade name Propecia, is
also given orally to treat male pattern baldness, but at a lower dose than that of
Proscar. The hormone dihydrotestosterone that causes BPH is also responsible
for causing male pattern baldness.

# Drug Alert!

Because dutasteride and finasteride are androgen inhibitor drugs, their drug inserts, packaging, and advertising warn women not to take these drugs or even handle them (see ■ **FIGURE 7–6**). This is because of the possibility that, if the woman is pregnant or might become pregnant with a male fetus, the drugs would block the normal male fetal development and cause birth defects.

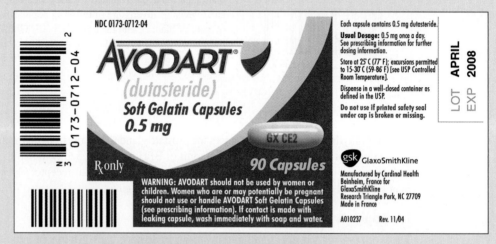

■ **FIGURE 7–6 Drug label for dutasteride (Avodart).**
This drug label is for the trade name drug Avodart (generic drug name dutasteride) that is used to treat BPH. This drug comes in the form of soft gelatin capsules in a dose of 0.5 mg. Notice the warning written at the bottom of the label.

### Alpha₁-Receptor Blocker Drugs for BPH

Alpha₁-receptor blocker drugs block alpha₁ receptors in the smooth muscle of the walls of the urethra and prostate gland. This causes the smooth muscle to relax and allows urine to flow more easily. Because there are only a few alpha₁ receptors in the neck of the bladder, these drugs do not relax the muscles in the bladder sphincter or cause incontinence.

alfuzosin (Uroxatral)          tamsulosin (Flomax)

doxazosin (Cardura)           terazosin (Hytrin)

## Drugs Used to Treat Prostatitis

Prostatitis is an acute or chronic bacterial infection of the prostate gland due to a urinary tract infection or a sexually transmitted disease. Prostatitis is treated with antibiotic and anti-infective drugs. Also see the previous section on combination drugs for UTIs that are also used to treat prostatitis.

ciprofloxin (Cipro)

levofloxacin (Levaquin)

norfloxacin (Noroxin)

## Did You Know?

The alpha$_1$-receptor blocker drugs doxazosin and terazosin, which are used to treat BPH, are also used to treat hypertension. Their drug effect relaxes the smooth muscle in the artery walls, causing them to dilate, and this lowers the blood pressure.

**Saw palmetto**, a small palm tree that is native to the coast of the southeastern United States, is effective in treating BPH. Its fruit was used by the Seminole Indians to treat genitourinary conditions. Today, it is available as an over-the-counter dietary supplement.

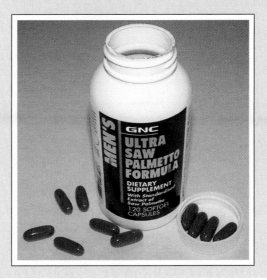

## Drugs Used to Treat Erectile Dysfunction

Erectile dysfunction (ED) is the inability of a man to achieve and maintain an erection during sexual intercourse. Through a series of steps, sexual stimulation in the male activates the chemical cGMP, which relaxes smooth muscle in the arteries of the penis, increases blood flow, and creates an erection. Afterwards, the enzyme PDE5 metabolizes cGMP, and the erection resolves. Phosphodiesterase type 5 (PDE5) inhibitor drugs and prostaglandin E$_1$ drugs are used to treat erectile dysfunction.

### PDE5 Inhibitor Drugs for ED

These drugs, which are given orally, inhibit the enzyme PDE5 that inactivates cGMP, and so an erection is sustained and sexual intercourse is possible (see ▥ **FIGURE 7–7**).

    sildenafil (Viagra)

    tadalafil (Cialis)

    vardenafil (Levitra)

### Prostaglandin E$_1$ Drugs for ED

These drugs act locally to relax the smooth muscle in the arteries of the penis, increase blood flow, and create an erection. After receiving training from a physician, the patient either injects the drug (Caverject, Edex) into the side of the penis or inserts a pellet (Muse) into the urethra.

    alprostadil (Caverject, Edex, Muse)

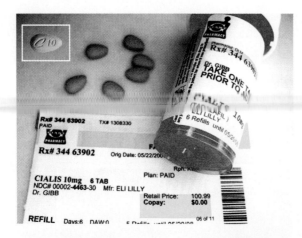

**■ FIGURE 7-7 Cialis**

Once a topic that men hesitated to discuss, even with their own physicians, erectile dysfunction (ED) and its treatment have become the subject of numerous newspaper articles and television and magazine advertisements. The mustard-colored, teardrop-shaped tablet of Cialis is unusual. Note that 6 tablets cost $100.99.

## Did You Know?

Viagra was the first drug for treating erectile dysfunction. It was approved in 1998 and, in the first 3 months it was on the market, physicians wrote 3 million prescriptions for it. Even former presidential candidate Bob Dole appeared in a television commercial, candidly discussing ED and urging viewers to ask their doctor about appropriate treatment. From 1998 to 2003, 20 million prescriptions were written for Viagra, for about 1 billion tablets! Following the success of Viagra, both Levitra and Cialis were introduced by other drug companies in 2003. The average age of a man using these drugs is 55. Because of the baby boomer generation, it is estimated that there will be 34 million men in this age range by 2010 and one in every 10 could have erectile dysfunction.

## Drug Alert!

Although the PDE5 inhibitor drugs for erectile dysfunction improve the quality and duration of an erection in men with erectile dysfunction, the drug inserts and advertisements warn that men experiencing an erection lasting longer than 4 hours should see their physician or go to the emergency room. This adverse effect might occur more often with Cialis because its duration of action is 36 hours, compared to 4 hours for Viagra and 5 hours for Levitra.

All of the PDE5 inhibitor drugs can also cause the side effect of a temporary loss of the ability to see blue/green colors!

## In Depth

Prostaglandin is a naturally occurring body substance that was first isolated from the prostate gland, from which it derives its name. Prostaglandins are present in many different tissues in the body and, when used as drugs, they have several different effects. Prostaglandin $E_1$ drugs cause vasodilation, which is useful in treating erectile dysfunction. Prostaglandin $E_1$ drugs are also used to keep open a patent ductus arteriosus to sustain life in a newborn with a congenital heart defect such as tetralogy of Fallot. Prostaglandin $E_2$ drugs stimulate smooth muscle in the wall of the uterus and are used to induce premature labor and terminate a pregnancy.

# Chapter Review

## Quiz Yourself

1. Describe the therapeutic effects of various diuretic drugs and how these drugs are useful for treating hypertension.
2. Why do so many potassium supplements contain the letter *K* in the trade name of the drug?
3. Why do patients on a diuretic drug often need to take a potassium supplement?
4. What is the most common cause of UTIs?
5. How does the action of sulfonamide drugs differ from that of antibiotic drugs in treating urinary tract infections?
6. What symptoms are urinary analgesic drugs prescribed to treat?
7. Give examples of two drugs that color the urine.
8. What disease is finasteride (Proscar) used to treat?
9. How do alpha$_1$-receptor blocker drugs work to treat BPH?
10. Compare the therapeutic effects of various drugs used to treat ED.
11. To what category of drugs does each of the following belong?
    a. dutasteride (Avodart)
    b. furosemide (Lasix)
    c. Kay Ciel
    d. metolazone (Zaroxolyn)
    e. phenazopyridine (Pyridium, Urogesic)
    f. sildenafil (Viagra)
    g. tamsulosin (Flomax)
    h. trospium (Sanctura)
    i. vardenafil (Levitra)

## Spelling Tips

| | |
|---|---|
| **Dyazide** | Spelled *Dy*, not *Di* as in *diuretic*. |
| **NegGram** | Unusual internal capitalization. |
| **HydroDIURIL** | Unusual use of all capital letters in the second part of the drug name. |
| **Kay Ciel** | When dictated by a physician, it is often not recognized as a trade name drug, but is mistaken for *KCl*, the abbreviation for the chemical name *potassium chloride*. |

## Clinical Applications

1. Look at this photograph and answer the following questions.
    a. What is the name of the drug on the left?
    b. Is this a generic or trade name?
    c. What is the name of the drug on the right?
    d. Is this a generic or trade name?
    e. To what category of drugs do both of these drugs belong?

**f.** How do the therapeutic effects of these drugs differ from each other?

**g.** If a patient was tested and was found to have a low blood potassium level, which of these drugs would be the most appropriate one for that patient to take? Why?

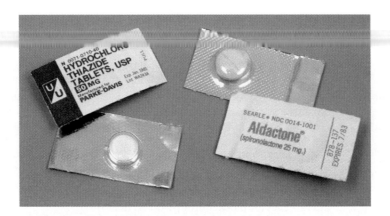

2. Look at this handwritten prescription and answer the following questions.

**a.** The prescribed drug is given as an abbreviation. What drug name does the abbreviation stand for?

**b.** What is the strength of the dose?

**c.** In what drug form is it given?

**d.** Translate the rest of the prescription into plain English.

**e.** What important piece of information is missing from this prescription?

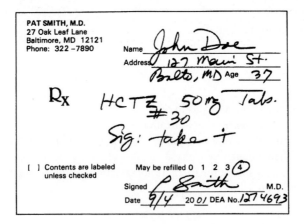

## Multimedia Extension Exercises

■ Go to www.pearsonhighered.com/turley and click on the photo of the cover of *Understanding Pharmacology for Health Professionals* to access the interactive Companion Website created for this textbook.

# Gastrointestinal Drugs

## CHAPTER CONTENTS

## Learning Objectives

After you study this chapter, you should be able to

1. Differentiate between the therapeutic effects of antacid drugs, $H_2$ blocker drugs, and proton pump inhibitor drugs in treating peptic ulcer disease.

2. Describe how anticholinergic drugs relieve gastrointestinal spasms from diseases such as irritable bowel syndrome.

3. Describe the effect of narcotic drugs that is useful in treating diarrhea.

4. Name five categories of laxative drugs and describe their differing therapeutic effects.

5. Describe the various ways in which antiemetic drugs treat nausea and vomiting caused by different conditions.

6. List four different categories of drugs that are used to treat hemorrhoids.

7. Describe the differing therapeutic effects of drugs used to treat obesity.

8. Given the generic and trade names of a gastrointestinal drug, identify what drug category they belong to or what disease they are used to treat.

9. Given a gastrointestinal drug category, identify several generic and trade name drugs in that category.

Gastrointestinal drugs are used to treat diseases of the esophagus, stomach, small intestine, large intestine, liver, and gallbladder (see ■ FIGURE 8–1). These diseases include peptic ulcer disease, *Helicobacter pylori* infection, gastroesophageal reflux disease, gastrointestinal spasms, diarrhea, hemorrhoids, constipation, ulcerative colitis, nausea and vomiting, hepatitis, gallstones, and obesity. Gastrointestinal drugs include antacid drugs, H₂ blocker drugs, proton pump inhibitor drugs, gastrointestinal stimulant drugs, antispasmodic drugs, antidiarrheal drugs, laxative drugs, gastric stimulant drugs, and antiemetic drugs.

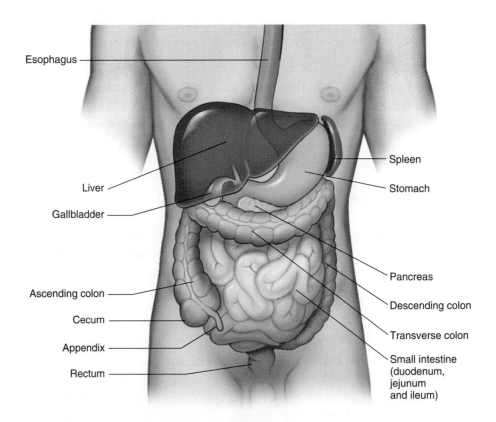

■ FIGURE 8–1  The gastrointestinal system.
The structures of the gastrointestinal system include the mouth and salivary glands (which are discussed in Chapter 19), the esophagus, stomach, small intestine (duodenum, jejunum, and ileum), large intestine (cecum, colon, and rectum), and the accessory organs of the liver and gallbladder, all of which are discussed in this chapter. Each of these structures can be affected by some gastrointestinal condition or disease that is treated with drugs.

## Drugs Used to Treat Peptic Ulcer Disease

A peptic ulcer is an ulcer located anywhere in the esophagus, stomach, or duodenum. Peptic ulcers in the stomach are specifically known as *gastric ulcers*. All peptic ulcers are caused by irritation of the mucous membranes that line the gastrointestinal tract. This irritation is caused by excessive amounts of hydrochloric acid, which strip away the protective mucus of the mucous membrane. Then the subsequent action of pepsin, a protein-digesting enzyme, begins to break down the underlying membrane.

Aspirin, nonsteroidal anti-inflammatory drugs (NSAIDs), alcohol, and caffeine also irritate the mucous membranes and can contribute to ulcer formation. Gastric ulcers can also be caused by a bacterial infection due to *Helicobacter pylori*. Treatment for peptic ulcer disease includes antacid drugs, $H_2$ blocker drugs, and proton pump inhibitor drugs. Drugs used to treat *H. pylori* infections are discussed in the next section.

### Antacid Drugs for Heartburn

Antacid drugs were the original, and for many years the only, treatment for peptic ulcers. They are weak bases that exert a therapeutic effect by neutralizing hydrochloric acid. This raises the pH of the stomach contents, which decreases mucous membrane irritation. This also inhibits the action of pepsin so that it does not break down exposed mucous membranes. Antacid drugs are only used now to prevent and treat heartburn and acid indigestion. They contain aluminum, magnesium, calcium, sodium, or a combination of these, as the active ingredients. Antacid drugs are available without a prescription.

These antacid drugs contain aluminum as their active ingredient.

AlternaGEL

Alu-Tab

Amphojel

These antacid drugs contain magnesium as their active ingredient.

Dulcolax

milk of magnesia (MOM, Phillips' Milk of Magnesia)

## Drug Alert!

A trade name drug is associated with just one generic name drug. An unusual exception to this is the trade name Dulcolax, which is associated with two different generic drugs. Dulcolax as a liquid contains the generic drug magnesium and is used as an antacid drug. Dulcolax as an enteric-coated tablet or suppository contains the generic drug bisacodyl and is an irritant/stimulant laxative drug.

These antacid drugs contain calcium as their active ingredient.

| | |
|---|---|
| Alka-Mints | Maalox Antacid Barrier |
| Chooz | Tums Ultra |

## Focus on Healthcare Issues

The use of calcium-containing antacid drugs can provide an additional benefit to women by supplementing calcium intake—so say the drug companies. One advertisement showed a woman taking an antacid drug for heartburn and saying, "And it's something my body needs anyway." In reality, the use of calcium-containing antacid drugs should not take the place of adequate calcium intake in the diet.

### Combination Antacid Drugs

These combination drugs contain several antacid drugs (aluminum, calcium, magnesium, or sodium bicarbonate). Some of these combination drugs also contain simethicone to relieve flatulence and gas; simethicone acts by changing the surface tension of air bubbles trapped in the GI tract and allowing them to be expelled. Some of these combination drugs also contain aspirin or acetaminophen for pain relief.

Alka-Seltzer (aspirin, sodium bicarbonate)

Bromo Seltzer (acetaminophen, sodium bicarbonate)

Di-Gel (aluminum, magnesium, simethicone)

Gaviscon (aluminum, magnesium, sodium bicarbonate)

Gelusil (aluminum, magnesium, simethicone)

Maalox (aluminum, magnesium, simethicone)

Mylanta (aluminum, magnesium, simethicone)

Riopan (aluminum, magnesium)

Rolaids (calcium, magnesium)

Titralac Plus (calcium, simethicone)

## Drug Alert!

Baking soda (sodium bicarbonate) dissolved in water is an old home remedy for indigestion and heartburn. Although sodium bicarbonate neutralizes acid, it is not recommended as a long-term treatment for heartburn because the large amounts of sodium it contains are absorbed systemically. Physicians recommend the moderate use of salt (sodium), even for patients without hypertension and other medical conditions. However, even over-the-counter antacid drugs contain large amounts of sodium. One dose of the antacid drug Regular Alka-Seltzer contains 1,700 mg of sodium, and one dose of Bromo Seltzer contains over 2,700 mg. For patients on a low-salt diet, this exceeds their recommended allowance of sodium for the entire day.

Simethicone is available as a drug to treat gas. It is often combined with antacid drugs, but it has no antacid action of its own.

Gas-X

Mylanta Gas

Mylicon

Phazyme

Charcoal also decreases gas and can be used to treat diarrhea as well. It is available either alone or in combination with simethicone.

CharcoCaps

Flatulex

## H₂ Blocker Drugs for Heartburn and/or Peptic Ulcer Disease

Histamine, a natural chemical produced by the body, activates special histamine receptors ($H_2$ receptors) located on the parietal cells of the stomach. This causes the release of hydrochloric acid. Drugs that block these receptors and prevent the release of acid are known as *$H_2$ blocker drugs* and are used to treat heartburn, peptic ulcers, gastroesophageal reflux disease (GERD), and are part of the treatment for *Helicobacter pylori* infections. $H_2$ blocker drugs are prescription drugs, but some are also available over the counter. Over-the-counter $H_2$ blocker drugs are only for heartburn.

cimetidine (Tagamet)

famotidine (Pepcid)

nizatidine (Axid)

ranitidine (Zantac)

*Note:* The suffix *-tidine* is common to generic $H_2$ blocker drugs.

# Drug Alert!

All $H_2$ blocker drugs originally were approved as prescription drugs. Then famotidine became the first to be approved by the FDA for over-the-counter use. Now each of the prescription $H_2$ blocker drugs has a corresponding over-the-counter version. Over-the-counter $H_2$ blocker drugs are only approved for preventing and treating heartburn and acid indigestion.

| Prescription Trade Name and Doses | Over-the-counter (OTC) Trade Name and Doses |
|---|---|
| Tagamet 300 mg, 400 mg, 800 mg | Tagamet HB 200 mg (see ■ **FIGURE 8–2**) |
| Pepcid 20 mg, 40 mg | Pepcid AC 10 mg, 20 mg (see ■ **FIGURE 8–3**) |
| Axid 150 mg, 300 mg | Axid AR 75 mg |
| Zantac 150 mg, 300 mg | Zantac 75 mg, 150 mg |

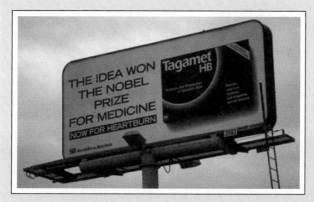

■ **FIGURE 8-2 Billboard advertisement for over-the-counter cimetidine (Tagamet HB).** The first drug in the $H_2$ blocker category was cimetidine (Tagamet), a prescription drug. The discovery of $H_2$ blocker drugs was awarded the Nobel Prize in Medicine in 1988. The over-the-counter strength of cimetidine, under the trade name Tagamet HB, was approved by the FDA to treat heartburn in 1999.

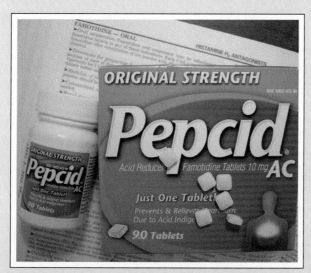

■ **FIGURE 8–3 Famotidine (Pepcid AC).** This box and tablet container are for the over-the-counter drug Pepcid AC, which comes in a dose strength of 10 mg tablets. Notice the background page from a drug reference, which categorizes famotidine under the header "Histamine $H_2$ Antagonists." An antagonist is another name for a drug that blocks a receptor. Famotidine is an $H_2$ blocker drug.

*(continued)*

## Drug Alert! *(continued)*

*Note:* The *HB* in Tagamet HB stands for *histamine blocker.* The *AC* in Pepcid AC stands for the Latin phrase *ante cibum,* which means *before meals,* as Pepcid AC is taken before meals. The *AR* in Axid AR stands for *acid reducer.*

### Combination H$_2$ Blocker Drugs for Peptic Ulcer Disease

This combination drug contains an H$_2$ blocker drug (famotidine) and two antacid drugs (calcium, magnesium).

Pepcid Complete (calcium, famotidine, magnesium)

### *Focus on Healthcare Issues*

An over-the-counter (OTC) drug is defined as one that can be purchased without a prescription and is generally considered safe for consumers to use if the label's directions and warnings are followed carefully. The FDA approves a prescription drug being reclassified as an OTC drug if the following criteria are met: (1) The indication for the drug's OTC use is similar to its use as a prescription drug, (2) the patient can easily monitor his or her own condition when using the OTC drug, (3) the OTC drug has a low rate of side effects/toxicity and a low potential for abuse, and (4) use of the OTC drug does not require the patient to have any special monitoring or ongoing tests. Over-the-counter H$_2$ blocker drugs meet all of these requirements.

### *Historical Notes*

For many years, it was known that histamine was released during an allergic reaction and that this caused red, itchy eyes, sneezing, and a runny nose. It was also known that histamine was released in the stomach, where it stimulated the production of hydrochloric acid, and that this was not related to any allergic reaction. Therefore, researchers realized that histamine must act on two different receptors in the body, and they named these *H$_1$ receptors* and *H$_2$ receptors.*

Because the therapeutic effect of antihistamine drugs (which block H$_1$ receptors) had been known since diphenhydramine (Benadryl) was introduced in 1945, researchers at the Smith, Kline & French drug company began to search for a drug that could block the action of histamine on H$_2$ receptors in the stomach. Such a drug would prevent the release of acid and would be useful in treating peptic ulcers. By rearranging the chemical structure of a molecule of histamine, they developed a drug that combined with H$_2$ receptors but would not activate them, thus effectively blocking the receptor and the release of acid. A drug that blocks a receptor is known as an *antagonist.* In 1977, the first H$_2$ blocker drug was created and given the generic name cimetidine. Syllables from the words *ant**ag**onist* and *c**imet**idine* were combined to make the drug's trade name Tagamet.

### Proton Pump Inhibitor Drugs for Peptic Ulcer Disease

Proton pump inhibitor drugs decrease gastric acid by blocking the final step of acid production within the gastric parietal cell. This final step involves an enzyme system known as the *proton pump,* hence the name of this drug category. Proton pump inhibitor drugs are used to treat heartburn and peptic ulcers.

> esomeprazole (Nexium) (see ▉ **FIGURE 8–4**)
>
> lansoprazole (Prevacid)
>
> omeprazole (Prilosec) (see ▉ **FIGURE 8–5**)

*Note:* For a complete list of proton pump inhibitor drugs, see the section "Drugs Used to Treat Gastroesophageal Reflux Disease" later in this chapter.

## *Did You Know?*

Horses get gastric ulcers too! Omeprazole is available in a cinnamon-flavored oral paste just for horses under the trade name GastroGard.

### Other Drugs for Peptic Ulcer Disease

Patients on long-term therapy with aspirin or nonsteroidal anti-inflammatory drugs (NSAIDs) can develop gastric ulcers. This is a common side effect because aspirin and NSAIDs inhibit the formation of prostaglandins. Prostaglandins normally protect the gastric mucosa. When aspirin and NSAIDs suppress the action of prostaglandins, they remove its protective action on the gastric mucosa. This drug is a synthetic prostaglandin drug that is given to protect the gastric mucosa when natural prostaglandins are inhibited by aspirin or NSAIDs.

> misoprostol (Cytotec)

This drug acts topically on the actual surface of the ulcer because it is attracted to areas of mucous membrane that are damaged or draining fluid that is high in protein. This drug binds directly to these areas, forming a protective layer or "bandage" over the ulcer, allowing it to heal.

> sucralfate (Carafate)

## Drugs Used to Treat *H. Pylori* Infection

*Helicobacter pylori* are helical (spiral) bacteria that have flagella (thin, whip-like tails). They live in the gastric or duodenal mucosa and are the cause of some peptic ulcers. Successful treatment of an *H. pylori* infection involves the use of a combination of antibiotic drugs, antiprotozoal drugs, bismuth, and either an $H_2$ blocker drug or a proton pump inhibitor drug. Antibiotic drugs, antiprotozoal drugs, and bismuth disrupt the cell wall that surrounds this bacterium, causing cell death.

### $H_2$ Blocker Drugs and Proton Pump Inhibitor Drugs for *H. Pylori* Infections

Only the $H_2$ blocker drug ranitidine and the proton pump inhibitor drugs esomeprazole (Nexium), lansoprazole (Prevacid), and omeprazole (Prilosec) are indicated for the treatment of *H. pylori* infections.

### Combination Drugs for *H. Pylori* Infection

These combination drugs contain an antibiotic drug (amoxicillin, clarithromycin, tetracycline), an anti-infective drug (bismuth), a proton pump inhibitor drug (lansoprazole), or an antiprotozoal drug (metronidazole).

> Helidac (bismuth, metronidazole, tetracycline)
>
> Prevpac (amoxicillin, clarithromycin, lansoprazole)

## Drug Alert!

Some drugs are used to treat a wide range of different types of diseases. It is important to mentally allow yourself to associate a drug with more than just a single therapeutic use. For example, the antiprotozoal drug metronidazole is used to treat many different diseases besides *H. pylori* infection of the stomach. Metronidazole (Flagyl) is taken orally to treat intestinal amebiasis and pelvic inflammatory disease. Metronidazole (MetroGel-Vaginal) is applied vaginally as a gel to treat vaginal bacteriosis. Metronidazole (MetroGel) is applied topically to the skin as a gel to treat acne rosacea.

## Drugs Used to Treat Gastroesophageal Reflux Disease

Gastroesophageal reflux disease (GERD) occurs when stomach acid refluxes or flows back into the esophagus, causing esophagitis with irritation, inflammation, and pain. GERD is treated with proton pump inhibitor drugs and gastrointestinal stimulant drugs.

### Proton Pump Inhibitor Drugs for GERD

Proton pump inhibitor drugs decrease the production of hydrochloric acid in the stomach and raise the pH of the stomach contents. Some of these proton pump inhibitor drugs are used to treat heartburn and peptic ulcer, as discussed in a previous section. All proton pump inhibitor drugs are used to treat esophagitis and GERD. The suffix *-prazole* is common to generic proton pump inhibitor drugs.

esomeprazole (Nexium) (see ■ FIGURE 8–4)       pantoprazole (Protonix)

lansoprazole (Prevacid)                                    rabeprazole (AcipHex)

omeprazole (Prilosec) (see ■ FIGURE 8–5)

*Note:* The trade name drug AcipHex refers to the drug's action on the pH of the stomach.

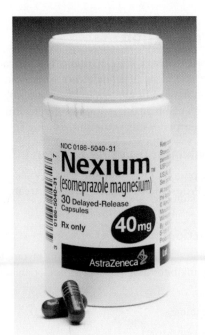

■ FIGURE 8–4 **Esomeprazole (Nexium).**
The prescription proton pump inhibitor drug Nexium is used to treat gastroesophageal reflux disease, esophagitis, and peptic ulcer disease. This drug is known by patients as "the purple pill." It is available in the drug forms of a delayed release capsule and a powder that is reconstituted to be a liquid that is given intravenously.

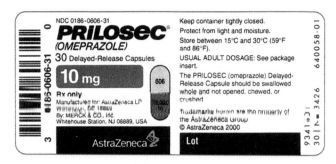

**■ FIGURE 8–5  Drug label for omeprazole (Prilosec).**
This drug label is for the prescription proton pump inhibitor drug
Prilosec, as indicated by the inscription *Rx only* on the drug label.
Interestingly, prescription Prilosec comes in a 10 mg, 20 mg, or
40 mg capsule, while over-the-counter Prilosec OTC—which can
be obtained without a prescription—comes in a 20 mg tablet.

### Combination Proton Pump Inhibitor Drugs for GERD

This combination drug contains a proton pump inhibitor drug (omeprazole) and an antacid drug
(sodium bicarbonate).

Zegerid, (omeprazole, sodium bicarbonate)

### *Did You Know?*

Following FDA approval of esomeprazole (Nexium), the drug company launched an extensive
advertising campaign on TV and in magazines. Patients were encouraged to ask their doctor
about "the purple pill." This drug even has its own Website: www.purplepill.com.

### Gastrointestinal Stimulant Drugs for GERD

This GI stimulant drug increases the rate of gastric emptying in order to keep excess hydrochloric
acid from accumulating in the stomach and refluxing into the esophagus.

metoclopramide (Maxolon, Reglan)

## Drugs Used to Treat Gastrointestinal Spasms

Intestinal conditions, such as irritable bowel syndrome, spastic colon, diverticulitis, and even peptic
ulcers, can be accompanied by abdominal pain due to spasms of the smooth muscle of the GI tract.
These spasms can be relieved by antispasmodic drugs, which are also known as *anticholinergic
drugs*. The neurotransmitter acetylcholine acts on cholinergic receptors to stimulate the release of
hydrochloric acid, to stimulate muscular contractions, and to begin peristalsis to move food through
the GI tract. Anticholinergic drugs can be given to block the effects of acetylcholine to decrease the
amount of acid and stop the spasms.

atropine (Sal-Tropine)

dicyclomine (Bentyl, Di-Spaz)

glycopyrrolate (Robinul)

L-hyoscyamine (Levbid, Levsin)

mepenzolate (Cantil)

methscopolamine (Pamine)

propantheline (Pro-Banthine)

### Combination Antispasmodic Drugs

These combination drugs contain an anticholinergic drug to decrease spasm (atropine, belladonna, clidinium, hyoscyamine, scopolamine), a central nervous system barbiturate sedative drug (butabarbital, phenobarbital), and/or an antianxiety drug (chlordiazepoxide).

Butibel (belladonna, butabarbital)

Donnatal (atropine, hyoscyamine, scopolamine, phenobarbital)

Librax (clidinium, chlordiazepoxide)

## Drugs Used to Treat Diarrhea

Antidiarrheal drugs produce a therapeutic effect by slowing peristalsis in the intestinal tract (anticholinergic drugs) or by absorbing extra water from diarrhea stools (absorbent drugs). Some antidiarrheal drugs exert their effect because they contain opium, a narcotic drug. When diarrhea is caused by an infection in the GI tract, an antibiotic or anti-infective drug is given.

### Anticholinergic Drugs for Diarrhea

This over-the-counter anticholinergic drug decreases the rate of peristalsis in the GI tract.

loperamide (Imodium A-D, K-Pek II) (see ■ FIGURE 8–6)

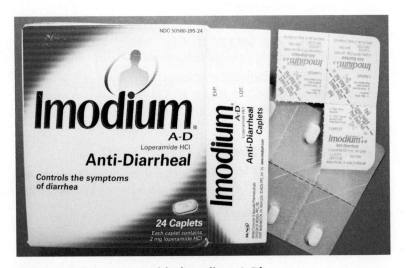

■ **FIGURE 8–6  Loperamide (Imodium A-D).**
This over-the-counter drug is used to treat diarrhea. It comes in the form of caplets, each of which is encased in an individual blister pak. The *A-D* in the trade name stands for *antidiarrheal*.

### Absorbent Drugs for Diarrhea

These over-the-counter drugs contain attapulgite, an absorbent drug to absorb excess water from diarrhea stools.

Kaopectate Maximum Strength

K-Pek

## Narcotic Drugs for Diarrhea

Antidiarrheal drugs that contain opium, a narcotic drug, are categorized as controlled substances (Schedule III drugs). As a category of drugs, narcotic drugs are most commonly used for their pain-relieving properties. However, a common side effect of these drugs is constipation, so this side effect then becomes the therapeutic effect in treating diarrahea.

opium (paregoric)

## Antibiotic and Anti-Infective Drugs for Diarrhea

These drugs are used to treat infection associated with bacterial, viral, or protozoal diarrhea, and traveler's diarrhea.

bismuth (Kaopectate, Pepto-Bismol)
  (see ■ FIGURE 8–7)
ciprofloxacin (Cipro)

doxycycline (Vibramycin, Vibra-Tabs)
trimethoprim/sulfamethoxazole (Bactrim, Septra)

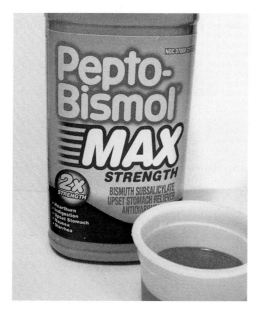

■ FIGURE 8–7  **Pepto-Bismol.**
This over-the-counter drug contains bismuth, an anti-infective drug that is active against bacteria and viruses that cause diarrhea. Bismuth is also included in combination drugs that are used to treat peptic ulcer disease caused by the bacterium *Helicobacter pylori.* In the drug name, *Pepto-* refers to the anatomic adjective *peptic,* while *Bismol* refers to the drug *bismuth.*

## Combination Drugs for Diarrhea

These combination drugs contain an anticholinergic drug to reduce the rate of peristalsis (atropine), an absorbent drug to absorb excess water from diarrhea stools (attapulgite, kaolin, pectin), an anti-infective drug (bismuth), and/or a Schedule IV or Schedule V narcotic drug to slow peristalsis (difenoxin, diphenoxylate).

Kaodene Non-Narcotic (bismuth, kaolin, pectin)
Kapectolin (kaolin, pectin)

Lomotil (atropine, diphenoxylate)
Motofen (atropine, difenoxin)

## Did You Know?

Attapulgite is an aluminum-magnesium compound found in clay soil. The soil in southwestern Georgia is particularly rich in attapulgite, as reflected in the name of the nearby town of Attapulgus, Georgia. Kaolin is a soft, white clay that is also mined in Georgia and is used to make fine china and porcelain. Pectin is a natural fiber derived from the cell walls of plants. It is added to foods to increase the amount of dietary fiber, and it is used as a plant-based jelling agent for making jam and jelly.

### Drugs for Treating Diarrhea and Wasting Disease in AIDS

These drugs are discussed in Chapter 20.

## Laxative Drugs

Laxative drugs are used for short-term treatment of constipation, with attention also being given to adequate water intake, dietary fiber/bulk, and other measures to promote bowel regularity. There are several categories of laxative drugs. These include osmotic laxative drugs, bulk-producing laxative drugs, stool softener laxative drugs, chloride channel laxative drugs, irritant/stimulant laxative drugs, and others.

### Osmotic Laxative Drugs

Osmotic laxative drugs use osmosis and osmotic pressure to attract water from the blood into the intestine to soften the stool. These are over-the-counter drugs, except for lactulose, which is only available by prescription.

Epsom salt

glycerin (Colace Suppository, Fleet Babylax)

lactulose (Cephulac)

milk of magnesia (MOM, Phillips' Milk of Magnesia)

### Bulk-Producing Laxative Drugs

Bulk-producing laxative drugs contain indigestible dietary fiber and other substances that absorb and hold water in the intestines to soften the stool. This action is the most natural and safest of all the laxative drugs.

methylcellulose (Citrucel)

polycarbophil (FiberCon)

psyllium (Fiberall, Metamucil, Perdiem)

### Stool Softener Laxative Drugs

Stool softener drugs are emulsifiers that allow fat in the stool to mix with water to soften the stool.

docusate (Colace, ex-lax Stool Softener, Surfak)

### Chloride Channel Laxative Drugs

Chloride channel laxative drugs stimulate chloride channels in the mucosa of the intestinal wall. This causes fluid to flow into the intestine to soften the stool.

lubiprostone (Amitiza)

### Irritant/Stimulant Laxative Drugs

Irritant/stimulant laxative drugs act directly on the intestinal mucosa to stimulate peristalsis.

bisacodyl (Correctol, Dulcolax, Feen-a-mint)

cascara

sennosides (Maximum Relief ex-lax, Fletcher's Castoria, Senokot)

### Other Laxative Drugs

Carbon dioxide gas in the form of a foam softens the stool. Oils soften the stool and increase its bulk. Misoprostol decreases the time that it takes for the stool to travel through the intestines; it is only available by prescription.

| | |
|---|---|
| carbon dioxide-releasing suppository (Ceo-Two) | mineral oil |
| castor oil (Emulsoil) | misoprostol (Cytotec) |

These laxative drugs are narcotic antagonist drugs. They are given to patients who are taking narcotic drugs for pain relief because they block the common side effect of constipation caused by narcotic drugs.

alvimopan (Entereg)

methylnaltrexone (Relistor)

### Combination Laxative Drugs

These combination drugs contain an osmotic laxative (magnesium), a bulk-producing laxative (psyllium), a stool softener (docusate), an irritant/stimulant laxative (senna/sennosides), and/or an oil laxative (mineral oil).

| | |
|---|---|
| Haley's M-O (magnesium, mineral oil) | Peri-Colace (docusate, senna) |
| Perdiem Overnight Relief (psyllium, senna) | Senokot-S (docusate, senna) |

### Bowel Evacuants/Enemas

These laxative drugs are given orally to evacuate the colon prior to surgery or endoscopic procedures. Most come as kits that also include a suppository or enema. The use of a bowel evacuant along with an enema is referred to as a *bowel prep*. All of these are prescription drugs.

| | |
|---|---|
| CoLyte | GoLYTELY |
| Fleet Prep Kit | polyethylene glycol (PEG, MiraLax) |

These drugs are given as enemas to evacuate the lower colon prior to an endoscopic or surgical procedure or to provide relief from constipation.

Fleet, Fleet Bisacodyl, Fleet Mineral Oil

Therevac-Plus

## Drugs Used to Treat Ulcerative Colitis or Crohn's Disease

Ulcerative colitis is a chronic disease of the colon and rectum that is characterized by diarrhea, abdominal pain, inflammation, and ulcers. The cause is unknown. Crohn's disease is a chronic disease of the ileum and colon with areas of inflammation followed by normal mucosa ("skip areas"). Symptoms are similar to those of ulcerative colitis and the cause is unknown. Besides the antispasmodic drugs described previously, ulcerative colitis and Crohn's disease are also treated with drugs to decrease inflammation.

Irritable bowel syndrome is a chronic disease of the colon that is characterized by severe spasms, cramping, abdominal pain, bloating, excessive mucus secretion, and diarrhea alternating with constipation. Irritable bowel syndrome is treated with drugs used to treat GI spasms as described previously, as well as with antianxiety drugs, antidiarrheal drugs, and laxative drugs.

## Aminosalicylic Acid Drugs for Ulcerative Colitis

Aminosalicylic acid (ASA) decreases intestinal inflammation by blocking the production of prostaglandins. These drugs contain 4-ASA or 5-ASA as the active ingredient or contain an ingredient that is metabolized to 5-ASA by bacteria in the colon. These drugs may be taken orally or administered rectally as a suppository or as a solution.

aminosalicylic acid (4-ASA, Pamisyl, Rezipas)

balsalazide (Colazal)

mesalamine (5-ASA, Asacol, Pentasa, Rowasa)

olsalazine (Dipentum)

sulfasalazine (Azulfidine)

### Did You Know?

Both olsalazine and sulfasalazine are converted in the colon to mesalamine. In the trade name drug Asacol, the *Asa-* refers to the drug *5-ASA,* and *-col* refers to *colon,* the site of the drug's action.

## Topical Corticosteroid Drugs for Ulcerative Colitis

This drug is a corticosteroid drug that exerts a more powerful anti-inflammatory effect than aminosalicylic acid. It is administered as an aerosol foam that is placed into the rectum.

hydrocortisone (Cortifoam)

## Other Drugs for Ulcerative Colitis and Crohn's Disease

Clonidine (Catapres) is an alpha-receptor blocker drug that is used to treat ulcerative colitis. Methotrexate is a chemotherapy drug that is used to treat severe ulcerative colitis and Crohn's disease.

clonidine (Catapres)

methotrexate (Rheumatrex Dose Pack)

thalidomide (Synovir, Thalomid)

These drugs are only used to treat Crohn's disease. Adalimumab, infliximab, and natalizumab are monoclonal antibody drugs. Budesonide is an oral corticosteroid drug. Etanercept is an immunomodulator drug. Certolizumab is an anti-tumor necrosis drug. Metronidazole is an antibiotic and antiprotozoal drug.

adalimumab (Humira)

budesonide (Entocort EC)

certolizumab (Cimzia)

etanercept (Enbrel)

infliximab (Remicade)

metronidazole (Flagyl)

natalizumab (Tysabri)

## Drugs for Irritable Bowel Syndrome

These antianxiety drugs are used to treat emotional stress, which can exacerbate the symptoms of irritable bowel syndrome. These are Schedule IV drugs with a limited potential for addiction.

alprazolam (Xanax)

chlordiazepoxide (Librium)

clorazepate (Tranxene)

diazepam (Valium)

lorazepam (Ativan)

oxazepam (Serax)

This serotonin receptor blocker drug is used to treat irritable bowel syndrome.

alosetron (Lotronex)

## Gastric Stimulant Drugs

Gastric stimulant drugs enhance the natural action of acetylcholine, a neurotransmitter that maintains normal peristalsis in the GI tract. Gastric stimulant drugs are used to treat gastroparesis (delayed gastric emptying in diabetic patients), to facilitate emptying of the intestines prior to x-rays, to facilitate excretion of barium after an x-ray, or to prevent distention and paralytic ileus from developing after major abdominal surgery.

dexpanthenol (Ilopan)

metoclopramide (Maxolon, Reglan)

## Antiemetic Drugs

Antiemetic drugs are used to control nausea and vomiting associated with many different diseases. Bacterial or viral illnesses can directly irritate the intestinal mucosa and cause nausea and vomiting. Chemotherapy drugs, radiation, and some other drugs irritate the intestinal mucosa and stimulate the chemoreceptor trigger zone and vomiting center in the brain. Surgery, particularly abdominal surgery, can temporarily stop peristalsis; then, as fluids accumulate in the GI tract, they cause distension and trigger postoperative nausea and vomiting. Patients who are actively vomiting and cannot take oral drugs can be given antiemetic drugs in the form of rectal suppositories.

Some antiemetic drugs used to treat nausea and vomiting block dopamine from activating receptors in the wall of the GI tract and in the chemoreceptor trigger zone and vomiting center in the brain.

| | |
|---|---|
| chlorpromazine (Thorazine) | perphenazine |
| cyclizine (Marezine) | phosphorated carbohydrate solution (Emetrol) |
| fluphenazine | prochlorperazine (Compazine) |
| haloperidol (Haldol) | promethazine (Phenergan) |
| palonosetron (Aloxi) | trimethobenzamide (Tigan) |

### *Did You Know?*

Chlorpromazine, fluphenazine, haloperidol, perphenazine, and prochlorperazine are antipsychotic drugs whose main therapeutic use is to treat psychosis, schizophrenia, or manic-depressive disorder.

### Antiemetic Drugs for Use with Chemotherapy Drugs

Certain antiemetic drugs are used specifically to treat the nausea and vomiting caused by chemotherapy drugs. These drugs are discussed in Chapter 21.

### Antiemetic Drugs for Motion Sickness or Vertigo

Motion sickness occurs when the repetitive but varying motions of a car, boat, or airplane overstimulate the inner ear and activate the vomiting center in the brain. Vertigo is a sensation of lightheadedness, dizziness, and whirling caused by irritation or infection in the inner ear that upsets the balance and stimulates the vomiting center. Drugs used to treat motion sickness or vertigo act either by blocking inner ear stimuli from reaching the chemoreceptor trigger zone and the vomiting center in the brain or by reducing the sensitivity of the inner ear to motion. All of these drugs are given orally with the exception of scopolamine (Transderm-Scōp), which is manufactured as a small transdermal patch that is worn behind the ear.

cyclizine (Marezine)                                    meclizine (Antivert) (see ■ FIGURE 8–9)

dimenhydrinate (Dramamine) (see ■ FIGURE 8–8)          promethazine (Phenergan)

diphenhydramine (Benadryl)                             scopolamine (Transderm-Scōp)

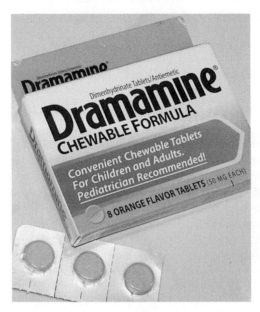

■ **FIGURE 8–8  Dramamine.**
Dramamine is a popular drug for preventing motion sickness. It is taken prior to riding in a car, boat, or airplane. The drug label states that it is an antiemetic drug. The prefix *anti-* means *against,* and the combining form *emet/o-* means *to vomit.* Dramamine comes as an over-the-counter drug in the form of orange-flavored, chewable tablets.

## Drug Alert!

Over-the-counter Dramamine contains the generic drug dimenhydrinate, but the over-the-counter drug Dramamine Less Drowsy Formula actually contains the generic drug meclizine.

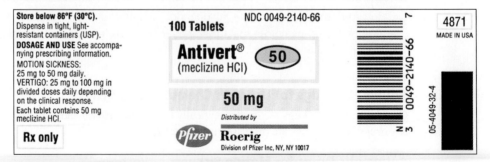

■ **FIGURE 8–9  Drug label for meclizine (Antivert).**
The prescription drug name Antivert combines the prefix *anti-* (against) from *antiemetic* and the letters *vert* from *vertigo* to show that the therapeutic effect of this drug is to prevent the symptoms of vertigo. Antivert is only available as a prescription drug, but its generic drug meclizine is available as both a prescription and an over-the-counter drug.

## Drugs Used to Treat Gallstones

Patients who are unable to undergo surgery to remove gallstones from the gallbladder can be given drugs to help dissolve the stones. These drugs are given orally or through a tube inserted directly into the gallbladder. Although these drugs are effective, gallstones do recur in 50 percent of the patients who are treated.

chenodiol (Chenix)

monoctanoin (Moctanin)

ursodiol (Actigall)

## Drugs Used to Treat Hemorrhoids

Hemorrhoids are enlarged, swollen veins that occur internally within the rectum or externally in the perianal area. Hemorrhoids can be itchy and painful, particularly when irritated by a bowel movement. Over-the-counter topical drugs used to treat hemorrhoids include anesthetic drugs to relieve pain (benzocaine, dibucaine, lidocaine, pramoxine), corticosteroid anti-inflammatory drugs to decrease inflammation (hydrocortisone), vasoconstrictor drugs to constrict the swollen veins (phenylephrine), and an astringent drug (zinc oxide). These drugs are over-the-counter or prescription drugs.

benzocaine (Lanacane)

dibucaine (Nupercainal)

hydrocortisone (Anusol, Cortifoam, Proctocort)

lidocaine

phenylephrine (Preparation H)

pramoxine (ProctoFoam NS, Tronolane, Tuks)

zinc oxide (Tronolane Suppository)

### Combination Drugs for Hemorrhoids

This combination drug contains a corticosteroid anti-inflammatory drug (hydrocortisone) and an anesthetic drug (lidocaine).

Xyralid (hydrocortisone, lidocaine)

## Drugs Used to Treat Obesity

Drugs used to treat obesity act in one of two ways: They keep dietary fat from being absorbed in the intestines or they suppress the appetite to decrease the total amount of food being eaten.

### Lipase Inhibitor Drugs for Obesity

Lipase inhibitor drugs chemically bond to the enzyme lipase so that it cannot break down dietary fat in the intestines. The fat is excreted rather than being absorbed into the blood.

orlistat (Alli, Xenical)

### Appetite Suppressant Drugs for Obesity

Appetite suppressant drugs are similar in chemistry to amphetamine drugs, but with less addictive properties. These drugs suppress the appetite by affecting dopamine or serotonin levels in the satiety center of the brain. Appetite suppressant drugs are also known as *anorexiant drugs*. The use of these drugs is limited to short-term treatment of obesity, in conjunction with dietary restrictions. Patients may develop drug dependence and experience withdrawal symptoms if these drugs are discontinued abruptly because they are Schedule III and Schedule IV drugs. Bupropion is an antidepressant drug that is used to treat obesity; it is not a schedule drug.

| | |
|---|---|
| benzphetamine (Didrex) | phendimetrazine (Prelu-2) |
| bupropion (Wellbutrin) | phentermine (Pro-Fast) |
| diethylpropion | sibutramine (Meridia) |

## Drug Alert!

Alli was the first over-the-counter, FDA-approved weight loss drug. It contains the same drug as the prescription weight-loss drug Xenical, but at a lower dose that allows it to be sold over the counter. Its advertising slogan is "You provide the will. We provide the way." The drug name is meant to imply that the drug is your ally or helper as you lose weight, and its Website is myalli.com. According to MSNBC health writer Melissa Dahl "Dieters have been flocking to the drugstores to pick up Alli...despite the scary warning: Stray too far from your low-fat diet and you just might poop in your pants." The drug company GlaxoSmith-Kline has been up front about the drug's side effects, suggesting that first-time users wear dark pants or bring a change of clothes to work. Because Alli acts to decrease the absorption of 25 percent of the fat in the diet, it produces stools that are fatty and can pass involuntarily. Some patients and counselors, however, see this as a positive effect in that the drug warns patients not to eat fatty foods and then penalizes them if they do—so that patients learn not to do that again! One Alli pill is taken with each meal. A 20-day supply costs $45 to $55.

## Historical Notes

Most consumers think of weight loss drugs as relatively safe and free of side effects. However, the popular appetite suppressant drugs Acutrim and Dexatrim were taken off the market because they contained phenylpropanolamine, a drug that caused hundreds of hemorrhagic strokes and some deaths.

In 1997, the FDA removed from the market the popular weight control drugs fenfluramine (Pondimin) and dexfenfluramine (Redux). The widely popular "fen-phen" combination treatment for weight loss (18 million prescriptions were written in 1996) consisted of fenfluramine (Pondimin) and another appetite suppressant, phentermine (Fastin), which was not taken off the market. Nearly 2 million Americans took dexfenfluramine (Redux) before it was removed from the market. Fenfluramine and dexfenfluramine were linked to cases of patients who developed primary pulmonary hypertension and valvular heart disease.

*Chapter Review*

## Quiz Yourself

1. Describe the therapeutic effect of H₂ blocker drugs.

2. What did the drug companies want to convey when they selected these drug trade names?

   Antivert       Pepto-Bismol

   Asacol        Tagamet

3. How do the therapeutic effects of antacid drugs, H₂ blocker drugs, proton pump inhibitor drugs, misoprostol (Cytotec), and sucralfate (Carafate) differ from each other in treating peptic ulcer disease?

4. What trade name drug is known by patients as "the purple pill"?

5. Describe why anticholinergic drugs are useful in treating gastrointestinal spasms associated with irritable bowel syndrome and other conditions.

6. Explain why narcotic drugs are useful in treating diarrhea.

7. Name five categories of laxative drugs, describe their therapeutic effects, and give examples of drugs in those categories.

8. Describe how aminosalicylic acid drugs are used to treat ulcerative colitis.

9. Describe the therapeutic effects of drugs used to treat motion sickness and vertigo.

10. Name two categories of drugs used to treat obesity and describe their therapeutic effects.

11. To what category of drugs does each of these drugs belong, or what is the therapeutic effect of each of these drugs?

    **a.** cimetidine (Tagamet)

    **b.** docusate (Colace, Surfak)

    **c.** Lomotil

    **d.** loperamide (Imodium A-D)

    **e.** lubiprostone (Amitiza)

    **f.** mesalamine (Asacol, Canasa, Pentasa, Rowasa)

    **g.** Mylanta

    **h.** nizatidine (Axid)

    **i.** omeprazole (Prilosec)

    **j.** orlistat (Alli, Xenical)

    **k.** prochlorperazine (Compazine)

    **l.** ranitidine (Zantac)

    **m.** scopolamine (Transderm-Scōp)

    **n.** ursodiol (Actigall)

## Spelling Tips

| | |
|---|---|
| **AcipHex** | Unusual internal capitalization. |
| **antacid** | Although antacid drugs have an anti-acid effect, the *i* is omitted in *antacid*. |
| **AlternaGEL** | But Ampho**jel** and Basal**jel**; unusual internal capitalization. |
| **CoLyte** | Unusual internal capitalization. |
| **GoLYTELY** | Unusual internal capitalization. |
| **MiraLax** | Unusual internal capitalization. |

## Clinical Applications

1. Look at the drug label and answer the following questions.
   a. What is the generic name of this drug?
   b. To what drug category does this drug belong?
   c. What is the dose contained in each tablet?
   d. Is this a prescription or over-the-counter drug?
   e. Give the trade name of the prescription drug that shares the same generic drug name.

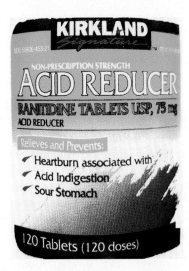

2. Look at the drug label and answer the following questions.
   a. What generic drug is in this product "Gas Relief"?
   b. In what drug form does this drug come?
   c. What is the dose?
   d. What is the therapeutic effect of this generic drug in relieving gas?

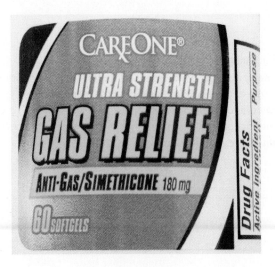

**3.** Look at the drug label and answer the following questions.
   **a.** What is the name of this trade name drug.
   **b.** The label says this drug is a stool softener. To what larger category of drugs does it belong?
   **c.** What is the generic name of this drug?
   **d.** In what drug form does it come?

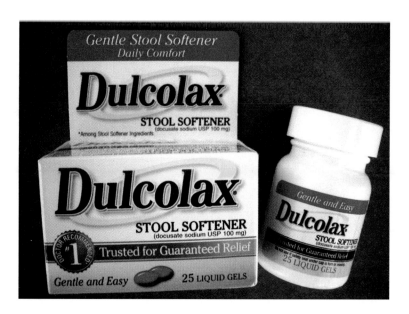

**4.** Read this handwritten prescription  Rewrite the information in words that could be understood by the patient.

PAT SMITH, M.D.
27 Oak Leaf Lane
Baltimore, MD  12121
Phone:  322 –7890          Name_____

                          Address_____

                                              Age_____

$R_x$   Zantac  150 mg  Tablets
              #100
        ÷ BID

[  ] Contents are labeled        May be refilled 0  1  2  3  4
     unless checked

                   Signed_____ M.D.

                   Date_____ 20___ DEA No._____

5. Look at the photograph of the drug label and answer the following questions.
   a. What is the trade name of this drug?
   b. What is the generic name of this drug?
   c. To what category of drugs does it belong?
   d. How can you tell that this drug form is not given orally?

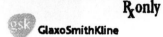

**Store below 30°C (86°F).** Do not freeze. Protect from light. Discard if markedly discolored. Each mL contains, in aqueous solution, prochlorperazine, 5 mg, as the edisylate; sodium biphosphate, 5 mg; sodium tartrate, 12 mg; sodium saccharin, 0.9 mg; benzyl alcohol, 0.75%, as preservative.
**Dosage:** For deep I.M. or I.V. injection.
See accompanying prescribing information.

LOT
EXP:
731780-AF

GlaxoSmithKline
Research Triangle Park, NC 27709

**10mL Multi-Dose Vial**
**5mg/mL**
NDC 0007-3343-01

**COMPAZINE**®
PROCHLORPERAZINE
*as the edisylate INJECTION*

R$_x$ only

gsk **GlaxoSmithKline**

## Multimedia Extension Exercises

■ Go to www.pearsonhighered.com/turley and click on the photo of the cover of *Understanding Pharmacology for Health Professionals* to access the interactive Companion Website created for this textbook.

# Musculoskeletal Drugs

## Learning Objectives

After you study this chapter, you should be able to

1. List several factors that contribute to the development of osteoporosis.

2. Describe the differing therapeutic effects of four categories of drugs used to treat osteoporosis.

3. Compare and contrast the therapeutic effects of the various types of drugs used to treat osteoarthritis.

4. Compare and contrast the types of drugs used to treat osteoarthritis with those used to treat rheumatoid arthritis.

5. Describe the ways in which drugs are used to treat elevated uric acid levels in patients with gout.

6. Given the generic and trade names of a musculoskeletal drug, identify what drug category they belong to or what disease they are used to treat.

7. Given a musculoskeletal drug category, identify several generic and trade name drugs in that category.

Musculoskeletal drugs are used to treat diseases of the muscles and bones. These diseases include osteoporosis, osteoarthritis, bursitis, tendinitis, rheumatoid arthritis, muscle spasms, fibromyalgia, and gout. Musculoskeletal drugs include bone resorption inhibitor drugs, selective estrogen receptor modulator drugs, aspirin and other salicylate drugs, nonsteroidal anti-inflammatory drugs (NSAIDs), gold compound drugs, corticosteroid drugs, skeletal muscle relaxant drugs, and other drugs.

## Drugs Used to Treat Osteoporosis

Most people think of bone as a hard, unchanging substance when, in fact, it is not. Although mature bone is hard, it is also a living tissue that undergoes change. Each year, about 10 percent of the entire bony skeleton is rebuilt. Two types of bone cells are constantly at work: Osteoblasts deposit new bone and osteoclasts break down and remove areas of old or damaged bone. Normal bone maintains a healthy balance (homeostasis) between new bone deposition and bone resorption (breakdown) (see ■ FIGURE 9–1a). This balance is maintained by hormones that control the

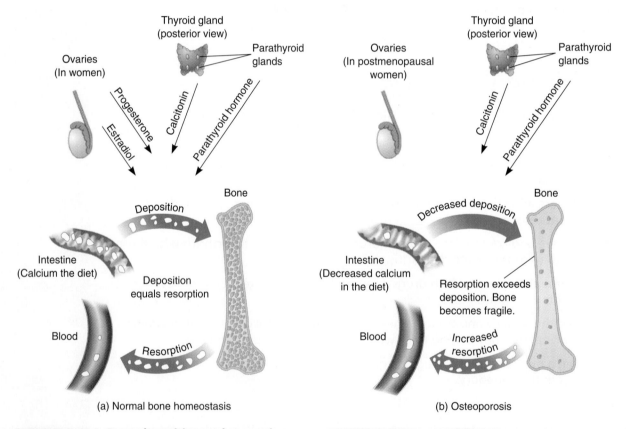

(a) Normal bone homeostasis

(b) Osteoporosis

■ **FIGURE 9–1 Bone deposition and resorption.**

(a) Normal bone homeostasis. Deposition of new bone by osteoblasts is balanced by bone resorption or breakdown by osteoclasts. Normal bone balance (or homeostasis) is maintained through the action of parathyroid hormone, calcitonin, dietary calcium, exercise, and (in women) by the hormones estradiol and progesterone. (b) Osteoporosis. In both older men and women, but particularly in postmenopausal women whose estradiol level has decreased, the rate of bone resorption (breakdown) exceeds that of bone deposition, and this leads to osteoporosis.

amount of calcium in the blood (parathyroid hormone from the parathyroid glands and calcitonin hormone from the thyroid gland), calcium (in the diet), vitamin D (in the diet and from exposure to the sun), exercise, and—in women—by the hormones progesterone and estradiol from the ovaries (progesterone stimulates osteoblasts to build new bone, while estradiol inhibits osteoclasts that break down bone).

Osteoporosis is a thinning of the bone at the cellular level. The combining form *oste/o* means *bone* and the combining form *por/o* means *small openings*. Risk factors for osteoporosis in both men and women include Caucasian or Asian race, slender build, smoking, alcohol use, and lack of exercise. Osteoporosis is more common in women than men, and most common in post-menopausal women. In postmenopausal women, decreasing levels of progesterone no longer stimulate new bone formation, while decreasing levels of estradiol allow osteoclasts to increase the breakdown of bone (see ■ **FIGURE 9–1(b)**). Osteoporosis is prevented or treated with drugs that decrease the rate of bone resorption, with supplemental estradiol and progesterone (in post-menopausal women), with supplemental calcium and vitamin D, and by increasing exercise (to increase weightbearing that stimulates bone growth).

## *Focus on Healthcare Issues*

Osteoporosis is a major public health problem. An estimated 44 million Americans who are 55 years of age or older have osteoporosis or are at risk for developing it. One in every two women and one in every four men over age 50 will have a fracture due to osteoporosis at some time in their lives. There were more than 2 million osteoporosis-related fractures in 2005, with the highest number being fractures of the vertebrae. Healthcare costs for osteoporosis-related fractures increased from $7 billion in 1995 to $19 billion in 2005.

Osteoporosis is treated with bone resorption inhibitor drugs, selective estrogen receptor modulator (SERM) drugs, estrogen drugs, other hormone drugs, calcium supplements, and other drugs.

### Bone Resorption Inhibitor Drugs for Osteoporosis

Bone resorption inhibitor drugs inhibit osteoclasts and this decreases the rate at which bone is resorbed (broken down).

| | |
|---|---|
| alendronate (Fosamax) (see ■ **FIGURE 9–2**) | risedronate (Actonel) |
| ibandronate (Boniva) | zoledronic acid (Reclast, Zometa) |
| pamidronate (Aredia) | (see ■ **FIGURE 9–3**) |

*Note:* The suffix *-dronate* is common to generic bone resorption inhibitor drugs.

## *Did You Know?*

Actress Sally Field had an active lifestyle and was involved in many sports when, just prior to her 60th birthday, she discovered she had osteoporosis. Now, she is a spokesperson and is featured in magazine and television advertisements for the bone resorption inhibitor drug ibandronate (Boniva), a tablet that only needs to be taken once a month.

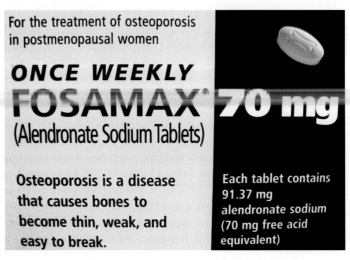

For the treatment of osteoporosis in postmenopausal women

*ONCE WEEKLY*

**FOSAMAX® 70 mg**
(Alendronate Sodium Tablets)

**Osteoporosis is a disease that causes bones to become thin, weak, and easy to break.**

Each tablet contains 91.37 mg alendronate sodium (70 mg free acid equivalent)

■ **FIGURE 9–2  Drug label for alendronate (Fosamax).**
This drug was the first bone resorption inhibitor drug approved for the treatment of osteoporosis. It is taken orally each week. It has a unique bone-shaped indentation on the tablet to remind patients that it is used to improve bone density.

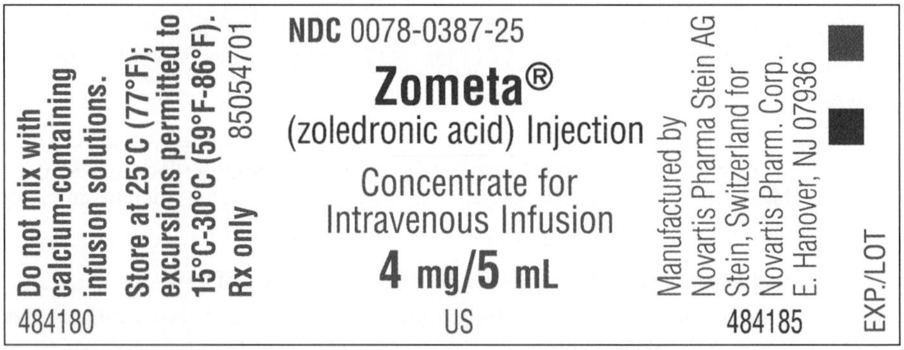

Do not mix with calcium-containing infusion solutions.
Store at 25°C (77°F); excursions permitted to 15°C-30°C (59°F-86°F).
Rx only
85054701
484180

**NDC** 0078-0387-25

**Zometa®**
(zoledronic acid) Injection

Concentrate for Intravenous Infusion

**4 mg/5 mL**

US

Manufactured by Novartis Pharma Stein AG Stein, Switzerland for Novartis Pharm. Corp. E. Hanover, NJ 07936

484185

EXP./LOT

■ **FIGURE 9–3  Drug label for zoledronic acid (Zometa).**
This bone resorption inhibitor drug is used to treat osteoporosis. Unlike oral drugs for osteoporosis which are taken every week or every month, this drug can only be given intravenously in the physician's office, but its advantage is that it only needs to be given once a year. The label indicates the route of administration as "intravenous infusion."

## *Drug Alert!*

Although all bone resorption inhibitor drugs are used to treat osteoporosis, their frequency of doses and their routes of administration are very different. Alendronate and risedronate tablets are taken orally every morning, 30 minutes before eating. Ibandronate is advertised as the osteoporosis drug that is the easiest to remember to take. It can be taken daily (the 2.5-mg tablet), but its selling point is that it can also be taken just once a month (the 150-mg tablet).

Zoledronic acid is now approved to treat osteoporosis in postmenopausal women with a single dose just once a year, but that dose can only be given intravenously, which necessitates a visit to the doctor's office or clinic. A study in the *New England Journal of Medicine* found that an annual intravenous dose was just as effective as the oral route in treating osteoporosis but had a slightly increased risk of causing a cardiac arrhythmia.

### Selective Estrogen Receptor Modulator Drugs for Osteoporosis

Selective estrogen receptor modulator (SERM) drugs bind to estradiol receptors on cells and stimulate the receptors in the same way that estradiol does. This drug is are used to prevent and treat osteoporosis.

raloxifene (Evista)

## *Historical Notes*

In the past, a selective estrogen receptor modulator (SERM) drug—tamoxifen—was being used to treat breast cancer. It was discovered that, in patients who took tamoxifen for breast cancer, there was a positive effect on the bones. Researchers then created another SERM drug that did not have the severe side effects of tamoxifen and was suitable for treating patients with osteoporosis; that drug was Evista.

### Estrogen Drugs for Osteoporosis

Estradiol, the female hormone secreted by the ovaries, inhibits the action of osteoclasts that break down bone. When estradiol levels naturally decline during menopause, the rate of bone resorption (breakdown) accelerates. Hormone replacement drugs are used to treat the symptoms of menopause, and some of the drugs in that category are also indicated for the prevention of osteoporosis in postmenopausal women.

conjugated estrogens (Premarin)

estradiol (Estrace, Estraderm, Vivelle)

estropipate (Ogen, Ortho-Est)

## *Drug Alert!*

In the past, hormone replacement therapy was commonly used for extended periods of time to treat the symptoms of menopause (hot flashes, vaginal dryness) in postmenopausal women, with a secondary effect of preventing osteoporosis. Now, however, it is known that this can increase the risk of endometrial cancer, breast cancer, stroke, and myocardial infarction; this has limited the use of these drugs for the long-term treatment of osteoporosis in postmenopausal women. Naturopathic physicians recommend the use of over-the-counter progesterone cream to treat the symptoms of menopause, prevent osteoporosis, and avoid the adverse effects of hormone replacement therapy with estrogen.

### Other Hormone Drugs for Osteoporosis

Calcitonin-salmon is the drug form of the hormone calcitonin; it takes excess calcium in the blood and deposits it in the bones. Teriparatide is the drug form of parathyroid hormone (created by recombinant DNA technology); it is used to stimulate new bone formation in patients who are at high risk for a fracture.

> calcitonin-salmon (Miacalcin)
>
> teriparatide (Forteo)

## *Did You Know?*

Calcitonin-salmon (Miacalcin) is actually derived from salmon fish. It can be injected or given as a nasal spray. Human calcitonin is also available (as an orphan drug), but its action is less potent and does not last as long.

### Calcium Supplements for Osteoporosis

Over-the-counter calcium supplements, as well as calcium with added vitamin D, are readily available. In addition, milk with added calcium is sold in supermarkets; soy and rice milks also have added calcium. Also, the antacid Tums, which uses calcium to neutralize stomach acid, has advertised that it has a secondary therapeutic effect of calcium supplementation for women, implying that it would be helpful in preventing osteoporosis.

### Combination Drugs for Osteoporosis

These combination drugs contain a bone resorption inhibitor drug (alendronate, risedronate) and calcium or vitamin D.

> Actonel with Calcium (risedronate, calcium)
>
> Fosamax Plus D (alendronate, vitamin D)

## Drugs Used to Treat Osteoarthritis

Osteoarthritis, also known as *degenerative joint disease,* occurs when cumulative damage ("wear and tear") causes degeneration of the cartilage pad and erosion of the bone ends inside a joint. The weightbearing joints (hips and knees), as well as those joints that are used constantly (fingers and toes), are the first to exhibit signs of osteoarthritis, which include pain, inflammation, and swelling. The synovial membrane of the joint can also be involved, and the damaged bone ends often form bony spurs that irritate adjacent tissues.

Drugs used to treat osteoarthritis include drugs that reduce pain and inflammation by inhibiting the production of prostaglandins. These drugs include salicylates (such as aspirin), acetaminophen, nonsteroidal anti-inflammatory drugs (NSAIDs), and COX-2 inhibitor drugs. In addition, corticosteroid drugs can be used. None of these drugs, however, can reverse the cartilage and bone damage that has already occurred in the joint.

### Salicylate Drugs for Osteoarthritis

Salicylate drugs used to treat osteoarthritis include aspirin, one of the oldest drugs known to man. Aspirin, or acetylsalicylic acid (ASA), is the most well-known drug in the salicylate class. The analgesic and anti-inflammatory effects of salicylate drugs are useful in treating the pain and inflammation of osteoarthritis, as well as minor conditions of the bones and muscles (such as bursitis, tendinitis, and muscle sprains).

aspirin (Bayer, Ecotrin)       magnesium salicylate (Doan's)

diflunisal (Dolobid)           salsalate (Salsitab)

Because salicylate drugs, such as aspirin, are irritating to the stomach, and long-term therapy with these drugs has been shown to cause gastric ulcers, some drug companies take precautions to reduce this irritation. Ecotrin is manufactured as an enteric-coated tablet that does not dissolve in the stomach; it dissolves only when it comes in contact with the higher pH environment of the duodenum. Aspirin can also be combined with an antacid drug, as described on page 144.

## Acetaminophen for Osteoarthritis

Although acetaminophen is an analgesic drug, as is aspirin, acetaminophen lacks the ability to inhibit the production of prostaglandins and has no anti-inflammatory action. However, the American College of Rheumatology recommends the use of acetaminophen to treat mild-to-moderate pain associated with osteoarthritis because it is the drug of choice for treating musculoskeletal pain in older patients and it has fewer gastric side effects than aspirin or NSAIDs, even though it cannot treat the inflammation associated with osteoarthritis.

acetaminophen (Tylenol)

## Nonsteroidal Anti-Inflammatory Drugs for Osteoarthritis

Nonsteroidal anti-inflammatory drugs (NSAIDs) inhibit the production of prostaglandins to produce an analgesic effect and anti-inflammatory effect. NSAIDs have less of a tendency than aspirin to cause gastric irritation or ulcers. NSAIDs are structurally similar enough to aspirin that some patients who are allergic to aspirin should not take NSAIDs. The following NSAIDs are used to treat the pain and inflammation of osteoarthritis and rheumatoid arthritis.

diclofenac (Cataflam, Voltaren)       meloxicam (Mobic)

etodolac                              nabumetone

fenoprofen (Nalfon)                   naproxen (Aleve, Naprosyn)

flurbiprofen (Ansaid)                 oxaprozin (Daypro)

ibuprofen (Advil, Motrin)             piroxicam (Feldene)

indomethacin (Indocin)                sulindac (Clinoril)

ketoprofen                            tolmetin

meclofenamate

*Note:* The suffix *-profen* is common to generic nonsteroidal anti-inflammatory drugs.

## Drug Alert!

The NSAID diclofenac (Voltaren) is available as a topical gel to treat the pain of osteoarthritis. It was the first prescription topical skin gel approved by the FDA for treating the pain of osteoarthritis.

Besides its use in treating osteoporosis, indomethacin (Indocin) has an unusual use: It is given intravenously to newborn infants to close a persistent patent ductus arteriosus, a part of the fetal circulation that normally closes after birth.

## Did You Know?

Cats and dogs with osteoarthritis are given the NSAID carprofen (Rimadyl). This drug belongs to the NSAID category of drugs, but it has never been approved for use in humans.

### COX-2 Inhibitor Drugs for Osteoarthritis

COX-2 inhibitor drugs, which also belong to the larger category of NSAIDs, selectively inhibit the enzyme cyclooxygenase-2 (COX-2). This decreases the production of prostaglandins that cause the pain and inflammation of osteoarthritis.

celecoxib (Celebrex) (see ■ FIGURE 9–4)

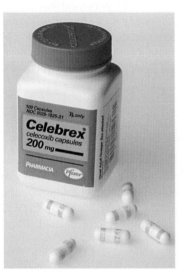

■ **FIGURE 9–4  Bottle and capsules of celecoxib (Celebrex).**
Celecoxib (Celebrex) belongs to the COX-2 inhibitor category of drugs. This drug is used to treat the pain and inflammation of osteoarthritis. Celecoxib (Celebrex) is only available from Pfizer drug company and is protected under patent until 2015. As a general rule, when a drug patent expires and another drug company makes its own generic version, that drug would be as effective as the original trade name drug, but is usually less expensive.

## Drug Alert!

COX-2 inhibitor drugs were hailed as a new, effective way to treat osteoarthritis when they first came on the market in 1999. In the past, the COX-2 category of drugs also included rofecoxib (Vioxx) and valdecoxib (Bextra), but these drugs were taken off the market in 2004 and 2005 because they greatly increased the risk of heart attacks and strokes. Celecoxib (Celebrex) is the only COX-2 inhibitor drug that remains on the market even though a study showed that patients who use this drug have an increased risk of heart problems. It is also used to treat dysmenorrhea and colon polyps.

## In Depth

Prostaglandins, which are present throughout the body and exert various effects, were so named because they were originally isolated from semen from the prostate gland in men.

Prostaglandins play a role in causing the pain and inflammation of osteoarthritis and rheumatoid arthritis. When body tissue is damaged, cells are destroyed, and the cell contents spill into the interstitial fluid. There, the enzyme cyclooxygenase (COX) converts these cellular contents into prostaglandins. The prostaglandins then stimulate pain receptors in that area. The greater the amount of tissue damage, the more prostaglandins are produced and the greater the sensation of pain. The joints have a large number of pain receptors and damage to the joints can cause chronic, severe pain. By inhibiting the cyclooxygenase (COX) enzyme, fewer prostaglandins are produced to activate pain receptors.

## Corticosteroid Drugs for Osteoarthritis

Glucocorticoid hormones, secreted by the cortex of the adrenal gland, have a powerful anti-inflammatory action. Corticosteroid drugs have this same anti-inflammatory effect and are given orally to treat acute episodes of osteoarthritis associated with inflammation of the synovial membrane. Because of the side effects associated with prolonged oral use, corticosteroid drugs are only prescribed to treat acute symptoms for a limited time.

Some corticosteroid drugs (betamethasone, dexamethasone, methylprednisolone, triamcinolone) can also be injected directly into a joint affected by osteoarthritis (intra-articular administration) to relieve inflammation. They can also be injected into the soft tissue near the joint to relieve bursitis and tendinitis.

| | |
|---|---|
| betamethasone (Celestone) | methylprednisolone (Depo-Medrol, Medrol) |
| cortisone | prednisolone (Orapred, Prelone) |
| dexamethasone (Decadron) | prednisone (Deltasone, Meticorten) |
| hydrocortisone (Cortef, Solu-Cortef) | triamcinolone (Aristospan Intra-articular, Kenalog) |

## Topical Drugs for Osteoarthritis

These over-the-counter topical drugs are used to treat the pain of osteoarthritis. Menthol is an analgesic drug. Methyl salicylate and trolamine salicylate are salicylate analgesic drugs. Capsaicin is a natural substance derived from chile pepper plants; it makes the skin and joint less sensitive to pain by diminishing sensory nerve signals. These combination drugs are also used to treat the pain of minor muscle injuries.

| | |
|---|---|
| Absorbine Power Gel (menthol) | Icy Hot (menthyl salicylate, menthol) |
| Aspercreme Cream (trolamine salicylate) | Musterole Deep Strength Rub (methyl salicylate, menthol) |
| Ben-Gay (methyl salicylate, menthol) | Therapeutic Mineral Ice (methyl salicylate, menthol) |
| capsaicin (Capsin, Zostrix) | |

## Other Drugs for Osteoarthritis

Hyaluronic acid is secreted by the synovial membrane of a joint and helps to maintain the lubricating quality of the synovial fluid. This drug, a derivative of hyaluronic acid, is injected into the joints of patients with osteoarthritis to improve the viscosity and lubricating quality of the synovial fluid.

hyaluronic acid (Hyalgan, Synvisc)

## Did You Know?

Hyaluronic acid (Hyalgan, Synvisc) is derived from the combs of chickens! Hyaluronic acid, under the trade names Hylaform and Restylane, is a gel-type filler that is injected under the skin to provide fullness and minimize wrinkle lines on the face. A related drug, sodium hyaluronate (Amvisc, Healon), is injected into the anterior chamber of the eye to maintain its shape during eye surgery.

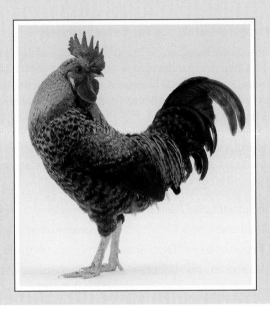

### Combination Drugs for Osteoarthritis

These combination drugs contain a salicylate drug (aspirin, magnesium salicylate), a nonsteroidal anti-inflammatory drug (diclofenac), an antacid drug (aluminum, calcium, magnesium), and/or a prostaglandin drug (misoprostol) to protect the mucous membranes of the stomach. A barbiturate sedative drug (phenyltoloxamine) can be added.

Arthritis Pain Formula (aspirin, aluminum, magnesium)

Arthrotec (diclofenac, misoprostol)

Ascriptin (aspirin, aluminum, calcium, magnesium)

Bayer Buffered Aspirin (aspirin, calcium, magnesium)

Bufferin (aspirin, calcium, magnesium)

Mobigesic (magnesium salicylate, phenyltoloxamine)

## In Depth

Although prostaglandins in the tissues cause pain and inflammation, they actually have a protective action on the mucous membranes of the stomach. However, when drugs are given to decrease pain and inflammation from osteoarthritis, they also decrease the prostaglandins present in the stomach and this can lead to gastric ulcers.

# Drugs Used to Treat Rheumatoid Arthritis

Rheumatoid arthritis produces symptoms of pain, inflammation, swelling, joint deformity, and loss of joint function. Rheumatoid arthritis is caused by an autoimmune reaction in which the body's own antibodies target and destroy cartilage, connective tissue, and joints. Rheumatoid arthritis is thought to be triggered by a virus. Rheumatoid arthritis is treated with salicylate drugs, NSAIDs, COX-2 inhibitor drugs, gold compound drugs, corticosteroid drugs, and other drugs.

## Salicylate Drugs, NSAIDs, and COX-2 Inhibitor Drugs for Rheumatoid Arthritis

Rheumatoid arthritis is treated with many of the same drugs used to treat osteoarthritis. All of the salicylate drugs, NSAIDs, and COX-2 inhibitor drugs described previously are the first line of treatment for rheumatoid arthritis. (Acetaminophen is not used to treat rheumatoid arthritis because it is not effective against inflammation.) If these drugs fail to control the symptoms of rheumatoid arthritis, gold compound drugs may be added to the treatment regimen.

## Gold Compound Drugs for Rheumatoid Arthritis

Gold compound drugs contain actual gold (from 29 percent to 50 percent of the total drug) in capsules or in a solution for injection. Gold compound drugs are used to treat active rheumatoid arthritis. These drugs inhibit macrophages from the immune system that attack the joints, but they cannot reverse joint damage that has already occurred.

auranofin (Ridaura)

aurothioglucose (Solganal)

gold sodium thiomalate (Aurolate)

## Corticosteroid Drugs for Rheumatoid Arthritis

Corticosteroid drugs were discussed previously. These drugs are given orally or as intra-articular injections into specific joints to decrease the inflammation associated with rheumatoid arthritis.

## Other Drugs for Rheumatoid Arthritis

Dapsone is used to treat leprosy. Hydroxychloroquine is used to kill the parasite that causes malaria. Both drugs have an immune system-modulating effect that is effective in treating rheumatoid arthritis.

dapsone

hydroxychloroquine (Plaquenil)

These immunosuppressant drugs suppress the immune system in patients with active, uncontrolled rheumatoid arthritis.

azathioprine (Azasan, Imuran)

cyclosporine (Gengraf, Neoral, Sandimmune)

tacrolimus (Prograf)

### Did You Know?

The immunosuppressant drugs azathioprine, cyclosporine, and tacrolimus are commonly given to patients following organ transplant surgery. They suppress the immune system and prevent the patient's body from forming antibodies against the donor organ (such as a kidney).

These drugs have a variety of actions that are effective in reducing joint and tissue damage, inflammation, pain, and swelling. Anakinra blocks interleukin-1 from binding with receptors on cartilage cells and destroying them. Abatacept inhibits T lymphocytes that attack joint tissues. Adalimumab and etanercept are monoclonal antibody drugs that bind with tumor necrosis factor to prevent inflammation. Alemtuzumab, infliximab, and rituximab are monoclonal antibody drugs that prevent lymphocytes from making antibodies against joint tissues. Interleukin-1 receptor antagonist blocks the growth of T and B lymphocytes. Leflunomide modulates the response of the immune system. Methotrexate is a chemotherapy drug used to treat many different types of cancer; its exact action in treating rheumatoid arthritis is not known.

| | |
|---|---|
| abatacept (Orencia) | infliximab (Remicade) |
| adalimumab (Humira) | interleukin-1 receptor antagonist (Antril) |
| alemtuzumab (Campath) | leflunomide (Arava) |
| anakinra (Kineret) | methotrexate (Rheumatrex Dose Pack) |
| etanercept (Enbrel) | rituximab (Rituxan) |

## Drug Alert!

Leflunomide (Arava) has a very long half-life. Traces of the drug can still be found in the body six months after the last dose. This drug is not recommended for patients who have decreased liver function and cannot metabolize the drug normally, as this prolongs the half-life even more and can result in toxic levels of the drug.

## Did You Know?

Phenylbutazone (Butazolidin) is commonly used in race horses to reduce inflammation. Its slang name is *bute*. It is illegal to race a horse that is being treated with phenylbutazone, and post-race urine tests are done to detect this drug. In the past, this drug was used to treat osteoarthritis in humans, but was replaced by NSAIDs.

## Muscle Relaxant Drugs

Acute muscular conditions, such as strains, sprains, and "pulled muscles," are treated with analgesic drugs and nonsteroidal anti-inflammatory drugs, as previously described. However, a muscle relaxant drug may also be used, along with rest and physical therapy. Muscle relaxant drugs specifically relieve muscle spasm and stiffness, but cannot relieve pain or inflammation.

| | |
|---|---|
| carisoprodol (Soma) | metaxalone (Skelaxin) |
| chlorzoxazone (Paraflex, Parafon Forte DSC) | methocarbamol (Robaxin) |
| cyclobenzaprine (Flexeril) | (see ■ FIGURE 9–5) |
| diazepam (Valium) | orphenadrine (Norflex) |

## Drug Alert!

Diazepam (Valium) belongs to the benzodiazepine category of antianxiety drugs, a different class of drugs from the other muscle relaxant drugs. Diazepam is best known for its use in treating anxiety and neurosis. It is also used to prevent epileptic seizures and to treat agitation and tremor in patients who are undergoing detoxification from alcohol.

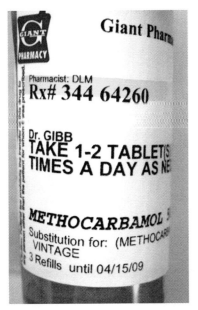

**■ FIGURE 9–5 Prescription bottle of methocarbamol.**
This muscle relaxant drug, available as the trade name drug Robaxin, has been on the market for many years. It relaxes sore, bruised, or strained muscles without causing drowsiness.

These muscle relaxant drugs are used to treat severe muscle spasticity in patients with multiple sclerosis, cerebral palsy, stroke, or spinal cord injury.

baclofen (Lioresal)    L-baclofen (Neuralgon)

dantrolene (Dantrium)    tizanidine (Zanaflex)

diazepam (Valium)

### Combination Muscle Relaxant Drugs

These combination drugs contain a muscle relaxant drug (carisoprodol, orphenadrine), a salicylate analgesic drug (aspirin), and/or a narcotic analgesic drug (codeine).

Norgesic (orphenadrine, aspirin)

Soma Compound (carisoprodol, aspirin)

Soma Compound with Codeine (carisprodol, aspirin, codeine)

## Drugs Used to Treat Fibromyalgia

Fibromyalgia is a disease in which specific, small trigger points along the neck, back, or hips are firm and very tender to the touch. The cause of fibromyalgia is unknown. Drugs used to treat fibromyalgia include a muscle relaxant drug (cyclobenzaprine), a local anesthetic drug (lidocaine, procaine) injected into the trigger points, or an anticonvulsant drug (pregabalin).

cyclobenzaprine (Flexeril)    pregabalin (Lyrica)

lidocaine (Xylocaine)    procaine (Novocain)

## Drugs Used to Treat Gout

Gout is caused by a metabolic defect that allows uric acid to accumulate in the blood. The kidneys are unable to excrete the excess uric acid, and it crystallizes within the joints, causing pain and inflammation. Drugs used to treat gout and gouty arthritis act either by increasing the excretion of uric acid in the urine or by inhibiting enzymes that produce uric acid in the blood.

allopurinol (Zyloprim)    sodium thiosalicylate

colchicine    sulfinpyrazone (Anturane)

probenecid

In addition, several nonsteroidal anti-inflammatory drugs (NSAIDs) have been found to be of particular benefit in treating gout and gouty arthritis.

indomethacin (Indocin)

naproxen (Aleve, Naprosyn)

sulindac (Clinoril)

This drug increases the pH of the urine to help prevent the formation of uric acid stones in the kidneys in patients who have gout.

potassium citrate (Urocit-K)

# Chapter Review

## Quiz Yourself

1. Name six things that support the normal balance between new bone deposition and bone resorption.
2. Which bone cells are inhibited by bone resorption inhibitor drugs?
3. Describe the various routes of administration and timing of doses for the different bone resorption inhibitor drugs.
4. Why are hormone (estrogen) replacement drugs not used as often for the long-term treatment of osteoporosis as they once were?
5. Give the meaning of the abbreviations *ASA, COX,* and *NSAID.*
6. Name the categories of drugs used to treat osteoarthritis and give examples of drugs from each category.
7. Contrast the therapeutic effect of aspirin with those of acetaminophen.
8. How does enteric-coated aspirin help prevent gastric ulcers in patients with osteoarthritis?
9. Indocin is an NSAID that is used to treat osteoarthritis in the elderly and patent ductus arteriosus in newborn infants. True or false?
10. Why are gold compound drugs useful in treating rheumatoid arthritis but not osteoarthritis?
11. List the medical conditions for which a muscle relaxant drug might be prescribed.
12. To what category of drugs does each of these drugs belong?
    a. abatacept (Orencia)
    b. alendronate (Fosamax)
    c. allopurinol (Zyloprim)

     **d.** auranofin (Ridaura)

     **e.** capsaicin (Capsin, Zostrix)

     **f.** carisoprodol (Soma)

     **g.** celecoxib (Celebrex)

     **h.** diclofenac (Cataflam, Voltaren)

     **i.** ibandronate (Boniva)

     **j.** oxaprozin (Daypro)

     **k.** raloxifene (Evista)

     **l.** triamcinolone (Aristospan Intra-articular)

     **m.** zoledronic acid (Reclast, Zometa)

## Spelling Tips

Several gold compound drug names contain *Au,* the chemical symbol for gold: **au**ranofin, **Au**rolate, **au**rothioglucose, Rid**aura**.

## Clinical Applications

**1.** Look at this photograph and answer the following questions.

     **a.** What is the generic name of this drug?

     **b.** To what category of drugs does it belong?

     **c.** What is the drug form of this drug?

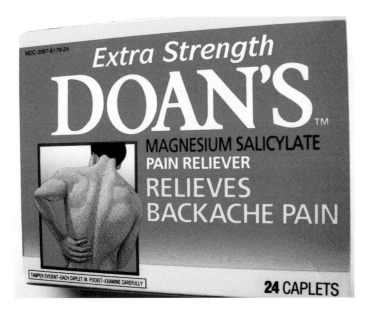

2. Look at this handwritten prescription and answer the following questions.
   a. What drug is prescribed here?
   b. What is the generic name of this drug?
   c. To what category of drugs does it belong?
   d. What is the strength of the dose?
   e. In what drug form is it given?
   f. Translate the rest of the prescription into plain English.

---

PAT SMITH, M.D.
27 Oak Leaf Lane
Baltimore, MD 12121
Phone: 322 –7890

Name_____

Address_____

Age_____

Rx   Motrin 400 mg Tabs
         #40
   Sig: 400 mg to 800mg TID
        w/ food prn pain

[  ] Contents are labeled          May be refilled 0  1  2  3  4
     unless checked

Signed _____ M.D.

Date_____ 20___ DEA No._____

---

3. Look at this handwritten prescription and answer the following questions.
   a. What drug is prescribed here?
   b. What is the generic name of this drug?
   c. To what category of drugs does it belong?
   d. What is the strength of the dose?
   e. In what drug form is it given?
   f. Translate the rest of the prescription into plain English.

---

PAT SMITH, M.D.
27 Oak Leaf Lane
Baltimore, MD 12121
Phone: 322 –7890

Name_____

Address_____

Age_____

Rx   Caps. Feldene 20 mg
            #30
      Sig. ⊤ q d w/ food or milk.

[  ] Contents are labeled          May be refilled 0  1  2  3  4
     unless checked

Signed _____ M.D.

Date_____ 20___ DEA No._____

4. Look at this electronic prescription and translate it into English.

> *Robaxin 500 mg 1-2 po QID PRN #40 #3 RFs*

5. Look at this drug label and answer the following questions.
   a. What is the generic name of this drug?
   b. To what category of drugs does it belong? *Hint:* The drug category is mentioned on the label.
   c. The consumer is invited to compare this over-the-counter generic drug to what other competitor trade name drug that is mentioned on the label?
   d. If a consumer did make this comparison, and the dose of both drugs was the same and the active ingredient of both drugs was the same, what difference would a consumer notice between this drug as compared to that trade name drug?
   e. Besides the trade name drug mentioned on the label, what is another common trade name for this generic drug?

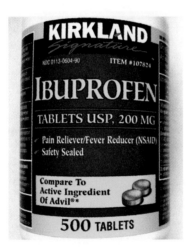

## Multimedia Extension Exercises

■ Go to www.pearsonhighered.com/turley and click on the photo of the cover of *Understanding Pharmacology for Health Professionals* to access the interactive Companion Website created for this textbook.

# 10 Pulmonary Drugs

## Learning Objectives

After you study this chapter, you should be able to

1. Compare and contrast the differing therapeutic effects of bronchodilator drugs and corticosteroid drugs.

2. Name several types of inhaler devices and describe how they work.

3. Describe the therapeutic effects of leukotriene receptor blocker drugs, monoclonal antibody drugs, and mast cell stabilizer drugs.

4. Name several drugs from the fluoroquinolone category of antibiotic drugs that are used to treat Legionnaire's disease.

5. Explain why tuberculosis must be treated with several different antitubercular drugs at the same time.

6. Describe the therapeutic effects of expectorant drugs.

7. Describe the differing therapeutic effects of drugs to help a person stop smoking.

8. Given the generic and trade names of a pulmonary drug, identify what drug category they belong to or what disease they are used to treat.

9. Given a pulmonary drug category, identify several generic and trade name drugs in that category.

Pulmonary drugs are used to treat diseases of the bronchi, bronchioles, and lung. These diseases include asthma (reversible obstructive airway disease), bronchitis, chronic obstructive pulmonary disease (COPD), bacterial and viral infections of the lung, tuberculosis, Legionnaire's disease, and respiratory distress syndrome (see ■ FIGURE 10–1). Pulmonary drugs include bronchodilator drugs, corticosteroid drugs, leukotriene receptor blocker drugs, monoclonal antibody drugs, mast cell stabilizer drugs, expectorant drugs, and drugs used to stop smoking

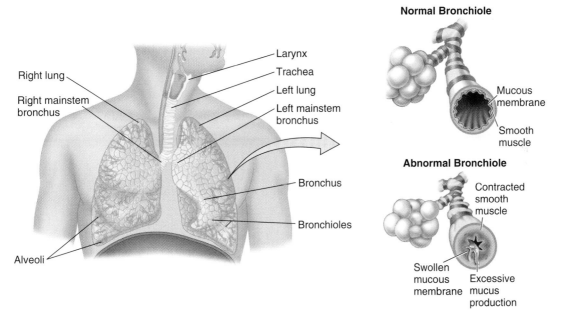

**■ FIGURE 10–1  The respiratory system.**
The bronchi and bronchioles of the respiratory system normally have an open inner air passageway that is surrounded by a layer of relaxed smooth muscle. In asthma, the smooth muscle layer is contracted, the air passageway is narrowed, the mucous membranes are edematous, and there is an excessive amount of mucus production. In chronic bronchitis and chronic obstructive pulmonary disease, the mucous membranes are inflamed and there is an excessive amount of mucus production.

## Bronchodilator Drugs

Bronchodilator drugs are used to prevent or treat asthma, bronchospasm, exercise-induced bronchospasm, chronic obstructive pulmonary disease (COPD), and emphysema. Bronchodilator drugs relax the smooth muscle that surrounds the bronchioles, allowing the bronchioles to dilate to increase air flow. There are several categories of bronchodilator drugs, each of which causes the smooth muscle around the bronchioles to relax and dilate. These categories include the following.

- Sympathomimetic bronchodilator drugs stimulate beta$_2$ receptors in the smooth muscle around the bronchioles (they mimic the action of epinephrine from the sympathetic division of the nervous system).
- Xanthine derivative bronchodilator drugs act directly on smooth muscle around the bronchioles and stimulate the respiratory centers in the brain.
- Anticholinergic bronchodilator drugs block the action of acetylcholine on muscarinic receptors in the smooth muscle around the bronchioles.

albuterol (ProAir HFA, Proventil HFA, Ventolin HFA) (see ■ FIGURE 10–2)
aminophylline

arformoterol (Brovana)
bitolterol (Tornalate)
dyphylline (Lufyllin)

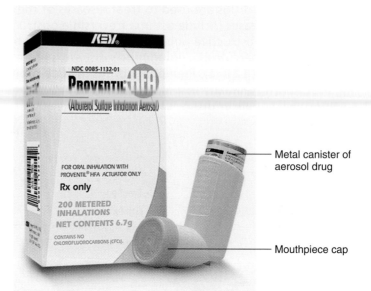

**FIGURE 10–2 Box and metered-dose inhaler for albuterol (Proventil).**
The bronchodilator drug albuterol (Proventil) is administered through a metered-dose inhaler device. It delivers a premeasured puff of the aerosol drug, which is inhaled through the mouth and into the lungs.

ephedrine
epinephrine (microNefrin, Primatene Mist)
formoterol (Foradil Aerolizer)
ipratropium (Atrovent HFA)
isoetharine
levalbuterol (Xopenex HFA)
metaproterenol (Alupent)
pirbuterol (Maxair Autohaler)

salmeterol (Serevent Diskus)
 (see ■ FIGURE 10–3)
terbutaline (Brethine)
theophylline (Bronkodyl,
 Elixophyllin, Uniphyl)
tiotropium (Spiriva)
 (see ■ FIGURE 10–4)

*Note:* The suffixes *-terol* and *-phylline* are common to generic bronchodilator drugs.

## Drug Alert!

Be careful to distinguish between these two sound-alike generic bronchodilator drugs: arformoterol and formoterol.

## Focus on Healthcare Issues

In the past, asthma inhalers contained the propellant chlorofluorocarbon (CFC). When CFC was banned as a pollutant under the U.S. Clean Air Act, drug companies switched to the propellant hydrofluoroalkane, which appears as HFA in the trade names of bronchodilator drugs (see ■ FIGURE 10–2).

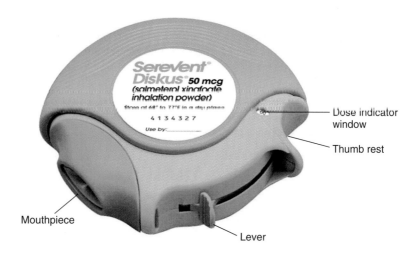

**■ FIGURE 10–3  Diskus inhaler device for salmeterol (Serevent).**
This Diskus inhaler device contains the bronchodilator drug salmeterol (Serevent)
in the form of a powder and in a dose strength of 50 mcg per actuation. The small
dose indicator window shows the number of doses remaining in the Diskus.
Pulling the lever releases a premeasured dose of powdered drug, which is inhaled
through the mouth and into the lungs.

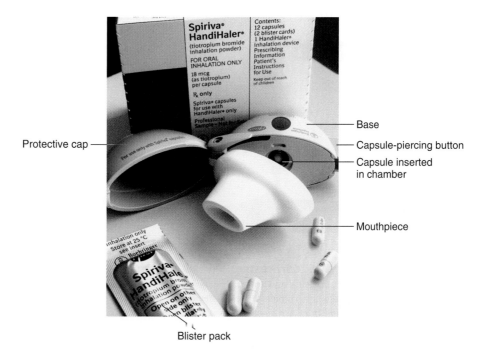

**■ FIGURE 10–4  Box and Handihaler device for tiotropium (Spiriva).**
The bronchodilator drug tiotropium (Spiriva) is administered through a Handihaler device that
crushes a capsule that contains the powdered drug. The powder is then inhaled through the
mouth and into the lungs.

## Corticosteroid Drugs

Glucocorticoid hormones (mainly cortisol), which are secreted by the adrenal cortex, suppress the inflammatory response of the immune system. Corticosteroid drugs act in the same way to reduce inflammation and tissue edema that is associated with asthma and other chronic lung diseases and thereby prevent acute attacks. Corticosteroid drugs do not dilate the bronchioles, and so they cannot be used to treat acute attacks, so the patient must also take a bronchodilator drug. Most of these corticosteroid drugs are given by an inhaler device, and the dose is prescribed in numbers of puffs or actuations, but methylprednisolone is given intramuscularly and prednisolone is given orally.

beclomethasone (QVAR)

budesonide (Pulmicort) (see ■ FIGURE 10–5a)

ciclesonide (Alvesco)

flunisolide (AeroBid, AeroSpan)

fluticasone (Flovent)

methylprednisolone (Depo-Medrol)

mometasone (Asmanex)
   (see ■ FIGURE 10–5b)

prednisolone (Orapred, Pediapred)

triamcinolone (Azmacort)

*Note:* The suffixes *-lide, -nide, -lone,* and *-sone* are common to generic corticosteroid drugs.

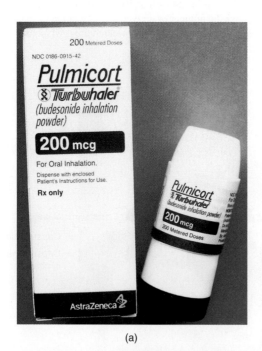

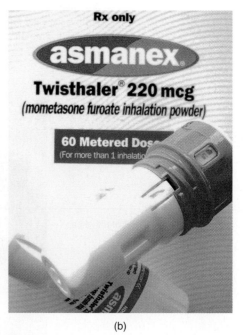

(a)  (b)

■ **FIGURE 10–5 Corticosteroid drugs and inhaler devices.**
(a) The generic corticosteroid drug budesonide is available as the trade name Pulmicort. This powdered drug is administered with a Turbuhaler inhaler device. (b) The generic corticosteroid drug mometasone is available as the trade name drug Asmanex. This powdered drug is administered with a Twisthaler inhaler device.

### Combination Drugs

These combination drugs contain a bronchodilator drug (albuterol, dyphylline, ephedrine, formoterol, ipratropium, salmeterol, theophylline), a corticosteroid drug (budesonide, fluticasone), an expectorant drug (guaifenesin, potassium iodide), an antihistamine drug to dry up secretions (hydroxyzine), and/or a sedative drug (phenobarbital).

Advair (salmeterol, fluticasone)
(see ■ FIGURE 10–6)

Combivent (albuterol, ipratropium)

Elixophyllin-GG (theophylline, guaifenesin)

Elixophyllin-KI (theophylline, potassium iodide)

Lufyllin-EPG (dyphylline, ephedrine, guaifenesin, phenobarbital)

Lufyllin-GG (dyphylline, guaifenesin)

Marax (theophylline, ephedrine, hydroxyzine)

Quibron (theophylline, guaifenesin)

Symbicort (formoterol, budesonide)

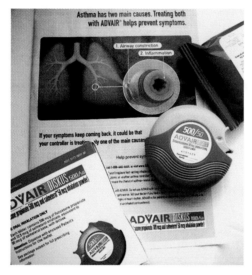

■ **FIGURE 10–6** **Advair drug advertisement and inhaler device.**
The combination drug Advair contains the bronchodilator drug salmeterol and the corticosteroid anti-inflammatory drug fluticasone. Notice the background magazine advertisement that points out that asthma has two main causes: airway constriction and inflammation. A combination drug such as Advair treats both at the same time to prevent acute attacks.

## *Drug Alert!*

Bronchodilator drugs and corticosteroid drugs come in a variety of inhaler devices that deliver a premeasured dose of drug into the lungs. The drug doses are measured in puffs or **actuations**. A **metered-dose inhaler (MDI)** is an L-shaped device (see Figure 10–2). The top of the device holds a small, removable metal canister that contains the drug in an aerosol form. The patient holds the device in an upright "L" position, puts the mouthpiece in the mouth, presses down on the canister, and then inhales the aerosol drug. A **spacer** is a long plastic chamber that can be attached at one end to the inhaler mouthpiece and has its own mouthpiece at the other end. A spacer makes it easier to coordinate the steps involved in using an MDI and keeps the drug from being deposited in the mouth and throat rather than in the lungs. A **Diskus** is a round device that contains the drug in a powdered form (see Figure 10–3 and Figure 10–6). The patient holds the Diskus in a horizontal position, slides the lever to release one dose of drug, puts the mouthpiece into the mouth, and then inhales the powdered drug. The thumb rest is then used as leverage to help rotate the outer case into a closed position and keep the mouthpiece clean. A **Handihaler** contains three pieces: a base that holds a capsule that contains the powdered drug, a mouthpiece, and a protective upper cap (see Figure 10–4). After a capsule is inserted into a small chamber in the base, the

*(continued)*

# Drug Alert! (continued)

mouthpiece is snapped into place over the base, and the capsule-piercing button is pushed to break open the capsule and release the powder. The patient puts the mouthpiece into the mouth and inhales the powdered drug. Printed on the cap is a reminder to only use Spiriva capsules in the device. Because the Spiriva capsule looks very similar to capsules that are taken orally, the FDA has issued an advisory to patients taking Spiriva not to swallow the capsule. A **Turbuhaler** and a **Twisthaler** (see Figure 10–5) are similar in that each consists of a protective cap and a combination mouthpiece and base that contain the powdered drug. As the cap is twisted off from the base, a new dose of powdered drug is prepared. The patient holds the Turbuhaler vertically and the Twisthaler horizontally, inserts the mouthpiece into the mouth, and inhales the powdered drug. With the Twisthaler, a dose indicator window in the base tells exactly how many doses still remain in the device.

## Leukotriene Receptor Blocker Drugs

Leukotriene, a substance that is produced by the body in response to inhaled antigens, causes airway edema, bronchospasm, and inflammation. Leukotriene receptor blocker drugs block the action of leukotriene at the receptor level or block the production of leukotriene. These drugs are used to prevent and treat asthma, but are not used for other respiratory diseases.

> montelukast (Singulair) (see ▦ **FIGURE 10–7**)
>
> zafirlukast (Accolate)
>
> zileuton (Zyflo CR)

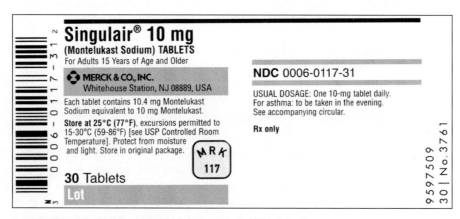

▦ **FIGURE 10–7  Montelukast (Singular) drug label.**
This leukotriene receptor blocker drug is used to prevent and treat asthma. It is given orally as a tablet.

## Monoclonal Antibody Drugs

Monoclonal antibody drugs keep immunoglobulin E (IgE) from binding to receptors on mast cells and basophils and triggering the release of histamine from them. These drugs are used to treat moderate-to-severe, persistent asthma. This drug is given by subcutaneous injection in the doctor's office.

> omalizumab (Xolair)

## Mast Cell Stabilizer Drugs

Mast cell stabilizer drugs stabilize the cell membrane of mast cells and prevent them from releasing histamine during the immune system's response to an antigen. This prevents bronchospasm in patients with asthma due to allergies. Mast cell stabilizer drugs are only effective in preventing asthma attacks, not in treating them once they have occurred. This drug is inhaled.

cromolyn (Intal)

## Drug Alert!

The names of all generic monoclonal antibody drugs end with the suffix –*mab* for **m**onoclonal **a**nti**b**ody.

With their sound-alike pronunciations, be careful not to confuse cromolyn, an inhaled mast cell stabilizer drug used to treat asthma, with Chromelin, a topical drug used to treat depigmented areas of skin (vitiligo).

## Drugs Used to Treat Respiratory Infections

Antibiotic drugs are used to treat lower respiratory tract infections and pneumonia. These include antibiotic drugs from the aminoglycoside, carbapenem, cephalosporin, fluoroquinolone, ketolide, macrolide, monobactam, penicillin, and tetracycline categories. Antiviral drugs are used to treat influenza and respiratory syncytial virus infection. These antibiotic and antiviral drug categories and their individual generic and trade name drugs are discussed in Chapter 20.

## Drugs Used to Treat Legionnaire's Disease

Legionnaire's disease, a serious and sometimes fatal pneumonia caused by the bacterium *Legionnella pneumophilia,* was named for its first recognized outbreak, which occurred in 1976 at an American Legion convention in Philadelphia. This gram-negative bacterium grew in standing water in the air conditioning system of the convention center and was distributed through ventilation ducts. The bacterium is especially attracted to the environment of the lungs, and so its full scientific name is *Legionnella* (based on where it originated) and *pneumophilia* (which means *thing that loves the lungs*). Legionnaire's disease is treated with these fluoroquinolone antibiotic drugs.

ciprofloxacin (Cipro)              moxifloxacin (Avelox)

levofloxacin (Levaquin)        ofloxacin (Floxin)

lomefloxacin (Maxaquin)

*Note:* The suffix *-floxacin* is common to generic fluoroquinolone antibiotic drugs.

## Drugs Used to Treat Tuberculosis

Tuberculosis (TB) is caused by the bacterium *Mycobacterium tuberculosis,* a gram-positive bacterium. Tuberculosis is spread by airborne droplets expelled by coughing. If the patient's immune system is strong, the infection can remain dormant for years without causing symptoms. Because of a unique waxy coating around its bacterial wall, *M. tuberculosis* is difficult to kill and is resistant to antibiotic drugs that are effective against other gram-positive bacteria. Treatment of tuberculosis is accomplished with a combination (not just one) of the following special antitubercular drugs over a period of nine months.

| | |
|---|---|
| ethambutol (Myambutol) | rifampin (Rifadin, Rimactane) |
| isoniazid (INH, Nydrazid) | rifapentine (Priftin) |
| pyrazinamide | streptomycin |

These secondary antitubercular drugs are most commonly used to treat multidrug resistant tuberculosis (MDRTB), which occurs when the tuberculosis bacterium has developed resistance to the primary antitubercular drugs, listed previously.

| | |
|---|---|
| aminosalicylic acid (Paser) | cycloserine (Seromycin Pulvules) |
| capreomycin (Capastat) | ethionamide (Trecator-SC) |

## Combination Drugs for Tuberculosis

Several antitubercular drugs are always given to treat each case of tuberculosis. These combination drugs contain antitubercular drugs (isoniazid, pyrazinamide, rifampin), which are combined into a single capsule or tablet for ease of dosing.

IsonaRif (isoniazid, rifampin)

Rifamate (isoniazid, rifampin)

Rifater (isoniazid, pyrazinamide, rifampin)

## *Focus on Healthcare Issues*

The tuberculosis bacterium has developed varying degrees of resistance to most antitubercular drugs. Resistant strains develop when the patient is not compliant and does not take the antitubercular drug for the prescribed length of time. To minimize the chance of resistant strains developing, antitubercular drugs are given in combination, and patients must continue drug treatment for a full nine months. Because tuberculosis is such a large and challenging public health problem, patients who refuse to (or are unable to) be compliant with drug treatment may be required to participate in **directly observed therapy (DOT)**, in which the patient must come to a clinic each day and be observed while actually taking each dose. In San Francisco (which has the highest TB rate on the West Coast), the attorney general can order noncompliant patients to remain in their homes (except for doctor visits) or even send them to jail (where their treatment is continued).

## *Historical Notes*

The microbiologist Selman Waksman (who discovered the antibiotic drug neomycin and the chemotherapy drug actinomycin D and who coined the word *antibiotic*) was a professor at Rutgers University where he studied soil bacteria. He was looking for a drug that would be effective against tuberculosis, because the newly discovered antibiotic drug penicillin was not. He and his students examined 10,000 different soil samples, looking for a substance that could kill the tuberculosis bacterium. They examined a clump of dirt taken from the throat of a sick chicken. On it was growing the mold that would be found to destroy the tuberculosis bacterium. They called it *streptomycin.* Just before their discovery, however, a financial officer at Rutgers suggested Waksman be fired to cut down on expenses, stating that Waksman's work was obscure and his research would never repay the money invested in it. After the discovery of streptomycin, Waksman was offered $10 million; he gave the money to Rutgers, which, at his suggestion, used it to build a microbiology laboratory.

## Expectorant Drugs

Expectorant drugs reduce the viscosity or thickness of mucus (sputum) in the lungs so that patients can more easily cough it up. Expectorant drugs are only prescribed for productive coughs.

guaifenesin (Humibid, Mucinex, Naldecon, Robitussin) (see ■ **FIGURE 10–8**)

potassium iodide (Pima, SSKI)

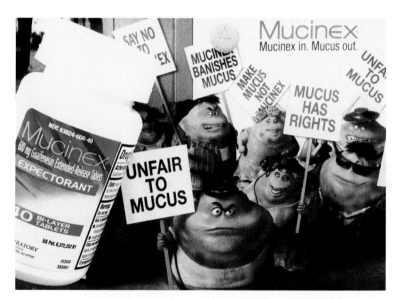

■ **FIGURE 10–8 Bottle and advertisement for guaifenesin (Mucinex).**
The expectorant drug guaifenesin is available as a prescription drug and in several over-the-counter drugs, one of which is Mucinex. Its drug advertisement personifies mucus as being upset about being expelled from the lungs by the expectorant action of the drug.

These drugs are used to break apart very thick mucus secretions in patients with acute or chronic pulmonary disease, such as pneumonia, asthmatic bronchitis, emphysema, cystic fibrosis, or tuberculosis. These drugs dissolve the chemical bonds of mucoproteins and thin the mucus so that it can be coughed up.

acetylcysteine (Mucomyst)

dornase alfa (Pulmozyme)

## Did You Know?

Acetylcysteine (Mucomyst) is also used as an antidote for acetaminophen (Tylenol) overdose. Dornase alfa is manufactured using recombinant DNA technology and ovary cells taken from Chinese hamsters.

## Drugs Used to Stop Smoking

Smoking has been linked to lung cancer, emphysema, bronchitis, and other pulmonary diseases. Nicotine is a strongly addictive substance that stimulates nicotine receptors in the frontal cortex to increase alertness and performance and stimulates nicotine receptors in the limbic lobe to provide pleasure; these two addicting effects make it difficult to quit smoking.

### Nicotine Drugs

Nicotine drugs provide a gradual withdrawal from nicotine, which diminishes the craving and helps persons to successfully stop smoking. These drugs supply a decreasing amount of nicotine in various drug forms: chewing gum, nasal spray, or transdermal patch.

Nicoderm CQ
Nicorette
Nicotrol

### Nicotine Antagonist Drugs

These drugs bind to nicotine receptors and block them from being activated by nicotine.

varenicline (Chantix)

### Other Drugs for Smoking Cessation

These drugs help persons to stop smoking and have various uses as well. Bupropion is an antidepressant drug. Clonidine, an adrenergic blocker drug, is used to treat hypertension, excessive sweating, alcohol withdrawal, and restless legs syndrome. Topiramate is an anticonvulsant drug that is also used to treat dependence behaviors (alcohol use, cocaine use, binge eating).

bupropion (Zyban)
clonidine (Catapres TTS-1)
topiramate (Topamax)

## Focus on Healthcare Issues

According to the Centers for Disease Control (CDC), nicotine addiction is the most common form of chemical dependence in the United States, and nicotine can be as addicting as heroin, cocaine, or alcohol. About 20 percent of Americans smoke, slightly more men than women. Cigarette smoking is the leading preventable cause of death in the United States, accounting for one out of every five deaths. Each day, more than 4,000 people under age 18 try smoking and more than 1,100 of these become daily smokers. Surveys indicate that 70 percent of smokers want to quit.

## Drugs Used to Treat Respiratory Distress Syndrome

Surfactant is a substance that is produced by the alveoli in the lungs. It is a protein-fat compound that reduces surface tension and keeps the walls of the alveolus from collapsing together during exhalation. Decreased levels of surfactant cause the alveoli to collapse.

A surfactant drug is used to supplement low levels of surfactant in the lungs of premature infants to prevent and treat respiratory distress syndrome (RDS). As the lungs mature, they begin to produce their own surfactant. Colfosceril and Procysteine are used to treat adult respiratory distress syndrome, in which severe infection or injury to the lungs damages the lungs and makes them unable to produce surfactant. Surfactant drugs are administered via an endotracheal tube.

beractant (Survanta)

calfactant (Infasurf)

colfosceril (Exosurf, Exosurf Neonatal)

poractant alfa (Curosurf)

Procysteine

This corticosteroid drug is used to decrease inflammation associated with respiratory distress syndrome.

dexamethasone (Decadron)

### Did You Know?

Surfactant drugs are derived from natural surfactant taken from ground-up cows' lungs. All of the trade name drugs contain the syllable *sur* or *surf,* referring to surfactant. Respiratory distress syndrome was formerly known as *hyaline membrane disease.* This disease first became a household word in the United States when the premature son of then-President John Kennedy died from it in 1963.

## Drugs Used to Treat Ventilator Patients

These neuromuscular blocker drugs are used to facilitate endotracheal intubation and to paralyze patients who are on mechanical ventilation so that they will not resist the inflow of air from the ventilator.

atracurium (Tracrium)

cisatracurium (Nimbex)

mivacurium (Mivacron)

pancuronium

rocuronium (Zemuron)

succinylcholine (Anectine, Quelicin)

vecuronium (Norcuron)

These drugs are used to sedate patients who are intubated and on the ventilator. Dexmedetomidine and propofol are sedative drugs. Sufentanil is a Schedule II narcotic drug.

dexmedetomidine (Precedex)

propofol (Diprivan)

sufentanil (Sufenta)

# Chapter Review

## Quiz Yourself

1. Describe the three categories of bronchodilator drugs and their therapeutic effects.
2. Corticosteroid drugs can be inhaled to provide relief from an acute asthma attack. True or false?
3. Describe how these inhaler devices are used and what categories of drugs they contain: metered-dose inhaler (MDI), Diskus, Handihaler, Turbuhaler, Twisthaler.
4. What condition is a mast cell stabilizer drug used to treat and what is its therapeutic effect?
5. What monoclonal antibody drug must be given by subcutaneous injection in the doctor's office to treat asthma?
6. What is the significance of the suffix -*mab* at the end of a generic drug?
7. How did the bacterium *Legionella pneumophilia* receive its name?
8. What is the name of the causative agent of tuberculosis?
9. Give the names of the six primary drugs used to treat tuberculosis.
10. What is *directly observed therapy?*
11. Mucomyst is used to treat patients with cystic fibrosis or acetaminophen overdose. True or false?
12. How do drugs such as Nicoderm CQ and varenicline (Chantix) help persons to quit smoking?
13. What is the significance of the syllable *sur* or *surf* in drugs used to treat respiratory distress syndrome?
14. To what category of drugs does each of these drugs belong?
    a. albuterol (Proventil)
    b. cromolyn (Intal)
    c. fluticasone (Flovent)
    d. isoniazid (INH, Nydrazid)
    e. montelukast (Singulair)
    f. pirbuterol (Maxair Autohaler)
    g. rifampin (Rifadin, Rimactane)
    h. tiotropium (Spiriva)
    i. triamcinolone (Azmacort)
    j. varenicline (Chantix)
    k. zileuton (Zyflo)

## Spelling Tips

| | |
|---|---|
| **AeroBid, AeroSpan** | Unusual internal capitalization. |
| **Asmanex** | Different spelling between the drug and the disease asthma. |
| **Azmacort** | Different spelling between the drug and the disease asthma. |
| **IsonaRif** | Unusual internal capitalization. |
| **microNefrin** | No initial capital letter. |
| **Pulmicort Turbuhaler** | *Pulmi-*, not *pulmo-* as in *pulmonary. Turbu-,* not *turbo-*. |
| **theophylline** | Final "e" in the generic name but not in the trade name Elixophyllin. |

## Clinical Applications

1. Look at this photograph and answer the following questions.
   a. What generic drug does this box contain?
   b. Give three trade names for this generic drug.
   c. To what category of drugs does this drug belong?
   d. What is the therapeutic effect of this drug?

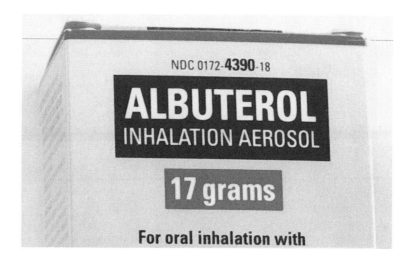

2. Look at this handwritten prescription and answer the following questions.
   a. What two drugs are prescribed here?
   b. Translate both prescriptions into plain English.

3. Compare these two metered-dose inhalers. Look at the photographs and answer the following questions.
   a. What generic drug name is on the label of the metered-dose inhaler on the left?
   b. What trade name is on the canister at the top of the metered-dose inhaler on the left?
   c. Is the patient inhaling two different drugs? Explain your answer.
   d. What is the name of the generic drug in the metered-dose inhaler on the right?
   e. What is the name of the trade name drug in the metered-dose inhaler on the right?
   f. What is the difference in the therapeutic effects of the drugs in these two different metered-dose inhalers?

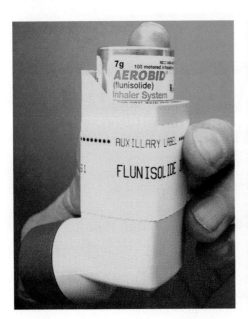 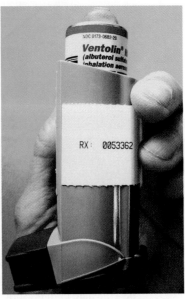

4. Compare these two photographs. Each is a photograph of a Diskus device produced by GlaxoSmithKline drug company. What three differences are there between these two devices, aside from the color difference?

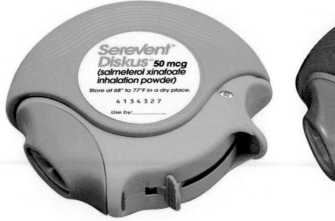 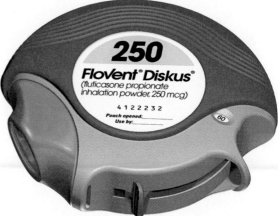

5. Look at this photograph and answer the following questions.
   a. What is the trade name of this combination drug?
   b. What two generic drugs does it contain?
   c. What is the therapeutic effect of each drug?
   d. What is the route of administration for this drug?
   e. How many puffs does the inhaler contain?

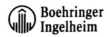

NDC 0597-0013-14

# Combivent®
(ipratropium bromide and
albuterol sulfate)

## Inhalation Aerosol

14.7 grams
200 metered actuations

Each actuation delivers 18 mcg ipratropium bromide and
103 mcg albuterol sulfate from the mouthpiece.

R$_x$ only

**Boehringer
Ingelheim**

## Multimedia Extension Exercises

■ Go to www.pearsonhighered.com/turley and click on the photo of the cover of *Understanding Pharmacology for Health Professionals* to access the interactive Companion Website created for this textbook.

# 11 Cardiovascular Drugs

## CHAPTER CONTENTS

## Learning Objectives

After you study this chapter, you should be able to

1. Compare and contrast the therapeutic effects of beta-blocker drugs, calcium channel blocker drugs, and ACE inhibitor drugs.

2. Name five different cardiac diseases that propranolol is used to treat.

3. Compare and contrast the therapeutic effects of bile acid sequestrant drugs versus "statin drugs."

4. Define the words and phrases *negative chronotropic effect, positive inotropic effect, therapeutic index, half life, preload, afterload,* and *asystole.*

5. List three ways in which digitalis toxicity can be treated.

6. Describe the therapeutic effect of nitrate drugs.

7. Describe how the drug epinephrine (Adrenalin) is used to treat cardiac arrest.

8. Given the generic and trade names of a cardiovascular drug, identify what drug category they belong to or what disease they are used to treat.

9. Given a cardiovascular drug category, identify several generic and trade name drugs in that category.

Cardiovascular drugs are used to treat diseases of the heart and blood vessels. These diseases include hypertension (HTN), hyperlipidemia, congestive heart failure (CHF), angina pectoris, myocardial infarction (MI), cardiac arrhythmias, peripheral vascular disease, and other diseases. Cardiovascular drugs include beta-blocker drugs, alpha/beta-blocker drugs, alpha-blocker drugs, calcium channel blocker drugs, ACE inhibitor drugs, angiotensin II receptor blocker drugs, renin inhibitor drugs, aldosterone receptor inhibitor drugs, bile acid sequestrant drugs, HMG-CoA reductase inhibitor drugs (statin drugs), digitalis drugs, nitrate drugs, peripheral vasodilator drugs, and other drugs.

## Drugs Used to Treat Hypertension

Hypertension (HTN) is characterized by an increase in the systolic and/or diastolic blood pressure. Hypertension is caused by arteriosclerosis, kidney disease, and other diseases, or it may have no identified cause (in which case, it is known as *essential hypertension*). Normal blood pressure is defined as being lower than 120/80 mm Hg. Prehypertension is defined as a systolic blood pressure between 120–139 mm Hg and a diastolic blood pressure between 80–89 mm Hg. Blood pressure readings higher than this are defined as hypertension. Over time, untreated hypertension can damage the heart, blood vessels, kidneys, and other organs.

### *Focus on Healthcare Issues*

The treatment of hypertension follows what is known as a *stepped-care approach.* Lifestyle changes are suggested first: Patients are asked to restrict the use of salt in cooking and at the table, or the physician may prescribe a low-salt diet to limit the total dietary sodium intake. In addition, the patient may be asked to lose weight, exercise, and stop smoking. If these measures cannot control the blood pressure, drugs are added to the treatment regimen. Often a diuretic drug is prescribed first. If a satisfactory reduction in blood pressure is not achieved, a beta-blocker drug is added. A beta-blocker drug can also be selected as the first step of treatment. Other drugs, such as calcium channel blocker drugs, ACE inhibitor drugs, angiotensin II receptor blocker drugs, or other antihypertensive drugs, can be added.

### Diuretic Drugs for Hypertension

By promoting the excretion of sodium and water in the urine, diuretic drugs decrease the total blood volume, which lowers the blood pressure. For a discussion of diuretic drugs, see Chapter 7.

### Beta-Blocker Drugs for Hypertension

Beta-blocker drugs block the action of epinephrine at all beta receptors to decrease the heart rate and dilate the blood vessels. Both of these effects lower the blood pressure. This category includes beta-blocker drugs and cardioselective beta-blocker drugs. For a detailed description of the therapeutic effects of these drugs, see the In Depth feature box on the next page.

| | |
|---|---|
| carteolol (Cartrol) | pindolol (Visken) |
| nadolol (Corgard) | propranolol (Inderal) (see ■ FIGURE 11–1) |
| penbutolol (Levatol) | timolol (Blocadren) |

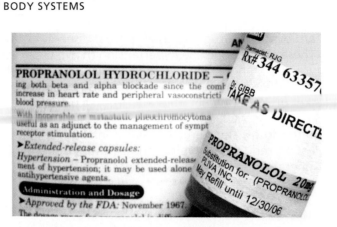

**■ FIGURE 11–1  Prescription bottle of propranolol.**
Propranolol was the first drug in the beta-blocker drug category. It
was approved by the FDA in 1967 for treating hypertension.
Currently, it is also indicated for angina pectoris, ventricular
tachycardia, atrial flutter/fibrillation, myocardial infarction, as
well as for migraine headaches, performance anxiety, and the
tremors of Parkinson's disease and familial tremors.

## *In Depth*

Beta receptors are special protein molecules located on the cell membranes of myocardial
cells in the heart and smooth muscle cells in the blood vessels and bronchi. Beta receptors
in the heart are designated as beta$_1$ receptors. Beta receptors in the smooth muscle of
blood vessels or bronchi are designated as beta$_2$ receptors. All beta receptors are stimulated by the hormone epinephrine in response to stress or danger (the so-called "fight or
flight" response). When beta$_1$ receptors in the heart are stimulated, they cause the heart
rate to increase. When beta$_2$ receptors in blood vessel smooth muscle are stimulated, they
cause the blood vessels to constrict. Both of these actions raise the blood pressure. When
beta$_2$ receptors in the smooth muscle of the bronchi are stimulated, they cause the bronchi
to relax, increasing air flow to the lungs.

In patients with hypertension, beta-blocker drugs block the action of epinephrine on beta
receptors and this slows the heart rate and dilates the blood vessels; both of these actions
decrease the blood pressure.

Beta-blocker drugs block all beta$_1$ and beta$_2$ receptors. Cardioselective beta-blocker
drugs are more selective in their action and block only beta$_1$ receptors in the heart and
beta$_2$ receptors in the blood vessels (but not in the bronchi).

Cardioselective beta-blocker drugs block the action of epinephrine at beta$_1$ receptors in the
heart and beta$_2$ receptors in the blood vessels. They do not block the action of beta$_2$ receptors in
the bronchi, so the bronchi remain dilated. Hypertensive patients with asthma are treated with
cardioselective beta-blocker drugs because they allow the bronchi to remain open.

| | |
|---|---|
| acebutolol (Sectral) | bisoprolol (Zebeta) |
| atenolol (Tenormin) | metoprolol (Lopressor, Toprol-XL) (see **■ FIGURE 11–2**) |
| betaxolol (Kerlone) | nebivolol (Bystolic) |

*Note:*  The suffix *-olol* is common to both types of generic beta-blocker drugs.

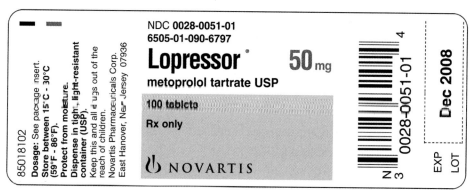

**■ FIGURE 11–2  Drug label for metoprolol (Lopressor).**
Metoprolol (Lopressor) is a cardioselective beta-blocker drug used to treat hypertension.

## *Did You Know?*

Several beta-blocker drugs (atenolol, metoprolol, nadolol, propranolol, and timolol) are pre-scribed to prevent migraine headaches. These drugs act on beta receptors in blood vessels in the brain to limit the tendency of the vessels to overdilate during a migraine.

Several beta-blocker drugs are prescribed to treat performance anxiety (stage fright). Some professional musicians, actors, and even professional golfers use beta-blocker drugs to block the effect of excess epinephrine (dry mouth, tremors, cold extremities, GI upset, inabil-ity to concentrate) that impairs their ability to perform.

## Alpha/Beta-Blocker Drugs for Hypertension

These drugs block both alpha receptors and beta$_2$ receptors in the smooth muscle of the blood ves-sels to lower the blood pressure.

> carvedilol (Coreg)
>
> labetalol (Normodyne, Trandate)

## Alpha-Blocker Drugs for Hypertension

These drugs block only alpha$_1$ receptors. Alpha$_1$ receptors are located in the peripheral blood vessels in both arteries and veins. Blocking these receptors causes both the arteries and veins to dilate, and this lowers the blood pressure.

> doxazosin (Cardura)          prazosin (Minipress)
>
> mecamylamine (Inversine)     terazosin (Hytrin)

*Note:* The suffix *azosin* is common to generic alpha-blocker drugs.

## *Did You Know?*

Some alpha-blocker drugs are also used to treat an enlarged prostate gland in men.

## Calcium Channel Blocker Drugs for Hypertension

Calcium channel blocker drugs block the movement of calcium ions into the heart muscle and smooth muscles in the blood vessels. This decreases the heart rate, dilates the arteries, and lowers the blood pressure. For a detailed description of this therapeutic effect see the In Depth feature box.

amlodipine (Norvasc)

clevidipine (Cleviprex)

diltiazem (Cardizem) (see ■ FIGURE 11–3)

felodipine (Plendil)

isradipine (DynaCirc)

nicardipine (Cardene)

nifedipine (Adalat CC, Procardia)

nisoldipine (Sular)

verapamil (Calan, Covera-HS)

*Note:* The suffix *-dipine* is common to generic calcium channel blocker drugs.

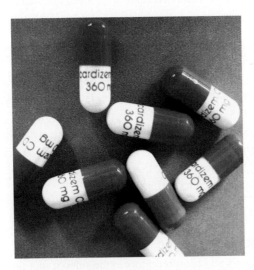

■ **FIGURE 11–3  Cardizem capsules.**
The capsule for the calcium channel blocker drug Cardizem is a distinctive blue and white color with the drug name and drug strength clearly printed on it. This is helpful for elderly patients who often take many different drugs at the same time. The generic name for this drug is diltiazem.

## *In Depth*

The pumping contraction of the heart muscle, as well as the contraction of smooth muscle in the blood vessels, depends on the flow of calcium ions from outside to inside each cell. These calcium ions move into the cell through calcium channels in the cell membrane. Calcium channel blocker drugs prevent the movement of calcium into the cell. With less calcium inside the cell, it contracts less strongly and less often. This causes the blood vessels to dilate, and the heart muscle contracts less forcefully and less frequently; both of these effects decrease the blood pressure.

## ACE Inhibitor Drugs for Hypertension

Angiotensin-converting enzyme (ACE) inhibitor drugs have an antihypertensive effect that is distinctly different from that of the other drugs described previously. ACE inhibitor drugs block an enzyme in the blood that converts angiotensin I to angiotensin II. Angiotensin II is a vasoconstrictor.

When the enzyme is blocked, angiotensin II is not produced, the blood vessels dilate, and this decreases the blood pressure. See the In Depth feature box on the next page.

benazepril (Lotensin)          moexipril (Univasc)

captopril (Capoten)          perindopril (Aceon)

enalapril (Vasotec)          quinapril (Accupril) (see ■ FIGURE 11-4)

fosinopril (Monopril)          ramipril (Altace)

lisinopril (Prinivil, Zestril)          trandolapril (Mavik) (see ■ FIGURE 11-5)

*Note:* The suffix *-pril* is common to generic ACE inhibitor drugs.

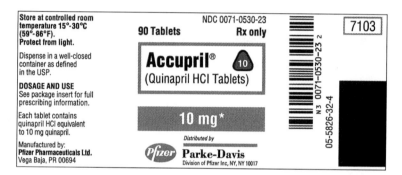

■ **FIGURE 11-4 Drug label for quinapril (Accupril).**
This ACE inhibitor drug blocks the production of angiotensin II, a vasoconstrictor. With less angiotensin II, the blood vessels dilate, which lowers the blood pressure. The dose strength for this form of the drug is 10 mg, although it also comes in other strengths.

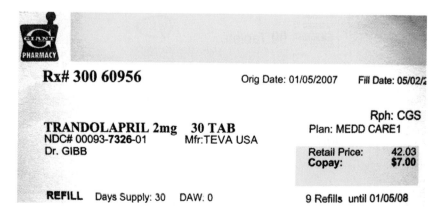

■ **FIGURE 11-5 Prescription label for trandolapril.**
This prescription was filled with the generic ACE inhibitor drug trandolapril, rather than with the trade name drug Mavik. This saves the patient money because the cost of a generic name drug is always less than a trade name drug.

## In Depth

The body has its own natural blood pressure-regulating system. In response to low blood pressure, the kidneys secrete renin, which then helps to produce angiotensin I. Angiotensin I is a relatively inactive substance, but when acted upon by angiotensin-converting enzyme (ACE), it becomes angiotensin II, a strong vasoconstrictor that raises the blood pressure.

ACE inhibitor drugs keep angiogensin-converting enzyme from changing angiotensin I into angiotensin II. Angiotensin II receptor blocker drugs keep angiotensin II from binding to and activating receptors on the smooth muscle of the blood vessels.

## Angiotensin II Receptor Blocker Drugs for Hypertension

Angiotensin II receptor blocker drugs keep angiotensin II from binding to and activating receptors on the smooth muscle of the blood vessel. This allows the smooth muscle to relax (vasodilation) and the blood pressure decreases.

candesartan (Atacand)                    olmesartan (Benicar)

eprosartan (Teveten)                      telmisartan (Micardis)

irbesartan (Avapro)                       valsartan (Diovan)

losartan (Cozaar) (see ■ FIGURE 11–6)

*Note:* The suffix *-sartan* is common to generic angiotensin II receptor blocker drugs.

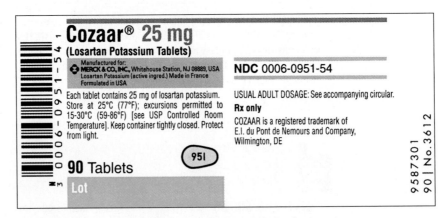

■ **FIGURE 11–6 Drug label for losartan (Cozaar).**
Losartin (Cozaar) is an angiotensin II receptor blocker drug that blocks angiotensin II from activating a receptor and causing vasodilation. This drug is used to treat hypertension.

## Renin Inhibitor Drugs for Hypertension

This drug blocks renin produced by the kidney. With less renin, less angiotension I is produced and so the smooth muscle in the blood vessels relaxes, the blood vessels dilate, and the blood pressure decreases.

aliskiren (Tekturna)

## Aldosterone Receptor Inhibitor Drugs for Hypertension

Aldosterone is produced by the cortex of the adrenal gland. Its action is to increase the reabsorption of sodium from the kidney tubules back into the blood. As sodium moves back into the blood, it brings water with it by the process of osmosis, and this increases the blood pressure. This drug blocks the action of aldosterone and this lowers the blood pressure.

eplerenone (Inspra)

## Peripheral Vasodilator Drugs for Hypertension

Peripheral vasodilator drugs relax the smooth muscle in the blood vessels and cause the blood vessels to dilate. This decreases the blood pressure.

hydralazine (Apresoline)

minoxidil

### *Did You Know?*

Minoxidil is also marketed under the trade name Rogaine and is used to treat thinning hair and baldness in men and women. Applied topically to the scalp, its vasodilator effect reestablishes blood flow to the hair follicles, resulting in new hair growth.

## Other Drugs for Hypertension

These drugs stimulate alpha$_2$ receptors in the vasomotor center of the brain. Stimulating these receptors decreases the number of nerve impulses sent by the sympathetic division of the nervous system to the adrenal medulla. The adrenal medulla secretes less epinephrine; this decreases the heart rate and allows the blood vessels to dilate, which lowers the blood pressure.

clonidine (Catapres)              guanfacine (Tenex)

guanabenz (Wytensin)              methyldopa

This drug depletes the store of epinephrine in the adrenal medulla so that it is not available to stimulate alpha and beta receptors in the heart and blood vessels.

reserpine

## Combination Drugs for Hypertension

These combination drugs contain an antihypertensive drug (from the categories listed below) and/or a diuretic drug (bendroflumethiazide, chlorthalidone, hydrochlorothiazide).

- beta-blocker drug (atenolol, bisoprolol, metoprolol, nadolol, propranolol, timolol)
- ACE inhibitor drug (benazepril, enalapril, fosinopril, lisinopril, quinapril, trandolapril)
- calcium channel blocker drug (amlodipine, verapamil)
- renin inhibitor drug (aliskiren)
- angiotensin II receptor blocker drug (candesartan, irbesartan, losartan, telmisartan, valsartan)

Accuretic (quinapril, hydrochlorothiazide)

Atacand HCT (candesartan, hydrochlorothiazide)

Avalide (irbesartan, hydrochlorothiazide)

Corzide (nadolol, bendroflumethiazide)

Diovan HCT (valsartan, hydrochlorothiazide)

Exforge (amlodipine, valsartan)

Hyzaar (losartan, hydrochlorothiazide)

Inderide (propranolol, hydrochlorothiazide)

Lopressor HCT (metoprolol, hydrochlorothiazide)

Lotensin HCT (benazepril, hydrochlorothiazide)

Lotrel (amlodipine, benazepril)

Micardis HCT (telmisartan, hydrochlorothiazide)

Monopril HCT (fosinopril, hydrochlorothiazide)

Prinzide (lisinopril, hydrochlorothiazide)

Tarka (trandolapril, verapamil)

Tekturna HCT (aliskiren, hydrochlorothiazide)

Tenoretic (atenolol, chlorthalidone)

Timolide (timolol, hydrochlorothiazide)

Vaseretic (enalapril, hydrochlorothiazide)

Zestoretic (lisinopril, hydrochlorothiazide)

Ziac (bisoprolol, hydrochlorothiazide)

*Note:* Combination drugs that include hydrochlorothiazide often reflect this by including the abbreviation *HCT* in their trade names.

## Drugs Used to Treat Hyperlipidemia

Hyperlipidemia is a category that encompasses both hypercholesterolemia (an increased level of serum cholesterol) and hypertriglyceridemia (an increased level of serum triglycerides). Hyperlipidemia is one of several well-defined risk factors for atherosclerosis.

Dietary therapy rather than drug therapy is the first choice of treatment for hyperlipidemia. In addition, these lifestyle changes may be recommended: exercise, weight loss, decreased alcohol consumption, or cessation of smoking. If diet and lifestyle changes are not enough to decrease the cholesterol level, then drug therapy is added. Hypercholesterolemia is treated with bile acid sequestrant drugs and HMG-CoA reductase inhibitor drugs. Hypertriglyceridemia is treated with other drugs.

### *In Depth*

Cholesterol is produced by the liver, and a certain amount of cholesterol is needed by the body for the production of hormones and bile and as a component of skin and nerve fibers. However, excess dietary intake of cholesterol can cause an elevated serum cholesterol level. Dietary sources of cholesterol include foods of animal origin, such as meats, egg yolks, bacon, shrimp, cream, lard, and so forth. Some patients develop an extremely high serum cholesterol level, not because of excess dietary intake, but because they have a genetic disorder with too few receptors on the cell membranes for cholesterol to bind to, and so the cholesterol level in the blood remains high.

Triglycerides are produced by the liver and are used to make subcutaneous fat to cushion and protect the body. However, excess dietary intake of nonanimal fats can result in excessive storage of fat in the body and a high triglyceride level in the blood. Dietary sources of triglycerides include oils and margarines. Also of interest is that an excess dietary intake of sugar is converted into triglycerides. Alcoholics often have an extremely elevated serum triglyceride level. Alcoholic beverages contain no nutrients except sugar. The large number of calories contained in alcoholic beverages is converted to triglycerides.

Just as water and oil do not mix, so fats and lipids (cholesterol and triglycerides) do not mix with the serum portion of the blood. To be transported through the blood, cholesterol and triglycerides must bind to certain carrier molecules, which are known as **lipoproteins**. There are three types of lipoproteins. High-density lipoproteins (HDLs) carry cholesterol to the liver where it is excreted in the bile. High levels of HDL are desirable. Low-density lipoproteins (LDLs) carry cholesterol to the cells where it is metabolized for energy. However, they also deposit cholesterol on artery walls to form arteriosclerotic plaques. High levels of LDL are undesirable. Very low-density lipoproteins (VLDLs) carry triglycerides. High levels of VLDL are undesirable.

## Bile Acid Sequestrant Drugs for Hypercholesterolemia

Cholesterol from the blood is used by the liver to produce bile. Bile is stored in the gallbladder and released to digest dietary fats in the intestine. Most of the bile is then reabsorbed from the intestine back into the blood and reused by the liver. If the serum cholesterol level is elevated, bile acid sequestrant drugs are given orally; they bind with bile, forming an insoluble complex that is excreted in the feces, taking the cholesterol with it. *Sequester* means *to remove and keep hidden*. Because the bile is not reabsorbed, the liver must draw cholesterol from the blood to produce a new supply of bile. This lowers the level of cholesterol in the blood.

cholestyramine (Prevalite, Questran)

colesevelam (WelChol)

colestipol (Colestid)

### *Did You Know?*

Oatmeal is effective in lowering the cholesterol level in the blood. The oat fiber binds to bile in the intestine and keeps it from being reabsorbed back into the blood. This is the same action as some bile acid sequestrant prescription drugs! In 1997, the FDA allowed companies to submit research that showed the health benefits of their food products. So for 10 years, the Quaker Oats company has been able to publicize the cholesterol-lowering effects of oatmeal, when coupled with a healthy diet and exercise.

## HMG-CoA Reductase Inhibitor Drugs for Hypercholesterolemia

HMG-CoA reductase is an enzyme that is involved in one of the steps in the production of cholesterol in the body. HMG-CoA reductase inhibitor drugs block this enzyme. These drugs also increase the level of high-density lipoproteins (HDL) that carry cholesterol to the liver, where it can be excreted in the bile. These drugs are also known as *statin drugs* because their generic drug names end in the suffix *-statin*. Patients taking statin drugs are tested periodically for liver function abnormalities.

atorvastatin (Lipitor) (see ▨ FIGURE 11–7)       pravastatin (Pravachol)

fluvastatin (Lescol)                              rosuvastatin (Crestor)

lovastatin (Mevacor)                              simvastatin (Zocor) (see ▨ FIGURE 11–8)

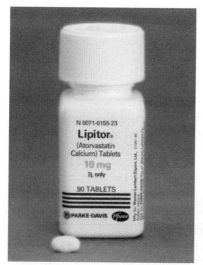

▨ **FIGURE 11–7  Bottle of atorvastatin (Lipitor).**
Atorvastatin (Lipitor) is an HMG-CoA reductase inhibitor drug used to treat hypercholesterolemia. In the past, Lipitor television advertisements featured Dr. Robert Jarvik, the inventor of the artificial heart, who takes Lipitor.

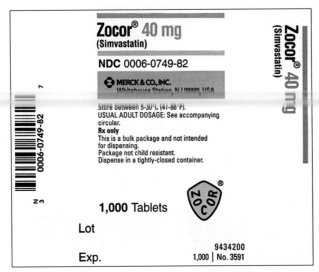

■ **FIGURE 11–8  Drug label for simvastatin (Zocor).**
Simvastatin (Zocor) is an HMG-CoA reductase inhibitor drug used to treat an elevated level of serum cholesterol.

## *Did You Know?*

In 2001, the drug company that makes lovastatin (Mevacor) asked the FDA to allow this drug to be offered as an OTC drug, but the FDA would not approve this change. By law, an over-the-counter drug must be one for which the patient can easily monitor his or her own condition, one that has a low rate of side effects/toxicity, and one that does not require any special monitoring or ongoing tests. Lovastatin did not meet these criteria.

There is an over-the-counter food supplement (brand name Cholestin) that contains red yeast fermented either on rice or honeybee pollen. Its active ingredient is a naturally occurring form of the cholesterol-lowering prescription drug lovastatin. The food supplement has been used in China under the name Hong Qu for over 2,000 years to promote cardiovascular health.

## Drugs for Hypercholesterolemia and Hypertriglyceridemia

These drugs reduce the serum level of cholesterol, reduce the amount of the lipoprotein carrier LDL, and reduce the serum level of triglycerides. They also increase the amount of the lipoprotein carrier HDL.

ezetimibe (Zetia)

fenofibrate (Tricor)

niacin (Niacor, Niaspan)

omega-3 fatty acids (Promega Pearls)

## Other Drugs for Hyperlipidemia

This drug decreases the production of triglycerides in the liver and inhibits the synthesis of the lipoprotein carrier VLDL, as well as accelerating its breakdown. This results in a lower serum level of triglycerides and less VLDL to carry triglycerides in the blood.

gemfibrozil (Lopid)

## *Did You Know?*

Omega-3 fatty acids are found in the oil of cold water fish. While the American Heart Association recommends eating fish, it does not endorse the use of fish oil supplements.

## Combination Drugs

This combination drug contains a calcium channel blocker drug (amlodipine) to treat hypertension and an HMG-CoA reductase inhibitor drug (atorvastatin) to lower the serum cholesterol level.

Caduet (amlodipine, atorvastatin)

These combination drugs contain an HMG-CoA reductase inhibitor drug (lovastatin, simvastatin) and another drug (ezetimibe, niacin), both of which lower the serum cholesterol level.

Advicor (lovastatin, niacin)

Simcor (simvastatin, niacin)

Vytorin (ezetimibe, simvastatin)

# Drugs Used to Treat Congestive Heart Failure

Congestive heart failure (CHF) occurs when the heart muscle is weakened by disease or a structural defect (leaky valve) and is unable to adequately pump blood. Right-sided heart failure causes a backup of blood from the right ventricle into the venous circulation, producing distended neck veins, liver enlargement, and peripheral edema in the extremities. Left-sided heart failure causes a backup of blood from the left ventricle into the pulmonary circulation, producing pulmonary edema in the lungs. Drugs used to treat congestive heart failure help the heart to beat more slowly but contract more forcefully. Diuretic drugs can also be given to help the body excrete the excess fluid of edema in the urine. Drugs used to treat congestive heart failure include digitalis drugs, ACE inhibitor drugs, angiotensin II receptor blocker drugs, and other drugs.

## Digitalis Drugs for Congestive Heart Failure

Digitalis drugs make the heart pump more slowly, but more strongly. Digitalis drugs are also known as *cardiac glycoside drugs* because they have a molecular structure that consists of chains of glucose sugars known as *glycosides* and they are used to treat the heart (cardiac). For a detailed description of their therapeutic effect, see the In Depth feature box. This digitalis drug is used to treat congestive heart failure.

digoxin (Digitek, Lanoxicaps, Lanoxin) (see ■ **FIGURE 11–9**)

## *In Depth*

Digitalis drugs cause the release of acetylcholine, a neurotransmitter that depresses the SA node in the heart; this slows the electrical conduction and the heart rate. This action is known as a **negative chronotropic effect**. (*Chron/o-* means *time.*) Digitalis drugs also inhibit the flow of positive sodium ions into the cell; instead, positive calcium ions flow in and this results in a stronger, more forceful contraction of the myocardial cells. This action is known as a **positive inotropic effect**. (*In/o-* means [cardiac muscle] *fibers.*) The negative chronotropic effect in combination with the positive inotropic effect allows the heart to pump more slowly, to fill completely with blood before the next contraction—an important therapeutic effect for patients with congestive heart failure—and then to contract strongly.

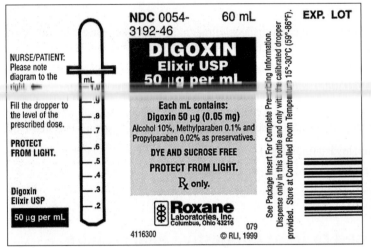

■ **FIGURE 11–9 Drug label for digoxin.** Although most cases of congestive heart failure occur in the elderly, some children with heart defects can also develop congestive heart failure. As is common with many pediatric drugs, this liquid digoxin elixir is administered with a special dropper calibrated in 0.1 mL increments. The drug strength of 50 µg/mL on the label is equal to 0.05 mg/mL.

## Did You Know?

In the past, the dried foxglove plant was used to treat congestive heart failure. This plant was given the Latin name *Digitalis lanata* because its flowers resembled digits or fingers, and the drug derived from it was called digitalis. The modern drug digoxin is the only digitalis drug that remains on the market. Physicians often use a slang term—*dig* (pronounced "dij")—to refer to digoxin.

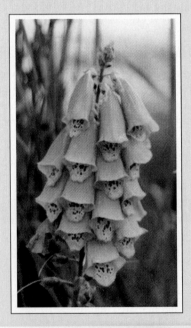

## Historical Notes

Foxglove was given its botanical name *Digitalis* in the 1500s. In the 1780s, an English physician stated, "My opinion was asked concerning a family recipe for the cure of dropsy [an old word for *congestive heart failure*]. I was told that it had long been kept a secret by an old woman in Shropshire who had sometimes made cures after the regular practitioners had failed . . . This medicine was composed of 20 or more different herbs; but it was not very difficult for one conversant in these subjects to perceive that the active herb could be none other than foxglove." Michael C. Gerald, *Pharmacology: An Introduction to Drugs,* 2nd ed. (Englewood Cliffs, NJ: Prentice Hall, 1981), p. 402, out of print.

## *Focus on Healthcare Issues*

Digitalis toxicity is a serious adverse effect. Nearly one-third of patients taking a digitalis drug develop symptoms of digitalis toxicity. This is because these drugs have a low **therapeutic index** (i.e., there is a narrow margin between the therapeutic dose and the toxic dose) and a long **half-life**, which is even more prolonged in elderly patients with decreased kidney function. Symptoms of toxicity include a pulse rate below 60 beats per minute, confusion, restlessness, nausea and vomiting, diarrhea, hallucinations, or seeing yellow-green halos around lights (see ■ **FIGURE 11–10**). To prevent toxic effects, physicians periodically order blood tests to monitor the drug level. These tests are often referred to as "dig levels" (pronounced "dij"). Symptoms of toxicity can be treated in one of three ways: (1) Decrease the dose of the digitalis drug, (2) give the digitalis drug less frequently, or, in severe cases, (3) administer an antidote drug to reverse the toxic effects of the digitalis drug.

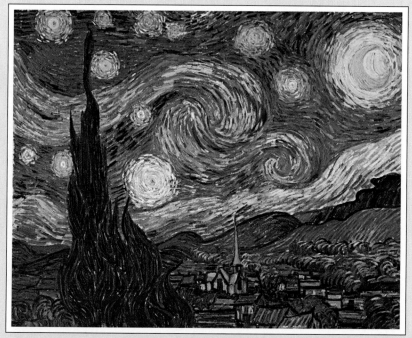

■ **FIGURE 11–10 Digitalis toxicity.**
Vincent van Gogh's *The Starry Night* (1889) is felt by some to show evidence of digitalis toxicity in the way the Dutch painter depicted yellow-green halos around the stars. Van Gogh (1853–1890) suffered from mania and epilepsy and may have been given digitalis for lack of a more specific drug therapy.

Vincent van Gogh, "The Starry Night," 1889. Oil on Canvas, 29 × 36 1/4 in. The Museum of Modern Art/Licensed by Scala-Art Resource, NY. Acquired through the Lillie P. Bliss Bequest. (472.1941) Photograph © 2000 The Museum of Modern Art, New York.

## Drugs for Digitalis Toxicity

Bile acid sequestrant drugs (cholestyramine, colestipol) bind with digitalis in the intestine and cause it to be excreted in the feces. The other use of bile acid sequestrant drugs, to decrease the serum cholesterol level, was discussed previously. Digoxin immune Fab is an antibody drug that is given intravenously; it binds with and inactivates a digitalis drug in the blood, forming an antibody-antigen complex that is excreted in the urine.

cholestyramine (Prevalite, Questran)

colestipol (Colestid)

digoxin immune Fab (Digibind, Digidote)

These drugs are specifically used to treat ventricular arrhythmias caused by digitalis toxicity.

edetate (Endrate)

propranolol (Inderal)

## Did You Know?

Digoxin immune Fab is an antigen-binding fragment obtained from sheep that have been treated to produce antibodies against the basic molecule of digoxin. The word *Fab* in the generic drug name stands for *fragment, antibody binding*. The trade names Digibind and Digidote come from *digi-* for *digitalis* and *-bind* (to describe its binding action) or *-dote* for *antidote*.

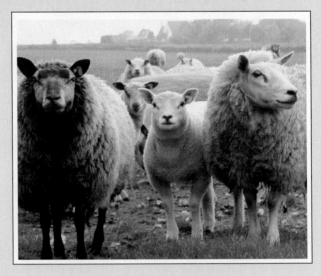

## Diuretic Drugs for Congestive Heart Failure

Diuretic drugs are often used in conjunction with digitalis drugs to treat patients with congestive heart failure. Diuretic drugs increase the excretion of sodium and water to reduce edema, a common symptom of congestive heart failure. For a complete discussion of diuretic drugs, see Chapter 7.

Unlike other diuretic drugs which treat edema associated with many different diseases, this diuretic drug is only used to treat the edema associated with congestive heart failure.

acetazolamide (Diamox Sequels)

### ACE Inhibitor Drugs for Congestive Heart Failure

Angiotensin-converting enzyme (ACE) inhibitor drugs block the enzyme that converts angiotensin I to angiotensin II, a vasoconstrictor. By blocking this enzyme, ACE inhibitor drugs cause vasodilation and decrease the blood pressure, the resistance against which the heart must pump. This allows the heart to pump with less effort. ACE inhibitor drugs (captopril, enalapril, fosinopril, lisinopril, quinapril, ramipril, and trandolapril) are used to treat hypertension and are used in conjunction with digitalis drugs and diuretic drugs to treat congestive heart failure. These drugs were discussed in a previous section.

### Angiotensin II Receptor Blocker Drugs for Congestive Heart Failure

Angiotensin II receptor blocker drugs block the action of angiotensin II, which allows the smooth muscle in the blood vessels to dilate and the blood pressure decreases. This allows the heart to pump with less effort. Only these angiotensin II receptor blocker drugs are specifically indicated for congestive heart failure.

> candesartan (Atacand)
>
> valsartan (Diovan)

### Other Drugs for Congestive Heart Failure

This drug blocks both alpha receptors, $beta_1$ receptors in the heart, and $beta_2$ receptors in the smooth muscle of the blood vessels to lower the blood pressure against which the heart must pump.

> carvedilol (Coreg)

This aldosterone receptor inhibitor drug blocks the action of aldosterone and this lowers the blood pressure against which the heart must pump.

> eplerenone (Inspra)

### Drugs for Severe Congestive Heart Failure

These drugs are used to treat severe congestive heart failure that has not responded to digitalis drugs, diuretic drugs, and other drugs. These drugs are only given intravenously.

These inotropic drugs increase the strength of contraction of the heart muscle.

> inamrinone
>
> milrinone (Primacor)

These vasopressor drugs stimulate $beta_1$ receptors in the heart to increase the heart rate in patients with severe congestive heart failure.

> dobutamine
>
> dopamine

This human B-type natriuretic peptide drug binds to receptors on the smooth muscle of both arteries and veins and causes them to relax, decreasing the blood pressure and the pressure against which the heart must pump. This drug is manufactured from *E. coli* bacteria using recombinant DNA technology.

> nesiritide (Natrecor)

## Drugs Used to Treat Angina Pectoris

The pain of angina pectoris occurs when cells of the myocardium receive insufficient oxygenated blood to meet their needs. This can occur during exercise or stress, when the need for oxygen increases. Angina pectoris can be caused by plaques in the coronary arteries that occlude the flow of blood, spasm of the coronary arteries, or vasoconstriction of the arteries due to smoking. It can also be due to an increased **afterload** (the pressure of the arterial system against which the heart must pump) or an increased **preload** (the pressure of the pulmonary circulatory system and the pressure in the left ventricle during diastole). The pain of angina pectoris denotes cellular ischemia but not cellular death of the heart muscle cells. If untreated, however, this ischemia can progress to cellular death (i.e., a myocardial infarction). Drugs used to treat angina pectoris include nitrate drugs, beta-blocker drugs, calcium channel blocker drugs, and other drugs.

## Nitrate Drugs for Angina Pectoris

Nitrate drugs dilate the coronary arteries and increase the flow of oxygenated blood to the myocardium. They also dilate arteries and veins throughout the circulatory system. By dilating the arteries, they decrease arterial blood pressure and afterload. By dilating the veins, these drugs reduce preload and decrease the need of the myocardium for oxygen. The most frequently prescribed nitrate drug is nitroglycerin.

amyl nitrite

isosorbide dinitrate (Isordil)

isosorbide mononitrate (Imdur, ISMO)

nitroglycerin (Minitran, Nitro-Dur, Nitrostat)

Nitrate drugs can be administered in several different ways: sublingually as a tablet, translingually as a spray, inhaled as vapors through the nose, orally as a sustained-release capsule or tablet, transdermally as a patch, topically as an ointment (measured in inches), or intravenously. However, not every nitrate drug can be administered by every route.

### *Did You Know?*

In the mid-1890s, physicians observed that the pain of angina pectoris seemed to be relieved in those patients who worked in dynamite factories where nitroglycerin was an ingredient in the manufacturing process. This led to prescribing nitroglycerin for angina, a practice that has continued to the present time.

Physicians often dictate "nitro paste" when the correct drug form is actually nitroglycerin ointment. Topical nitroglycerin (Nitro-Bid, Nitrol) is an ointment that is applied to the skin using an applicator paper that has a measuring line on it. The ointment dose is measured in inches.

## Beta-Blocker Drugs for Angina Pectoris

Although nitrate drugs, particularly nitroglycerin, are the standard for antianginal therapy, beta-blocker drugs may also be prescribed. Beta-blocker drugs decrease the heart rate, which decreases the need of the myocardium for oxygen; this decreases the pain of angina. Only the beta-blocker drugs atenolol, metoprolol, nadolol, and propranolol are used to treat angina pectoris. This category of drugs was previously discussed in the section on hypertension.

## Calcium Channel Blocker Drugs for Angina Pectoris

Calcium channel blocker drugs are used in conjunction with nitrate drugs or beta-blocker drugs to treat angina. Calcium channel blocker drugs cause the smooth muscle in the coronary arteries to dilate, and this allows more blood to flow through them to the myocardium. Only the calcium channel blocker drugs amlodipine, diltiazem, nicardipine, nifedipine, and verapamil are used to treat angina pectoris. This category of drug was previously discussed in the section on hypertension.

### Other Drugs for Angina Pectoris

Anticoagulant drugs, such as warfarin, platelet aggregation inhibitor drugs (including low-dose aspirin), and thrombin inhibitor drugs are used in patients with angina pectoris to prevent a blood clot that would cause a myocardial infarction. These drugs are discussed in Chapter 12.

This drug increases blood flow to the heart. The exact action by which it treats angina pectoris is not known.

ranolazine (Ranexa)

### Combination Drugs for Angina Pectoris

This combination drug contains a peripheral vasodilator drug (hydralazine) and a nitrate drug to dilate the coronary arteries.

BiDil (hydralazine, isosorbide dinitrate)

## Drugs Used to Treat Myocardial Infarction

When myocardial cell ischemia associated with angina pectoris is not treated, it may progress to cellular death, which is known as a *myocardial infarction*. Once the tissue has died, this process cannot be reversed. However, drugs can be given to limit the extent of the area of dead tissue and to improve the survival rate following a myocardial infarction.

Thrombolytic drugs can be given to dissolve clots in the coronary arteries at the time of a myocardial infarction to prevent more cells from dying. Thrombolytic drugs are discussed in Chapter 12.

Some beta-blocker drugs (atenolol, metoprolol, propranolol, timolol), some alpha/beta-blocker drugs (carvedilol), some ACE inhibitor drugs (captopril, lisinopril), an angiotensin II receptor blocker drug (valsartan), and an aldosterone receptor inhibitor drug (eplerenone) are used to improve survival rates after a myocardial infarction.

Platelet aggregation inhibitor drugs are used to prevent blood clots in patients who have already had a myocardial infarction. These drugs are discussed in Chapter 12.

## Drugs Used to Treat Arrhythmias

Cardiac arrhythmias are caused by abnormalities in the conduction of electrical impulses from the SA node through the rest of the conduction system of the heart. Disruptions in the conduction path, as well as changes in the normal period of time between beats, can result in various arrhythmias involving the atria or ventricles. Arrhythmias include bradycardia (abnormally slow heart rate), heart block, tachycardia (abnormally fast heart rate), atrial flutter and fibrillation (very rapid contractions of the atria that are not coordinated with the ventricles), ventricular flutter (very rapid contractions of the ventricles), ventricular fibrillation (ineffective, extremely rapid twitching of the ventricle), or asystole (no heart contractions).

### Drugs for Bradycardia

Bradycardia is a heart rate of less than 60 beats per minute. Normally, the vagus nerve (of the parasympathetic division of the nervous system) releases the neurotransmitter acetylcholine to keep the heart in a slow, normal rhythm. This drug blocks acetylcholine receptors in the heart, and the heart rate increases.

atropine

## Drugs for Heart Block

These drugs are used to treat heart block, in which only some or none of the electrical impulses from the SA node are able to travel through the conduction system to the ventricles.

ephedrine

isoproterenol (Isuprel)

## Drugs for Tachycardia

These drugs are used to treat ventricular tachycardia, a fast but regular heart rate of up to 200 beats per minute. Some of these drugs are also used to treat premature ventricular contractions (PVCs).

Beta-blocker drugs block beta receptors in the heart from responding to epinephrine. Epinephrine, which is normally secreted by the adrenal medulla through the action of the sympathetic division of the nervous system, increases the heart rate. By blocking epinephrine, beta-blocker drugs slow the heart rate.

| | |
|---|---|
| acebutolol (Sectral) | propranolol (Inderal) |
| esmolol (Brevibloc) | sotalol (Betapace) |

Calcium channel blocker drugs slow the movement of calcium in and out of the SA node, which causes the heart to beat more slowly.

diltiazem (Cardizem)

verapamil (Calan, Covera-HS)

These drugs are also used to treat ventricular tachycardia.

| | |
|---|---|
| adenosine (Adenocard) | moricizine (Ethmozine) |
| amiodarone (Cordarone) | procainamide (Pronestyl) |
| disopyramide (Norpace) | propafenone (Rythmol) |
| flecainide (Tambocor) | quinidine |
| mexiletine (Mexitil) | |

## Drugs for Atrial Flutter and Fibrillation

These antiarrhythmic drugs are used to treat atrial flutter or atrial fibrillation. Clonidine stimulates alpha$_2$ receptors in the brain; this decreases sympathetic nerve impulses and slows the heart rate. Digoxin, also used to treat congestive heart failure, stimulates the release of acetylcholine from the vagus nerve, which slows the heart rate. Dofetilide blocks the flow of potassium ions into the heart cell, and this delays the contraction of the heart muscle. Ibutilide prolongs the refractory period (time between beats when the heart muscle is normally unresponsive) by causing sodium ions to move into the heart cells.

| | |
|---|---|
| clonidine (Catapres) | dofetilide (Tikosyn) |
| digoxin (Lanoxicaps, Lanoxin) | ibutilide (Corvert) |

Beta-blocker drugs block epinephrine from reaching and stimulating beta receptors in the heart, and this slows atrial flutter and fibrillation.

propranolol (Inderal)

Calcium channel blocker drugs slow the movement of calcium in and out of the SA node, to treat atrial flutter and atrial fibrillation.

| | |
|---|---|
| diltiazem (Cardizem) | verapamil (Calan, Covera-HS) |

These drugs are also used to treat atrial flutter and atrial fibrillation.

| | |
|---|---|
| flecainide (Tambocor) | quinidine |
| propafenone (Rythmol) | |

*Did You Know?*

The antiarrhythmic drug Corvert takes its name from the Latin word *cor* (meaning *heart*) and the letters *-vert* (that stand for *convert* [the arrhythmia]).

### Drugs for Ventricular Fibrillation

Ventricular fibrillation is a very fast, but uncoordinated, quivering of the heart. This is a life-threatening emergency in which the heart is not able to pump blood to the body. These drugs are used to treat ventricular fibrillation, but they have no effect if the heart has already stopped (asystole, cardiac arrest).

> amiodarone (Cordarone) (see ▇ **FIGURE 11–11**)
>
> bretylium
>
> lidocaine (Xylocaine)

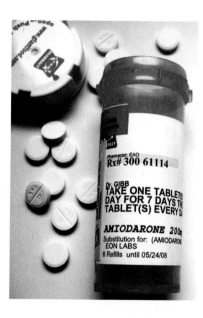

▇ **FIGURE 11–11  Prescription bottle for amiodarone.** Amiodarone (Cordarone) is an antiarrhythmic drug that is used only to treat ventricular tachycardia and ventricular fibrillation.

*Did You Know?*

The antiarrhythmic drug lidocaine (Xylocaine) is also a topical anesthetic drug. It inhibits the flow of sodium into nerve cells. This stops electrical impulses along sensory nerves, and then there is no transmission/perception of pain.

### Drugs for Asystole

In the body, the hormone epinephrine secreted by the adrenal medulla has the following actions:

- Stimulate alpha receptors to constrict the peripheral blood vessels and raise the blood pressure
- Stimulate beta$_1$ receptors in the heart to increase the heart rate and cardiac output
- Stimulate beta$_2$ receptors in the lungs to relax bronchial smooth muscle, dilate the bronchi, and increase air flow to the lungs.

The drug epinephrine (Adrenalin) has these same effects (see ■ FIGURE 11–12). In cardiac arrest (asystole), epinephrine can actually stimulate contractions of the myocardium. Epinephrine also makes the myocardium more responsive to the electrical impulse of a defibrillator to restore a normal rhythm. As epinephrine stimulates the heart to beat, it helps to maintain blood pressure and blood flow to the heart and brain to improve the chances of a successful resuscitative effort.

epinephrine (Adrenalin)

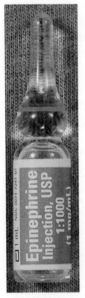

■ **FIGURE 11–12  Ampule of epinephrine.**
Epinephrine is given during resuscitation for a patient in cardiac arrest. This ampule of epinephrine contains a single dose. Once the ampule is broken open, it must be used or discarded because it contains no preservative.

## Drug Alert

The hormone epinephrine from the adrenal gland (it is also a neurotransmitter of the sympathetic division of the nervous system) is also known as *adrenaline* (a combination of the combining form *adrenal/o-* meaning *adrenal gland* and the suffix *-ine* meaning *substance pertaining to*). As a drug, epinephrine is the generic name drug, but Adrenalin (without a final "e") is the trade name drug. The slang word for the generic drug epinephrine is "epi."

## Drugs Used to Treat Peripheral Vascular Disease

Peripheral vasodilator drugs are used to increase peripheral blood flow to treat diseases such as arteriosclerosis obliterans, Buerger's disease, Raynaud's disease, and diabetic peripheral vascular insufficiency. These drugs selectively dilate blood vessels in the skeletal muscles.

isoxsuprine (Vasodilan)

papaverine

Patients with peripheral vascular disease often experience intermittent claudication (calf pain caused by ischemia) when they exercise. These drugs improve blood flow by keeping platelets from sticking together to block blood flow or by decreasing the thickness of the blood and increasing red blood cell flexibility.

cilostazol (Pletal)

pentoxifylline (Trental)

## Drugs Used to Treat Pulmonary Arterial Hypertension

Pulmonary arterial hypertension is characterized by hypertension within the lungs, arising from a variety of causes. The heart, as it pumps blood into the pulmonary arteries, is forced to work against this increased pressure and often develops right-sided congestive heart failure. Patients with this condition can require heart-lung transplantation. Calcium channel blocker drugs (amlodipine, diltiazem, felodipine, nifedipine) used to treat pulmonary arterial hypertension were previously discussed in the section on hypertension. These drugs relax the smooth muscle in the pulmonary arteries in the lungs, which allows the arteries to dilate and this lowers the pulmonary arterial pressure.

ambrisentan (Letairis)

beraprost

bosentan (Tracleer)

epoprostenol (Flolan)

iloprost (Ventavis)

sildenafil (Revatio)

treprostinil (Remodulin)

### Did You Know?

Sildenafil (Revatio) for pulmonary arterial hypertension is also available under the trade name Viagra and is used to treat erectile dysfunction in men. The underlying mechanism of action is the same: increase the blood flow to the affected organ.

## Drugs Used to Treat Hypertensive Crisis

A patient in hypertensive crisis exhibits an extremely high blood pressure. This can occur with malignant hyperthermia (caused by a reaction to an anesthetic drug) or because of severe preeclampsia during pregnancy, or because of untreated, severe hypertension. This is a life-threatening emergency. Most beta-blocker drugs, calcium channel blocker drugs, and peripheral vasodilator drugs, as described previously, can be given intravenously to quickly lower the blood pressure. In addition, these drugs are used exclusively to treat hypertensive crisis.

diazoxide (Hyperstat)

fenoldopam (Corlopam)

mecamylamine (Inversine)

nitroprusside (Nitropress)

phentolamine

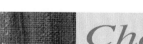

# Chapter Review

## Quiz Yourself

1. Describe the difference between the therapeutic effects of beta-blocker drugs versus cardio-selective beta-blocker drugs.
2. Name the categories of drugs used to treat hypertension and give an example of a drug from each category.
3. How do bile acid sequestrant drugs exert a therapeutic effect in patients with hyperlipidemia?
4. What two basic therapeutic effects do digitalis drugs exert on the heart?
5. As a student of both pharmacology and art history, what insightful comment might you make concerning Vincent van Gogh's painting, *The Starry Night*?
6. If a patient exhibits symptoms of digitalis toxicity, what three interventions can the physician choose from?

7. Given these suffixes, tell which category of drugs they are related to: *-olol, -pril, -sartan, -azosin,* and *-statin.*

8. Name five routes by which nitroglycerin can be administered.

9. Name the categories of drugs used to treat angina pectoris.

10. Fill in the blank. Foxglove : digoxin as sheep's antibodies : _____.

11. What drug used to treat ventricular arrhythmias is also used as a local anesthetic drug?

12. To what category does each of these drugs belong and what diseases are they used to treat?

a. atenolol (Tenormin)
b. atorvastatin (Lipitor)
c. atropine
d. Caduet
e. digoxin (Lanoxin)
f. diltiazem (Cardizem)
g. epinephrine (Adrenalin)

h. lidocaine (Xylocaine)
i. losartan (Cozaar)
j. nebivolol (Bystolic)
k. nitroglycerin (Nitrostat)
l. simvastatin (Zocor)
m. trandolapril (Mavik)
n. Vytorin

13. Define the abbreviations *ACE, CHF,* "*dig,*" "*epi,*" *Fab, HTN.*

## Spelling Tips

| | |
|---|---|
| **Catapres, Minipress, Nitropress** | One or two of the letter *s.* |
| **Cozaar, Hyzaar** | Unusual double *a.* |
| **DynaCirc** | Unusual internal capitalization. |
| **Nitro-Dur** | Unusual internal capitalization. |
| **Rythmol** | Does not have an *h* like the word *rhythm.* |
| **Vaseretic, Vasotec** | *Vase-* or *Vaso-.* |
| **WelChol** | Unusual internal capitalization. |

## Clinical Applications

1. Look at these photographs and answer the following questions.
   a. Research has shown that eating oatmeal can benefit your heart in what way?
   b. What category of prescription drugs has a similar action?

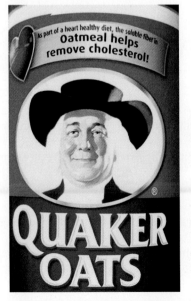

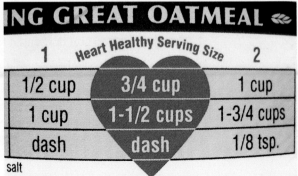

2. This patient is being admitted to the hospital to Dr. Smith's service. Review this patient's admission Physician's Order Sheet and answer the following questions.
   a. What is this patient's diagnosis?
   b. Does the patient have any drug allergies?
   c. The first drug prescribed for the patient is furosemide, a diuretic drug. What is its therapeutic effect in a patient with this diagnosis? Translate the drug order into English.
   d. What is the second drug that is ordered?
   e. What is the therapeutic effect of the second drug?
   f. For the second drug, write the dose strength and dose schedule in plain English.
   g. Translate the drug order for the third drug.
   h. Translate the drug order for the fourth drug.
   i. What a.m. blood work from the laboratory was ordered?

| PATIENT: | **MEMORIAL HOSPITAL** |
|---|---|
| AGE: | BALTIMORE, MARYLAND |
| SEX: | **PHYSICIAN'S ORDER RECORD** |
| RACE: | |
| CHART NO. | BEAR DOWN ON HARD SURFACE WITH BALL POINT PEN |

GENERIC EQUIVALENT IS AUTHORIZED UNLESS CHECKED IN THIS COLUMN

| ALLERGY OR SENSITIVITY | DIAGNOSIS | | COMPLETED OR DISCONTINUED |
|---|---|---|---|
| TO___ | | | |
| NONE KNOWN ☐   SIGNED:___ | | | |

| DATE | TIME | ORDERS | PHYSICIAN'S SIG. | NAME | DATE | TIME |
|---|---|---|---|---|---|---|
| | | Admit to Dr. Smith | Med C | | | |
| | | DX - CHF | | | | |
| | | Condition - Good | | | | |
| | | Diet: 500mg Na, 1200 Cal ADA fluid restrict to 1200 cc/d | | | | |
| | | allergies: Ø | | | | |
| | | Meds furosemide 20mg IV BID | | | | |
| | | Dig 0.25 mg on even days | | | | |
| | | NitroPaste - 1" q 6° | | | | |
| | | Isosorbide 2.5mg SL TID | | | | |
| | | Send urine for U/A Send pt. for CXR | | | | |
| | | AM Labs: Dig level | | | | |

PHARMACY COPY

3. Look at this photograph and answer the following questions.
   a. What is the name of this drug?
   b. To what category of drugs does it belong?
   c. What dose strength are the tablets in this prescription bottle?
   d. Give the trade name associated with this drug.
   e. List four cardiac diseases/conditions that this drug is used to treat.

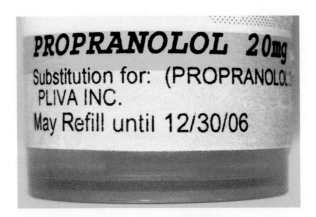

4. Look at this photograph and answer the following questions.
   a. What is the trade name of this drug?
   b. What is the generic name of this drug?
   c. To what category of drugs does it belong?
   d. What dose strength are the tablets of this drug?

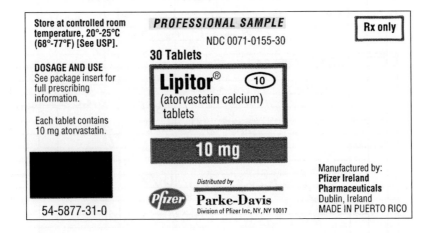

**5.** Look at this photograph and answer the following questions.
   **a.** What is the trade name of this drug?
   **b.** What is the generic name of this drug?
   **c.** To what category of drugs does it belong?
   **d.** What dose strength are the tablets of this drug?

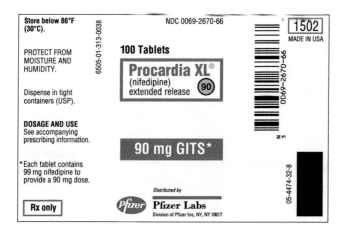

**6.** Look at these two photographs. These prescription bottles look alike, but they are not. How are they different?

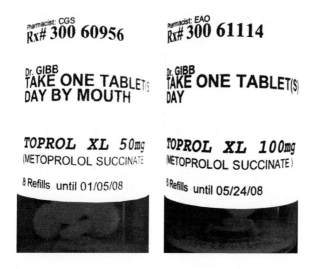

7. Look at this Physician's Order Sheet and answer the following questions.
   a. List the name of each prescribed drug. (There are six.)
   b. If the name is a generic name, give the trade name of the drug. (You do not need to do this for the last drug in the list.)
   c. Two of these drugs are not specifically given for patients with heart diseases. Identify those two drugs. (Hint: Look in Appendix D.)
   d. For the other four drugs, state what cardiac diseases they are used to treat.
   e. Translate the entire written prescription for those six drugs into plain English.

**GENERAL HOSPITAL** | MEDICINE

## FACE SHEET
### Page 1 of 2

NO ABBREVIATIONS

THIS FORM SHOULD BE COMPLETED PRIOR TO PATIENT'S DISCHARGE

| ADMISSION DATE | DISCHARGE DATE |
|---|---|
| 5/24/07 | 5/31/07 |

**PATIENT INSTRUCTI**

| ACTIVITY | ☑ NO RESTRICTIONS | ☐ RESTRICTIONS |
|---|---|---|

| DIET | ☐ NO RESTRICTIONS | ☑ RESTRICTIONS |
|---|---|---|

per recommendations for patients taking Coumadin

MEDICATIONS: Take all your medications in the manner prescribed. Carry your medication list with you at all times.

Amiodarone 200 mg twice a day for 1 week then once a day thereafter

Zoloft 25 mg once a day

MAVIK 2 mg once a day

Cardizem CD 360 mg once a day

Iron sulfate 325 mg once a day

Toprol XL 100 mg once a day

## Multimedia Extension Exercises

- Go to www.pearsonhighered.com/turley and click on the photo of the cover of *Understanding Pharmacology for Health Professionals* to access the interactive Companion Website created for this textbook.

# Hematologic Drugs

## CHAPTER CONTENTS

## Learning Objectives

After you study this chapter, you should be able to

1. Compare and contrast the therapeutic effect and route of administration of heparin with that of other anticoagulant drugs.

2. Explain how patients taking certain oral anticoagulant drugs must restrict their diet.

3. Differentiate between the therapeutic effects of anticoagulant drugs versus thrombolytic drugs.

4. Describe several different ways in which drugs are used to treat anemia.

5. Given the generic and trade names of a hematologic drug, identify what drug category they belong to.

6. Given a hematologic drug category, identify several generic and trade name drugs in that category.

Hematologic drugs are used to treat diseases of the blood. Hematologic drugs include anticoagulant drugs (heparin and oral anticoagulant drugs) to prevent clot formation, thrombolytic drugs to dissolve blood clots that have already formed, topical hemostatic drugs to stop bleeding, drugs to treat anemia, and drugs to treat hemophilia.

## Anticoagulant Drugs

Blood coagulates to form a blood clot following a complex cascading series of steps involving clotting factors, thromboplastin, and platelets. The liver produces clotting factors I through XIII. The formation of many of these clotting factors is dependent on the presence of vitamin K. When an injury occurs, the injured tissue releases tissue thromboplastin, and clotting factors in the blood are activated. Platelets stick to the damaged tissue to form clumps, a process known as *platelet aggregation.* The clotting factors eventually produce thrombin, then fibrinogen, and finally strands of fibrin. These strands trap red blood cells, and this forms a blood clot. Blood clots that form in arteries are mainly composed of platelet clumps. Blood clots that form in veins are mainly composed of fibrin strands and red blood cells.

Anticoagulant drugs are used to prevent a blood clot in patients with arteriosclerosis of the arteries, atrial fibrillation, acute coronary syndrome (unstable angina and myocardial infarction), a history of a previous myocardial infarction or stroke, or an artificial heart valve. Anticoagulant drugs are also used to prevent deep venous thrombosis (DVT) or pulmonary embolism in patients who are undergoing abdominal or joint replacement surgery and in patients who have sluggish blood flow because of poor mobility. Anticoagulant drugs are also used to provide anticoagulation during hemodialysis for patients in chronic renal failure or for patients on cardiopulmonary bypass during open heart surgery.

Anticoagulant drugs inhibit the action of clotting factors in the blood, or they inhibit the formation of those clotting factors in the liver that require the presence of vitamin K. Other anticoagulant drugs prevent platelets from adhering to the site of injury or prevent platelets from clumping together to begin the formation of a clot. Other anticoagulant drugs decrease the viscosity (thickness) of the blood and increase red blood cell flexibility to promote the flow of blood.

Anticoagulant drugs include heparin and low molecular weight heparin drugs, warfarin, platelet aggregation inhibitor drugs, thrombin inhibitor drugs, and factor Xa inhibitor drugs.

### Heparin and Low Molecular Weight Heparin Drugs

Heparin was the first anticoagulant drug. Heparin inhibits clotting factor X in the blood, which stops the series of steps needed to form a blood clot (see ■ FIGURE 12–1). Heparin is composed of large molecules that are not easily absorbed, and so only about 20 to 30 percent of a dose of heparin exerts a therapeutic effect. Heparin is always measured in units. Heparin is given subcutaneously or intravenously, never orally.

Low molecular weight heparin (LMWH) drugs (dalteparin, enoxaparin, and tinzaparin) were created by breaking apart the heparin molecule and decreasing the size of the molecule. These smaller molecules mean that almost the entire dose of low molecular weight heparin is absorbed and exerts a therapeutic effect. Low molecular weight heparin drugs also inhibit clotting factor X in the blood. Dalteparin and tinzaparin are measured in units (like heparin), but enoxaparin is measured in milligrams (mg). Low molecular weight heparins are given subcutaneously, never orally.

Both heparin and low molecular weight heparins are prepared from cows' or pigs' intestines. Patients receiving subcutaneous heparin or a low molecular weight heparin drug administered by a nurse in the hospital are switched to an oral anticoagulant drug before being discharged to home.

dalteparin (Fragmin)        heparin

enoxaparin (Lovenox)       tinzaparin (Innohep)

*Note:* The suffix *-parin* is common to generic heparin and low molecular weight heparin drugs.

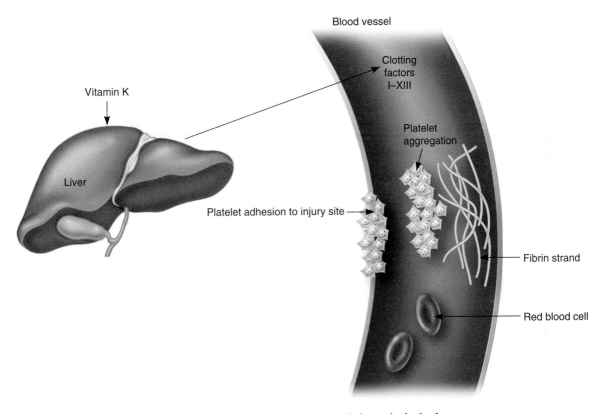

**■ FIGURE 12–1** **Therapeutic effects of anticoagulant and thrombolytic drugs.**
Heparin and low molecular weight heparins inhibit clotting factor X in the blood. Warfarin inhibits vitamin K that the liver uses to produce certain clotting factors. Platelet aggregation inhibitor drugs keep platelets from adhering to the site of injury and clumping together. Thrombin inhibitor drugs inhibit thrombin (activated factor II) in the blood from forming a clot. Factor Xa inhibitor drugs inhibit clotting factor Xa in the blood. Thrombolytic drugs break apart fibrin strands to dissolve already formed blood clots.

## *Clinical Applications*

A saline or heparin lock is a device that provides access for administering intravenous drugs without having intravenous fluids running continuously. The lock contains a reservoir of saline or heparin to keep the vein free of clots. Heparin was commonly used in the past but, because it can cause hemorrhaging and is incompatible with some drugs, saline is now most often used.

## Focus on Healthcare Issues

An increasingly large number of drugs and drug ingredients are manufactured outside the United States. In February 2008, Baxter International, which supplies one-half of the heparin used in the United States, announced it would discontinue its heparin product. This was because 350 serious allergic reactions or deaths were associated with Baxter's heparin product in the preceding three months. Baxter had obtained the active ingredient in its heparin product from a Chinese manufacturing plant. The FDA approved this company without inspecting it because it confused its name with that of another Chinese manufacturing plant that had already been inspected.

### Warfarin

The anticoagulant drug warfarin blocks vitamin K and keeps the liver from producing clotting factors that are dependent on the presence of vitamin K (see Figure 12–1). Without adequate levels of those clotting factors, the series of steps needed to form a blood clot is interrupted. Warfarin is measured in milligrams (mg) and is given orally (see ■ FIGURE 12–2).

warfarin (Coumadin, Jantoven)

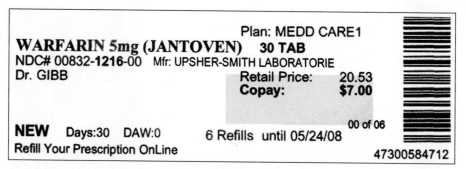

■ FIGURE 12–2 Label for prescription drug warfarin.
This patient's physician prescribed warfarin, a generic anticoagulant drug. The pharmacy filled the prescription with Jantoven, one of the trade names for warfarin. Coumadin is another trade name for the generic drug warfarin. The pharmacy could have filled the prescription with generic warfarin, Coumadin, or Jantoven. All of these drugs have the same anticoagulant effect, but there would be a difference in price between the generic name drug and the trade name drugs.

## Drug Alert!

Patients taking warfarin (Coumadin, Jantoven) for long-term anticoagulant therapy should monitor their dietary intake of certain types of foods. Leafy green vegetables (broccoli, Brussels sprouts, spinach, bok choi, kale, parsley, turnip greens), beef liver, garbanzo beans (chickpeas), and soy products (soybeans, soy milk, tofu) contain large amounts of vitamin K that can decrease the therapeutic effect of an anticoagulant drug. This is known as **antagonism**. On the other hand, garlic has its own natural anticoagulant effect that can multiply the effect of an anticoagulant drug. This is known as **synergism**.

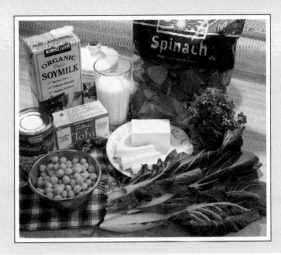

### Platelet Aggregation Inhibitor Drugs

Platelet aggregation inhibitor drugs prevent platelets from adhering to the site of injury or from clumping together (platelet aggregation) to begin the formation of a clot (see Figure 12–1). Some of these drugs block a receptor (glycoprotein IIb/IIIa) on the platelets to prevent the platelets from binding to fibrinogen (factor I).

Some platelet aggregation inhibitor drugs are used to prevent a blood clot in patients who are undergoing angioplasty, stent placement, or cardiac valve surgery. Others are used to prevent a blood clot in patients who have had a myocardial infarction or stroke, or to treat patients with acute coronary syndrome. One drug (cilostazol) is also a vasodilator and is used to treat peripheral vascular disease and intermittent claudication. Dipyridamole is given in conjunction with other anticoagulant drugs to enhance their effectiveness by specifically preventing platelets from adhering to artificial heart valves. These drugs are given orally, except for abciximab, ebtifibatide, and tirofiban, which are given intravenously.

abciximab (ReoPro)

aspirin (Bayer Children's Aspirin, Ecotrin Adult Low Strength)

cilostazol (Pletal)

clopidogrel (Plavix)

dipyridamole (Persantine)

eptifibatide (Integrilin)

tirofiban (Aggrastat)

### Combination Platelet Aggregation Inhibitor Drugs

This combination drug contains two platelet aggregation inhibitor drugs. It is given orally.

Aggrenox (aspirin, dipyridamole)

### Other Anticoagulant Drugs

This drug decreases blood viscosity (thickness) to prevent clots and increases red blood cell flexibility to improve blood flow.

pentoxifylline (Trental)

### Thrombin Inhibitor Drugs

Thrombin inhibitor drugs inhibit the action of thrombin. They bind to receptor sites on both circulating thrombin and thrombin already incorporated in a blood clot (see Figure 12–1). These drugs are used to prevent blood clots in patients with unstable angina who are undergoing coronary artery angioplasty or to prevent deep venous thrombosis in patients undergoing joint replacement surgery. Argatroban and lepirudin are used to prevent blood clots in patients with heparin-induced thrombocytopenia. These drugs are given intravenously, except for desirudin, which is given subcutaneously.

| | |
|---|---|
| argatroban | desirudin (Iprivask) |
| bivalirudin (Angiomax) | lepirudin (Refludan) |

*Note:* The suffix *–rudin* is common to generic thrombin inhibitor drugs.

### Factor Xa Inhibitor Drugs

Factor Xa inhibitor drugs inhibit the action of factor Xa, a subset of clotting factor X, in the blood (see Figure 12–1). They have no effect on thrombin or platelets. They are used to prevent or treat deep venous thrombosis or pulmonary embolism in patients undergoing joint replacement surgery or abdominal surgery. This drug is given subcutaneously.

fondaparinux (Arixtra)

## Thrombolytic Drugs

Because anticoagulant drugs can only prevent blood clots from forming (or enlarging once they are formed), but are not effective in dissolving blood clots, thrombolytic enzyme drugs and tissue plasminogen activator drugs are used to lyse (break apart) a blood clot once it has formed (see Figure 12–1). These drugs bind to fibrin strands in the clot and then convert plasminogen in the clot to plasmin. Plasmin (also known as *fibrinolysin*) is an enzyme that lyses fibrin. As the fibrin strands break apart, the clot dissolves.

### Thrombolytic Enzyme Drugs and Tissue Plasminogen Activator Drugs

Thrombolytic enzyme drugs were the first drugs that could actually dissolve a clot. Their appearance revolutionized the treatment of myocardial infarction and stroke. Only one of those original thrombolytic enzyme drugs is still on the market: streptokinase. Tissue plasminogen activator (tPA) drugs were created using recombinant DNA technology, although their action is essentially the same as that of a thrombolytic enzyme drug.

These drugs are given at the time of a myocardial infarction, stroke, or pulmonary embolism to dissolve a blood clot that has already formed in the coronary artery or within arteries to the brain or lung. Some of these drugs are used to treat deep venous thrombosis. Cathflo Activase is used to break up a blood clot that has formed within a central venous catheter. These drugs are given intravenously.

| | |
|---|---|
| alteplase (Activase, Cathflo Activase) | streptokinase (Streptase) |
| reteplase (Retavase) | tenecteplase (TNKase) |

*Note:* The suffix *–ase* (which means *enzyme*) is common to both the generic and trade names of thrombolytic drugs.

## Topical Hemostatic Drugs

Topical hemostatic drugs contain gelatin, collagen fibers, cellulose, fibrin, or thrombin in a liquid sealant or powder form. They are applied topically during surgery or dental procedures to control bleeding.

absorbable gelatin (Gelfilm, Gelfilm Ophthalmic, Gelfoam)

fibrin (Evicel)

microfibrillar collagen hemostat (Hemopad, Hemotene)

oxidized cellulose (Oxycel, Surgicel)

thrombin (Thrombogen, Thrombostat)

*Note:* The suffix *–cel* is common to trade name topical hemostatic drugs that contain cellulose.

## Drugs Used to Treat Anemia

Anemia is a decrease in the number of red blood cells (erythrocytes) produced by the red bone marrow. This can be due to insufficient amounts of amino acids, folic acid, iron, or vitamin $B_{12}$, all which are needed to form red blood cells. Anemia can also be caused by disease, cancer, radiation, or chemotherapy drugs that damage the red bone marrow where red blood cells are produced. Anemia can also result from excessive blood loss due to trauma or hemophilia. Anemia can also be caused by increased destruction of fragile red blood cells, as in sickle cell anemia.

Cyanocobalamin and hydroxocobalamin are vitamin $B_{12}$ drugs that are used to treat pernicious anemia. Darbepoetin alfa, epoetin alfa, and epoetin beta are erythropoietin-like drugs created with recombinant DNA technology; like natural erythropoietin (a hormone produced by the kidneys), these drugs stimulate red blood cell production and are used to treat various types of anemia. All of the generic drugs that have *ferrous* or *iron* in their names are iron supplements that are used to treat iron deficiency anemia. Folic acid is a B vitamin that is used to treat folic acid anemia (megaloblastic anemia). Oxymetholone is an anabolic steroid drug that is used to treat various types of anemia, as well as anemia caused by chemotherapy. These drugs are given by various routes.

cyanocobalamin (Cyomin, Nascobal)

darbepoetin alfa (Aranesp)

epoetin alfa (Epogen, Procrit) (see ■ FIGURE 12–3)

epoetin beta (Marogen)

epoetin beta-methoxy polyethylene glycol (Mircera)

ferrous fumarate (Ferro-Sequels, Hemocyte)

ferrous gluconate (Fergon)

ferrous sulfate (Feosol, Fer-In-Sol, Slow FE)

folic acid (Folvite)

hydroxocobalamin (Hydro-Crysti-12)

iron dextran

iron sucrose (Venofer)

oxymetholone (Anadrol-50)

sodium ferric gluconate (Ferrlecit)

## *Did You Know?*

The chemical symbol for *iron* is *Fe.* The adjective form for *iron* is *ferrous.*

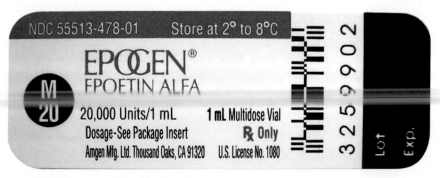

**■ FIGURE 12–3  Epoetin alfa (Epogen).**
The generic drug epoetin alfa (trade name Epogen) was created by DNA recombinant technology to mimic the action of erythropoietin, a hormone produced by the kidneys, that stimulates red blood cell production. Information on the label tells you the trade name and generic name of the drug, that Epogen comes in a vial, and that it contains 20,000 units per 1 mL.

## Drugs Used to Treat Hemophilia

Hemophilia is an inherited genetic abnormality that causes a deficiency of a specific clotting factor. Hemophilia A, caused by a lack of clotting factor VIII, is the most common type. Hemophilia B is caused by a lack of factor IX. Hemophilia C is caused by a lack of factor XI. Patients with hemophilia continue to bleed for long periods of time following even a minor injury. Bleeding into body cavities, organs, and joints causes pain and can cause death.

The drug Coagulin-B is the actual cellular gene that directs the liver to produce clotting factor IX. Factor VIIa, VIII, and IX are the actual blood clotting factors in a drug form. Other drugs specifically block inhibitor substances that some hemophiliac patients produce against factor VIII. Hemophiliac patients are also given blood transfusions or clotting factors derived from donated blood (see ■ **FIGURE 12–4**). These drugs are given intravenously.

anti-inhibitor coagulant complex (Feiba VH)

Coagulin-B

factor VIIa (NovoSeven)

factor VIII (Hemofil M, Recombinate, Xyntha)

factor IX (Bebulin VH, Mononine, Proplex T)

tranexamic acid (Cyklokapron)

### Combination Drugs for Hemophilia

This combination drug contains blood clotting factor VII plus von Willebrand factor to treat hemophilia A and von Willebrand disease.

Humate-P (factor VIII, von Willebrand factor)

## *Historical Notes*

The political climate we live in today was the indirect result of someone with hemophilia. Czar Nicholas of Russia and his wife Alexandra had four female children before they finally had Alexei, the heir to the throne. Unfortunately, Alexei had hemophilia (his mother was the carrier of the hemophilia gene) and was frequently near death. Obsessed with their son's illness, Czar Nicholas and Alexandra paid little attention to the affairs of state, the widespread economic depression, and the rising call for political reform. Because of this, the entire family was executed during the Bolshevik Revolution, thus ending the czarist form of government forever in Russia and paving the way for Lenin and the communist system of government.

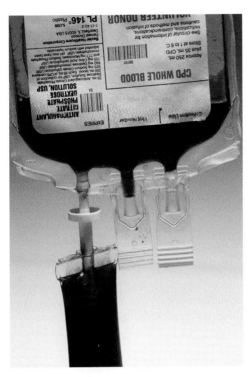

■ **FIGURE 12–4 Blood and blood products.**
Blood (units of whole blood) and blood products (plasma, packed red blood cells, clotting factors, and so forth) are often given to treat hematologic diseases such as anemia and hemophilia. The various types of blood and blood products are discussed in Chapter 24.

## Clinical Applications

Phytonadione (Mephyton) is a vitamin K drug that is given prophylactically to all newborns to prevent hemorrhagic disease of the newborn. Newborns' blood levels of vitamin K are less than 60 percent of normal. However, a one-time, intramuscular dose is sufficient to temporarily correct the deficiency until vitamin K levels become normal by six weeks of age. This drug is also used to treat bleeding disorders in patients whose livers do not make enough factor II, VII, IX, or X. It is also used to treat patients who have received an overdose of an anticoagulant drug.

Protamine sulfate is a heparin antagonist drug that binds with heparin to neutralize its anticoagulant effect. This drug is used to treat an overdose of heparin or reverse the therapeutic effect of heparin when it is administered during surgery.

# Chapter Review

## Quiz Yourself

1. Why do patients go home on oral anticoagulant drugs instead of heparin when discharged from the hospital?
2. What is the difference between heparin and low molecular weight heparin drugs?
3. What drug is given to reverse the therapeutic effect of heparin?
4. Describe the difference between the therapeutic effect of oral anticoagulant drugs and that of thrombolytic enzymes.
5. What suffix is common to generic thrombolytic drugs?
6. Name six foods that decrease the effectiveness of the oral anticoagulant drug warfarin (Coumadin, Jantoven).

7. Name several topical hemostatic trade name drugs that are used to control bleeding during surgery or dental procedures.
8. What is the difference between the source of erythropoietin and the source of the drug epoetin alfa?
9. What is the name of the vitamin B drug that is used to treat megaloblastic anemia?
10. The suffix *–parin* is common to generic drug names in what category of drugs?
11. What drug is given to newborn infants to prevent hemorrhagic disease of the newborn?
12. To what category of drugs does each of the following belong?
    a. iron sucrose (Venofer)
    b. bivalirudin (Angiomax)
    c. clopidogrel (Plavix)
    d. reteplase (Retavase)
    e. absorbable gelatin (Gelfilm, Gelfilm Ophthalmic, Gelfoam)
    f. enoxaparin (Lovenox)
    g. epoetin alfa (Epogen, Procrit)
    h. streptokinase (Streptase)

## Spelling Tips

**Cyklokapron**  Unusual spelling of syllable *cyclo-*.
**Retavase**  With an *a*, but **reteplase** (the generic name drug) with an *e*.

## Clinical Applications

1. Review this patient's Physician's Order Sheet and answer the following questions. Use Appendix C to help you define the abbreviations.
    a. What drug did the physician prescribe?

| PATIENT: | | MEMORIAL HOSPITAL |
|---|---|---|
| AGE: | | BALTIMORE, MARYLAND |
| SEX: | | **PHYSICIAN'S ORDER RECORD** |
| RACE: | | |
| CHART NO. | | |

BEAR DOWN ON HARD SURFACE WITH BALL POINT PEN

GENERIC EQUIVALENT IS AUTHORIZED UNLESS CHECKED IN THIS COLUMN

| ALLERGY OR SENSITIVITY | DIAGNOSIS | | COMPLETED OR DISCONTINUED |
|---|---|---|---|
| TO | | | |
| NONE KNOWN ☐  SIGNED: | | | |

| DATE | TIME | ORDERS | PHYSICIAN'S SIG. | NAME | DATE | TIME |
|---|---|---|---|---|---|---|
| | | Bolus c̄ 3,000 u heparin IV over ½ h. | | | | |
| | | PTT @ 8 PM. Call H.O. with results | | | | |
| | | Turn off heparin drip in 1 h for 1 h and restart @ 950 u per h. VO Dr. Smith | | | | |

   **b.** What dose was prescribed (in the first line)?
   **c.** What measurement is used for this dose?
   **d.** What is the prescribed route of administration?
   **e.** What is the meaning of the word *bolus?*
   **f.** What is the meaning of the abbreviation *VO?*

2. Look at this photograph and answer the following questions.
   **a.** What is the generic name of this drug?
   **b.** What hematologic disease is it used to treat?
   **c.** Name three trade name drugs associated with this generic name drug.
   **d.** The strength of the dose in one tablet is measured in two different ways. Give the number and the unit of measurement for each way.

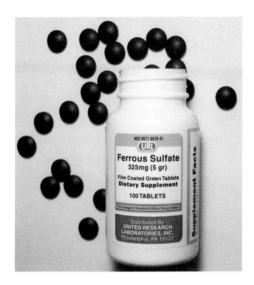

3. A nurse noticed that the physician had written a new drug order on the Physician's Order Sheet in the patient's medical record. The order was for vitamin K 5 mg. The nurse then proceeded to go to the medication cart in the nurses' station and select a vial of potassium chloride from which to administer the drug. What error in critical thinking did the nurse make?

4. This is an excerpt from a hospital discharge drug order form. Answer the following questions.
   **a.** What drug(s) did the physician order?
   **b.** Why did the physician put a slash between the two drug names?
   **c.** What tablet strength was ordered?
   **d.** What quantity of tablets was ordered?
   **e.** How many tablets should the patient take at a time and how often?
   **f.** By what route is this drug taken?
   **g.** How many refills were ordered?

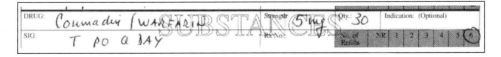

## Multimedia Extension Exercises

■ Go to www.pearsonhighered.com/turley and click on the photo of the cover of *Understanding Pharmacology for Health Professionals* to access the interactive Companion Website created for this textbook.

# Gynecologic and Obstetric Drugs

13

## Learning Objectives

After you study this chapter, you should be able to

1. Describe the difference between monophasic, biphasic, and triphasic oral contraceptive drugs.

2. Describe the therapeutic effect of ovulation-stimulating drugs used to treat infertility.

3. Describe two different actions of drugs that result in abortion of a fetus.

4. Describe how endometriosis develops and how hormone drugs are used to treat it.

5. Compare and contrast the symptoms of and the drugs used to treat premenstrual syndrome versus premenstrual dysphoric disorder.

6. Describe the types of drugs used to treat vaginal infections and sexually transmitted diseases.

7. Discuss the risks involved with taking hormone replacement therapy drugs for the symptoms of menopause.

8. Given the generic and trade names of an OB-GYN drug, identify what drug category they belong to or what disease they are used to treat.

9. Given an OB-GYN drug category, identify several generic and trade name drugs in that category.

Gynecologic and obstetric drugs are used to prevent pregnancy, to treat infertility, to stop premature labor, to induce labor, to treat postpartum hemorrhage, to produce abortion, and to treat endometriosis, dysmenorrhea, premenstrual syndrome, premenstrual dysphoric disorder, abnormal menstruation, vaginal infections, sexually transmitted diseases, and menopause. These drugs include birth control pills and devices, ovulation-stimulating drugs, prenatal vitamins, drugs to stop premature labor, uterine-stimulating drugs to induce labor, treat postpartum hemorrhage or induce abortion, hormone drugs to suppress endometriosis, drugs to treat dysmenorrhea, anti-infective drugs to treat vaginal infections and sexually transmitted diseases, and hormone drugs to treat the hot flashes and vaginal dryness of menopause.

## Drugs Used to Prevent Pregnancy

Pregnancy occurs at the moment that an ovum from the female is fertilized by a spermatozoon from the male. Drugs used to prevent pregnancy act in one of several different ways: They change the hormonal environment of the female reproductive tract so that a mature ovum is not produced or released by the ovary, they kill spermatozoa from the male, or they keep a fertilized ovum from implanting in the endometrium.

### Oral Contraceptive Drugs

Oral contraceptive drugs or **birth control pills** exert a hormonal influence to prevent pregnancy and are 99 percent effective, if taken as directed (see ■ FIGURE 13–1). These drugs change the hormonal environment of the female reproductive tract (see In Depth). Oral contraceptive drugs are divided into three groups: monophasic, biphasic, and triphasic. Oral contraceptive drugs (OCPs) contain a combination of the hormone drug categories of progestins and estrogen, whose doses are fixed or varied.

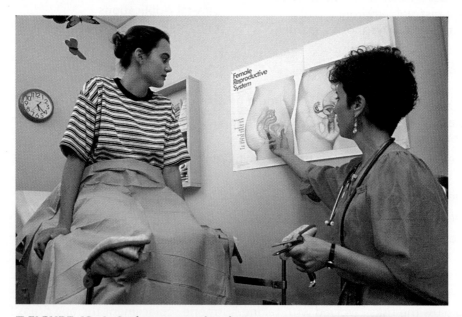

■ **FIGURE 13–1  Oral contraceptive drugs.**
This young adult female has requested a prescription for an oral contraceptive drug during her annual checkup. Her gynecologist is explaining how oral contraceptive drugs act on the ovaries and uterus to prevent pregnancy. She will also discuss with the patient the medical advantages and disadvantages of oral contraceptive drugs, as compared to other types of contraception (such as a diaphragm, cervical cap, rhythm, or abstinence).

## In Depth

Normally, the anterior pituitary gland secretes follicle-stimulating hormone (FSH), which stimulates a follicle in the ovary to develop a mature ovum. FSH also causes the follicle to secrete estradiol, the primary female hormone. Estradiol causes the endometrium to proliferate and thicken. Later, the anterior pituitary gland also secretes luteinizing hormone (LH), which causes the follicle to rupture and release the mature ovum (ovulation). LH also causes the corpus luteum (the remainder of the ruptured follicle) to secrete estradiol and progesterone. If the ovum is fertilized, the corpus luteum continues to secrete progesterone to prepare the endometrium to accept the fertilized ovum. If the ovum is not fertilized, the corpus luteum disintegrates and progesterone production stops. When this happens, the uterine lining sloughs off in the process of menstruation.

Oral contraceptive drugs supply hormone drugs from the progestins and estrogen categories. These drugs replace the hormones progesterone and estradiol. This supresses the release of FSH and LH from the anterior pituitary gland and so a mature ovum is never developed or released. Without an ovum, spermatozoa from the male have nothing to fertilize. Oral contraceptive drugs also cause changes in the cervical mucosa and endometrium that inhibit spermatozoa or keep a fertilized ovum from implanting in the endometrium. All of these actions work together to prevent conception and pregnancy.

## Focus on Healthcare Issues

Oral contraceptive drugs can cause serious adverse effects, such as blood clots, stroke, and heart attack, because of their estrogen content. Because of these risks, most physicians choose to prescribe an oral contraceptive drug that contains 35 mcg of estrogen or less in each tablet. The risk of these adverse effects increases significantly for patients who are older than 35 years of age and who smoke. All oral contraceptive drugs also carry the warning that they do not protect against sexually transmitted diseases, including HIV.

### Monophasic Oral Contraceptive Drugs

A monophasic oral contraceptive drug has one (*mon/o-* means *one*) phase of treatment with fixed doses of a progestin (levonorgestrel, norethindrone, norgestrel, norgestimate, and others) and an estrogen (ethinyl estradiol) in each hormone tablet of the pill pack (see ■ FIGURE 13–2).

Alesse (levonorgestrel, ethinyl estradiol)

Brevicon (norethindrone, ethinyl estradiol)

Demulen (ethynodiol, ethinyl estradiol)

Desogen (desogestrel, ethinyl estradiol)

Loestrin (norethindrone, ethinyl estradiol)

Lo/Ovral (norgestrel, ethinyl estradiol)

Lybrel (levonorgestrel, ethinyl estradiol)

Modicon (norethindrone, ethinyl estradiol)

Norinyl (norethindrone, ethinyl estradiol)

Ortho-Cept (desogestrel, ethinyl estradiol)

Ortho-Cyclen (norgestimate, ethinyl estradiol)

Ortho-Novum (norethindrone, ethinyl estradiol)

Ovcon (norethindrone, ethinyl estradiol)

Ovral (norgestrel, ethinyl estradiol)

Seasonale (levonorgestrel, ethinyl estradiol)

Yasmin (drospirenone, ethinyl estradiol)

YAZ (drospirenone, ethinyl estradiol)

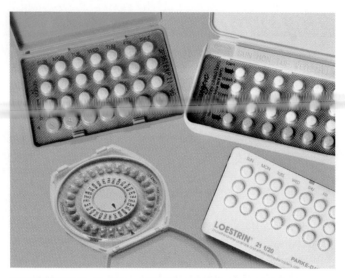

■ **FIGURE 13–2 Monophasic oral contraceptive pill packs.**
Monophasic oral contraceptive drugs in a 21-day pill pack contain 21 hormone tablets with fixed doses of progestin and estrogen hormones. The patient takes one tablet each day for 21 days and then takes no tablets for the remaining days of her menstrual cycle. Monophasic oral contraceptive drugs in a 28-day pill pack contain 21 hormone tablets with fixed doses of progestin and estrogen hormones, followed by 7 inert sugar tablets that contain no hormones (but may contain supplemental iron) to complete a 28-day menstrual cycle. The abrupt discontinuation of the hormones triggers the onset of menstruation.

## *Did You Know?*

Lybrel was the first oral contraceptive drug to eliminate menstrual periods. It comes as a 28-day pill pack in which every tablet contains fixed doses of a progestin and an estrogen. There are no tablets without hormones, and so the endometrium remains intact and menstruation does not occur. Lybrel was approved by the FDA in 2007. Studies show that nearly 50 percent of women would prefer not to menstruate at all.

YAZ is the only oral contraceptive drug that is approved by the FDA for treating acne and premenstrual dysphoric disorder.

Some women prefer a 21-day pill pack, while others prefer the 28-day pill pack because of the consistency of taking a tablet every day.

## *Drug Alert!*

There are many different trade names of oral contraceptive drugs. Some (but not all) include numbers after the trade name, and it is important to understand what those numbers mean. A monophasic oral contraceptive drug has one (*mon/o-*) phase of treatment with fixed amounts of hormones. For some monophasic oral contraceptive drugs, the doses of a progestin and an estrogen are designated by two numbers following the trade name of the drug.

For example, the trade name drugs Norinyl 1 + 35 and Ortho-Novum 1/35 contain 1 mg of a progestin drug and 35 mcg of an estrogen drug in each tablet. The trade name Ovcon-35 indicates only the amount of the estrogen drug in each tablet. A biphasic oral contraceptive drug has two (*bi-*) phases with changing doses of a progestin but a fixed dose of an estrogen. For some biphasic oral contraceptive drugs, this is reflected in the trade name of the drug. For example, Ortho-Novum 10/11 provides 35 mcg of an estrogen for all 21 days, but the dose of a progestin changes from 0.5 mg for the first 10 days, followed by 1 mg for the last 11 days. A triphasic oral contraceptive drug has three (*tri-*) phases of varying doses of hormones. For example, the trade name Ortho-Novum 7/7/7 shows that there are three phases of differing hormone doses and that each phase lasts for 7 days. Other triphasic oral contraceptive drugs (Ortho-TriCyclen, Triphasil) have the prefix *tri-* in their trade names to indicate the three phases.

## Biphasic Oral Contraceptive Drugs

Biphasic oral contraceptive drugs  have two phases of hormone tablets in each pill pack. The first phase provides fixed doses of a progestin (desogestrel, levonorgestrel, norethindrone) and an estrogen (ethinyl estradiol); the second phase provides an increased dose of a progestin but the same dose of an estrogen in each hormone tablet.

> Mircette (desogestrel, ethinyl estradiol)
>
> Otrtho-Novum 10/11 (norethindrone, ethinyl estradiol)
>
> Seasonique (levonorgestrel, ethinyl estradiol)

## *Drug Alert!*

These two oral contraceptive drugs sound very much alike: Seasonale and Seasonique. Seasonale is a monophasic oral contraceptive, while Seasonique is a biphasic oral contraceptive. These drugs are made by the same drug manufacturer. They are unique in that their hormone tablets are taken continuously for three 28-day cycles (84 tablets), followed by 7 inert tablets. This means that the patient has a menstrual period only 4 times a year, as opposed to every month when taking other oral contraceptive drugs. These drugs are known as *extended-regimen oral contraceptive drugs.* Their trade names make reference to the four seasons of the year, with menstruation occurring just once each season.

## Triphasic Oral Contraceptive Drugs

Triphasic oral contraceptive drugs  have three phases of hormone tablets in each pill pack. The first phase provides fixed doses of a progestin (desogestrel, levonorgestrel, norethindrone, norgestimate) and an estrogen (ethinyl estradiol); in the second phase, either one or both of the hormone doses increases in each hormone tablet; in the third phase, either one or both of the hormone doses increases or decreases in each hormone tablet in the pill pack.

> Cyclessa (desogestrel, ethinyl estradiol)
>
> Estrostep (norethindrone, ethinyl estradiol)
>
> Ortho-Novum 7/7/7 (norethindrone, ethinyl estradiol)
>
> Ortho Tri-Cyclen (norgestimate, ethinyl estradiol)
>
> Tri-Levlen (levonorgestrel, ethinyl estradiol)
>
> Triphasil (levonorgestrel, ethinyl estradiol)

## Other Hormone Contraceptive Drugs

These contraceptive drugs provide daily fixed doses of a progestin (etonogestrel, norelgestromin) and an estrogen (ethinyl estradiol), but they are not given orally. Instead, they are in the form of a ring (NuvaRing) inserted into the vagina or a transdermal patch (Ortho Evra) applied to the skin.

NuvaRing (etonogestrel, ethinyl estradiol)

Ortho Evra (norelgestromin, ethinyl estradiol) (see ■ FIGURE 13–3)

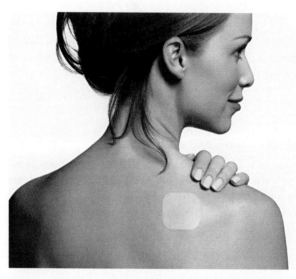

**■ FIGURE 13–3 Ortho Evra transdermal patch.**
A transdermal patch is a convenient way to take a birth control drug without having to remember to take a tablet each day.

This oral contracepetive drug contains a progestin (levonorgestrel) and an estrogen (ethinyl estradiol), but only two tablets are taken orally after unprotected intercourse to prevent pregnancy.

Preven (levonorgestrel, ethinyl estradiol)

### *Did You Know?*

Ortho Evra, introduced in 2001, was the first transdermal patch contraceptive drug. It is produced by the same drug company that introduced the very first oral contraceptive drug in 1931. NuvaRing, introduced in 2001, was the first contraceptive vaginal ring. It is a flexible, clear, 3-inch polymer ring that is inserted into the vagina for 3 weeks of every month.

## Progestin-Only Contraceptive Drugs

These oral contraceptive drugs only contain a progestin (norethindrone, norgestrel). They are slightly less effective in preventing pregnancy than combination oral contraceptive drugs, particularly if the patient forgets to take even one daily tablet. Progestin-only oral contraceptive drugs contain no estrogen, and so the risk of blood clots and other adverse effects of estrogen are avoided. These contraceptive drugs are also useful for mothers who have just given birth and want to breastfeed, as the drug does not interfere with milk production.

Ortho Micronor (norethindrone)

Ovrette (norgestrel)

These progestin-only (etonogestrel, levonorgestrel, progesterone) contraceptive drugs are contained within an implant that is inserted under the skin or within a T-shaped device that is inserted into the uterus. The contraceptive effect lasts from one to five years depending on the amount of drug in the device.

Implanon (etonogestrel)

Mirena (levonorgestrel) (see ▓ **FIGURE 13–4**)

Progestasert (progesterone)

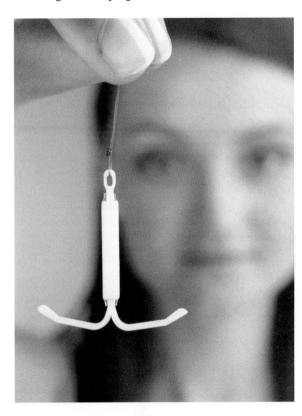

▓ **FIGURE 13–4 Mirena contraceptive device.**
This contraceptive drug is contained within a T-shaped intrauterine device. The shape of the device irritates the endometrium to prevent implantation of a fertilized ovum. The device reservoir contains the progestin drug levonorgestrel, which suppresses the release of FSH and LH from the anterior pituitary gland, and so a mature ovum is never developed or released. This contraceptive device can be kept in the uterine cavity for up to five years.

This progestin-only contraceptive drug is injected subcutaneously during the first five days of the menstrual cycle, during the first five days after giving birth, or, for breastfeeding mothers, six weeks after giving birth. The contraceptive effect lasts for three months.

medroxyprogesterone (Depo-Sub Q Provera)

This progestin-only (levonorgestrel) contraceptive drug is taken orally but only after unprotected intercourse to prevent pregnancy.

Plan B (levonorgestrel)

## Drug Alert!

The herb St. John's wort, which is often taken for depression, can cause serum hormone levels to decrease in patients taking oral contraceptive drugs, and this increases the chance of pregnancy.

### Spermicidal Drugs for Contraception

These over-the-counter drugs (nonoxynol-9, octoxynol-9) are inserted in the vagina prior to intercourse to kill spermatozoa and prevent pregnancy.

Contraceptrol (nonoxynol-9)

Gynol II (nonoxynol-9)

Ortho Gynol (octoxynol-9)

## Drugs Used to Treat Infertility

Drugs used to treat infertility either stimulate the ovaries to produce ova, prepare the endometrium to receive a fertilized ovum, or correct hormonal imbalances. These drugs are often used as part of a program of assisted reproductive technology (ART).

### Ovulation-Stimulating Drugs for Infertility

Ovulation-stimulating drugs stimulate a nonovulating ovary to develop multiple follicles and then release several mature ova. Ovulation-stimulating drugs are appropriate for patients with anovulation (failure to ovulate), but are not appropriate for patients with infertility due to blocked fallopian tubes or problems that require surgical intervention. Some ovulation-stimulating drugs act by stimulating the hypothalamus and anterior pituitary gland; this causes the release of follicle-stimulating hormone (FSH) that causes the ovary to develop follicles, and the release of luteinizing hormone (LH) that causes the follicles to release mature ova. Other ovulation-stimulating drugs act in the same manner as follicle-stimulating hormone or luteinizing hormone.

choriogonadotropin alfa (Ovidrel)

clomiphene (Clomid) (see ■ FIGURE 13–5)

follitropin alfa (Gonal-f)

follitropin beta (Follistim AQ)

human chorionic gonadotropin (Pregnyl, Profasi)

lutropin alfa (Luveris)

menotropins (Repronex)

sermorelin (Geref)

somatropin (Norditropin)

urofollitropin (Bravelle)

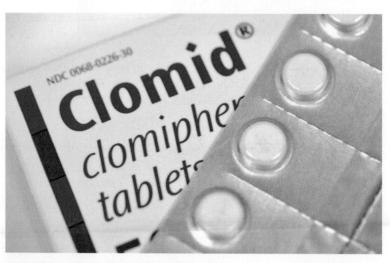

■ FIGURE 13–5  **Clomiphene (Clomid).**
Patients who have difficulty becoming pregnant often take an ovulation-stimulating drug, such as Clomid, to help their ovaries develop mature ova.

## Did You Know?

Follitropin alfa and follitropin beta are manufactured using recombinant DNA technology. Human chorionic gonadotropin (HCG) is a hormone normally produced by the placenta in pregnant women. Urofollitropin is extracted from the urine of postmenopausal women.

Bobbi McCaughey, age 29, of Carlisle, Iowa, took human chorionic gonadotropin for infertility; she became pregnant and subsequently gave birth to the world's only surviving set of septuplets on November 20, 1997. The four boys and three girls were born at 30 weeks' gestation and weighed from 2 pounds, 5 ounces, to 3 pounds, 4 ounces. They celebrated their tenth birthday in November 2007.

## Focus on Healthcare Issues

Ovulation-stimulating drugs cause several mature ova to be released from the ovary at the same time. This increases the chances that an infertile woman will become pregnant. However, a pregnancy with multiple babies can endanger the life of the mother and/or the babies. Some obstetricians recommend elective removal of one or more of the growing fetuses prior to delivery, but this creates an ethical and moral dilemma. For *in vitro* fertilization as part of an assisted reproductive technology program, the release of multiple mature ova increases the chance for successful harvesting of ova from the mother, fertilization of several ova, and successful implantation of fertilized ova back in the mother. However, using only some of the fertilized ova, while the rest are frozen (or possibly used in research), also creates ethical and moral issues.

### Progesterone Drugs for Infertility

This progesterone drug prepares the endometrium to receive fertilized ova. This drug is used in conjunction with other drugs for infertility in women.

progesterone (Crinone, Prochieve)

### Other Drugs for Infertility

These drugs decrease excessive amounts of gonadotropin-releasing hormone that can be secreted by the hypothalamus in patients who are on ovulation-stimulating drugs.

cetrorelix (Cetrotide)

ganirelix

These drugs are used to treat type 2 diabetes mellitus. They are also used to stimulate ovulation in women with polycystic ovaries.

metformin (Glucophage)

rosiglitazone (Avandia)

This growth hormone drug is used to stimulate ovulation.

somatropin (Norditropin)

## Drugs Used During Pregnancy

Few drugs are prescribed during pregnancy, particularly during the first trimester, because of the increased risk of causing birth defects in the developing fetus. Drugs for chronic diseases, such as hypothyroidism, diabetes mellitus, or hypertension, or antibiotic drugs for acute infections, are given during pregnancy, as determined by the physician, to protect the health of both the mother and fetus. Pregnant women are prescribed prenatal vitamins, iron, and folic acid.

### *Focus on Healthcare Issues*

The U.S. Public Health Service recommends the use of folic acid supplements for all women of childbearing age. Folic acid significantly decreases the incidence of babies who have neural tube defects (spina bifida, myelomeningocele). Since 1988, some breads, cereals, and pastas have had supplemental folic acid added to them for this reason.

### *Historical Notes*

Most women dread the morning sickness that often accompanies early pregnancy and wish there was a drug to relieve this excessive nausea and vomiting caused by changing hormone levels. In the late 1950s, the drug thalidomide was developed in West Germany and used extensively to treat morning sickness. The FDA refused to approve its use in the United States without further studies. Before these additional studies could be completed, evidence against the safety of the drug began to accumulate. Over 8,000 babies were born in Europe with deformed extremities ("seal limbs," or phocomelia). The FDA has established five categories of drugs (Category A through E) to indicate a drug's potential to cause birth defects, if taken by a woman while she is pregnant.

## Drugs Used to Treat Premature Labor

Premature or preterm labor and delivery greatly increase disease and death rates in newborn infants. Premature labor contractions can be inhibited by using uterine-relaxing drugs. These drugs act on beta$_2$ receptors in the smooth muscle of the uterus to decrease both the frequency and strength of uterine contractions. These drugs are known as **tocolytic drugs**. The word *tocolytic* contains the combining form *toc/o-* (labor and childbirth), the combining form *lyt/o-* (break down), and the suffix *-ic* (pertaining to); the word means *pertaining to breaking down labor and childbirth*.

### *Focus on Healthcare Issues*

In the past, the drug ritodrine (Yutopar) was widely used to treat preterm labor. However, it was taken off the market in 2000 due to safety reasons. Currently, there is no drug specifically approved by the FDA to treat preterm labor. Other drugs that inhibit contractions of the uterus have been used and are still being used to treat preterm labor. These are prescribed at the physician's discretion, and this is known as an "unlabeled use" as it is unofficial, but legal. Such drugs include terbutaline (FDA-approved bronchodilator drug used to treat asthma), magnesium sulfate (FDA-approved drug used to treat seizures caused by toxemia during pregnancy), isoxsuprine (FDA-approved vasodilator drug), and indomethacin (FDA-approved nonsteroidal anti-inflammatory drug).

## Drugs Used to Induce Labor

Women in labor may be given a uterine stimulant if their uterine contractions are too weak (uterine inertia) to produce delivery or if complications such as preeclampsia or diabetes mellitus necessitate induction of labor for the safety of the mother. Normally, the hormone oxytocin (secreted by the posterior pituitary gland) stimulates the uterus by binding to special oxytocin receptors on the smooth muscle cells of the uterus. The drug oxytocin works in the same way to increase both the frequency and strength of uterine contractions. Oxytocin is not used when prolonged labor is due to cephalopelvic disproportion in which the fetus's skull is too large to fit through the mother's bony pelvis.

oxytocin (Pitocin)

## Did You Know?

Skeletons of prehistoric women have been discovered with the head of the fetus wedged into the mother's pelvic bones (cephalopelvic disproportion).

Labor consists of uterine contractions as well as dilatation (widening) and effacement (thinning) of the cervix of the uterus. Prostaglandins secreted by the placenta help to widen and thin the cervix as labor begins. They cause smooth muscle fibers in the cervix to dilate and the collagen fibers to break down. This process of dilatation and effacement is known as *cervical ripening*. When the cervix does not dilate and thin during labor, these prostaglandin drugs can be given. Dinoprostone is applied topically. Misoprostol is taken orally.

dinoprostone (Cervidil, Prepidil)

misoprostol (Cytotec)

## Did You Know?

Prostaglandin is a naturally occurring body substance that was first isolated from semen from the prostate gland of men, from which it derives its name.

Prostaglandins in the body have many actions. Not only do they act on the cervix to prepare it for labor, they also normally protect the gastric mucosa. Aspirin and nonsteroidal anti-inflammatory drugs taken for pain and inflammation suppress the action of prostaglandins in the body, decrease its protective action on the gastric mucosa, and may cause gastric ulcers. Prostaglandin drugs such as misoprostol are given to protect the gastric mucosa in patients taking long-term aspirin or nonsteroidal anti-inflammatory drugs.

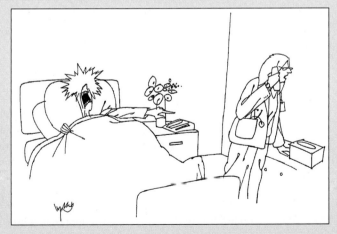

*"Pharmacy? . . . Hi! . . . I have a patient in labor here, . . . and she's demanding your entire inventory of narcotics."*

## Drugs Used to Treat Postpartum Bleeding

Normally after delivery of a baby and the placenta, the uterine muscle contracts strongly. This closes bleeding blood vessels at the site of placental separation. Postpartum bleeding is due to uterine relaxation or atony, which results in increased bleeding at the site of placental separation. These drugs stimulate the uterine muscle to contract and are used to treat postpartum bleeding.

carboprost (Hemabate)                    misoprostol (Cytotec)

ergonovine (Ergotrate)                   oxytocin (Pitocin)

methylergonovine (Methergine)

### Clinical Applications

During any pregnancy, some of the fetus's red blood cells enter the mother's blood via the placenta. If the fetus is Rh-positive and the mother is Rh-negative, the mother develops antibodies against Rh-positive RBCs. This does not affect the first fetus while it is in the uterus. However, during any subsequent pregnancy with an Rh-positive fetus, the mother's antibodies will attack the RBCs of the fetus. This fetus then develops hemolytic disease of the newborn. MICRhoGAM or RhoGAM are immunoglobulin drugs that are given to an Rh-negative mother after the birth of an Rh-positive newborn. These drugs prevent the mother from making antibodies during any subsequent pregnancies with an Rh-positive fetus. These drugs are also given to women who have had a miscarriage, spontaneous or induced abortion, or an amniocentesis. These drugs are never given to the newborn.

## Drugs Used to Treat Postpartum Depression

The hormonal changes of pregnancy and delivery can cause depression in some women. Drugs used to treat postpartum depression are discussed in Chapter 16.

## Drugs Used to Produce Abortion

Drugs that produce abortion cause the uterus to contract strongly enough to spontaneously abort a fetus while they also cause the cervix to dilate. Other abortion drugs inhibit progesterone from the corpus luteum (or later from the placenta) that keeps the thickened endometrium intact; without the action of progesterone, the endometrium deteriorates and the pregnancy is aborted. These drugs are given by various routes: carboprost is injected intramuscularly, dinoprostone is given as a vaginal suppository, mifepristone and misoprostol are given orally, and urea is injected into the amniotic fluid.

carboprost (Hemabate)                    misoprostol (Cytotec)

dinoprostone (Prostin E2)                urea (Ureaphil)

mifepristone (Mifeprex)

## Focus on Healthcare Issues

Carboprost is used to abort a fetus and terminate the pregnancy, but it is also used to treat postpartum hemorrhage and save the life of the mother after delivery. Dinoprostone is used to produce abortion, but it is also used (under the trade names Cervidil and Prepidil) to cause the cervix to dilate and efface in preparation for delivery of a baby. Dinoprostone (prostaglandin $E_2$, Prostin E2) is used to abort a fetus, but a related drug alprostadil (prostaglandin $E_1$, Prostin VR) is used to save the lives of infants born with congenital heart defects; it keeps open the ductus arteriosus that normally closes at birth so that these infants can maintain adequate oxygenation, in spite of their heart defects, until surgical correction can be performed.

## Drugs Used to Treat Endometriosis

Endometriosis develops when endometrial tissue from the uterus travels through the fallopian tubes and implants on the outer surface of the ovaries and other abdominal organs and on the walls of the pelvic cavity. This abnormal condition occurs when endometrial tissue sloughs off during menstruation but is forced upward through the fallopian tubes by uterine contractions (because of a retroflexed position of the uterus) instead of downward through the cervix. This tissue remains alive and sensitive to hormonal changes. During each menstrual cycle, this tissue thickens and then sloughs off, forming more implants in the abdominal cavity, along with old blood and tissue debris. The tissue also forms adhesions between the abdominal organs. Endometriosis causes pelvic pain and inflammation, cyst formation on the ovaries, and can block the fallopian tubes. These hormone drugs are used to suppress the menstrual cycle for several months, during which time the endometrial implants shrink and fade.

| | |
|---|---|
| danazol | nafarelin (Synarel) |
| goserelin (Zoladex) | norethindrone (Aygestin) |
| leuprolide (Lupron Depot) | |

## Did You Know?

Danazol is also used to treat fibrocystic breast disease, precocious puberty, and gynecomastia in males. Goserelin is also used to treat breast and prostate cancer. Leuprolide is also used to treat uterine fibroids.

## Drugs Used to Treat Dysmenorrhea, Premenstrual Syndrome, and Premenstrual Dysphoric Disorder

Dysmenorrhea (painful menstrual cramps) is caused by an increase in prostaglandins that causes the uterus to contract painfully. It is treated with over-the-counter or prescription analgesic drugs (nonsteroidal anti-inflammatory drugs [NSAIDs] or COX-2 inhibitor drugs) that inhibit the action of prostaglandins.

| | |
|---|---|
| celecoxib (Celebrex) | meclofenamate |
| diclofenac (Cataflam, Flector, Voltaren) | mefenamic acid (Ponstel) |
| ibuprofen (Advil, Motrin) | naproxen (Aleve, Midol Extended Relief, Naprosyn) |
| ketoprofen | |

Premenstrual syndrome (PMS) is characterized by dysmenorrhea, breast tenderness, edema from fluid retention ("bloating"), and mild mood changes. It is treated with combination drugs that contain an analgesic drug for dysmenorrhea, a diuretic drug to treat fluid retention and an antihistamine drug with a weak diuretic effect and a sedative effect. These over-the-counter trade name combination drugs include Midol, Pamprin, Premsyn, and Women's Tylenol Multi-Symptom Menstrual Relief.

Premenstrual dysphoric disorder (PMDD) includes similar physical and emotional symptoms, but to a much greater degree than PMS, with depression, anxiety, and sleep disturbances that significantly interfere with life. PMDD is considered a mood disorder caused by an alteration in the level of brain neurotransmitters. The antianxiety drugs alprazolam and buspirone and the antidepressant drugs citalopram, clomipramine, desipramine, fluoxetine, nortriptyline, paroxetine, and sertraline are used to treat premenstrual dysphoric disorder. Venlafaxine is for depression and anxiety. The oral contraceptive drug YAZ has also been approved to treat premenstrual dysphoric disorder.

| | |
|---|---|
| alprazolam (Xanax) | nortriptyline (Aventyl, Pamelor) |
| buspirone (BuSpar) | paroxetine (Paxil) |
| citalopram (Celexa) | sertraline (Zoloft) |
| clomipramine (Anafranil) | venlafaxine (Effexor) |
| desipramine (Norpramin) | YAZ |
| fluoxetine (Sarafem) | |

## Drug Alert!

Midol is a well-known, over-the-counter trade name drug for treating dysmenorrhea. However, it is important to note that different trade names of Midol actually contain different generic drugs. Midol Maximum Strength Cramp Formula contains the analgesic drug ibuprofen. Midol Extended Relief contains the analgesic drug naproxen. Midol Maximum Strength Menstrual, Midol Maximum Strength PMS, and Midol Teen Maximum Strength are combination drugs that contain the analgesic drug acetaminophen and a diuretic drug to decrease edema.

## Drugs Used to Treat Abnormal Menstruation

Amenorrhea (the absence of menstruation) and abnormal uterine bleeding are treated with progestin drugs that act directly on the tissues of the endometrium to restore a normal menstrual cycle.

medroxyprogesterone (Provera) (see ■ FIGURE 13–6)

norethindrone (Aygestin)

progesterone (Crinone)

Primary hypothalamic amenorrhea—the absence of menstruation due to decreased levels of gonadotropin-releasing hormone (GnRH) from the hypothalamus—is treated with a drug that mimics the action of GnRH and stimulates the release of the FSH and LH from the anterior pituitary gland. A special pump is needed to administer this drug intravenously so that it can be given in pulses that mimic the natural release of GnRH from the hypothalamus.

gonadorelin (Lutrepulse)

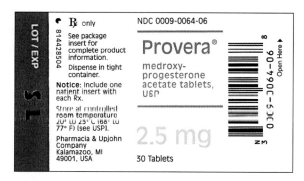

**■ FIGURE 13–6 Drug label for medroxyprogesterone (Provera).**
This drug corrects an underlying hormone imbalance (a lack of progesterone) that causes amenorrhea. Notice that the generic drug name medroxyprogesterone contains the name of the natural hormone progesterone.

## Drugs Used to Treat Vaginal Infections

Drugs used to treat vaginal infections are applied vaginally and are manufactured in the form of creams, ointments, suppositories, or vaginal tablets.

Vaginal yeast infections are caused by *Candida albicans*, and the infection is known as *candidiasis*. It causes a cheesy, white discharge and vaginal itching. Vaginal yeast infections are treated with these over-the-counter drugs.

| | |
|---|---|
| butoconazole (Gynazole-1, Mycelex-3) | nystatin |
| clotrimazole (Gyne-Lotrimin, Mycelex) | sulfanilamide (AVC) |
| miconazole (Monistat 3, Monistat 7, Vagistat-3) (see ■ **FIGURE 13–7**) | terconazole (Terazol) |
| | tioconazole (Monistat 1, Vagistat-1) |

*Note:* Many drugs used to treat candidiasis end in the suffix *-azole*. Many antifungal drugs also end with this suffix. This is because yeast and fungi are closely related, and drugs that are effective against one often are effective against the other.

## Drug Alert!

Did you notice that the trade name drugs Monistat 3 and Monistat 7 are listed with the generic drug miconazole, but the trade name drug Monistat 1 is listed with the generic drug tioconazole? This can be a source of confusion. The generic drug tioconazole is a stronger antifungal drug than miconazole, and only one day of treatment is needed as compared to three or seven days of treatment with miconazole. The drug company that manufactures Monistat chose to keep the same trade name on all these products (even though the generic drugs are different). The same is true for the drug company that makes Vagistat.

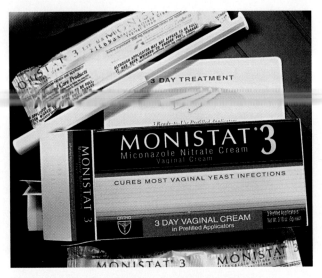

■ **FIGURE 13–7 Miconazole (Monistat 3).**
This topical antifungal drug is a cream that is inserted into the
vagina by means of an applicator tube. The patient takes one dose
for three consecutive days to treat a vaginal yeast infection. Other
antifungal drugs require seven days of treatment (miconazole
[Monistat 7]) or just one day of treatment (tioconazole [Monistat 1]).

## Did You Know?

Nystatin was discovered in 1950 by two physicians who named the drug for their employer—
the **N**ew **Y**ork **Stat**e Department of Health. Nystatin is given vaginally to treat vaginal yeast
infections; it is also given orally ("swish and swallow") to treat yeast infections in the mouth
and throat (oral candidiasis).

Bacterial vaginal infections (bacterial vaginosis) are caused by several different bacteria, including *Haemophilus*, *Gardnerella*, and *Corynebacterium*. These topical anti-infective drugs are applied
vaginally to treat bacterial vaginal infections.

clindamycin (Cleocin)

metronidazole (MetroGel-Vaginal)

## Did You Know?

Metronidazole is both an antibacterial and an antiprotozoal drug. It is taken orally to treat pelvic
inflammatory disease and amebiasis. It is used to treat serious infections caused by anaerobic bacteria. In combination with other anti-infective drugs, it is taken orally to treat peptic ulcers caused
by *Helicobacter pylori*. Metronidazole (MetroGel) is also applied topically to treat acne rosacea.

# Drugs Used to Treat Sexually Transmitted Diseases

Common sexually transmitted diseases (STDs) include gonorrhea, syphilis, chlamydia, acquired immunodeficiency syndrome (AIDS), genital herpes, and genital warts.

## Drugs for Gonorrhea

Gonorrhea is caused by the gram-negative coccus *Neisseria gonorrhoeae*. It can cause painful urination and a thick, yellow vaginal discharge. Oral antibiotic drugs from several different categories (penicillins, cephalosporins, tetracyclines, fluoroquinolones) are effective in treating gonorrhea. These categories of oral antibiotic drugs are discussed in Chapter 20.

## Drugs for Syphilis

Syphilis is caused by the gram-negative spirochete *Treponema pallidum*. It can cause a fever and rash with a lesion (chancre) in the genital area that ulcerates and forms a crust. Oral antibiotic drugs from several different categories (penicillins, tetracyclines) are effective in treating syphilis. These categories of oral antibiotic drugs are discussed in Chapter 20.

## *Historical Notes*

In the early 1900s, Paul Ehrlich, a German chemist, tested 605 separate arsenic compounds before finding the first drug known to cure syphilis. This drug was nicknamed "the magic bullet" because of its ability to cure syphilis, a common but until-then incurable disease.

## Drugs for Chlamydial Infections

Chlamydial vaginal infections are caused by *Chlamydia trachomatis*, a gram-negative coccus. It can cause painful urination with a thin discharge. Oral antibiotic and anti-infective drugs from several different categories (penicillins, macrolides, tetracyclines, fluoroquinolones, sulfonamides) are used to treat chlamydia. These categories of oral drugs are discussed in Chapter 20.

## Drugs for Acquired Immunodeficiency Syndrome

Acquired immunodeficiency syndrome (AIDS) is caused by the human immunodeficiency virus (HIV), a retrovirus. HIV causes fever, night sweats, weight loss, enlarged lymph nodes, and diarrhea. HIV invades CD4 lymphocytes in order to reproduce. Large numbers of CD4 lymphocytes are destroyed during this process. With the balance between CD4 and CD8 lymphocytes upset, the CD8 lymphocytes then suppress the immune system, leaving the patient defenseless against infection and cancer. Oral antiviral drugs used to treat HIV and AIDS are discussed in Chapter 20.

## Drugs for Genital Herpes

Genital herpes is caused by a herpes simplex virus type 2 infection in the genital area; this is a sexually transmitted disease. (*Note:* Herpes simplex virus type 1 infections involve other areas of the body, particularly the mouth, and are known as *cold sores*; they are not a sexually transmitted disease.) Genital herpes lesions are treated topically and with oral antiviral drugs that are discussed in Chapter 17.

## Drugs for Genital Warts

The human papillomavirus causes both common warts (verrucae) and genital or venereal warts (condylomata acuminata). Topical drugs used to treat genital warts are discussed in Chapter 17.

This drug is a vaccine that is used to prevent infection in females ages 9 to 26 from several strains of the human papillomavirus. It also can prevent cervical cancer caused by those same strains, but it does not protect against all strains of the virus.

Gardisil

## Drugs Used to Treat Menopause

As a woman enters menopause, the ovaries secrete decreasing amounts of estradiol and progesterone. This causes symptoms of vaginal dryness, hot flashes, and fatigue, which can be treated by hormone replacement therapy (HRT). Estrogen hormone replacement therapy corrects this deficiency of estradiol. Combination progestin and estrogen replacement therapy is also used. The long-term use of hormone replacement therapy may also reduce the risk of osteoporosis and keep cholesterol levels low; however, estrogen is associated with an increased risk of breast and endometrial cancer, blood clots, stroke, heart attack and dementia. Most doctors now recommend hormone replacement therapy drugs only for short-term treatment in younger women who are experiencing severe menopausal symptoms.

### Estrogen Hormone Replacement Therapy for Menopause

These drugs replace decreased levels of the hormone estradiol.

| | |
|---|---|
| conjugated estrogens (Premarin) | estradiol (Climara, Estraderm, Evamist, Vivelle) |
| esterified estrogens (Menest) | estropipate (Ogen, Ortho-Est) |

### Did You Know?

The trade name Premarin indicates the source of the drug: **pre**gnant **mar**es' ur**in**e. Animal rights activists claim that the horse is treated inhumanely by being confined to a stall with a catheter in its bladder to collect the urine. Over 40 billion Premarin tablets have been sold since it was approved by the FDA in 1942. Other hormone replacement therapy drugs are derived from yams or soybeans (Climara, Estrace, Estraderm, Menest, Ogen, Ortho-Est, and Vivelle) or are manufactured synthetic hormone drugs.

The trade name Climara refers to *climacteric,* the physiologic and psychological changes that occur as a woman enters menopause. *Climacteric* is from a Greek word that means *the rungs of a ladder,* because menopause represents moving toward a different stage of life.

### Combination Drugs for Menopause

These drugs combine a progestin (drospirenone, levonorgestrel, medroxyprogesterone, methyltestosterone, norethindrone, norgestimate) and an estrogen (conjugated estrogens, esterified estrogens, ethinyl estradiol, estradiol). These drugs (except for Angeliq, CombiPatch, and Estratest) are also indicated for the prevention of osteoporosis in postmenopausal women.

| | |
|---|---|
| Activella (norethindrone, estradiol) | Estratest (methyltestosterone, esterified estrogens) |
| Angeliq (drospirenone, estradiol) | Femhrt (norethindrone, estradiol) |
| ClimaraPro (levonorgestrel, estradiol) | Premphase (medroxyprogesterone, conjugated estrogens) |
| CombiPatch (norethindrone, estradiol) (see ■ FIGURE 13–8) | Prempro (medroxyprogesterone, conjugated estrogens) |

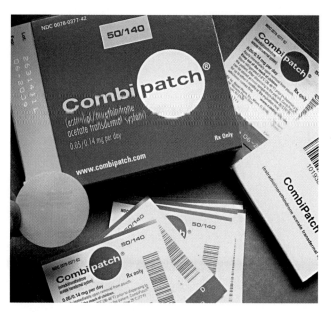

■ **FIGURE 13–8  CombiPatch.**
CombiPatch is one of only two combination hormone replacement
drugs for menopause that come in the drug form of a transdermal
patch that is applied to the skin. The other drug is ClimaraPro.
The transdermal patch needs to be changed only once every three
or four days. All other combination hormone replacement drugs
are in a tablet form that must be taken daily.

## *Did You Know?*

The *hrt* in the trade name Femhrt refers to its use as **h**ormone **r**eplacement **t**herapy.

### Other Drugs for Menopause

This drug stimulates alpha$_2$ receptors in the brain and is used to treat the hot flashes of menopause.
It is also used to treat many other conditions, most commonly hypertension.

    clonidine (Catapres)

These antidepressant drugs are usually used to treat depression, but are also used to treat the hot
flashes of menopause.

    fluoxetine (Sarafem)

    paroxetine (Paxil)

    venlafaxine (Effexor)

This over-the-counter drug contains the herb black cohosh that has been used for years to treat
the symptoms of menopause; it is effective in some women. It is available without a prescription
and, because it does not contain estrogen, does not have the risk of blood clots, stroke, or heart
attack.

    Remifemin (see ■ **FIGURE 13–9**)

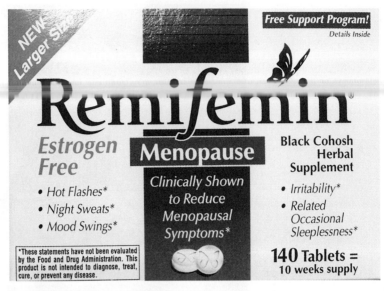

**■ FIGURE 13–9  Remifemin.**
This over-the-counter drug contains black cohosh, an herb which also is known
as *black snakeroot* or *bugbane* and is a garden perennial flower known as
*Cimicifuga racemosa.* Notice that the box states that it is clinically proven to
reduce menopausal symptoms, but the warning box at the bottom left states that
"These statements have not been evaluated by the Food and Drug
Administration. This product is not intended to diagnose, treat, cure, or prevent
any disease."

## Drugs Used to Treat Postmenopausal Osteoporosis

Nonhormonal drugs that inhibit bone resorption and are used to treat postmenopausal osteoporosis
are discussed in Chapter 9.

# *Chapter Review*

## Quiz Yourself

1. Describe the actions of these body hormones: estradiol, progesterone, oxytocin, follicle-stimulating hormone (FSH), and luteinizing hormone (LH).
2. Name the three categories of oral contraceptive drugs (birth control pills). Describe the difference between the categories. Give examples of generic and trade name drugs from each
   category.
3. Explain why patients taking the oral contraceptive drugs Seasonale and Seasonique only have
   four menstrual periods a year.
4. What types of drugs are prescribed during pregnancy?

5. Describe the historical events that occurred when the drug thalidomide was used in Europe to treat morning sickness in pregnant women.
6. Describe how endometriosis develops and how hormone drugs are used to treat it.
7. What are the pros and cons of hormone replacement therapy (HRT)?
8. Discuss the moral and ethical issues that arise from the use of ovulation-stimulating drugs that result in multiple fertilized ova or multiple fetuses.
9. What is the therapeutic effect of RhoGAM, and to whom is this drug given?
10. List the symptoms of premenstrual syndrome and contrast them to the symptoms of premenstrual dysphoric disorder. What categories of drugs are used to treat these two disorders?
11. What is unique about these contraceptive drugs: Implanon, Mirena, NuvaRing, and Ortho Evra?
12. To what category of drugs does each of these drugs belong, or what is the therapeutic effect of each of these drugs?

   **a.** conjugated estrogens (Premarin)
   **b.** Cyclessa
   **c.** dinoprostone (Cervidil, Prepidil)
   **d.** estradiol (Climara)
   **e.** Lybrel
   **f.** metronidazole (MetroGel-Vaginal)

   **g.** miconazole (Monistat 3)
   **h.** Ortho-Novum
   **i.** oxytocin (Pitocin)
   **j.** Prempro
   **k.** YAZ

## Spelling Tips

| | |
|---|---|
| **BuSpar** | Unusual internal capitalization. |
| **ClimaraPro** | Unusual internal capitalization. |
| **CombiPatch** | Unusual internal capitalization. |
| **Femhrt** | Unusual word ending that actually is the abbreviation *hrt* (for *hormone replacement therapy*). |
| **MetroGel-Vaginal** | Unusual internal capitalization. |
| **MICRhoGAM** | Unusual internal capitalization. |
| **NuvaRing** | Unusual internal capitalization. |
| **RhoGAM** | Unusual internal capitalization. |
| **YAZ** | All capital letters. |

## Clinical Applications

1. Look at this handwritten prescription and answer the following questions.
   **a.** What is the name of the drug that the physician ordered?
   **b.** To what category of drugs does this belong?
   **c.** What is the meaning of this drug strength: 0.125/2.5?
   **d.** How many tablets should the pharmacist give the patient?
   **e.** Translate the section for "Sig:" into plain English.
   **f.** What condition is this drug used to treat?

| **Rx** | | Strength | Dispense | Sig: | Refills |
|---|---|---|---|---|---|
| 1 | Prempro | 0.125/2.5 | 30 | T po 5 day | 10 |

2. Look at this photograph and answer the following questions.
   a. What is the name of this drug?
   b. Which type of drug form is it?
   c. What is the name of its generic drug?
   d. To what category of drugs does it belong?

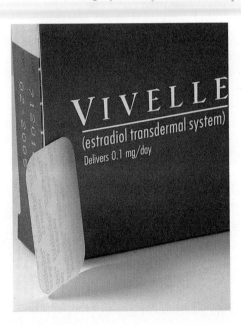

## Multimedia Extension Exercises

■ Go to www.pearsonhighered.com/turley and click on the photo of the cover of *Understanding Pharmacology for Health Professionals* to access the interactive Companion Website created for this textbook.

# Endocrine Drugs

## Learning Objectives

After you study this chapter, you should be able to

1. Compare and contrast the causes and treatments of diabetes mellitus type 1 versus diabetes mellitus type 2.

2. Differentiate between the therapeutic effects of insulin and oral antidiabetic drugs.

3. Describe the therapeutic effects of several categories of antidiabetic drugs besides insulin.

4. Name drugs used to treat hyperthyroidism and hypothyroidism.

5. Compare and contrast the therapeutic effects of drugs used to treat growth failure versus acromegaly.

6. Differentiate between the therapeutic effects of corticosteroid drugs and anabolic steroid drugs.

7. Given the generic and trade names of an endocrine drug, identify what drug category they belong to.

8. Given an endocrine drug category, identify several generic and trade name drugs in that category.

The endocrine system consists of many glands that secrete hormones into the blood (see ■ FIGURE 14–1). When these glands malfunction, they secrete either a decreased or an increased amount of hormone. Endocrine drugs are used as replacement therapy to treat diseases that occur when an endocrine gland secretes too little hormone; other endocrine drugs are used to suppress an endocrine gland when it secretes too much hormone.

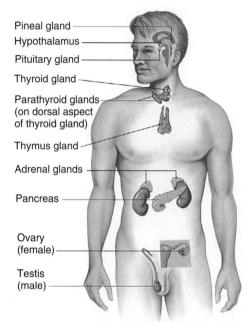

Pineal gland
Hypothalamus
Pituitary gland
Thyroid gland
Parathyroid glands
(on dorsal aspect
of thyroid gland)
Thymus gland
Adrenal glands
Pancreas
Ovary
(female)
Testis
(male)

■ FIGURE 14–1 Glands of the endocrine system.
The glands of the endocrine system include the pineal gland, hypothalamus, and anterior and posterior pituitary gland in the brain; the thyroid gland and parathyroid glands in the neck; the thymus in the chest; the adrenal glands superior to each kidney; the pancreas in the abdominal cavity; the female ovaries in the pelvic cavity; and the male testes in the scrotum. When these glands malfunction, endocrine drugs can be used to correct the resulting disease.

## *Did You Know?*

A number of famous people have suffered from endocrine disorders: boxer Sugar Ray Robinson and blues guitarist B. B. King have diabetes mellitus; former President and Barbara Bush, as well as Olympic gold medalist Gail Devers, have hyperthyroidism; and former President John F. Kennedy had Addison's disease, which gave his skin its unusually bronzed and tanned appearance.

## Insulin

Insulin is secreted by beta cells in the islets of Langerhans in the pancreas (see ■ FIGURE 14–2). Insulin plays an essential role in glucose (sugar) metabolism. Insulin lowers the blood glucose level by enabling cells to utilize glucose. Insulin transports glucose to the cell, binds with an insulin receptor on the cell membrane, and transports glucose inside the cell where the glucose is metabolized to provide energy.

Diabetes mellitus is a disease of the pancreas and body cells. It occurs when

■ the pancreas does not produce any insulin (type 1 diabetes mellitus)
■ the pancreas produces too little insulin (type 2 diabetes mellitus)
■ the number of or sensitivity of insulin receptors on body cells is decreased (type 2 diabetes mellitus).

Type 1 diabetes mellitus was previously known as *insulin-dependent diabetes mellitus (IDDM)* or *juvenile-onset diabetes mellitus* (see ■ TABLE 14–1). Type 1 diabetes mellitus is

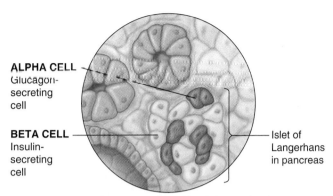

Glucagon—raises blood glucose level
Insulin—lowers blood glucose level

**■ FIGURE 14–2  Alpha and beta cells of the pancreas.**
In a healthy person, the alpha and beta cells of the pancreas work together to control the blood glucose level. When the blood glucose level is low, the alpha cells of the pancreas secrete glucagon, which stimulates the liver to break down glycogen (stored glucose) and release it into the blood. On the other hand, when the blood glucose level is high, the beta cells of the pancreas secrete insulin, which transports glucose from the blood into the cells where it is metabolized to produce energy.

**■ TABLE 14–1  Comparison of type 1 and type 2 diabetes mellitus.**

| Type | Type 1 | Type 2 |
|------|--------|--------|
| Former Names | Insulin-dependent diabetes mellitus (IDDM) | Non–insulin-dependent diabetes mellitus (NIDDM) |
| | Juvenile-onset diabetes mellitus | Adult-onset diabetes mellitus |
| Onset | Childhood, young adulthood | Middle age |
| Contributing Factors | Viral trigger, heredity | Obesity, heredity |
| Treatment | Diabetic diet, weight control, exercise, insulin | Diabetic diet, weight control, exercise, antidiabetic drugs, sometimes insulin |

treated with subcutaneously injected insulin. Type 2 diabetes mellitus was previously known as *non–insulin-dependent diabetes mellitus (NIDDM)* or *adult-onset diabetes mellitus*. Type 2 diabetes mellitus is treated with antidiabetic drugs, but insulin may also be needed. A diet with controlled amounts of calories from carbohydrates and fats, weight control, and exercise are also very important components of managing both types of diabetes mellitus.

Untreated or uncontrolled diabetes mellitus results in a blood glucose level that is constantly elevated. This eventually leads to the diabetic complications of diabetic retinopathy, diabetic neuropathy, arteriosclerosis, ketoacidosis, and even death.

## *Historical Notes*

The word *insulin* is derived from the Latin word *insula* meaning *island,* a reference to the islets of Langerhans. Before the discovery of the drug insulin, diabetic patients were kept on extremely low-calorie diets (often to the point of starvation), as this was the only known treatment to keep the blood glucose level within the normal range.

The drug insulin was first isolated in the 1920s. The first insulin was extracted from the ground-up pancreases of cows and pigs, and the injected liquid was thick and muddy brown due to impurities. Later, insulin was purified, refined, and a standardized measurement, the unit, was adopted for insulin doses.

New insulin drugs have been created using recombinant DNA technology. This technology inserts the gene for human insulin into bacteria or yeasts, which then multiply rapidly and produce large amounts of insulin drug. Other insulin drugs created by recombinant DNA technology include the insulin analog drugs. An analog is structurally similar to the original molecule (human insulin) but is not entirely the same.

The yeast used to make one type of insulin is the same as baker's yeast used in the kitchen!

Humulin insulin was the first recombinant DNA drug of any type to be marketed. NovoLog was the first insulin to be approved by the FDA specifically for use with an external insulin pump.

Exubera, the first powdered insulin that could be inhaled, was approved by the FDA in 2006 but was removed from the market in 2007.

Regardless of the original source of the insulin (whether from an animal or created by recombinant DNA or other technology), all insulin drugs are grouped according to

- how quickly they act in the body to lower the blood glucose level (this depends on the size of the insulin crystal)
- how many hours their therapeutic effect continues (this depends on the amount of protamine and zinc added to the insulin).

Insulin drug groups include rapid-acting insulin, intermediate-acting insulin, and long-acting insulin.

### Rapid-Acting Insulin Drugs

Rapid-acting insulin drugs are taken in the morning or before eating. The onset of their therapeutic effect is almost immediate. Rapid-acting insulin drugs can begin to lower the blood glucose level in as little as 15 minutes. The therapeutic effect of these drugs lasts from 2 to 12 hours. Rapid-acting insulin drugs are also known as *regular insulin*, and this is sometimes reflected in the drug's trade name as the abbreviation *R*.

The three different types of rapid-acting insulin drugs are

- derived from pig pancreas (Regular Iletin II) (see ■ FIGURE 14–3)
- created by recombinant DNA technology (Humulin R, Novolin R) (see ■ FIGURE 14–4)
- insulin analog drugs created by recombinant DNA technology (insulin aspart, insulin glulisine, and insulin lispro).

| | |
|---|---|
| Humulin R | insulin lispro (Humalog) |
| insulin aspart (NovoLog) | Novolin R |
| insulin glulisine (Apidra) | Regular Iletin II |

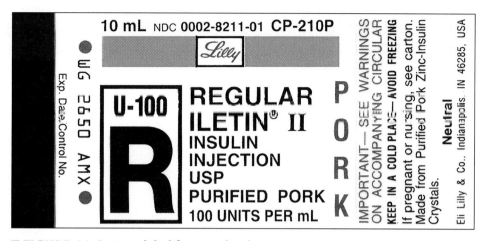

■ **FIGURE 14–3 Drug label for Regular Iletin II insulin.**
Regular Iletin II is a regular insulin drug with a rapid onset of action. The label shows a large capital *R* that stands for *regular insulin.* Doses are measured in 100 units/mL. U-100 or the equivalent 100 units/mL is a universal standard of measurement for insulin. The label clearly indicates in red capital letters that the source of this insulin is from pork.

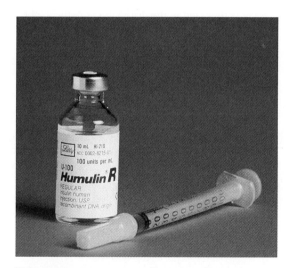

■ **FIGURE 14–4 Humulin R insulin and insulin syringe.**
Humulin R insulin is a rapid-acting regular insulin drug created with recombinant DNA technology. The *R* in its trade name stands for *regular insulin.* Insulin drugs come in a standardized concentration of 100 units/mL and are administered in a special insulin syringe that is calibrated in units.

## In Depth

A molecule of human insulin consists of an A and a B chain of amino acids. When analog insulin drugs are created, one or more of the amino acids in the human insulin molecule is changed. In the analog insulin drug named insulin aspart, aspartic acid is inserted at site B28 on the B chain. In insulin glulisine, glutamic acid and lysine are substituted. In insulin lispro, the amino acids lysine and proline are reversed at sites B28 and B29. Can you see how the names of the changed amino acids are used to create the name of the analog insulin drug? In insulin detemir (described on page 235), myristic acid is substituted on the B chain. In insulin glargine (described on page 235), the amino acids glycine and arginine are substituted. Some of the trade names (Humalog, Novolog) of these analog insulin drugs contain parts of the word *analog* to indicate how the drug was created.

### Intermediate-Acting Insulin Drugs

Intermediate-acting insulin drugs have a slower onset but a longer effect than rapid-acting insulin drugs. The onset of the therapeutic effect of intermediate-acting insulin drugs is within 1 to 2 hours. The therapeutic effect of these drugs lasts for 24 hours.

There are two types of intermediate-acting insulin drugs: those with added protamine and zinc (NPH insulin drugs) to prolong the therapeutic effect of the insulin and those with different sizes of insulin crystals (lente insulin drugs) to slow down the onset of action of the insulin.

The NPH insulin drugs Humulin N and Novolin N are produced by recombinant DNA technology. NPH is reflected in the drug's trade name as the abbreviation *N*.

The insulin drug Lente Iletin II is derived from pig pancreas.

Humulin N

Lente Iletin II

Novolin N

## Did You Know?

The abbreviation *NPH* stands for *neutral protamine Hagedorn*. Hans Christian Hagedorn (1888–1971), a Scandinavian physician, took animal insulin and added protamine, a substance from the semen of river trout, to prolong the therapeutic effect of insulin. He then adjusted the solution until it had a neutral pH so that the drug could be injected into the tissues.

## Focus on Healthcare Issues

Beef and beef/pork insulin drugs are no longer on the market in the United States because of the risk that they might transmit bovine spongiform encephalopathy (a fatal disease in cows) that has been linked to outbreaks of a fatal neurologic condition in humans known as Creutzfeldt-Jakob disease. Some diabetic patients who have tried to switch from beef or beef/pork insulin to other types of insulin have found that they have poorly controlled blood glucose levels. Some diabetic patients have tried to obtain beef or beef/pork insulin from other countries. Only pork insulin is available in the United States.

## Long-Acting Insulin Drugs

Long-acting insulin drugs have large insulin crystals and contain added zinc. Long-acting insulin drugs do not begin to lower the blood glucose level for over an hour. The therapeutic effect of long-acting insulin drugs lasts a full 24 hours after just one dose. Long-acting insulin drugs are also known as *ultralente insulin.* In the past, the ultralente category was reflected in some drugs' trade names that contained the abbreviation *U.* However, there currently are no ultralente long-acting insulin drugs on the market whose trade name contain a *U.*

These long-acting insulin drugs belong to the category of insulin analog drugs.

insulin detemir (Levemir)

insulin glargine (Lantus)

## Combination Insulin Drugs

These combination drugs contain a mixture of an intermediate-acting insulin (NPH insulin drug or insulin analog drug) and a rapid-acting insulin (regular insulin drug or insulin analog drug). The percentage of the intermediate-acting insulin drug is the number listed first in the trade name.

Humalog Mix 75/25                   Novolin 70/30

Humulin 50/50                        NovoLog Mix 70/30

Humulin 70/30 (see ■ **FIGURE 14–5**)

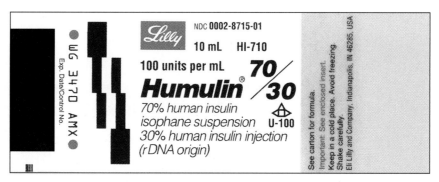

■ **FIGURE 14–5  Drug label for Humulin 70/30 insulin.**
This insulin is a mixture of 70% intermediate-acting NPH insulin (isophane is another name for NPH insulin) and 30% rapid-acting regular insulin. The designation *rDNA origin* indicates that this drug is manufactured using recombinant DNA technology.

## *Clinical Applications*

Because the insulin molecule is broken down by digestive enzymes, insulin can never be given orally. Patients with type 1 diabetes mellitus inject insulin subcutaneously once or several times a day at various sites on the upper arms, thighs, or abdomen where there is some subcutaneous fat (see ■ **FIGURE 14–6**).

*(continued)*

*Clinical Applications (continued)*

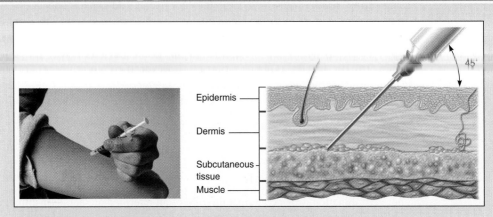

■ **FIGURE 14–6  Subcutaneous insulin injection.**
Insulin must be injected subcutaneously into the fat layer beneath the skin. The needle is inserted at a
45-degree angle so that it does not go into the muscle layer. The upper arms, thighs, abdomen, and
other sites can be used for insulin injections. A new site must be selected for each injection to avoid
tissue damage. This process is known as *site rotation.*

An insulin syringe is used to administer insulin drugs (see ■ **FIGURE 14–7**). This syringe
is never used to administer any other type of liquid drug. Its calibrations are unique because they
are in units, a standard measurement for insulin doses.

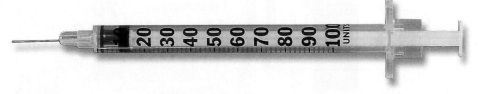

■ **FIGURE 14–7  An insulin syringe.**
Any amount of insulin from 1 unit to 100 units can be drawn up in this syringe. The pre-attached
needle on an insulin syringe is shorter than other needles so that it will deposit the drug into the
subcutaneous fat, not in the deeper muscle layer.

Insulin can also be administered directly into the blood via tubing connected to a portable
insulin pump that is attached to a belt or carried in a pocket (see ■ **FIGURE 14–8**). A totally
implantable computerized insulin pump is also available for patients who have poorly controlled
diabetes mellitus. The pump is implanted in the abdomen, and the patient programs the insulin dose
via remote control.

## Oral Antidiabetic Drugs

The pancreas of a patient with type 2 diabetes mellitus is still producing insulin, but in a smaller
amount than normal. There is also resistance by the body cells to allowing the insulin that is

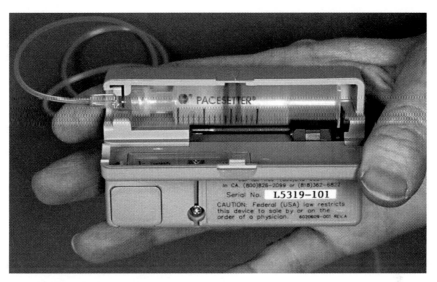

**█ FIGURE 14–8 Insulin pump.**
This insulin pump, which is attached to a belt or carried in a pocket, runs on batteries. It can deliver as little as 0.1 unit of insulin and has alarms to alert the patient if the tubing becomes blocked or if the insulin reservoir is empty.

produced to enter the cells. With diet control, exercise, and weight loss, the amount of available insulin can be sufficient to keep the blood glucose level in a normal range. If not, the physician will prescribe an oral antidiabetic drug. Contrary to popular opinion, oral antidiabetic drugs are not insulin and are not effective in treating patients with type 1 diabetes mellitus. Oral antidiabetic drugs stimulate the beta cells of the pancreas to produce more insulin; these drugs also increase the number of insulin receptors so that the cells are not resistant to the effects of any insulin that is present. There are six categories of oral antidiabetic drugs: sulfonylurea drugs, meglitinide drugs, thiazolidinedione drugs, alpha-glucosidase inhibitor drugs, biguanide drugs, and DPP-4 inhibitor drugs.

## Sulfonylurea Oral Antidiabetic Drugs

The sulfonylurea class of oral antidiabetic drugs was the first type of antidiabetic drugs that could be given orally. They are structurally derived from anti-infective sulfonamide drugs (the source of their name), but do not have any anti-infective action. The first generation of sulfonylurea oral antidiabetic drugs was produced in the 1950s. Their generic drug names end in the suffix *-amide*. A second and more powerful generation of sulfonylurea oral antidiabetic drugs was introduced in the early 1970s; their generic drug names end in the suffix *-ide*. All sulfonylurea oral antidiabetic drugs stimulate the beta cells of the pancreas to produce more insulin.

chlorpropamide (Diabinese)

glimepiride (Amaryl)

glipizide (Glucotrol, Glucotrol XL)
  (see █ FIGURE 14–9)

glyburide (DiaBeta, Micronase)

tolazamide

tolbutamide (Orinase)

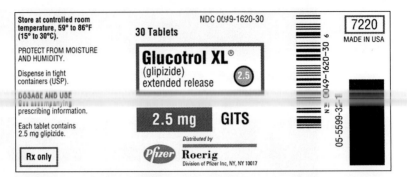

■ **FIGURE 14–9  Drug label for glipizide (Glucotrol XL).**
Glucotrol is the trade name of the generic drug glipizide. Glucotrol comes in
tablets, and Glucotrol XL comes in extended-release tablets that extend the
length of the therapeutic effect. The abbreviation *XL* stands for *extended length.*

## Did You Know?

The trade name DiaBeta is a combination of the words *diabetes* and *beta*, in reference to the
beta cells of the islets of Langerhans of the pancreas that produce insulin to treat diabetes.

### Meglitinide Oral Antidiabetic Drugs

The meglitinide class of oral antidiabetic drugs stimulates the beta cells of the pancreas to produce
more insulin.

  nateglinide (Starlix)

  repaglinide (Prandin)

### Thiazolidinedione Oral Antidiabetic Drugs

The thiazolidinedione class of oral antidiabetic drugs increases the sensitivity of the cell to any
insulin produced by the pancreas and suppresses the release of stored glucose from the liver. Both
of these actions help to maintain the normal level of blood glucose, without actually increasing
insulin production.

  pioglitazone (Actos)

  rosiglitazone (Avandia)

### Alpha-Glucosidase Inhibitor Oral Antidiabetic Drugs

The alpha-glucosidase inhibitor class of oral antidiabetic drugs inhibits the action of certain
enzymes that digest carbohydrates (the enzyme alpha-glucoside hydrolase from the small intestine
and the enzyme amylase from the pancreas). This means less glucose enters the blood, and the pancreas does not need to produce as much insulin to keep the blood glucose level low.

  acarbose (Precose)

  miglitol (Glyset)

### Biguanide Oral Antidiabetic Drugs

The biguanide class of oral antidiabetic drugs decreases the absorption of glucose from the intestine, suppresses the release of stored glucose from the liver, and improves the ability of cells to use the insulin that is produced by the pancreas. Biguanide oral antidiabetic drugs have an additional benefit. Because they do not stimulate the pancreas to produce more insulin, the diabetic patient is not at risk for developing hypoglycemia (low blood glucose), as with some oral antidiabetic drugs. This unique combination of effects and benefits makes biguanide oral antidiabetic drugs a good choice for pairing with other oral antidiabetic drugs in a combination drug.

metformin (Glucophage, Glucophage XR)

### DPP-4 Inhibitor Oral Antidiabetic Drugs

The DPP-4 inhibitor class of oral antidiabetic drugs prolongs the action of the hormones GLP-1 and GIP that stimulate the beta cells of the pancreas to make more insulin (see In Depth).

sitagliptin (Januvia)

## In Depth

GLP-1 and GIP are two hormones that are normally released by the intestine when food is present in the stomach. Both GLP-1 and GIP stimulate the beta cells of the pancreas to make more insulin. GLP-1 also suppresses the release of stored glucose from the liver. DPP-4, which stands for *dipeptidyl peptidase-4*, is an enzyme that normally breaks down and inactivates these hormones (GLP-1 and GIP). DPP-4 inhibitor oral antidiabetic drugs inhibit the enzyme DPP-4 and so prolong the desirable action of GLP-1 and GIP.

### Combination Oral Antidiabetic Drugs

These combination drugs contain a sulfonylurea oral antidiabetic drug (glimepiride, glyburide, glipizide), a meglitinide oral antidiabetic drug (repaglinide), a thiazolidinedione oral antidiabetic drug (pioglitazone, rosiglitazone), a biguanide oral antidiabetic drug (metformin), or a DPP-4 inhibitor oral antidiabetic drug (sitagliptin).

| | |
|---|---|
| ActoPlus Met (metformin, pioglitazone) | Glucovance (metformin, glyburide) |
| Avandamet (metformin, rosiglitazone) | Janumet (metformin, sitagliptin) |
| Avandaryl (glimepiride, rosiglitazone) | Metaglip (metformin, glipizide) |
| Duetact (glimepiride, pioglitazone) | PrandiMet (metformin, repaglinide) |

## Other Antidiabetic Drugs

These categories of drugs have therapeutic effects that are different from those of insulin or oral antidiabetic drugs. These drugs are used to treat type 2 diabetes mellitus and sometimes type 1 diabetes mellitus. Some of these drugs stimulate the release of insulin from the pancreas only when the blood glucose level is high. Others decrease the appetite, slow the emptying of food from the stomach, and suppress the release of stored glucose from the liver. Some of these drugs are given subcutaneously, while others are given orally.

### Amylin Analog Antidiabetic Drugs

The amylin analog class of antidiabetic drugs is based on the action of amylin, a substance in the body that is secreted from the beta cells of the pancreas at the same time as insulin. Amylin and the amylin analog class of antidiabetic drugs slow the rate at which food leaves the stomach, suppress the release of stored glucose from the liver, and work in the brain to decrease the appetite. All of these effects make amylin analog antidiabetic drugs useful for treating both type 1 and type 2 diabetes mellitus. This drug is given subcutaneously.

pramlintide (Symlin)

### Bile Acid Sequestrant Antidiabetic Drugs

Bile acid sequestrant drugs are commonly used to treat an elevated level of cholesterol in the blood. Now these bile acid sequestrant drugs have been approved to improve blood glucose control in patients with type 2 diabetes mellitus. This drug is given orally.

colesevelam (WelChol)

### Incretin Mimetic Antidiabetic Drugs

The incretin mimetic class of antidiabetic drugs is based on the action of incretins, a group of substances in the body that stimulate the beta cells of the pancreas to produce insulin only when the blood glucose level is high. Incretin mimetic antidiabetic drugs are used to treat type 2 diabetes mellitus. This drug is given subcutaneously. It is derived from Gila monster saliva.

exenatide (Byetta)

## Did You Know?

The antidiabetic drug Byetta is a synthetic version of a protein found in the saliva of the poisonous Gila monster, a lizard that lives in the Sonoran Desert of the southwestern United States and in Mexico. The saliva is secreted from grooves in the teeth. Gila monsters are about 2 feet long and weigh about 5 pounds.

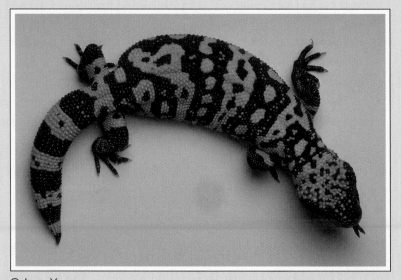

© Jerry Young

## Historical Notes

Dr. John Eng, an endocrinologist in New York in the early 1980s noticed that persons bitten by venous animals often developed pancreatitis because the venom overstimulated the pancreas. Dr. Eng remembers, "So we ordered up a whole variety of venoms—from snakes and other animals, including the Gila monster—and started looking for the compound that stimulated the pancreas." Dr. Eng worked on this research for 20 years until he discovered a compound in Gila monster saliva that stimulates the pancreas to secrete insulin. "The Gila monster is a beautiful reptile. All I can say is, without the Gila monster, this would never have happened and, to me, that is kind of humbling."

Carla McClain, "Gila monster spit aids diabetics," *Arizona Daily Star,* May 9, 2005.

# Drugs Used to Treat Thyroid Gland Dysfunction

Thyroid gland dysfunction includes hypothyroidism, in which too little thyroid hormone is secreted, and hyperthyroidism, in which too much thyroid hormone is secreted.

### Drugs for Hypothyroidism

The thyroid gland secretes the hormones triiodothyronine ($T_3$) and thyroxine ($T_4$). Decreased levels of these hormones cause hypothyroidism. Drugs used to treat hypothyroidism act by supplementing existing levels of $T_3$ and/or $T_4$. These drugs are obtained from natural sources, such as desiccated (dried) animal thyroid glands, or they are synthetically manufactured.

This thyroid hormone drug contains only $T_3$.

liothyronine (Cytomel, Triostat)

This thyroid hormone drug contains only $T_4$.

levothyroxine (Levothroid, Synthroid)

These thyroid hormone drugs contain both $T_3$ and $T_4$.

desiccated thyroid (Armour Thyroid)        liotrix (Thyrolar) (see ■ **FIGURE 14–10**)

### Drugs for Hyperthyroidism

Increased levels of $T_3$ and $T_4$ cause hyperthyroidism. Antithyroid drugs treat hyperthyroidism (thyrotoxicosis) by inhibiting the production of $T_3$ and $T_4$ in the thyroid gland. These drugs can also be given prior to a thyroidectomy. Radioactive sodium iodide 131 is used to treat both hyperthyroidism and thyroid cancer; the low-level radiation emitted by this drug destroys both hyperactive benign thyroid tissue and cancerous thyroid tissue.

iodine (ThyroShield)        propylthiouracil
methimazole (Tapazole)        sodium iodide 131 (Iodotope)

# Drugs Used to Treat Pituitary Gland Dysfunction

Pituitary gland dysfunction includes growth failure, in which too little growth hormone is secreted, and acromegaly, in which too much growth hormone is secreted. It also includes diabetes insipidus, in which too little antidiuretic hormone is secreted, and syndrome of inappropriate antidiuretic hormone (SIADH), in which too much antidiuretic hormone is secreted.

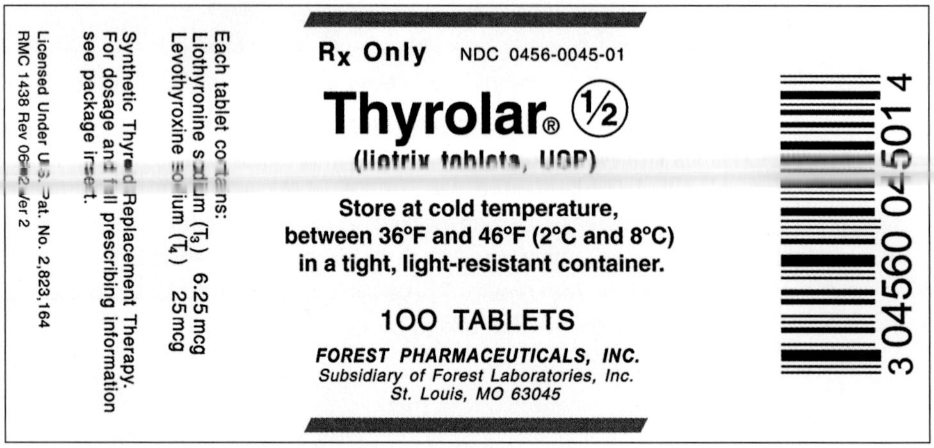

Each tablet contains:
Liothyronine sodium ($T_3$) 6.25 mcg
Levothyroxine sodium ($T_4$) 25 mcg

Synthetic Thyroid Replacement Therapy.
For dosage and full prescribing information
see package insert.

Licensed Under U.S. Pat. No. 2,823,164
RMC 1438 Rev 06/02 Ver 2

**Rx Only** NDC 0456-0045-01

# Thyrolar® ½

**(liotrix tablets, USP)**

**Store at cold temperature,
between 36°F and 46°F (2°C and 8°C)
in a tight, light-resistant container.**

**100 TABLETS**

**FOREST PHARMACEUTICALS, INC.**
Subsidiary of Forest Laboratories, Inc.
St. Louis, MO 63045

3 04560 04501 4

**■ FIGURE 14–10  Drug label for liotrix (Thyrolar).**
This Thyrolar label shows both the apothecary system of measurement with the dose in grains
(1/2 grain) and the metric system of measurement with the dose in micrograms ($T_3$, 6.25 mcg;
$T_4$, 25 mcg) (on the left side of the panel). Thyrolar is one of the few drugs in current use in
which the dose is still given in the apothecary system of measurement.

## Growth Hormone Replacement Drugs

The anterior pituitary gland secretes growth hormone, and growth hormone stimulates the production of
insulin-like growth factor-1. Children with a failure to grow in height can have an abnormality in any of
these areas: a decreased amount of growth hormone, antibodies against growth hormone, abnormalities
of the growth hormone receptors on cells, or a decreased amount of insulin-like growth factor-1. These
drugs are used as replacement therapy for growth hormone.

mecasermin (Increlex, Iplex)          somatrem (Protropin)

sermorelin (Geref)          somatropin (Humatrope, Nutropin)

## Did You Know?

Both somatrem and somatropin were created using recombinant DNA technology. The combining form *somat/o-* means *body* in Greek.

## Drugs for Acromegaly

In adults, an overproduction of growth hormone by the anterior pituitary gland causes acromegaly,
a widening and enlargement of the facial features, hands, and feet. These drugs decrease the production of growth hormone by the anterior pituitary gland or block growth hormone from activating
receptors on the cell membrane.

bromocriptine (Parlodel)          octreotide (Sandostatin)

lanreotide (Somatuline Depot)          pegvisomant (Somavert)

## Did You Know?

Octreotide is also used to treat severe diarrhea associated with VIPomas and AIDS.
Interestingly, this drug's side effect of decreased peristalsis is used as a therapeutic effect in
treating diarrhea and other disorders of peristalsis in the GI tract.

### Drugs for Diabetes Insipidus

Insufficient levels of antidiuretic hormone (ADH) cause diabetes insipidus with its symptoms of excessive, dilute urine, and thirst. These drugs treat diabetes insipidus by acting as replacement therapy for ADH. Desmopressin is a synthetic analog of ADH; its route of administration is unusual in that it is given as an intranasal spray. Vasopressin is actual antidiuretic hormone (ADH) in a drug form.

> desmopressin (DDAVP, Stimate)
>
> vasopressin (Pitressin)

### Drugs for Syndrome of Inappropriate Antidiuretic Hormone

The posterior pituitary gland secretes antidiuretic hormone (ADH), which decreases the amount of water excreted by the kidneys (an antidiuretic effect). If the posterior pituitary gland secretes excessive amounts of ADH, too little urine is produced. Conivaptan is an antagonist drug that blocks ADH from joining with certain receptors that it normally stimulates. The mechanism of the therapeutic effect of lithium in treating syndrome of inappropriate ADH (SIADH) is not well understood.

> conivaptan (Vaprisol)
>
> demeclocycline (Declomycin)
>
> lithium (Lithobid)

## Drugs Used to Treat Adrenal Gland Dysfunction

Adrenal gland dysfunction includes Cushing's syndrome, in which too much adrenal gland hormone is secreted, and Addison's disease, in which too little adrenal gland hormone is secreted.

### Drugs for Cushing's Syndrome

The adrenal cortex secretes the hormone cortisol. If a tumor causes the adrenal cortex to secrete increased amounts of cortisol, this causes Cushing's syndrome. This drug inhibits pregnenolone (the precursor to all the hormones secreted by the adrenal cortex). Decreasing the amount of pregnenolone lowers an elevated level of cortisol and treats Cushing's syndrome.

> aminoglutethimide (Cytadren)

### Drugs for Addison's Disease

Addison's disease is an autoimmune disease in which the body's own antibodies destroy the adrenal cortex and too little cortisol is secreted. Addison's disease causes fatigue, weight loss, and decreased ability to tolerate stress, disease, or surgery. In addition, patients have an unusual bronzed color to the skin. Corticosteroid drugs are used as cortisol replacement therapy to treat patients with Addison's disease.

> cortisone
>
> fludrocortisone (Florinef)
>
> hydrocortisone (Cortef)

## Corticosteroid Drugs

The adrenal cortex secretes the glucocorticoid hormones hydrocortisone and cortisol, both of which are powerful anti-inflammatory hormones. Glucocorticoid hormones available as drugs are known as *corticosteroid drugs* because they act in the same way as the natural hormones secreted

## Historical Notes

A researcher at the Mayo Clinic was attempting to identify hormones in the adrenal gland. He found five substances that he called Substances A, B, C, D, and E. To obtain just 2 ounces of Substance E, he had to grind 300,000 pounds of animal adrenal glands. In 1941, the United States received an intelligence report that Germany was giving adrenal gland extract to its pilots to enable them to fly at high altitudes. Although this report was false, it stimulated financial backing for adrenal gland research. Substance E later became known as *cortisone.*

by the adrenal cortex (*cortic/o-*), and their chemical structure is that of a steroid. Corticosteroid drugs are used as replacement therapy to treat Addison's disease, as described in the previous section. Other corticosteroid drugs (listed here) are given by mouth or injection to treat inflammatory reactions in various parts of the body. Corticosteroid drugs are also used to treat systemic inflammation caused by autoimmune diseases (rheumatoid arthritis, multiple sclerosis, lupus erythematosus, and so forth).

betamethasone (Celestone)

dexamethasone (Decadron)

hydrocortisone (Cortef, Solu-Cortef)

methylprednisolone (Medrol, Solu-Medrol)

prednisolone (Pediapred, Prelone) (see ■ **FIGURE 14–11**)

prednisone (Deltasone, Meticorten)

triamcinolone (Aristocort, Kenalog)

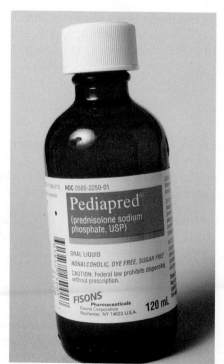

■ **FIGURE 14–11  Drug bottle of prednisolone (Pediapred).**
Corticosteroid drugs commonly come in the drug form of a tablet. However, Pediapred is in a liquid form that can be given more easily to pediatric patients, as the trade name implies.

Topical corticosteroid drugs used to treat inflammation of the skin are discussed in Chapter 17. Topical corticosteroid drugs used to treat inflammation of the ears, nose, and eyes are discussed in Chapter 18 and in Chapter 19.

## Drug Alert!

Patients who must take prolonged or high doses of a corticosteroid drug such as prednisone develop a unique appearance that is just like the appearance of patients who have hyper-secretion of glucocorticoids from the adrenal cortex (Cushing's syndrome). These patients have increased deposition of fat in the face (moon face) and back of the neck (buffalo hump); they have a thinning of facial connective tissue which allows the blood vessels to show through, giving their cheeks a reddened appearance; they also have an increased blood glucose level, as well as wasting of the muscles of the extremities and weakness from depressed protein synthesis.

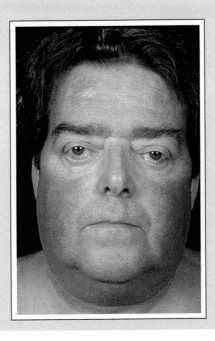

## Anabolic Steroid Drugs

Anabolic steroid drugs change the natural balance between anabolism (tissue building) and catabolism (tissue breakdown) in the body. Anabolic steroid drugs are prescribed for AIDS patients to counteract the loss of muscle mass and strength that occurs with AIDS wasting syndrome. These drugs are also prescribed to promote weight gain following extensive surgery or trauma, to increase the RBC count and treat anemia, or to increase muscle mass in patients with muscular dystrophy. Oxandrolone is also used to treat bone pain in patients with osteoporosis and to treat a lack of growth in patients with Turner syndrome. Both of these are Schedule III drugs.

oxandrolone (Oxandrin)

oxymetholone (Anadrol-50)

## Focus on Healthcare Issues

Although the use of anabolic steroid drugs to increase muscle mass, strength, and endurance is illegal in amateur and professional sports competitions, their use continues. Athletes discontinue the use of these drugs before a competition to avoid detection during random drug testing. The use of two or more anabolic steroids at the same time is referred to as "stacking." Often the dose taken is 10 to 100 times the dose that would be written for the prescription use of the drug. The continued use of anabolic steroid drugs can cause decreased sperm count, shrunken testicles, baldness, and irreversible breast enlargement in men. In women, these drugs can cause baldness and excessive growth of facial hair. The serious side effects of anabolic steroid drugs include aggressive behavior, atherosclerosis, and even liver cancer. All anabolic steroid drugs are classified as Schedule III controlled substances because of their high potential for addiction and abuse.

# Chapter Review

## Quiz Yourself

1. Name some endocrine drugs that are derived from animal sources.
2. List some of the differences between type 1 and type 2 diabetes mellitus with respect to former names, onset, contributing factors, and treatment.
3. How are doses of insulin measured?
4. Name two ways that insulin is administered.
5. Oral antidiabetic drugs contain a special type of insulin that can be taken orally. True or false?
6. Why were beef and beef/pork insulins removed from the market? What is the significance of this to some diabetic patients?
7. List some of the generic and trade names for insulin drugs that are produced using recombinant DNA technology.
8. Why are oral antidiabetic drugs not given to patients with type 1 diabetes mellitus?
9. Name several categories of antidiabetic drugs (besides insulin) and describe their therapeutic effects in treating diabetes mellitus.
10. Name an endocrine drug whose dose is still measured using the apothecary system of measurement.
11. List four trade names of drugs used to treat hypothyroidism.
12. What type of drug is used to treat children with failure to grow? To treat adults with acromegaly?
13. Name two powerful natural anti-inflammatory hormones secreted by the adrenal cortex.
14. Describe some of the physical changes that occur in a patient who takes a prolonged or high dose of a corticosteroid drug.
15. Describe the therapeutic effects of the legal use of anabolic steroid drugs and the detrimental side effects of the illegal use of anabolic steroid drugs.
16. What endocrine disease is each of these drugs used to treat?
    a. insulin aspart (NovoLog)
    b. gyburide (DiaBeta, Micronase)
    c. liothyronine (Cytomel, Triostat)
    d. hydrocortisone (Cortef)
    e. sitagliptin (Januvia)
    f. somatrem (Protropin)

   **g.** glipizide (Glucotrol)
   **h.** vasopressin (Pitressin)
   **i.** levothyroxine (Levothroid, Synthroid)
   **j.** rosiglitazone (Avandia)

## Spelling Tips

| | |
|---|---|
| **DiaBeta** | Unusual internal capitalization. |
| **Humalog** | Spelled with an *a* versus Humulin spelled with a *u*. |
| **NovoLog** | Unusual internal capitalization. |
| **Levothroid** | Although *thyroid* has a y in it, there is no *y* in this drug name. |
| **PrandiMet** | Unusual internal capitalization. |
| **Synthroid** | Although *thyroid* has a *y* in it, there is no *y* in this drug name. |

## Clinical Applications

1. Look at these two drug labels and then answer the following questions.
   **a.** What is the trade name of the generic drug levothyroxine?
   **b.** In what dose (tablet strength) is this drug being prescribed?
   **c.** What are five cautions or warnings that must be observed when taking this drug?
   **d.** What quantity of tablets did the pharmacist dispense in this prescription bottle?
   **e.** Who is the manufacturer of this particular version of the generic drug levothyroxine?
   **f.** When did the pharmacist fill this prescription?
   **g.** How many refills did the physician say were allowed?
   **h.** The directions "Take one tablet by mouth one time daily" were translated by the pharmacist from the original prescription so that the patient could understand the directions. Use medical language to rewrite these words as the physician actually wrote them on the original prescription.

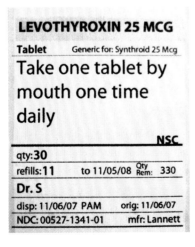

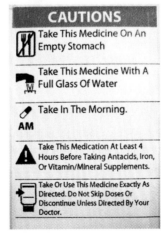

2. Read this handwritten prescription. Rewrite the information in words that could be understood by the patient.

**EDWIN ADAMS, M.D.**
Chartwell Professional Group
300 Medical Way
Pittsburgh, PA 13228
Phone: 312-569-1000

NAME _Joan R. Johnson_
Address _____
Age _62_

℞    Synthroid   0.125 mg tablet
         #60
     Sig: Take ī QAM 1 hr before breakfast

[✓] Do not substitute     Refills 0 (1) 2 3 4 5
Generic drug

Signature: _Edwin Adams_ M.D.
Date: _09/06/08_ DEA # _____

3. A diabetic patient in the emergency department takes a tablet from her purse when you ask her what drug she takes. She does not know the name of it. Look at this drug tablet. Based on your study of this chapter, can you determine which oral antidiabetic drug she is taking?

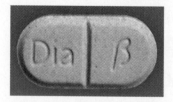

## Multimedia Extension Exercises

■ Go to www.pearsonhighered.com/turley and click on the photo of the cover of *Understanding Pharmacology for Health Professionals* to access the interactive Companion Website created for this textbook.

# Neurologic Drugs

## Learning Objectives

After you study this chapter, you should be able to

1. Describe the therapeutic effects of various categories of drugs used to treat epilepsy, Alzheimer's disease, and Parkinson's disease.

2. Explain the difficulties physicians face in treating the lack of dopamine that characterizes Parkinson's disease.

3. Describe the therapeutic effects of various categories of drugs used to treat neuralgia and neuropathy.

4. Describe the therapeutic effects of various categories of drugs used to treat insomnia and narcolepsy.

5. Given the generic and trade names of a neurologic drug, identify what category they belong to or what disease they are used to treat.

6. Given a neurologic drug category, identify several generic and trade name drugs in that category.

Neurologic drugs are used to treat diseases of the brain and nerves. These diseases include epilepsy, dementia and Alzheimer's disease, Parkinson's disease, myasthenia gravis, insomnia, neuralgia and neuropathy, and narcolepsy. Neurologic drugs include anticonvulsant drugs, cholinesterase inhibitor drugs, dopamine agonist drugs, MAO inhibitor drugs, anticholinergic drugs, COMT inhibitor drugs, cellular implants, hypnotic drugs, benzodiazepine drugs, barbiturate drugs, and others.

## Drugs Used to Treat Epilepsy

An epileptic seizure originates in the brain when a group of neurons spontaneously begins to send out impulses in an abnormal, uncontrolled way. These impulses then spread from neuron to neuron. Symptoms of epilepsy range from barely noticeable staring or a lack of attention to a full tonic-clonic seizure with unconsciousness, muscle jerking, tongue biting, and incontinence. The type of symptoms depends on the number and location of the affected neurons. Drugs used to treat epilepsy are known as **anticonvulsant drugs** because epilepsy is characterized by seizures or convulsions.

### *Historical Notes*

Efforts to control epilepsy were largely in vain for centuries. Epilepsy was attributed to supernatural forces, poison, and so forth. The treatment could involve trephining (boring a hole in the skull), prayers, or herbal remedies. Phenobarbital (Luminal), the first drug found to be effective for epilepsy, was introduced in 1912.

In 1923, Tracy Putnam was a resident in neurology. He became intrigued with the possibility that epilepsy might be caused by a chemical abnormality in the brain. He noted, for example, that patients who "rebreathed" their own carbon dioxide by putting a bag over their heads got some relief [from seizures]. He asked himself, "Might an institution for the treatment of epilepsy be established adjacent to a brewery, and the content of carbon dioxide in the atmosphere metered so as to be tolerable and yet sufficient to prevent attacks?" Putnam later abandoned this idea and instead began searching for drugs that might be effective for epilepsy. "I combed the catalog," Putnam later wrote, "for suitable compounds that were not obviously poisonous." He was looking for drugs in particular that contained a benzene ring because, among the barbitals, only phenobarbital, which also had a benzene ring, possessed the ability to suppress epilepsy. "Parke-Davis . . . wrote back to me that it had on hand samples of 19 different compounds analogous to phenobarbital and that I was welcome to them." Of the 19 compounds in the shipment, all were inactive and ineffective against epilepsy except one—phenytoin (Dilantin)—which was introduced in 1938 and is still the drug of choice for treating adult tonic-clonic seizures.

Edward Shorter, *The Health Century.* New York: Doubleday, 1987, pp. 110–111.

### Hydantoin Drugs for Epilepsy

Hydantoin drugs act on the cell membrane of neurons in the motor cortex of the brain. These drugs affect the flow of sodium in and out of the cell, thereby preventing the neuron from depolarizing and repolarizing (i.e., sending out an impulse) too rapidly or repeatedly.

> fosphenytoin (Cerebyx)
>
> phenytoin (Dilantin) (see ■ **FIGURE 15–1**)

*Note:* The suffix *-phenytoin* is common to generic hydantoin drugs.

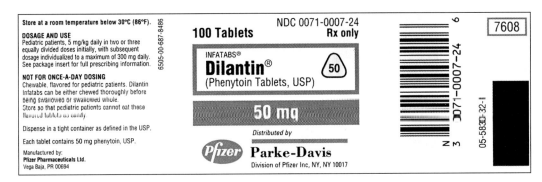

**■ FIGURE 15–1** **Drug label for phenytoin (Dilantin).**
Dilantin is one of the oldest drugs on the market. It has stood the test of time and patient safety for treating tonic-clonic seizures and has not been replaced by newer drugs, as is the case with many other drugs. This drug label is for Dilantin in the form of Infatabs, a chewable tablet that can be given to children.

## Succinimide Drugs for Epilepsy

Succinimide drugs depress the motor cortex of the brain and raise the seizure threshold.

> ethosuximide (Zarontin)
>
> methsuximide (Celontin)

*Note:* The suffix -*suximide* is common to generic succinimide drugs.

## Benzodiazepine Drugs for Epilepsy

Benzodiazepine drugs are Schedule IV drugs that act on several different types of receptors throughout the body to affect memory, emotion, and muscles. This makes them useful drugs in treating a variety of psychiatric and muscular diseases. In addition, some benzodiazepine drugs exert an anticonvulsant effect on receptors in the brainstem.

> clonazepam (Klonopin)
>
> diazepam (Valium)

## Barbiturate Drugs for Epilepsy

Barbiturate drugs have a sedative and anticonvulsant effect. Barbiturate drugs inhibit conduction of nerve impulses in the cerebral cortex and motor areas of the brain. Barbiturates are Schedule IV drugs.

> mephobarbital (Mebaral)
>
> phenobarbital (Luminal)

*Note:* The suffix -*barbital* is common to generic barbituate drugs.

## Other Drugs for Epilepsy

These anticonvulsant drugs are structurally related to gamma-aminobutyric acid (GABA), a substance in the brain that inhibits nerve impulses.

> gabapentin (Neurotin)    topiramate (Topamax) (see **■ FIGURE 15–2**)
> tiagabine (Gabitril)    valproic acid (Depakene, Depakote, Stavzor)

Sulfonamide drugs are usually used to treat bacterial infections. This sulfonamide drug, however, only acts as an anticonvulsant drug, although its mechanism of action is not understood.

> zonisamide (Zonegran)

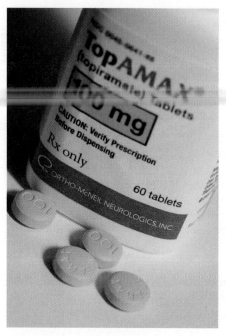

■ **FIGURE 15–2 Drug label for topiramate (Topamax).**
Topiramate (Topamax) has many different uses. As an anticonvulsant drug, it is used to treat tonic-clonic seizures and simple partial and complex partial seizures. It is also one of the most commonly prescribed drugs to treat migraine headaches. It is also used to treat the psychiatric conditions of bipolar disorder, alcohol and cocaine dependence, and bulimia, and is used as an aid to lose weight and stop smoking.

Carbonic anhydrase inhibitor drugs are usually used to treat glaucoma. They inhibit the enzyme carbonic anhydrase in the eye, which decreases the rate at which aqueous humor is formed in the eye. As anticonvulsant drugs, they inhibit carbonic anhydrase in the central nervous system. This causes a buildup of bicarbonate which makes the tissues slightly acidic, and this change in the pH suppresses stray electrical impulses that could trigger a seizure.

    acetazolamide (Diamox)

These anticonvulsant drugs are chemically unrelated to any other anticonvulsant drugs, and their mechanism of action is not understood. Some of these drugs are also used to treat painful nerve conditions. Some of these drugs are also used to treat the psychiatric condition of bipolar disorder.

    carbamazepine (Tegretol)      oxcarbazepine (Trileptal)
    lamotrigine (Lamictal)        primidone (Mysoline)
    levetiracetam (Keppra)

This anticonvulsant drug is only used if other anticonvulsant drugs have failed to control seizues.

    felbamate (Felbatol)

## *In Depth*

The choice of drug therapy for epilepsy depends on the proper classification of the type of seizure, and this is based on the patient's clinical symptoms and EEG pattern. Each type of epilepsy displays a specific EEG pattern during a seizure. No one drug has a therapeutic effect against all types of seizures. Some drugs that are effective for controlling one type of seizure may actually provoke another type of seizure. In patients with poorly controlled seizures, the physician will try different anticonvulsant drugs to find the one that best controls the patient's seizures. If the patient's seizures had been treated with a drug and were under control but then recurred, the physician would order a blood test to check that there was a therapeutic level of the drug in the blood. If the drug level was subtherapeutic, the physician would increase the dose. If the drug level was therapeutic, the physician would prescribe a different anticonvulsant drug.

There are four common types of seizures: (1) **tonic-clonic** (also known as *grand mal*), (2) **absence** (also known as *petit mal*), (3) **complex partial** (also known as *psychomotor*), and (4) **simple partial** (also known as *focal motor*).

### Drugs for Tonic-Clonic/Grand Mal Seizures

Tonic-clonic seizures are characterized by unconsciousness, with excessive motor activity in which the body alternates between muscle rigidity (tonic) and jerking muscle contractions (clonic) in the extremities, with tongue biting with jaw movements.

These are also known as *grand mal seizures.* These drugs are used to treat tonic-clonic seizures.

| | |
|---|---|
| carbamazepine (Tegretol) | phenobarbital (Luminal) |
| lamotrigine (Lamictal) | phenytoin (Dilantin) |
| levetiracetam (Keppra) | primidone (Mysoline) |
| mephobarbital (Mebaral) | topiramate (Topamax) |

Tonic-clonic seizures resistant to other drugs are treated with this orphan drug.

antiepilepsirine

### Drugs for Absence/Petit Mal Seizures

Absence seizures are characterized by impaired consciousness but with little or no muscle activity. There is vacant staring, repetitive blinking, or facial tics, all of which last about 10 seconds. These are also known as *petit mal seizures.* These drugs are used to treat absence seizures.

| | |
|---|---|
| clonazepam (Klonopin) | mephobarbital (Mebaral) |
| ethosuximide (Zarontin) | methsuximide (Celontin) |
| lamotrigine (Lamictal) | valproic acid (Depakene, Depakote, Stavzor) |

### Drugs for Complex Partial/Psychomotor Seizures

Complex partial seizures are characterized by some impairment of consciousness with involuntary contractions of one or more muscle groups (lip smacking, extremity movement). These are also known as *psychomotor seizures.* These drugs are used to treat complex partial seizures.

| | |
|---|---|
| carbamazepine (Tegretol) | primidone (Mysoline) |
| gabapentin (Neurontin) | tiagabine (Gabitril) |
| lamotrigine (Lamictal) | topiramate (Topamax) |
| phenobarbital (Luminal) | valproic acid (Depakene, Depakote, Stavzor) |
| phenytoin (Dilantin) | zonisamide (Zonegran) |

### Drugs for Simple Partial/Focal Motor Seizures

Simple partial seizures are characterized by no impairment of consciousness, but involuntary contractions of one or more muscle groups (jerking of one hand, turning of the head). These are also known as *focal motor seizures*. These drugs are used to treat simple partial seizures.

gabapentin (Neurontin)       primidone (Mysoline)

lamotrigine (Lamictal)       tiagabine (Gabitril)

levetiracetam (Keppra)       topiramate (Topamax)

oxcarbazepine (Trileptal)     valproic acid (Depakene, Depakote, Stavzor)

phenobarbital (Luminal)       zonisamide (Zonegran)

pregabalin (Lyrica)

### Drugs for Other Types of Seizures

These drugs are used to treat myoclonic seizures, which occur in the morning and during times of stress in children and adolescents.

clonazepam (Klonopin)

levetiracetam (Keppra)

These drugs are used to treat seizures associated with preeclampsia/eclampsia during pregnancy.

magnesium sulfate

phenytoin (Dilantin)

### Drugs for Status Epilepticus

Status epilepticus is a state of prolonged, continuous seizure activity or frequently repeated individual seizures that occur without the patient regaining consciousness. Seizures lasting over 30 seconds can cause brain damage. Therefore, status epilepticus is a medical emergency. It is treated with one or more of the following drugs.

diazepam (Diastat)        lorazepam (Ativan)

fosphenytoin (Cerebyx)     pentobarbital

## Drugs Used to Treat Alzheimer's Disease

Alzheimer's disease is the most common form of dementia. It is an irreversible, progressive disease caused by the destruction of neurons in the cerebral cortex and hippocampus. The levels of acetylcholine, a neurotransmitter, are greatly reduced. Beta-amyloid protein plaques accumulate between the neurons, while neurofibrillary tangles occur within the neurons. As the disease progresses, the loss of neurons causes difficulties with memory, judgment, and reasoning, that eventually progress to dementia. The more neurons that are destroyed, the greater the degree of cognitive impairment.

*Focus on Healthcare Issues*

Currently, over 5 million Americans have Alzheimer's disease—one in every eight people over age 65—and, in just a few years, the first of the baby boomers will begin to turn 65. In 2005, Medicare paid $91 billion to care for Alzheimer's patients. This is expected to increase by 75 percent to $160 billion by 2010. No drug currently on the market is able to reverse the symptoms of or cure Alzheimer's disease.

## Cholinesterase Inhibitor Drugs for Alzheimer's Disease

Drugs that inhibit the enzyme cholinesterase (which breaks down acetylcholine) effectively raise the acetylcholine level in the brain and help available acetylcholine to continue to function without being broken down. These drugs cannot reverse the underlying destruction of neurons.

donepezil (Aricept)
  (see ■ FIGURE 15–3)

galantamine (Razadyne)

rivastigmine (Exelon)
  (see ■ FIGURE 15–4)

tacrine (Cognex)

### Did You Know?

Galantamine was originally derived from an unusual strain of daffodil bulbs, but extracting it proved to be too expensive, and so now it is now produced synthetically.

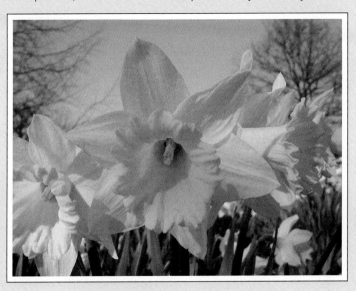

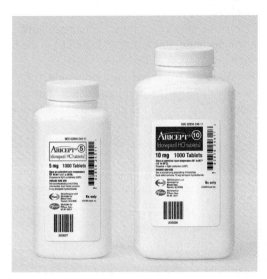

**■ FIGURE 15–3  Donepezil (Aricept).**
Donepezil (Aricept) is the most prescribed drug for Alzheimer's disease. It was first approved by the FDA in 1996 for treating mild-to-moderate Alzheimer's disease. In 2006, it became the first FDA-approved drug for treating all stages of Alzheimer's disease.

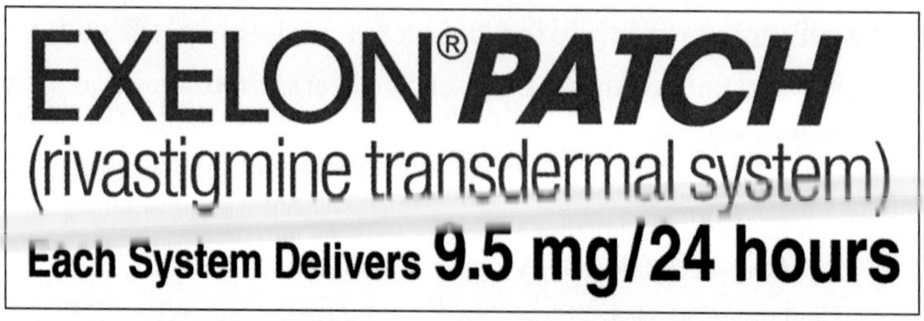

## EXELON®*PATCH*
(rivastigmine transdermal system)
Each System Delivers **9.5 mg/24 hours**

■ **FIGURE 15–4** **Transdermal patch of rivastigmine (Exelon).**
This is the only drug for Alzheimer's disease that comes in the form of a transdermal patch. It is indicated for the treatment of mild-to-moderate Alzheimer's disease. A new patch is applied each day. This drug form is convenient for caregivers to use, especially for dementia patients who can be uncooperative with taking oral drugs.

### Other Drugs for Alzheimer's Disease

This drug blocks NMDA receptors, which are overstimulated in Alzheimer's disease. This drug is used to treat moderate-to-severe Alzheimer's disease.

> memantine (Namenda)

This drug increases blood flow to improve cognitive skills and mental capacity.

> ergoloid mesylates

## Drugs Used to Treat Parkinson's Disease

The symptoms of Parkinson's disease were first described in 1817 by the English physician James Parkinson. Parkinson's disease is a chronic, degenerative condition affecting the brain. Its early symptoms, first appearing usually in late middle age, include muscle rigidity, tremors, and a slowing of voluntary movements. Parkinson's disease follows a progressively downhill clinical course. Later symptoms include a mask-like facial expression, drooling from rigidity of the facial muscles, resting tremor, and loss of the ability to ambulate.

The symptoms of Parkinson's disease are caused by an imbalance between dopamine and acetylcholine, two neurotransmitters in the brain. It is a lack of dopamine in the brain and a relative increase in acetylcholine that lead to the symptoms of Parkinson's disease.

Drug therapy for Parkinson's disease is divided into two main categories: drugs that increase or enhance the action of dopamine in the brain and drugs that inhibit the action of acetylcholine. The goal of drug therapy is to restore the natural balance between dopamine and acetylcholine.

### Dopamine Agonist Drugs for Parkinson's Disease

These drugs directly stimulate dopamine receptors to produce an effect that is similar to that of the neurotransmitter dopamine.

| | |
|---|---|
| amantadine (Symmetrel) | pramipexole (Mirapex) |
| apomorphine (Apokyn) | ropinirole (Requip) |
| bromocriptine (Parlodel) | rotigotine (Neupro) |

## MAO Inhibitor Drugs for Parkinson's Disease

These drugs inhibit MAO, an enzyme in the brain that breaks down dopamine. When MAO is inhibited, this results in increased levels of dopamine.

> rasagiline (Azilect)
>
> selegiline (Eldepryl, Emsam)

*Note:* The suffix *-giline* is common to generic MAO inhibitor drugs.

## Drug Alert!

Amantadine was originally used as an antiviral drug to treat influenza. It was given to a patient with influenza at Harvard Medical School who also, by coincidence, had Parkinson's disease, and his Parkinson's disease improved. Today, amantadine (Symmetrel) is still given to high-risk patients to prevent influenza A virus respiratory infections, but is also used to treat Parkinson's disease.

Pramipexole (Mirapex) was approved by the FDA in 1997 to treat Parkinson's disease. In 2006, it was also approved to treat restless legs syndrome (RLS). Even before its approval to treat RLS, a study by the Mayo Clinic warned that the drug might cause compulsive gambling. An article in the *Archives of Neurology* noted that the FDA's Adverse Event Reporting System database contained reports of Mirapex users developing gambling addictions at a rate that was "380 times greater than expected." Since that time, there have been more reports that the drug also causes other impulse control disorders, such as excessive, compulsive shopping and compulsive eating. Another drug in this category that can have similar adverse effects is ropinirole.

## Anticholinergic Drugs for Parkinson's Disease

These anticholinergic drugs inhibit the action of acetylcholine at cholinergic receptors in the brain to balance the relative abundance of acetylcholine compared to the scarcity of dopamine. They also help to prolong the action of any dopamine that is present.

> benztropine (Cogentin)    procyclidine
>
> biperiden (Akineton)    trihexyphenidyl (Trihexy)

## COMT Inhibitor Drugs for Parkinson's Disease

Catechol-O-methyltransferase (COMT) is the main enzyme that metabolizes the drug levodopa in the blood (levodopa is in the combination drugs described later). COMT inhibitor drugs inhibit the enzyme COMT, and this increases the level of levodopa in the blood so that more is available to cross the blood-brain barrier. The trade name Comtan reflects that this is a COMT inhibitor drug.

> entacapone (Comtan)
>
> tolcapone (Tasmar)

*Note:* The suffix *-capone* is common to generic COMT inhibitor drugs.

## Other Drugs for Parkinson's Disease

These drugs are specifically used to treat the tremors and rigidity of Parkinson's disease. Nadolol and propranolol are beta-blocker drugs most commonly used to treat hypertension and angina.

> atropine (Sal-Tropine)    nadolol (Corgard)
>
> L-hyoscyamine    propranolol (Inderal)

This drug is used to treat the slowed, abnormal muscle movements that characterize Parkinson's disease. Clonazepam is commonly used as an antianxiety drug and an anticonvulsant drug.

clonazepam (Klonopin)

These drugs are actually composed of millions of cells that, when implanted in the brain, produce levodopa or dopamine. They are currently approved by the FDA as orphan drugs. NeuroCell-PD contains nerve cells from fetal pigs (the *PD* stands for *Parkinson's disease*), while Spheramine contains pigment cells from human retinas.

NeuroCell-PD

Spheramine

## Combination Drugs for Parkinson's Disease

These combination drugs contain Parkinson's disease drugs that are no longer available as individual drugs (carbidopa, levodopa) and a COMT inhibitor drug (entacapone).

Duodopa (carbidopa, levodopa)          Sinemet (carbidopa, levodopa)

Parcopa (carbidopa, levodopa)          Stalevo (carbidopa, levodopa, entacapone)
                                       (see ■ FIGURE 15–5)

## In Depth

Early attempts to increase the diminished supply of dopamine in the brain were unsuccessful because dopamine as a drug in the blood cannot cross the blood–brain barrier and enter the brain. It was discovered, however, that the metabolic precursor of dopamine—the drug levodopa—could penetrate the blood–brain barrier. Once in the brain, levodopa is converted by the action of the enzyme dopa decarboxylase into dopamine. The drawbacks of levodopa were that (1) a very large oral dose of levodopa had to be given because 99 percent of the levodopa in the blood was converted into dopamine before it could reach the brain and (2) this extra dopamine in the blood caused side effects. It was found that if levodopa was given with carbidopa that the carbidopa would inhibit the enzyme dopa decarboxylase. This allowed more levodopa to cross the blood–brain barrier. The use of carbidopa also allowed the initial dose of levodopa to be smaller by at least 75 percent. Also, carbidopa cannot cross the blood–brain barrier to inhibit the enzyme dopa decarboxylase in the brain. Interestingly, carbidopa has no therapeutic effect of its own at all, unless it is taken with levodopa. Levodopa and carbidopa are no longer available as individual drugs, but are available in combination drugs.

None of the aforementioned drugs can cure Parkinson's disease. In fact, over time, tolerance to a drug's therapeutic effect can develop. A larger drug dose is then required to maintain control of parkinsonian symptoms; however, this larger dose also produces more side effects. When the dose can no longer be increased or side effects become intolerable, the physician will gradually withdraw the drug, placing the patient on a **drug holiday** for a few days. When drug therapy is again initiated, the patient will respond to lower doses of antiparkinsonian drugs.

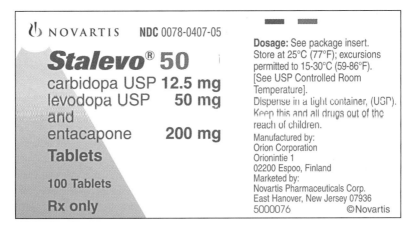

**FIGURE 15–5 Drug label for the combination drug Stalevo.**
Combination drugs for Parkinson's disease contain carbidopa and levodopa. Now, Stalevo also contains the COMT inhibitor drug entacapone. COMT inhibitor drugs inhibit the enzyme COMT that metabolizes levodopa in the blood. All three of these drugs raise the level of dopamine in the brain in different ways.

## Drugs Used to Treat Myasthenia Gravis and Multiple Sclerosis

Myasthenia gravis is characterized by excessive fatigue of the voluntary muscles. On a cellular level, patients produce antibodies against their own acetylcholine receptors that are on the cell membranes of voluntary muscle cells. These antibodies destroy many of the receptors. There are normal levels of acetylcholine, but too few receptors on the muscles. Normally, acetylcholine is released in the synapse between a neuron and a muscle cell, briefly acts on a receptor, and is then broken down by the enzyme cholinesterase. Drugs used to treat myasthenia gravis block cholinesterase so that the acetylcholine is not broken down and can activate the remaining receptors for a longer period of time. These anticholinesterase drugs are used to treat myasthenia gravis.

| | |
|---|---|
| ambenonium (Mytelase) | neostigmine (Prostigmin) |
| ephedrine | pyridostigmine (Mestinon) |
| mycophenolate (CellCept) | |

Multiple sclerosis is an autoimmune disease in which the body makes antibodies against the myelin covering around certain nerves. There is acute inflammation with chronic, progressive interruption of nerve conduction between the brain and the spinal cord. Symptoms include double vision, large muscle weakness, uncoordinated gait, muscle spasticity, tremors, and neuralgia. Drugs used to treat multiple sclerosis include monoclonal antibody drugs (alemtuzumab, natalizumab), muscle relaxant drugs (baclofen, L-baclofen, tizanidine), anticonvulsant drugs (gabapentin), immunosuppressant drugs (glatiramer, interferon), corticosteroid drugs (methylprednisolone, prednisone), and chemotherapy drugs (methotrexate, mitoxantrone)

| | |
|---|---|
| alemtuzumab (Campath) | interferon beta-1a (Avonex, Rebif) |
| baclofen (Lioresal) | interferon beta-1b (Betaseron) |
| gabapentin (Neurontin) | L-baclofen (Neuralgon) |
| glatiramer (Copaxone) | methotrexate (Rheumatrex) |

methylprednisolone
   (Medrol, Solu-Medrol)

mitoxantrone (Novantrone)

natalizumab (Tysabri)

prednisone (Deltasone, Meticorten)

tizanidine (Zanaflex)

## Drugs Used to Treat Neuralgia and Neuropathy

Neuropathy is a disease of the nerves that often results in neuralgia or nerve pain. This can be associated with several different conditions that cause chronic pain and unusual sensations. Peripheral neuropathy is a general category that includes any type of disease or injury to the nerves in the extremities. Diabetic neuropathy is a chronic complication of diabetes mellitus that is caused by degenerative changes in the nerves of the lower extremities. It is characterized by pain and altered sensations (paresthesias) in both feet and legs. Postherpetic neuralgia is caused by shingles, a herpesvirus infection originally from chickenpox that reappears in the elderly or at times of stress or illness and causes a chronic, painful skin eruption along the inflamed nerve pathways (dermatomes). Phantom limb pain is characterized by pain and unusual sensations that seem to come from an extremity that has been amputated. Restless legs syndrome is characterized by restlessness and twitching of the muscles of the legs, particularly the calf muscles, along with an indescribable tingling, aching, or crawling-insect sensation. The symptoms occur mainly at night and may be severe enough to prevent sleep.

This antianxiety drug is used to treat neuralgia and neuropathy.

clonazepam (Klonopin)

These antidepressant drugs are used to treat neuralgia and neuropathy. They elevate the mood and are useful in treating chronic pain conditions. They also have an antihistamine effect that relieves skin sensations and produces mild sedation.

amitriptyline

amoxapine

desipramine (Norpramin)

doxepin (Sinequan)

duloxetine (Cymbalta)

imipramine (Tofranil)

nortriptyline (Aventyl, Pamelor)

paroxetine (Paxil)

protriptyline (Vivactil)

These anticonvulsant drugs are used to treat neuralgia and neuropathy.

carbamazepine (Tegretol)

gabapentin (Neurontin)

oxcarbazepine (Trileptal)

pregabalin (Lyrica) (see ■ FIGURE 15–6)

This ACE inhibitor drug for hypertension is also used to treat neuralgia and neuropathy.

benazepril (Lotensin)

These topical irritant/anesthesia drugs are applied to the skin to treat neuralgia and neuropathy.

capsaicin (Capsin, Zostrix)

lidocaine (Lidoderm)

These drugs are specifically used to treat restless legs syndrome. Carbamazepine is an anticonvulsant drug. Clonidine blocks alpha$_2$ receptors to increase blood flow and also causes changes in

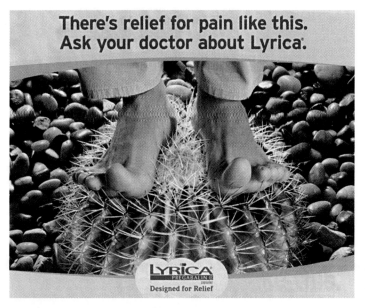

■ **FIGURE 15–6** **Drug advertisement for pregabalin (Lyrica).**
This drug advertisement graphically shows the sensation that some patients have who have neuralgia: a stabbing pain or shooting sensation in the feet. Other symptoms include burning pain, tingling, or numbness. Other Lyrica advertisements show ants crawling on the feet or thumbtacks pricking the feet.

brain chemistry. Pramipexole and ropinirole are dopamine-like drugs that are also used to treat Parkinson's disease.

| | |
|---|---|
| carbamazepine (Tegretol) | pramipexole (Mirapex) |
| clonidine (Catapres) | ropinirole (Requip) |

## Drugs Used to Treat Insomnia

Insomnia is characterized by difficulty falling asleep, awakening during the night, and/or difficulty getting back to sleep. This can be exacerbated by anxiety, stress, or pain. **Hypnotic drugs** are used to induce sleep. The word *hypnotic* is from the Greek word *hypnos*, for *sleep*. Hypnotic drugs are used on a short-term basis to treat insomnia, and they include nonbarbiturate drugs, benzodiazepine drugs, and barbiturate drugs.

### Nonbarbiturate Drugs for Insomnia

Nonbarbiturate drugs depress the central nervous system to produce sedation and sleep. Nonbarbiturate drugs are Schedule IV drugs with some potential for addiction.

| | |
|---|---|
| chloral hydrate | zaleplon (Sonata) |
| eszopiclone (Lunesta) (see ■ FIGURE 15–7) | zolpidem (Ambien) (see ■ FIGURE 15–8) |
| ramelteon (Rozerem) | |

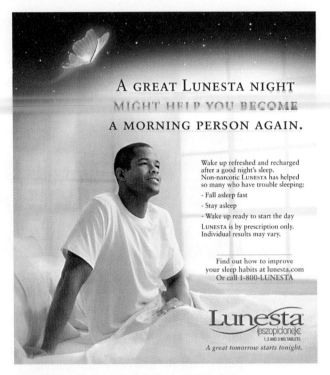

**■ FIGURE 15–7 Eszopiclone (Lunesta).**
The trade name Lunesta is a reference to the luna moth that only
comes out at night. The moth's name is derived from a Latin
word that refers to the moon. In drug advertisements for Lunesta,
this large, pale moth is seen flying in a bedroom window and
putting a person to sleep as it comes near or hovering nearby as a
person wakes up in the morning, feeling refreshed after a good
night's sleep.

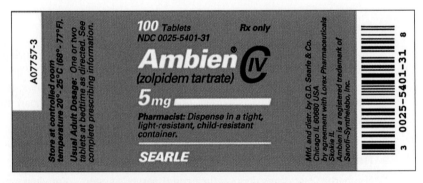

**■ FIGURE 15–8 Drug label for zolpidem (Ambien).**
Zolpidem (Ambien) is a Schedule IV drug with a limited potential for addiction. The
schedule symbol of a capital C with the Roman numeral IV inside it can be seen on
the label. All of the nonbarbiturate hypnotic drugs for insomnia are Schedule IV
drugs, except for ramelteon (Rozerem).

## Did You Know?

Melatonin is a hormone secreted by the pineal body in the brain. Melatonin maintains the body's internal clock, the 24-hour wake-sleep cycle (the circadian rhythm), and regulates the onset and duration of sleep. Melatonin is available as an over-the-counter drug. The prescription drug ramelteon (Rozerem) stimulates melatonin receptors in the brain to induce sleep and treat insomnia.

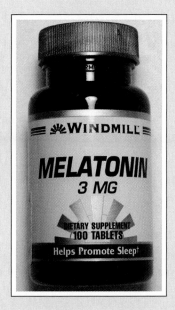

## Drug Alert!

Ambien is the most popular drug for insomnia. There were 26 million prescriptions written for Ambien in 2007. Some patients taking zolpidem (Ambien) have reported unusual adverse effects of amnesia (not being aware or remembering) while working, eating, and even while driving. This usually occurs when a patient takes Ambien but continues to stay awake or takes Ambien but does not get a full 8 hours of sleep before becoming active. There are reports of this occurring with other drugs in this category as well.

### Benzodiazepine Drugs for Insomnia

Benzodiazepine drugs are commonly used to treat anxiety and also have a sedative effect because they enhance the action of gamma-aminobutyric acid (GABA), a neurotransmitter in the brain that inhibits nerve impulses. Benzodiazepine drugs are Schedule IV drugs with some potential for addiction.

estazolam (ProSom)       temazepam (Restoril) (see ■ **FIGURE 15–9**)

flurazepam (Dalmane)    triazolam (Halcion)

quazepam (Doral)

*Note:*  The suffix -*azepam* and -*azolam* are common to generic benzodiazepine drugs.

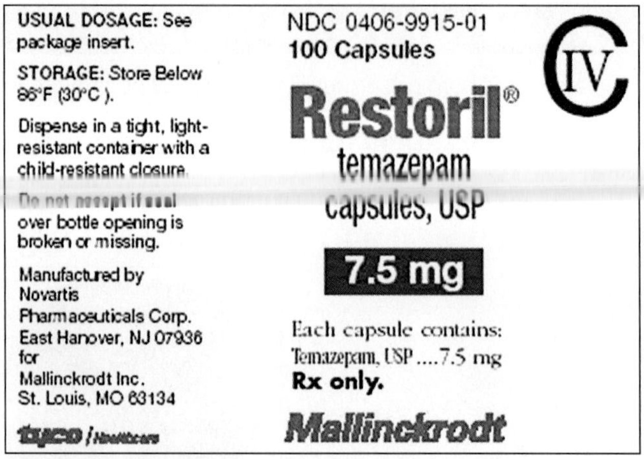

■ FIGURE 15–9 **Drug label for temazepam (Restoril).**
This benzodiazepine drug is used to treat insomnia. It is a Schedule IV drug, as are all of the other benzodiazepine drugs used to treat insomnia.

## Barbiturate Drugs for Insomnia

Some barbiturate drugs are useful in preventing epileptic seizures, but these barbiturate drugs have no anticonvulsant activity and are only used to provide sedation. These drugs exert a general depressing action on the central nervous system and cause sedation. They were once popular drugs for insomnia, but because they are Schedule II, III, and IV drugs and because of their higher potential to cause addiction, they are now used infrequently for treating insomnia.

amobarbital (Amytal)     phenobarbital (Luminal)

butabarbital (Butisol)     secobarbital (Seconal)

pentobarbital

*Note:* The suffix *-barbital* is common to generic barbiturate drugs.

## Other Drugs For Insomnia

Over-the-counter (OTC) sleep aids contain an antihistamine drug. These drugs use the antihistamine's side effect of drowsiness as the therapeutic effect to induce sleep.

diphenhydramine (Compoz Nighttime, Nytol, Sominex)

doxylamine (Unisom)

## Combination Drugs for Insomnia

These combination sleep aid drugs contain an antihistamine drug (diphenhydramine) with an analgesic drug (acetaminophen, ibuprofen) to treat pain that causes insomnia. To help the body adjust to disrupted sleep patterns or jet lag, some other OTC drugs include melatonin to regulate the wake–sleep cycle.

Advil PM (diphenhydramine, ibuprofen)

Excedrin P.M. (diphenhydramine, acetaminophen)

Extra Strength Tylenol PM (diphenhydramine, acetaminophen)

## Drugs Used to Treat Narcolepsy

Narcolepsy is characterized by brief, involuntary episodes of falling asleep and extreme daytime sleepiness. Patients with narcolepsy often fall asleep at work, at school, or while driving. Narcolepsy is caused by an abnormality in rapid-eye movement (REM) sleep, the deepest level of sleep during which the body rests and repairs itself. There is also a hereditary component to narcolepsy, and this condition may be a type of autoimmune disorder. Narcolepsy and the related disorder cataplexy are treated with drugs from many different categories. Some of these drugs are central nervous system stimulant drugs with a high potential for addiction. Others are stimulant drugs with a low potential for addiction.

| | |
|---|---|
| armodafinil (Nuvigil) | methylphenidate (Ritalin) |
| dextroamphetamine (Dexedrine) | modafinil (Provigil) |
| ephedrine | oxybate (Xyrem) |
| gamma hydroxybutyrate (GHB) | viloxazine (Catatrol) |

### Combination Drugs for Narcolepsy

This combination drug contains two stimulant drugs (amphetamine, dextroamphetamine).

Adderall XR (amphetamine, dextroamphetamine)

### Did You Know?

Gamma hydroxybutyrate (GHB) was previously an illegal drug known as the "date-rape drug." Female victims were given a liquid dose mixed with a beverage and when they became incapacitated, they were then raped. GHB is an orphan drug that is currently the only Schedule I drug that has a legal, medical use.

Methylphenidate (Ritalin) is also used to treat attention-deficit/hyperactivity disorder, depression in elderly stroke patients, and behavior associated with traumatic brain disorder.

## Drugs Used to Treat Migraine Headaches

Drugs used to prevent and treat migrane headaches are discussed in Chapter 22.

# Chapter Review

## Quiz Yourself

1. The choice of a drug for treating epilepsy in a specific patient is based on what two clinical criteria?
2. Name and describe four different types of seizures.
3. Name four categories of anticonvulsant drugs.
4. Name five different uses for the drug topiramate (Topamax).
5. Describe the therapeutic effect of cholinesterase inhibitor drugs used to treat Alzheimer's disease.
6. Which two hormones are out of balance in patients with Parkinson's disease?
7. Explain the meaning of the phrase *drug holiday*.
8. Why is levodopa administered with carbidopa in a combination drug for patients with Parkinson's disease?
9. Describe the symptoms of restless legs syndrome and name four drugs used to treat it.
10. Why are barbiturate drugs seldom used now to treat insomnia?
11. What is the action of the hormone and the drug melatonin?
12. If a patient needs to take a prescription drug to treat insomnia but is concerned about the potential for becoming addicted, which drug would be the most appropriate choice?
13. To what category of drugs does each of these drugs belong, and what disease are they used to treat?

   **a.** benztropine (Cogentin)
   **b.** capsaicin (Capsin, Zostrix)
   **c.** donepezil (Aricept)
   **d.** entacapone (Comtan)
   **e.** eszopiclone (Lunesta)
   **f.** ethosuximide (Zarontin)
   **g.** flurazepam (Dalmane)
   **h.** gabapentin (Neurontin)
   **i.** levetiracetam (Keppra)
   **j.** memantine (Namenda)

   **k.** modafinil (Provigil)
   **l.** phenytoin (Dilantin)
   **m.** pramipexole (Mirapex)
   **n.** pregabalin (Lyrica)
   **o.** ropinirole (Requip)
   **p.** selegiline (Eldepryl, Emsam)
   **q.** tacrine (Cognex)
   **r.** valproic acid (Depakene, Depakote)
   **s.** zaleplon (Sonata)

## Spelling Tips

**CellCept**   Unusual internal capitalization.
**Cerebyx**   Easily confused with the sound-alike drug **Celebrex** (used to treat pain and arthritis).
**ProSom**   Unusual internal capitalization.

## Clinical Applications

1. Look at this photograph and answer the following questions.
   a. What is the generic name of this prescribed drug?
   b. What is the trade name of this prescribed drug?
   c. What condition is this drug used to treat?
   d. Why do you think the physician did not give the patient any refills?

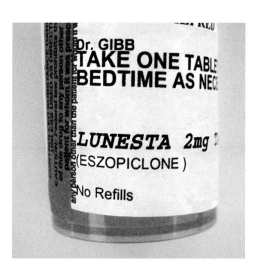

2. Look at this handwritten prescription and answer the following questions.
   a. What drug is prescribed here?
   b. What disease is this drug used to treat?
   c. What strength dose has been prescribed?
   d. How many capsules will be placed in the prescription bottle given to the patient?
   e. Use plain English to tell what is written on the rest of the prescription.

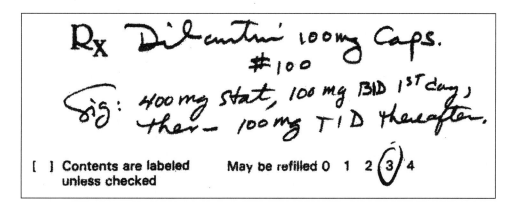

3. Look at this handwritten physician's order and answer the following questions.
   a. What drug is prescribed here?
   b. What condition is this drug used to treat?
   c. What dose strength has been prescribed?
   d. Use plain English to tell what is written on the rest of the prescription.

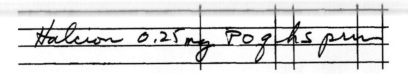

## Multimedia Extension Exercises

■ Go to www.pearsonhighered.com/turley and click on the photo of the cover of *Understanding Pharmacology for Health Professionals* to access the interactive Companion Website created for this textbook.

# Psychiatric Drugs

## CHAPTER CONTENTS

## Learning Objectives

After you study this chapter, you should be able to

1. Describe the therapeutic effects of various categories of drugs used to treat anxiety, psychosis, depression, and manic-depressive disorder.

2. List alternative names given to antianxiety and antipsychotic categories of drugs.

3. Describe the cause and symptoms of and the treatment for tardive dyskinesia.

4. Explain what dietary restrictions patients have when taking MAO inhibitor drugs and why.

5. Describe the types of drugs used to treat obsessive-compulsive disorder, social anxiety disorder, posttraumatic stress disorder, eating disorders, withdrawal from addiction, and attention-deficit/hyperactivity disorder.

6. Given the generic and trade names of a psychiatric drug, identify what drug category they belong to or what disease they are used to treat.

7. Given a psychiatric drug category, identify several generic and trade name drugs in that category.

Psychiatric drugs are used to treat diseases of the mind, otherwise known as *mental illnesses.* These include a variety of emotional disorders that involve abnormalities of personality, mood, or behavior. It is estimated that nearly 50 percent of all hospital admissions are in some way related to a mental health problem, such as anxiety, depression, suicide, postpartum depression, psychosis, psychosomatic illness, attention-deficit/hyperactivity disorder (ADHD), eating disorders, panic attacks, social phobias, obsessive-compulsive disorder (OCD), posttraumatic stress disorder (PTSD), drug addiction, or alcoholism. Psychiatric drugs include antianxiety drugs, antipsychotic drugs, antidepressant drugs, and others. Drugs, as well as psychotherapy, behavior modification, or educational programs, are used to treat mental illnesses.

## *Historical Notes*

During the 1800s, the treatment for mental illness included the use of the drugs digitalis, ipecac, alcohol, or opium. In 1903, barbiturate drugs were synthesized and used effectively as sedative drugs for agitated, mentally ill patients. Barbiturate drugs now have only limited use for treating insomnia and producing preoperative sedation before surgery; they are not used as psychiatric drugs. Before World War II, schizophrenic patients were treated in several ways: They were exposed to malaria to produce a high fever and delirium, injected with enough insulin to cause convulsions and coma, or given electroshock therapy. However, beginning in the early 1950s, advances were made in the treatment of mental illness with the introduction of new drugs to treat neurosis, psychosis, and depression.

## Drugs Used to Treat Anxiety and Neurosis

The symptoms of neurosis include anxiety, anxiousness, and tension—all at a more intense level than normal—as well as a feeling of apprehension with vague, unsubstantiated fears. A patient with anxiety or neurosis never experiences any loss of touch with reality. The treatment of neurosis involves the use of **antianxiety drugs,** which are also known as *anxiolytic drugs* or *minor tranquilizer drugs.*

## *Drug Alert!*

The phrase *minor tranquilizer drug* is somewhat of a misnomer in that it implies that this category of drugs is somehow less effective than the major tranquilizer drugs (which are used to treat psychosis) or that the minor tranquilizer drugs are just major tranquilizer drugs given at a lower dose. In fact, minor tranquilizer drugs are chemically unrelated to major tranquilizer drugs. Minor tranquilizer drugs are extremely effective drugs with a specific therapeutic effect for treating neurosis.

## *Historical Notes*

In 1945, researchers were looking for a new antibiotic drug to use against bacteria that were already becoming resistant to penicillin. One drug tested was found to produce muscle relaxation and exert a calming effect in animals. From this, the first minor tranquilizer drug was developed in 1955 and marketed as meprobamate (Miltown), which is still used. Also in 1955, a researcher at Hoffmann-La Roche laboratories was searching for a compound to make a commercial dye, but the chemicals he tested were not useful as dyes. A year and a half of research yielded no usable products. As he was doing his final cleanup of the project, he saw a single sample that he had forgotten to send for testing. He noted, "We were under great pressure by this time because my boss told us to stop these foolish things and go back to more useful work. I submitted it [the last sample] for animal testing. . . . I thought that it was just to finish up." That last sample, which was nearly forgotten, turned out to be chlordiazepoxide (Librium). It was approved for sale in 1960 and became the first of the benzodiazepine category of minor tranquilizer drugs that would come to revolutionize the treatment of neurosis. The same researcher continued to work with the basic molecular structure of chlordiazepoxide (Librium) and, in 1959, even before marketing of Librium had begun, he had synthesized the new drug diazepam (Valium) (see ■ FIGURE 16–1). The trade name *Valium* is derived from the Latin word *valere,* which means *to be healthy.* The wild European plant valerian has been known since the time of Hippocrates to calm the nerves. In 1970, Valium became the number one prescription drug in the United States. Ten years later, Hoffman-La Roche was still manufacturing 30 million Valium tablets every day. Librium and Valium are still in use today as antianxiety drugs.

Edward Shorter, *The Health Century.* New York: Doubleday, 1987, p. 127.

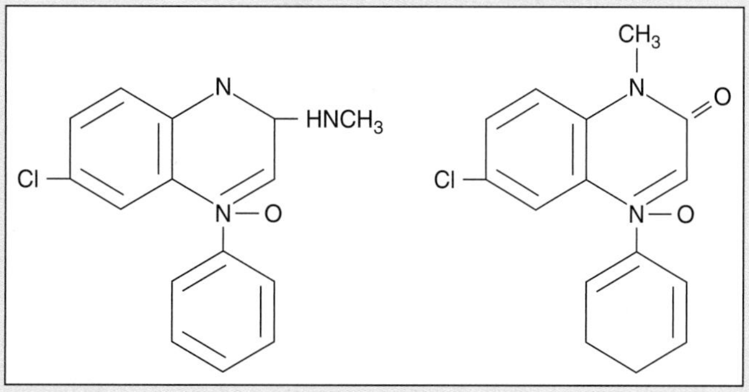

■ FIGURE 16–1 **Chemical structures of Librium and Valium.**
The similarity of the chemical structures of chlordiazepoxide (Librium) and diazepam (Valium) is evident. These were the first two benzodiazepine antianxiety drugs.

## Benzodiazepine Drugs for Anxiety

Benzodiazepine drugs are by far the most commonly prescribed drugs for the treatment of anxiety and neurosis. They bind to several specific types of receptor sites in the brain to provide sedation. They affect thought processes, and they affect emotional behavior by their action in the limbic system of the brain. They also decrease the muscle tension that comes with anxiety. All of the benzodiazepine drugs are Schedule IV drugs.

| | |
|---|---|
| alprazolam (Xanax) | diazepam (Valium) |
| chlordiazepoxide (Librium) | lorazepam (Ativan) |
| clorazepate (Tranxene) | oxazepam (Serax) |

*Note:* The suffix *-azepam* is common to generic benzodiazepine drugs.

## Antidepressant Drugs for Anxiety

These antidepressant drugs are specifically used to treat anxiety that also has a component of depression. Different categories of antidepressant drugs are effective in treating anxiety, including some of the tricyclic antidepressant drugs, selective serotonin reuptake inhibitor (SSRI) drugs, and serotonin and norepinephrine reuptake inhibitor (SNRI) drugs.

| | |
|---|---|
| citalopram (Celexa) | fluoxetine (Prozac) |
| doxepin (Sinequan) | paroxetine (Paxil) |
| duloxetine (Cymbalta) (see ■ FIGURE 16–2) | venlafaxine (Effexor) |
| escitalopram (Lexapro) | |

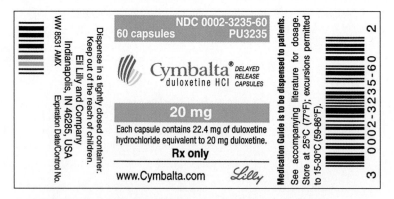

■ **FIGURE 16–2 Drug label for duloxetine (Cymbalta).**
Duloxetine (Cymbalta), a serotonin and norepinephrine reuptake inhibitor (SNRI) drug, is used to treat depression and several other conditions: anxiety, diabetic neuropathy, and fibromyalgia. It comes in the drug form of a delayed-release capsule.

## Other Drugs for Anxiety

Other drugs used to treat anxiety come from a variety of different drug categories. Buspirone stimulates serotonin receptors. Hydroxyzine is an antihistamine drug with a side effect of sedation to decrease anxiety. Meprobamate acts on the thalamus and limbic system to decrease anxiety; it is a Schedule IV drug. Prochlorperazine is an antipsychotic drug that is also used to control nausea and vomiting. Propranolol is a beta-blocker drug that is also used to treat hypertension as well as anxiety. Trifluoperazine is an antipsychotic drug.

| | |
|---|---|
| buspirone (BuSpar) | prochlorperazine (Compazine) |
| hydroxyzine (Vistaril) | propranolol (Inderal) |
| meprobamate (Miltown) | trifluoperazine |

## Drugs Used to Treat Psychosis

The symptoms of psychosis include a loss of touch with reality, resulting in delusions, hallucinations, inappropriate mood, and bizarre behaviors. Psychotic symptoms are based, in part, on an overactivity of the neurotransmitter dopamine in the brain, either from an overproduction of dopamine or from a hypersensitivity of dopamine receptors. Imbalances in the neurotransmitters serotonin, acetylcholine, and norepinephrine, and the chemical histamine are also thought to play a role in psychosis. Schizophrenia is the most common form of psychosis. Some of these drugs are also used to treat the psychosis with agitation that commonly occurs in patients with dementia, Alzheimer's disease, or Parkinson's disease.

The treatment of psychosis involves the use of **antipsychotic drugs,** which are also known as *neuroleptic drugs* or *major tranquilizer drugs.* These drugs block dopamine receptors in many areas of the brain, including the limbic system that controls emotions. Antipsychotic drugs decrease psychotic symptoms of hostility, agitation, and paranoia, without causing confusion or sedation. Unlike antianxiety drugs, these drugs are not schedule drugs and so they are not addictive.

## *Historical Notes*

Prior to the introduction of modern antipsychotic drugs, barbiturate drugs were used to sedate agitated, psychotic patients. Barbiturate drugs have been replaced by the phenothiazine group of antipsychotic drugs. Phenothiazine was the original parent drug for this group. It was first manufactured in 1883 as a wormer for livestock. Some minor changes in its chemical structure resulted in the creation of two large, but very different categories of phenothiazine drugs. One category is composed of phenothiazine drugs that act as antihistamine drugs and are used to treat allergies, itching, nausea, and vomiting. The second category is composed of phenothiazine drugs that are used to treat psychosis and schizophrenia. Chlorpromazine (Thorazine), the first of the modern antipsychotic drugs developed from the original parent molecule, is still one of the most widely used antipsychotic drugs.

### Phenothiazine Drugs for Psychosis

This is the largest, chemically related category of drugs used to treat psychosis and schizophrenia. These drugs block dopamine, histamine, alpha, and serotonin receptors in the brain.

| | |
|---|---|
| chlorpromazine (Thorazine) | prochlorperazine (Compazine) |
| fluphenazine | thioridazine |
| perphenazine | trifluoperazine |

*Note:* The suffix *-azine* is common to generic phenothiazine antipsychotic drugs.

### Dibenzapine Drugs for Psychosis

These drugs all belong to the dibenzapine category of antipsychotic drugs. These drugs mainly block dopamine and serotonin receptors in the brain. Their most common use is in treating schizophrenia.

clozapine (Clozaril)      olanzapine (Zyprexa)

loxapine (Loxitane)      quetiapine (Seroquel)

*Note:* The suffix *-apine* is common to generic dibenzapine drugs.

## Drug Alert!

Zyprexa Zydis is the trade name for a special tablet form of Zyprexa that dissolves in the mouth within 5 to 15 seconds. Because of their mental illness, many psychotic patients are noncompliant in taking their drugs as they do not understand the importance of the drugs or they feel someone is trying to poison them. One study found that up to 75 percent of schizophrenic patients do not take their drugs regularly, or at all. Psychotic patients commonly refuse a drug or hide a tablet in their mouths and later discard it. This drug form assures patient compliance, as the entire dose dissolves quickly in the mouth. These antipsychotic drugs are available as orally disintegrating tablets: aripiprazole, clozapine, olanzapine, and risperidone.

### Benzisoxazole Drugs for Psychosis

These drugs belong to the benzisoxazole category of antipsychotic drugs. These drugs block dopamine and serotonin receptors in the brain. They are used to treat schizophrenia.

paliperidone (Invega)      ziprasidone (Geodon)

risperidone (Risperdal)

*Note:* The suffix *-idone* is common to generic benzisoxazole drugs.

### Other Drugs for Psychosis

Other drugs used to treat psychosis are often chemically unrelated drugs. These drugs block dopamine and serotonin receptors in the brain. For convenience, these drugs are grouped together because each drug category only includes one or two drugs. These include the dihydroindolone, phenylbutylpiperadine, quinolinone, and thioxanthene categories of antipsychotic drugs. The drug clonidine, however, does not belong to any of these categories. Instead, it stimulates alpha$_2$ receptors in the brain and is used to treat hypertension, atrial fibrillation, severe pain in cancer patients, restless legs syndrome, and is used as an aid to stop smoking, as well as its use as an antipsychotic drug to treat schizophrenia.

aripiprazole (Abilify)                    molindone (Moban)

clonidine (Catapres)                      thiothixene (Navane)

haloperidol (Haldol) (see ■ FIGURE 16–3)

## Did You Know?

Haloperidol is also used to treat the symptoms of Tourette's syndrome, which include involuntary muscle tics (shrugging, winking, twisting), hyperactivity, obsessive-compulsive disorder (OCD), and involuntary, spontaneous vocalizations, sometimes with cursing.

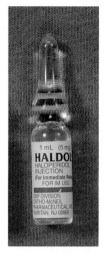

**■ FIGURE 16–3  An ampule of haloperidol (Haldol).**
This ampule contains the liquid drug form of Haldol that is given intramuscularly to treat acute, severe episodes of schizophrenia or agitation and psychosis in patients with Alzheimer's disease. For less urgent situations, the oral tablet form is given. To access the liquid in the ampule, an alcohol swab is placed over the neck (narrow part) of the ampule, and the ampule is quickly snapped into two pieces. A syringe and attached needle are then used to withdraw the liquid drug from the ampule.

These antipsychotic drugs are specifically used to treat agitation that occurs in patients with dementia, Alzheimer's disease, or Parkinson's disease.

| | |
|---|---|
| clozapine (Clozaril) | risperidone (Risperdal) |
| haloperidol (Haldol) | thiothixene (Navane) |
| olanzapine (Zyprexa) | ziprasidone (Geodon) |
| quetiapine (Seroquel) | |

## *Focus on Healthcare Issues*

The antipsychotic drugs, particularly the phenothiazine drugs, cause a group of adverse effects known collectively as **tardive dyskinesia**. Symptoms of tardive dyskinesia include involuntary, repetitive movements of the face (grimacing, smacking the lips, chewing, blinking the eyes, sticking out the tongue, rocking back and forth, marching in place, humming, or grunting), but can also include athetoid (writhing) movements of the arms, legs, and fingers. The phrase *tardive dyskinesia* was introduced in 1964. The word *tardive* means *late* and refers to the fact that these symptoms do not appear when treatment is first begun. The physician may recommend that the patient take a **drug holiday** from his or her antipsychotic drug to lessen the symptoms of tardive dyskinesia.

These drugs are used to treat tardive dyskinesia.

lithium (Lithobid)
reserpine
tetrabenazine (Xenazine)

## Drugs Used to Treat Depression

Depression is a mood disorder that is characterized by insomnia, crying, lack of pleasure in any activity, increased or decreased appetite, lack of ability to act or concentrate, feelings of guilt, helplessness, hopelessness, worthlessness, and thoughts of suicide and death. These symptoms occur daily, interfere with life activities, and last longer than two weeks. Depression is caused by decreased levels of the neurotransmitters norepinephrine and serotonin in the brain. The treatment for depression involves the use of antidepressant drugs.

**Antidepressant drugs,** also known as *mood-elevating drugs,* not only alleviate the symptoms of depression, but also increase mental alertness, normalize sleep patterns, normalize the appetite, and decrease suicidal ideation. There are several categories of antidepressant drugs: tricyclic antidepressant drugs, tetracyclic antidepressant drugs, selective serotonin reuptake inhibitor (SSRI) drugs, serotonin and norepinephrine reuptake inhibitor (SNRI) drugs, monoamine oxidase (MAO) inhibitor drugs, and others.

## Historical Notes

Originally, amphetamine drugs were used to treat depression; they acted to stimulate the central nervous system and mask the patient's depressive symptoms. However, amphetamine drugs have a high potential for abuse and do not correct the underlying chemical imbalance causing the depression. Therefore, they are no longer used to treat depression.

In 1951, while evaluating a drug for its effectiveness in treating tuberculosis, researchers noted that even seriously ill and dying patients developed a happy, optimistic attitude despite a lack of clinical improvement in their tuberculosis. This drug was identified as a monoamine oxidase (MAO) inhibitor, and it formed the basis for the first category of drugs used to treat depression—MAO inhibitor drugs.

In 1958, a drug being tested as an antipsychotic drug showed significant antidepressant effects. That drug was imipramine (Tofranil), and it was the first of the tricyclic antidepressant category of drugs.

### Tricyclic Antidepressant Drugs

Tricyclic antidepressant (TCA) drugs inhibit the reuptake of and prolong the action of norepinephrine or serotonin released by neurons in the brain. This helps to correct the low levels of these neurotransmitters that are found in patients with depression. Also, tricyclic antidepressant drugs increase the sensitivity of receptors on the neurons to available norepinephrine and serotonin. Thus, these drugs both prolong and enhance the action of norepinephrine and serotonin. Tricyclic antidepressant drugs also affect the levels of histamine and acetylcholine, and this produces the side effects of dry mouth, dry eyes, blurry vision, constipation, and urinary retention that are common to tricyclic antidepressant drugs. Tricyclic antidepressant drugs are so named because of the triple-ring configuration of their chemical structure (see ■ FIGURE 16–4).

| | |
|---|---|
| amitriptyline | imipramine (Tofranil) |
| amoxapine | nortriptyline (Aventyl, Pamelor) |
| desipramine (Norpramin) | protriptyline (Vivactil) |
| doxepin (Sinequan) | trimipramine (Surmontil) |

*Note:* The suffixes *-triptyline* and *-ipramine* are common to tricyclic antidepressant drugs.

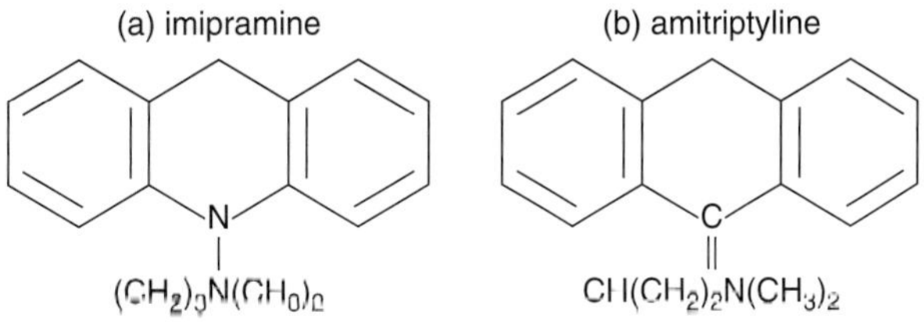

(a) imipramine          (b) amitriptyline

$(CH_2)_3N(CH_3)_2$          $CH(CH_2)_2N(CH_3)_2$

**FIGURE 16–4  Chemical structures of two tricyclic antidepressant drugs.**
The chemical structures of the tricyclic antidepressant drugs imipramine (Tofranil) and amitriptyline show the three-ring structure from which the drug category derives its name.

# Drug Alert!

Tricyclic antidepressant drugs and tetracyclic antidepressant drugs are indicated for the treatment of major depressive disorder. In the past, these drugs were used to treat a number of different conditions, such as migraine headaches, diabetic neuropathy, anorexia nervosa, and phantom limb pain. However, their use in treating any of these conditions has been found to be associated with an increased risk of suicidal thoughts and suicide attempts in children and teenagers, and so these drugs are prescribed less frequently than previously. Desipramine is the only one of these drugs that is still used for some other conditions.

## Tetracyclic Antidepressant Drugs

Although slightly different in chemical structure, tetracyclic antidepressant drugs have essentially the same therapeutic effect as the tricyclic antidepressant drugs described previously.

maprotiline

mirtazapine (Remeron)

## Selective Serotonin Reuptake Inhibitor Drugs for Depression

Selective serotonin reuptake inhibitor (SSRI) drugs block the normal reuptake of free serotonin by neurons. When serotonin levels are low (in patients with depression), these drugs allow the available serotonin to bind with more receptors for a longer period of time before it is broken down and recycled. These drugs do not affect histamine or acetylcholine levels, and so they do not cause the side effects that are seen with tricyclic antidepressant drugs.

citalopram (Celexa)               fluvoxamine (Luxor)

escitalopram (Lexapro)            paroxetine (Paxil)

fluoxetine (Prozac)               sertraline (Zoloft)
   (see **FIGURE 16–5**)

*Note:* The suffixes *-talopram* and *-oxetine* are common to generic SSRI drugs.

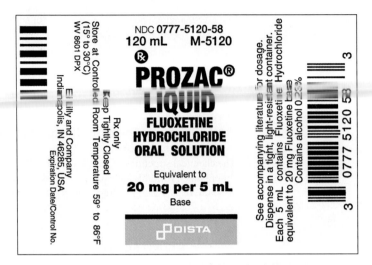

**■ FIGURE 16–5 Drug label for fluoxetine (Prozac).**
Prozac is used to treat depression but also a number of other mental illnesses, such as generalized anxiety disorder, obsessive-compulsive disorder, panic attacks, posttraumatic stress disorder, and bulimia.

## Did You Know?

Fluoxetine (Prozac) is used to treat depression, obsessive-compulsive disorder, panic disorder, premenstrual dysphoric disorder, and can also be used to treat anxiety and posttraumatic stress disorder. The book *Prozac Nation: Young and Depressed in America* (1994) described one woman's experience with depression, but the book quickly became the symbol of a generation of disillusioned, depressed young people in America.

### Serotonin and Norepinephrine Reuptake Inhibitor Drugs for Depression

Serotonin and norepinephrine reuptake inhibitor (SNRI) drugs block the normal reuptake of serotonin and norepinephrine by neurons. When serotonin and norepinephrine levels are low in patients with depression, these drugs allow the available serotonin and epinephrine to activate more receptors for a longer period of time before they are broken down.

desvenlafaxine (Pristiq)

duloxetine (Cymbalta) (see Figure 16–2)

venlafaxine (Effexor)

### Monoamine Oxidase Inhibitor Drugs for Depression

The neurotransmitters epinephrine, norepinephrine, dopamine, and serotonin are collectively known as *monoamines* because of their chemical structure. Monoamine oxidase (MAO) is an enzyme in the body that breaks down these monoamine neurotransmitters. Monoamine oxidase (MAO) inhibitor drugs prevent the enzyme monoamine oxidase from breaking down the neurotransmitters norepinephrine and serotonin in the brain. MAO inhibitor drugs are an older group of antidepressant drugs that are prescribed less frequently than other antidepressant drugs because of the possibility of severe side effects from drug–food interactions (see In Depth). MAO inhibitor drugs are not the drug of choice for initiating treatment for depression; they are only used to treat depression that has not responded to other drugs.

isocarboxazid (Marplan)

phenelzine (Nardil)

tranylcypromine (Parnate)

## In Depth

The enzyme monoamine oxidase (MAO) breaks down norepinephrine and serotonin in the brain, but in the intestine, it also breaks down tyramine in the foods we eat. When a patient takes an MAO inhibitor drug, the MAO enzyme is blocked and tyramine is not broken down in the intestine, but is absorbed into the blood. In the blood, large amounts of tyramine stimulate the release of norepinephrine, and this causes violent headaches, severe hypertension, and can even cause a stroke. This reaction occurs even more quickly if a patient on an MAO inhibitor drug eats foods that are high in tyramine; these include aged cheese, red wine, beer, chicken liver, bananas, bologna, salami, sausage, avocados, sauerkraut, raspberries, dried fruits, anchovies, caviar, meat tenderizer, soy sauce, ginseng, coffee, tea, colas, and chocolate.

## Other Drugs for Depression

These antidepressant drugs are chemically unrelated to other antidepressant drugs. Their mechanism of action in treating depression is not clearly understood.

bupropion (Aplenzin, Wellbutrin)
(see ■ FIGURE 16–6)

nefazodone

trazodone

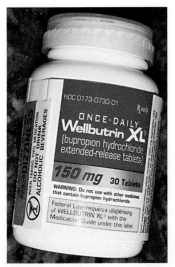

■ **FIGURE 16–6  Bottle of bupropion (Wellbutrin).**
Wellbutrin comes in the form of a tablet, as well as an extended-release tablet (Wellbutrin XL) that only needs to be taken once a day for depression. This generic drug bupropion is also available as the trade name Zyban and is used as a non-nicotine stop-smoking aid.

### Combination Drugs for Depression and Anxiety

These combination drugs contain an antidepressant drug (amitriptyline), a benzodiazepine antianxiety drug (chlordiazepoxide), or an antipsychotic drug (perphenazine).

Etrafon (amitriptyline, perphenazine)

Limbitrol (amitriptyline, chlordiazepoxide)

## Drug Alert!

In 2005, the FDA urged drug companies that make antidepressant drugs to put a warning label on these drugs, stating that patients taking antidepressant drugs can become suicidal. Persons being treated with an antidepressant drug can still feel sad but have a change in that they become more irritable, restless, and impulsive, and this can cause suicidal ideation that leads to suicide attempts, particularly in teens and young adults.

## Drugs Used to Treat Premenstrual Dysphoric Disorder

Premenstrual dysphoric disorder (PMDD) is a mood disorder that includes the physical and emotional symptoms of premenstrual syndrome, but also includes depression, anxiety, and sleep disturbances that significantly interfere with life. Drugs that are used to treat premenstrual dysphoric disorder are discussed in Chapter 13.

## Drugs Used to Treat Manic-Depressive Disorder

Manic-depressive disorder is characterized by two opposite emotions: mania and depression. The manic patient exhibits hyperactivity, agitation, and euphoria; thinks and talks rapidly; and devises many grandiose plans, but shows poor judgment. Mania is associated with increased levels of norepinephrine in the brain. Manic-depressive disorder is also known as **bipolar disorder** because the patient's moods swing between these two opposite poles of emotion. A more common, but less well known, type of bipolar disorder is characterized by mood swings between depression and anger and impulsiveness. Drugs used to treat manic-depressive disorder lessen the severity and frequency of these mood swings. The phrase **mood-stabilizing drug** applies to lithium, as well as to the anticonvulsant drugs used to treat manic-depressive disorder. Manic-depressive disorder is treated with drugs from these drug categories: antipsychotic drugs, anticonvulsant drugs, and antidepressant drugs, as well as other drugs that effectively treat only the mania phase of manic-depressive disorder.

These antipsychotic drugs are used to treat manic-depressive disorder.

chlorpromazine (Thorazine)

lithium (Lithobid)

These anticonvulsant drugs are used to treat manic-depressive disorder.

| | |
|---|---|
| carbamazepine (Equetro) | oxcarbazepine (Trileptal) |
| gabapentin (Neurotin) | topiramate (Topamax) |
| lamotrigine (Lamictal) (see ■ FIGURE 16–7) | valproic acid (Stavzor) |
| levetiracetam (Keppra) | |

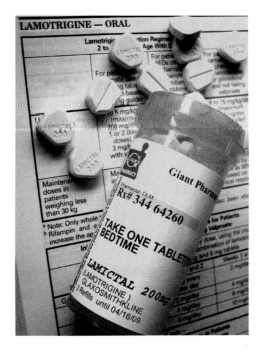

■ FIGURE 16–7 **Prescription bottle for lamotrigine (Lamictal).**
This anticonvulsant drug has been found to be useful in treating some forms of manic-depressive disorder in which the patient swings between depression and impulsiveness/anger rather than mania.

These drugs are effective for treating just the manic phase of manic-depressive disorder. They are benzodiazepine antianxiety drugs, anticonvulsant drugs, or antipsychotic drugs.

aripiprazole (Abilify)

olanzapine (Zyprexa)

chlorpromazine (Thorazine)

quetiapine (Seroquel)

clonazepam (Klonopin)

risperidone (Risperdal)

clozapine (Clorazil)

ziprasidone (Geodon)

This antidepressant drug is particularly useful for treating just the depression phase of manic-depressive disorder.

maprotiline

### Combination Drugs for Manic-Depressive Disorder

This combination drug contains a benzodiazepine antianxiety drug (olanzapine) to treat the mania of manic-depressive disorder and a selective serotonin reuptake inhibitor (SSRI) antidepressant drug (fluoxetine) to treat depression and anxiety.

Symbyax (olanzapine, fluoxetine)

## Drugs Used to Treat Obsessive-Compulsive Disorder

Obsessive-compulsive disorder (OCD) is characterized by thoughts that cause anxiety, followed by repetitive actions to relieve or escape the anxiety of a perceived threatening situation. These repetitive actions typically occupy hours of each day and involve repetitive cleaning, checking, hoarding, arranging, labeling, or even praying.

Although the person knows the behavior is excessive and unreasonable, he or she is unable to stop it. This disorder is treated with these antidepressant drugs and antipsychotic drugs.

citalopram (Celexa)

clomipramine (Anafranil)

duloxetine (Cymbalta)

fluoxetine (Prozac)

fluvoxamine (Luxor)

olanzapine (Zyprexa)

paroxetine (Paxil)

risperidone (Risperdal)

sertraline (Zoloft)

## Drugs Used to Treat Panic Disorder

Panic disorder, also known as *panic attacks*, is characterized by a sudden, overwhelming sense of great fear in the absence of any situation or reason that would create anxiety or fear. The physical symptoms are intense and can even mimic a heart attack. This disorder is treated with various types of antianxiety drugs and antidepressant drugs.

This antianxiety drug is used to treat panic disorder. It is a Schedule IV drug.

alprazolam (Xanax)

These antidepressant drugs are used to treat panic disorder.

citalopram (Celexa) (see ■ FIGURE 16–8)

clomipramine (Anafranil)

clonazepam (Klonopin)

desipramine (Norpramin)

duloxetine (Cymbalta)

escitalopram (Lexapro)

fluoxetine (Prozac)

fluvoxamine (Luxor)

imipramine (Tofranil)

nortriptyline (Aventyl, Pamelor)

paroxetine (Paxil)

sertraline (Zoloft)

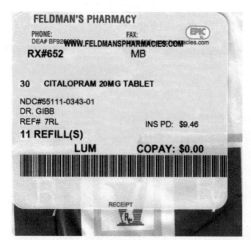

■ FIGURE 16–8 Prescription label for citalopram.
This prescription was filled with the generic drug citalopram. There was no cost (copay) to the patient because of good insurance coverage. However, if the prescription had been for the trade name drug Celexa, there would have been a cost to the patient.

## Drugs Used to Treat Social Anxiety Disorder

Social anxiety disorder, also known as *social phobia*, is characterized by fear in social situations (in crowds, stores, meetings, parties) and personal encounters (on the telephone or meeting or greeting a new person). There is also a fear of speaking to strangers or authority figures or speaking in front of a group. Physical symptoms include extreme nervousness, sweating, blushing, tremors, nausea, stammering, inability to think clearly, and the fear that everyone is looking at you. The person with social anxiety disorder knows that the fear is out of proportion to the situation, but cannot control the anxiety. This disorder is treated with these SSRI or SNRI antidepressant drugs.

| | |
|---|---|
| fluvoxamine (Luxor) | sertraline (Zoloft) |
| paroxetine (Paxil) | venlafaxine (Effexor) |

Professional actors, musicians, singers, and others in the public eye can experience temporary *performance anxiety* that is limited to that occasion. Instead of taking daily SSRI antidepressant drugs, these individuals usually take the following drug just prior to the performance to block the physical effects of excess epinephrine that is released in response to anxiety. Propranolol is a beta-blocker drug.

propranolol (Inderal)

## Drugs Used to Treat Posttraumatic Stress Disorder

Posttraumatic stress disorder (PTSD) is caused by exposure to life-threatening events or trauma, such as war, natural disasters, rape, or physical/mental abuse. This disorder is characterized by both physical and mental changes. Brainwave activity is altered. There are increased levels of epinephrine and norepinephrine and decreased levels of cortisol. Sleep abnormalities, headaches, nausea, dizziness, and chest pain are common. These symptoms may be mild or severe, constant or intermittent. This disorder also impairs personal and family relationships, activities of daily living, and employment. This disorder is treated with SSRI or SNRI antidepressant drugs.

| | |
|---|---|
| citalopram (Celexa) | paroxetine (Paxil) |
| duloxetine (Cymbalta) | sertraline (Zoloft) |
| fluoxetine (Prozac) | |

## Drugs Used to Treat Anorexia Nervosa and Bulimia Nervosa

Anorexia nervosa is a psychiatric illness in which the patient weighs much less than expected for his or her age and height, but cannot recognize this. The patient continues to diet, decreasing food intake to the point of starvation, denies being thin, and actually feels fat. Bulimia nervosa, on the other hand, is a psychiatric illness in which the patient is of normal weight, but wishes to be thinner. The patient diets, vomits, and uses laxatives to lose weight. Alternatively, the patient binges or eats large quantities of food. These mental illnesses are treated with tricyclic and SSRI antidepressant drugs, as well as lithium, a drug also used to treat mania, and topiramate, an anticonvulsant drug.

| | |
|---|---|
| amitriptyline | imipramine (Tofranil) |
| desipramine (Norpramin) | lithium (Lithobid) |
| fluoxetine (Prozac) | topiramate (Topamax) |
| fluvoxamine (Luxor) | |

## Drugs Used to Treat Withdrawal from Addiction

Addiction is a psychiatric substance-related disorder that is characterized by the frequent or constant use and abuse of drugs or chemicals to achieve a desired physical or emotional effect (a "high," sedation, or hallucinations). After a brief period of abuse, the person experiences dependence (the need for the drug to prevent withdrawal symptoms). Later, the person exhibits tolerance (decreasing effect even with increasing amounts of the drug). Addiction is a state of complete physical and psychological dependence on a drug. Schedule drugs, such as heroin, cocaine, narcotic drugs, barbiturate drugs, and antianxiety drugs, as well as alcohol, are commonly abused by addicts. The withdrawal process can be painful, both emotionally and physically, as the addict experiences withdrawal symptoms, such as irritability, sweating, runny nose, abdominal cramps, nausea and vomiting, diarrhea, confusion, tremors, muscle aches, and so forth.

These narcotic drugs are used to treat withdrawal from addiction to heroin, cocaine, or narcotic drugs. Buprenorphine, a Schedule III drug, is a narcotic agonist-antagonist drug. The agonist effect prevents withdrawal symptoms in the addict. The antagonist effect blocks the euphoria of any narcotic drug doses the addict may take because the administration of buprenorphine is unsupervised.

Methadone, a Schedule II drug, is a narcotic agonist drug that can be used to relieve severe pain or to treat narcotic addiction. It does not produce the degree of euphoria of other narcotic drugs, but because it has no antagonist effect, it cannot be given unsupervised. Recovering addicts must go to a clinic to obtain a daily dose of methadone.

buprenorphine (Buprenex, Subutex)

methadone (Diskets, Dolophine) (see ■ FIGURE 16–9)

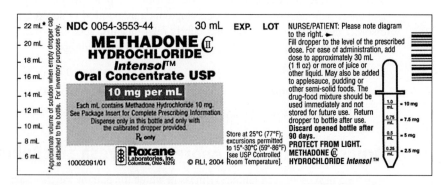

■ FIGURE 16–9 **Drug label for methadone.**
Methadone is used to treat withdrawal from addiction to heroin, cocaine, or narcotic drugs. It is available as tablets (trade name Dolophine), as orally dissolving tablets (trade name Diskets), and as an oral liquid (trade name Methadose, Methadone Intensol). This oral liquid is concentrated (hence its name Intensol) with 10 mg/mL, as compared to the regular strength of 10 mg/5 mL.

This combination drug contains a narcotic drug (buprenorphene) and a narcotic antagonist drug (naloxone).

Suboxone (buprenorphine, naloxone)

This narcotic antagonist drug blocks the effect of narcotics drugs to treat narcotic addiction. It is also used to treat alcohol dependence.

naltrexone (ReVia, Trexan, Vivitrol)

These antidepressant drugs are used to treat withdrawal from addiction to heroin, cocaine, or narcotic drugs. They are not schedule drugs.

desipramine (Norpramin)

imipramine (Tofranil)

trazodone

These antianxiety drugs are used to treat withdrawal from alcohol. These are Schedule IV drugs.

| | |
|---|---|
| chlordiazepoxide (Librium) | diazepam (Valium) |
| clonazepam (Klonopin) | oxazepam (Serax) |
| clorazepate (Tranxene) | |

This anticonvulsant drug is used to treat withdrawal from cocaine and alcohol.

topiramate (Topamax)

This alpha$_2$ receptor stimulating drug is used to treat withdrawal from heroin.

guanfacine (Tenex)

These drugs are used to treat withdrawal from alcohol. Clonidine is an alpha receptor blocker drug. Lithium is an antipsychotic drug. Topiramate is an anticonvulsant drug. They are not schedule drugs.

clonidine (Catapres)

lithium (Lithobid)

topiramate (Topamax)

These drugs are used as a deterrent to prevent drinking alcohol. They are given to alcoholic patients who want to remain sober, to prevent them from consuming alcohol.

acamprosate (Campral)

disulfiram (Antabuse)

## Drug Alert!

Disulfiram (Antabuse) inhibits an enzyme that normally metabolizes one of the breakdown products (acetaldehyde) of alcohol in the blood. If the patient drinks while taking this drug, the alcohol is changed to acetaldehyde but cannot be further metabolized. As acetaldehyde levels increase, the patient experiences flushing, headache, dizziness, and nausea, and can even have severe hypotension and cardiac arrhythmias. These adverse reactions are supposed to keep alcoholic patients from taking a drink. However, patients must first express a desire to remain sober and cannot be placed on this drug without being forewarned of these adverse effects and giving their consent to treatment. Patients must also be warned to avoid using cough syrups and mouthwashes that contain alcohol.

## Historical Notes

Disulfiram was originally used in the commercial production of rubber. In 1948, two Danish researchers began testing this compound for its effectiveness in treating intestinal worms. To study its safety in humans, they both took the compound. When each became ill after consuming alcohol, they concluded that the disulfiram alcohol combination had produced the reaction. The trade name drug Antabuse (*Ant-* for *anti*, meaning *against,* plus *abuse.*) was developed and first prescribed for treating alcoholism that same year.

## Drugs Used to Treat Attention-Deficit/Hyperactivity Disorder

Hyperactive children exhibit symptoms of restlessness, short attention span, distractibility, emotional lability, impulsiveness, and disruptive behavior. This complex of symptoms was previously known as *minimal brain dysfunction* and *attention deficit disorder* (ADD). With the added component of hyperactivity, it is now known as *attention-deficit/hyperactivity disorder (ADHD).* The cause of ADHD may be brain damage at birth, genetic factors, or other abnormalities. A 2007 study of progressive MRI scans of children with ADHD indicated that it is not a disease but a delay in brain development. It is five times more common in boys than in girls. Most children outgrow the symptoms of ADHD in late childhood. Drugs used to treat ADHD include amphetamines and other related CNS-stimulating drugs. These drugs regulate the levels of norepinephrine and dopamine; they exert what is known as a ***paradoxical effect*** in that they do not overstimulate but actually reduce impulsive behavior while lengthening the attention span. Drug therapy for ADHD is accompanied by psychological counseling, as well as special educational intervention, as needed.

### Amphetamine Drugs for ADHD

Amphetamine drugs are stimulant drugs that have a paradoxical (reverse) effect when given to patients with hyperactivity. Instead of increasing their hyperactivity, they actually lessen it. These drugs are categorized as Schedule II drugs and have a high potential for addiction.

>    dextroamphetamine (Dexedrine)
>    lisdexamfetamine (Vyvanse)
>    methamphetamine (Desoxyn)

## Historical Notes

Amphetamine was synthesized in the late 1920s. It was used during World War II to help soldiers keep alert and avoid battle fatigue. During the 1960s, methamphetamine ("speed") became a popular drug of abuse. In 1972, amphetamine drugs were categorized as Schedule II drugs because of their high potential for abuse.

### Other Stimulant Drugs for ADHD

These drugs stimulate the central nervous system but are not amphetamine drugs. They are, however, Schedule II drugs.

>    dexmethylphenidate (Focalin)
>    methylphenidate (Concerta, Daytrana, Ritalin) (see ■ **FIGURE 16–10**)

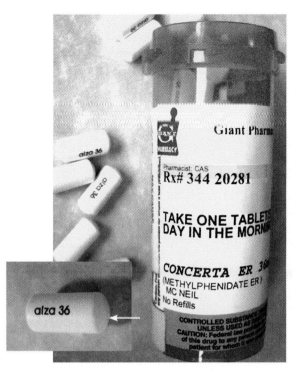

**■ FIGURE 16–10 Prescription bottle for methylphenidate (Concerta).**
Concerta is an extended-release form of methylphenidate. It comes as a special oblong tablet that has a new, patented drug-delivery technology. One end of the tablet contains a tiny, laser-drilled hole through which one quarter of the drug's daily dose is released immediately. Then, the other end of the tablet absorbs fluid from the intestine and expands internally, slowly forcing the rest of the drug dose through the hole over the next 12 hours. The printed "Alza" on the tablet refers to the name of the company who created this technology. The drug itself is manufactured by McNeil Pharmaceuticals. Concerta is a Schedule II drug. Its drug label has this printed on it as a capital C with a Roman numeral II inside it. However, the label for the prescription bottle does not have this. Instead, the pharmacist attached a red label at the bottom of the prescription bottle that warns that this is a controlled substance.

## *Focus on Healthcare Issues*

Methylphenidate was approved by the FDA in 1955. The American Academy of Pediatrics reported that, from 1990 to 1995, prescriptions for the drugs Ritalin and Prozac doubled in number for preschool children with ADHD in the United States. They attributed this to the managed care environment, parents wanting a quick diagnosis, the low cost of these drugs, and the fact that so many working parents do not have time to enforce a behavioral modification program. Other studies showed a 500 percent increase in prescriptions for Ritalin since 1996. In 2006, doctors wrote about 1 million prescriptions a month for Ritalin for children and adults, and nearly 10 percent of all 12-year-old boys are on Ritalin. One drawback of Ritalin was that its therapeutic effect lasted only 4 hours, so a dose had to be taken at breakfast, at lunch, and in the late afternoon. This was difficult to manage and embarrassing to children who had to take the drug during school. Now methylphenidate is available in a long-acting tablet (Ritalin LA), in an extended-release tablet (Concerta), and as a transdermal patch (Daytrana).

Dexmethylphenidate (Focalin) contains only the dextro isomer, the more active isomer, of the same chemical molecule that is in Ritalin.

## Other Drugs for ADHD

These drugs have a variety of effects. Atomoxetine inhibits the transport of norepinephrine in the synapses between neurons in the brain. Chlorpromazine is an antipsychotic drug. Clonidine stimulates alpha$_2$ receptors in the brain and is used to treat many medical diseases.

atomoxetine (Strattera) (see **■ FIGURE 16–11**)

chlorpromazine (Thorazine)

clonidine (Catapres)

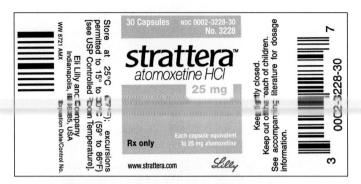

■ **FIGURE 16–11 Drug label for Strattera.**
Atomoxetine (Strattera) is used to treat attention-deficit/hyperactivity
disorder. Unlike other drugs for ADHD, Strattera is not a schedule drug
and carries no potential for addiction.

## Combination Drugs for ADHD

This drug combines two different forms of amphetamines and dextroamphetamines.
Dextroamphetamine is an isomer of amphetamine. An isomer is a drug that has the same chemical
formula and identical types and numbers of atoms as another drug, but those atoms are arranged dif-
ferently. In this case, the dextroamphetamine molecule is a right-handed (*dextr/o-* means *right*),
mirror image of the amphetamine molecule. This dextro isomer is several times more potent as a
stimulant drug.

Adderall (amphetamine, dextroamphetamine)

### Did You Know?

The name of the combination drug Adderall alludes to the abbreviation of the medical phrase
*attention-deficit disorder* (ADD).

# Chapter Review

## Quiz Yourself

1. Minor tranquilizers are the same drugs as major tranquilizers, but are given at a lower dose.
   True or false?
2. Antianxiety drugs are also known by what two other names?
3. Describe several different ways in which benzodiazepine drugs exert a therapeutic effect.
4. Describe the symptoms of psychosis.
5. Antipsychotic drugs are also known by what two other names?
6. Name the four types of receptors that are blocked by phenothiazine drugs for psychosis.

7. Describe the symptoms of tardive dyskinesia that occur due to antipsychotic drugs.
8. The words *tricyclic* and *tetracyclic* bring to mind what category of drugs? Why?
9. Why must certain foods be avoided when taking an MAO inhibitor drug? What foods are they?
10. Compare the therapeutic effect of SSRI versus SNRI drugs for depression.
11. What different categories of drugs are used to treat manic-depressive disorder?
12. What beta-blocker drug is used to treat performance anxiety?
13. What categories of drugs are used to treat PTSD?
14. Explain why amphetamine drugs can be used to treat ADHD in hyperactive children.
15. What is unique about the drug-delivery technology of Concerta?
16. What is the name of the transdermal patch drug used to treat ADHD?
17. To what category of drugs does each of these drugs belong?

   a. alprazolam (Xanax)
   b. chlorpromazine (Thorazine)
   c. diazepam (Valium)
   d. disulfiram (Antabuse)
   e. duloxetine (Cymbalta)
   f. fluoxetine (Prozac)
   g. haloperidol (Haldol)
   h. lithium (Lithobid)
   i. methylphenidate (Concerta, Daytrana)
   j. olanzapine (Zyprexa)
   k. risperidone (Risperdal)
   l. sertraline (Zoloft)

## Spelling Tips

| | |
|---|---|
| **Antabuse** | Not *Antiabuse;* there is no *i.* |
| **BuSpar** | Unusual internal capitalization. |
| **lisdexamfetamine** | Unusual spelling with an *f* rather than a *ph* for a drug in the amphetamine class. |
| **ReVia** | Unusual internal capitalization. |

## Clinical Applications

1. Look at this handwritten prescription and answer the following questions.
   a. What drug has the physician prescribed?
   b. What is the strength of the dose?
   c. In what drug form is it given?
   d. Translate the rest of the prescription into plain English.

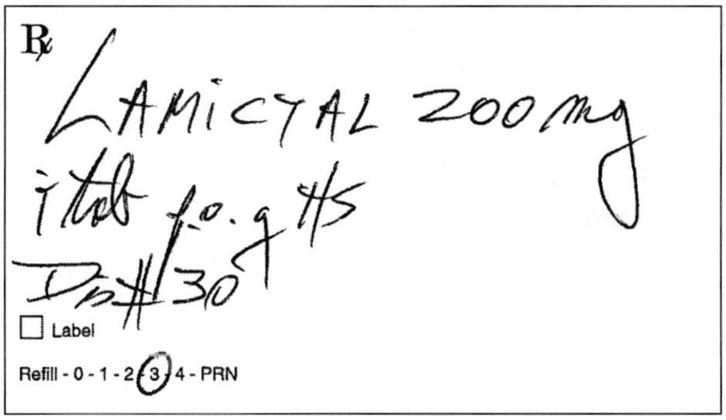

2. Look at this drug label and answer the following questions.
   a. What is the generic name of this drug?
   b. What is the trade name of this drug?
   c. To what category of drugs does this drug belong?

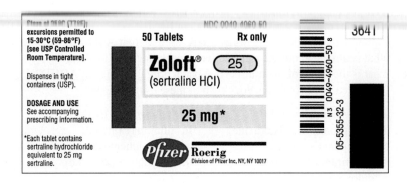

3. Look at this drug bottle and answer the following questions.
   a. What is the generic name of this drug?
   b. What is the trade name of this drug?
   c. What condition is this drug used to treat?
   d. What is the dose strength of each tablet?
   e. What schedule is this drug?

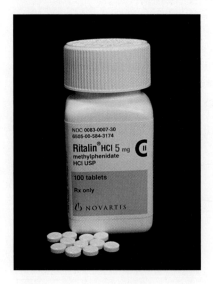

**4.** Look at this handwritten prescription and answer the following questions.
   **a.** What drug has the physician prescribed?
   **b.** What is the strength of the dose?
   **c.** In what drug form is it given?
   **d.** What is written inside the parentheses?
   **e.** Translate the rest of the prescription into plain English.

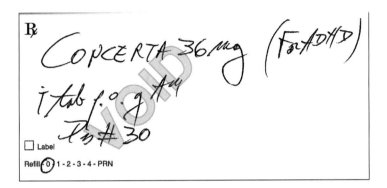

**5.** Look at this handwritten prescription and answer the following questions.
   **a.** What drug has the physician prescribed?
   **b.** What is the strength of the dose?
   **c.** How many will the hospital pharmacist send to the patient?
   **d.** Translate the rest of the prescription into plain English.

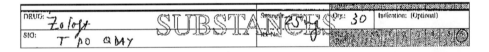

**6.** Look at this handwritten prescription and answer the following questions.
   **a.** What drug has the physician prescribed?
   **b.** To what category of drugs does this belong?
   **c.** What mental illness is it used to treat?
   **d.** What is the strength of the dose?
   **e.** How many tablets will be dispensed?
   **f.** Translate the rest of the prescription into plain English.
   **g.** At the end of the prescription, what does the physician warn the patient to avoid?

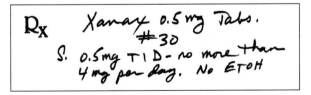

## Multimedia Extension Exercises

■ Go to www.pearsonhighered.com/turley and click on the photo of the cover of *Understanding Pharmacology for Health Professionals* to access the interactive Companion Website created for this textbook.

# 17 Dermatologic Drugs

## CHAPTER CONTENTS

## Learning Objectives

After studying this chapter, you should be able to

1. Explain the rationale behind using topical versus systemic drugs to treat skin conditions.

2. Compare and contrast the therapeutic effects of the various categories of drugs used to treat acne vulgaris.

3. Compare and contrast the therapeutic effects of the various categories of drugs used to treat psoriasis.

4. Compare and contrast the therapeutic effects of antibiotic drugs, antifungal drugs, antiyeast drugs, and antiviral drugs.

5. Explain how drugs are used to treat alopecia and wrinkles.

6. Describe the difference between the parasitic infections scabies and pediculosis, and the drugs used to treat them.

7. Describe various types of drugs used to treat burns, skin ulcers, and wounds.

8. Given the generic and trade names of a dermatologic drug, identify what drug category they belong to or what disease they are used to treat.

9. Given a dermatologic drug category, identify several generic and trade name drugs in that category.

ermatologic drugs are used to treat diseases of the skin. These diseases include acne vulgaris, acne rosacea, psoriasis, bacterial infections of the skin, fungal and yeast infections of the skin, viral infections of the skin, poison ivy, contact dermatitis, diaper rash, itching and inflammation, alopecia, wrinkles, scabies, pediculosis, burns, skin ulcers, wounds, vitiligo, and so forth. Because of the superficial nature and location of most dermatologic diseases, they respond well to topical drug therapy. Dermatologic drugs include many over-the-counter (OTC) as well as prescription drugs. Topical dermatologic drugs are available in these drug forms: cream, gel, liquid, lotion, mousse, ointment, and shampoo. Topical dermatologic drugs include keratolytic drugs, antibiotic drugs, vitamin A–type and vitamin D–type drugs, coal tar drugs, psoralen drugs, antifungal drugs, antiyeast drugs, antiviral drugs, corticosteroid drugs, antihistamine drugs, antipruritic drugs, anesthetic drugs, and others. However, when some dermatologic diseases become widespread, severe, or penetrate deeply below the skin, oral drugs that act systemically are given.

## Drugs Used to Treat Acne Vulgaris

Acne vulgaris is the form of acne that is commonly seen during adolescence. It is characterized by large amounts of oil that harden and block the pores, forming reddish papules. As bacteria feed on the oil, they cause infection. This draws white blood cells to the area, forming pustules (whiteheads). The hardened oil turns black as it is exposed to the air, forming comedos (blackheads). Topical drugs used to treat acne vulgaris cleanse away oil and dead skin (keratolytic action), close the pores (astringent action), and kill skin bacteria (anti-infective action). Ointments are not used to treat acne vulgaris because their high oil content clogs the pores.

### Topical Keratolytic Drugs for Acne Vulgaris

This over-the-counter drug has a keratolytic effect that removes oil and dead skin to cleanse the pores. The section on combination drugs lists several other topical keratolytic drugs (salicylic acid, sodium sulfacetamide, sulfur).

salicylic acid (Clearasil, Fostex, Stri-Dex)

## Did You Know?

Salicylic acid is used in stronger concentrations to remove corns, calluses, and warts from the skin.

### Topical Antibiotic Drugs for Acne Vulgaris

These antibiotic drugs kill bacteria on the skin and are used to treat the pustules of acne vulgaris. Except for ticlosan, these are prescription drugs.

azelaic acid (Azelex, Finacea)

benzoyl peroxide (Benzac, Desquam, PanOxyl)

clindamycin (Cleocin T)

erythromycin (Emgel, Eryderm)

triclosan (Clearasil, Oxy, Stri-Dex)

## Did You Know?

Triclosan is also found in deodorant, toothpaste, shaving cream, and mouthwash. It is the antibacterial component of Microban, a trade-name product that is incorporated into kitchen utensils and countertops, paints, spas, towels, flooring, bathroom fixtures, air filtration units, shoes, shopping carts, baby changing stations, food storage products, vacuum cleaners, and other products. Showering or bathing with triclosan is used to prevent outbreaks of bacterial infections, particularly due to methicillin-resistant *Staphylococcus aureus* (MRSA).

### Topical Combination Drugs for Acne Vulgaris

These combination drugs contain a keratolytic drug (salicylic acid, sodium sulfacetamide, sulfur) and an antibiotic drug (benzoyl peroxide, clindamycin, erythromycin). All of these are prescription drugs.

BenzaClin (benzoyl peroxide, clindamycin)

Benzamycin (benzoyl peroxide, erythromycin)

Clenia (sodium sulfacetamide, sulfur)

Duac (benzoyl peroxide, clindamycin)

Pernox (salicylic acid, sulfur)

Plexion (sodium sulfacetamide, sulfur)

Sulfoxyl (benzoyl peroxide, sulfur)

### Oral Antibiotic Drugs for Acne Vulgaris

These oral antibiotic drugs provide systemic treatment for severe cases of acne vulgaris. They travel through the blood to kill bacteria in the deeper layers of the skin. All of these prescription drugs belong to the tetracycline category of antibiotic drugs.

doxycycline (Vibramycin, Vibra-Tabs)

minocycline (Dynacin, Minocin)

tetracycline (Sumycin)

### Topical Vitamin A–Type Drugs for Acne Vulgaris

Vitamin A is known as *retinoic acid.* A deficiency of vitamin A can produce abnormal changes in the epithelial cells of the skin, such as those that occur with acne vulgaris. These drugs, which are known as **retinoid drugs,** are structurally similar to vitamin A or similar to metabolites of vitamin A. These drugs cause epidermal cells to multiply more rapidly. This rapid turnover prevents the pores from becoming clogged. These drugs also decrease the inflammation associated with acne vulgaris. These drugs are prescription drugs.

adapalene (Differin)

tazarotene (Avage, Tazorac)

tretinoin (Retin-A) (see ■ FIGURE 17–1)

## Did You Know?

Oral contraceptive drugs (birth control pills) have been found to be effective in treating acne vulgaris. Drug companies advertise this desirable effect along with these drugs' main therapeutic effect of birth control, and YAZ is FDA approved for treating acne.

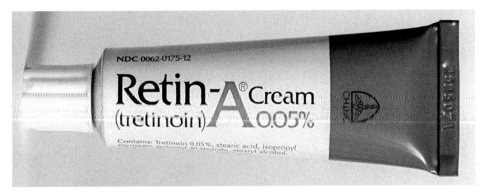

**■ FIGURE 17–1  Tretinoin (Retin-A).**
This retinoid drug is derived from vitamin A, and these two facts are reflected in the trade name of
the drug. Tretinoin (Retin-A) comes as a topical cream or gel to treat acne vulgaris. Under the trade
name Renova, tretinoin is also used to treat wrinkles.

## Oral Vitamin A–Type Drugs for Severe Acne Vulgaris

Severe cystic acne vulgaris that is unresponsive to other drugs is treated systemically with an oral
vitamin A–type drug. These drugs cause epithelial cells to multiply more rapidly, which prevents
clogged pores from becoming infected and forming cysts. This prescription drug is only used to
treat severe cystic acne vulgaris, not common acne vulgaris.

isotretinoin (Accutane)

# *Drug Alert!*

Isotretinoin (Accutane) has been linked to the unusual and severe adverse effects of
depression and suicide. The FDA has mandated that these adverse effects be brought to the
attention of the physician and patient with large warning boxes included with all literature
on the drug.

On that snowy January day, Brandon Troppman seemed to be loving life. He put on a
new shirt and combed his hair just so before heading to the mall to hang out with his
high school sweetheart . . . At 6:30 that evening, he talked on the phone with his
best friend, laughing and making his friend laugh, as always. An hour later, Brandon
hanged himself from a rod in his bedroom closet . . . [He] hadn't appeared
depressed, never abused drugs or alcohol, never talked of suicide. In the months
after his death, his parents reached a conclusion that now seems inescapable to
them: the popular acne drug Accutane, they believe, led to their son's suicide.
[Congressman Bart Stupak from Michigan] also publicly blamed the drug for his
17-year-old son's suicide. [During his own investigation], he found an internal 1988
FDA memo that stated: "Given all the pieces of evidence available, it is difficult to
avoid the conclusion that Accutane use . . . is associated with severe psychiatric
disease in some patients."

Gary Gately. "A Drug's Dark Side," *The Baltimore Sun,* March 4, 2001, p. N1.

## Drugs Used to Treat Acne Rosacea

Acne rosacea is an adult form of acne characterized by constant blotchy redness, dilated superficial blood vessels, and excessive amounts of oil on the face. It is exacerbated by heat, stress, and skin irritation. Drugs used to treat acne rosacea are topical antibiotic drugs. They are prescription drugs.

azelaic acid (Azelex, Finacea)

metronidazole (MetroCream, MetroGel) (see ■ FIGURE 17–2)

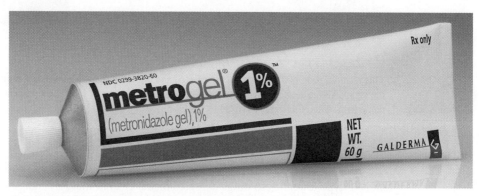

■ **FIGURE 17–2 Metronidazole (MetroGel).**
Metronidazole (MetroGel) is a topical drug that comes in the drug form of a gel. It has an antibiotic and antiprotozoal that kills bacteria on the skin of patients with acne rosacea.

### *Did You Know?*

Metronidazole has both an antibiotic and antiprotozoal effect and has many different uses. Topically, it is also used to treat infected decubitus ulcers. Metronidazole (Flagyl) is taken orally to treat dysentery and intestinal infections caused by protozoal organisms. Metronidazole (MetroGel-Vaginal) is applied topically in the vagina to treat vaginal infections caused by the bacteria *Hemophilus* and *Gardnerella*. Metronidazole in combination with bismuth and tetracycline (Helidac) is used to treat peptic ulcers caused by *Helicobacter pylori*, a spiral bacterium that is resistant to other antibiotic drugs.

## Drugs Used to Treat Psoriasis

Psoriasis is a chronic, autoimmune skin disorder that is characterized by scaly, raised, silvery-red patches on the skin. It is often resistant to treatment. In psoriasis, the skin is abnormal at the cellular level, exhibiting an abnormally accelerated rate of epithelial cell division and abnormality of the epithelial cells that produce keratin (keratinocytes). Topical coal tar drugs, vitamin A–type drugs, vitamin D–type drugs, and corticosteroid drugs are used to treat psoriasis.

### Topical Coal Tar Drugs for Psoriasis

Coal tar drugs decrease the rate of epithelial cell production, correct abnormalities of keratinocytes, cleanse away dead skin (keratolytic action), and decrease itching (antipruritic action). This is an over-the-counter drug.

coal tar (Balnetar, Neutrogena T/Gel, Zetar)

*Did You Know?*

Coal tar, a byproduct of the processing of bituminous coal, contains over 10,000 different chemicals. It has been used since the 1800s to treat psoriasis.

### Topical Vitamin A–Type Drugs for Psoriasis

A deficiency of vitamin A can produce abnormal changes in the epithelial cells of the skin, such as those that occur with psoriasis. This topical retinoid drug normalizes the abnormal production of epithelial cells. This is a prescription drug.

   tazarotene (Avage, Tazorac)

### Oral Vitamin A–Type Drugs for Psoriasis

This oral retinoid drug acts systemically to treat severe psoriasis that cannot be controlled with topical drugs. This is a prescription drug.

   acitretin (Soriatane)

### Topical Vitamin D–Type Drugs for Psoriasis

The red, scaly patches of psoriasis are caused by abnormal keratinocytes within the skin. This synthetic vitamin D-type drug activates vitamin D receptors in the keratinocytes and slows their abnormal cell growth. This is a prescription drug.

   calcipotriene (Dovonex)

### Topical Corticosteroid Drugs for Psoriasis

Topical corticosteroid drugs decrease the inflammation and itching associated with psoriasis. For a detailed discussion of topical corticosteroid drugs, see Drugs Used to Treat Inflammation and Itching.

### Other Topical Drugs for Psoriasis

These topical drugs for psoriasis either inhibit the production of cellular DNA or are toxic to epithelial cells; either action decreases the rate at which epithelial cells divide. Anthralin is a prescription drug; pyrithione zinc is an over-the-counter drug.

   anthralin (Dritho-Scalp, Psoriatec)

   pyrithione zinc (Denorex, Head and Shoulders)

### Oral Drugs for Psoriasis

These drugs are only used to treat moderate-to-severe, chronic psoriasis that has not responded to other drugs. These drugs either decrease the rate at which epithelial cells divide or act as an immunosuppressant to suppress the activity of T lymphocytes and the immune system. Adalimumab, efalizumab, and infliximab are monoclonal antibody drugs (as evidenced by the suffix -*mab*). Etanercept and tacrolimus are immunomodulator drugs. Methotrexate is a chemotherapy drug that kills rapidly dividing cells of many types (particularly cancerous cells).

| | |
|---|---|
| adalimumab (Humira) | infliximab (Remicade) |
| alefacept (Amevive) | methotrexate (Trexall) |
| cyclosporine (Gengraf, Neoral, Sandimmune) | sirolimus (Rapamune) |
| efalizumab (Raptiva) | tacrolimus (Protopic) |
| etanercept (Enbrel) (see ■ FIGURE 17–3) | thioguanine (Tabloid) |

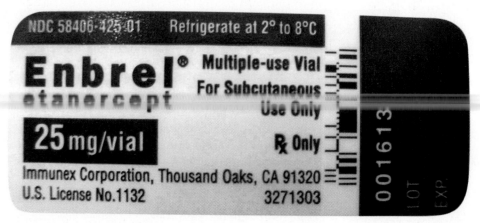

**■ FIGURE 17–3 Drug label for etanercept (Enbrel).**
Because psoriasis is an autoimmune disorder in which the body's immune system attacks skin cells, immunomodulator drugs such as etanercept (Enbrel) have been used to modulate (restore a normal balance) to the action of the immune system.

### Psoralen Drugs for Psoriasis

Severe, disabling psoriasis can also be treated by exposure to ultraviolet light in combination with a drug that sensitizes the skin to the effects of ultraviolet light. These drugs are collectively known as *psoralen drugs*. The treatment is known as **PUVA** (psoralen/ultraviolet wavelength A). This combined treatment damages cellular DNA and decreases the rate of cell division.

methoxsalen (Oxsoralen)

---

## *Did You Know?*

The word *psoralen* is derived from the name of the annual herb *Psoralea corylifolia,* which is known to cause sensitivity to light when eaten.

---

### Combination Drugs for Psoriasis

This topical prescription combination drug contains a vitamin D–type drug (calcipotriene) to slow the rate of abnormal epithelial cell growth and a corticosteroid drug (betamethasone) to control inflammation in psoriasis.

Taclonex, Taclonex Scalp (calcipotriene, betamethasone)

## Drugs Used to Treat Bacterial Infections of the Skin

Bacterial infections of the skin can occur anytime the skin is broken because there are always bacteria on the surface of the skin. Superficial abrasions, cuts, and burns that become infected are treated with topical antibiotic drugs. These drugs are also used to treat skin infections that develop as a result of skin diseases, such as acne vulgaris, contact dermatitis, or bacterial invasion into areas of fungal or viral skin infections.

## Topical Antibiotic Drugs

These over-the-counter and prescription antibiotic drugs are used topically to treat superficial bacterial skin infections. They inhibit the growth of bacteria (bacteriostatic action) or kill bacteria (bactericidal action) by blocking their ability to maintain a cell wall.

| | |
|---|---|
| bacitracin | mupirocin (Bactroban) |
| gentamicin | retapamulin (Altabax) |

### *Focus on Healthcare Issues*

Mupirocin (Bactroban) is active against a wide range of gram-positive bacteria, including methicillin-resistant *Staphylococcus aureus* (MRSA) (pronounced "MER-sah"). MRSA is a gram-positive bacterium that developed resistance to the penicillin category of drugs and the most common drug in the penicillin category, which was methicillin. MRSA causes serious and sometimes fatal infections in hospitalized patients. MRSA was found to exist as colonies in the noses of healthcare providers; they were not ill, but they inadvertently passed the bacterium to hospitalized patients whose immune systems were unable to combat it. Nonsymptomatic healthcare providers with MRSA colonies in the nose are treated with topical mupirocin (Bactroban) or retapamulin (Altabax), and hospitalized patients infected with MRSA are treated with the intravenous antibiotic drug vancomycin.

### *Historical Notes*

Retapamulin represents a new category of antibiotic drugs known as pleuromutilin drugs. Until retapamulin, there had not been a new category of antibiotic drugs discovered in the past 20 years.

Bacitracin was developed from a strain of *Bacillus subtilis,* a bacterium found growing in fluid draining from a wound in a patient named Margaret Tracy. The drug name *bacitracin* is a combination of the bacterium's name and the patient's name: ***Baci**llus subtilis* + ***Trac**y* + ***in***.

## Topical Antibiotic Combination Drugs

These over-the-counter combination drugs contain two or three topical antibiotic drugs (bacitracin, neomycin, polymyxin B).

Betadine First Aid (bacitracin, polymyxin B)

Neosporin Original (bacitracin, neomycin, polymyxin B) (see ■ **FIGURE 17–4**)

Polysporin (bacitracin, polymyxin B) (see ■ **FIGURE 17–4**)

Triple Antibiotic (bacitracin, neomycin, polymyxin B) (see ■ **FIGURE 17–4**)

These over-the-counter combination drugs contain three antibiotic drugs (bacitracin, neomycin, polymyxin B) and an anesthetic drug (lidocaine, pramoxine) to treat bacterial skin infections and control pain.

Lanabiotic (bacitracin, neomycin, polymyxin B, lidocaine)

Neosporin Plus Pain Relief (bacitracin, neomycin, polymyxin B, pramoxine)

This prescription combination drug contains an antibiotic drug (neomycin) and a corticosteroid drug (hydrocortisone) to treat bacterial skin infections and control inflammation.

Cortisporin (neomycin, hydrocortisone)

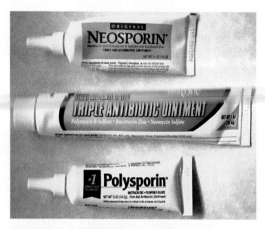

■ **FIGURE 17–4 Tubes of antibiotic ointment.**
These combination over-the-counter trade name antibiotic drugs—Neosporin, Triple Antibiotic, and Polysporin—contain two or three of these generic name antibiotic drugs (bacitracin, neomycin, and polymyxin B). All three of these tubes contain the drugs in the form of an ointment.

### Systemic Antibiotic Drugs

For serious or widespread bacterial infections of the skin, oral or intravenous antibiotic drugs that work systemically are prescribed. For a discussion of these drugs, see Chapter 20.

## Focus on Healthcare Issues

The Soap and Detergent Association reports that 45 percent of hand and body wash products contain antibacterial compounds. One study showed that 75 percent of liquid soaps and 30 percent of bar soaps contain antibacterial compounds. Small amounts of antibacterial compounds are present in a wide variety of products. Widespread use of antibacterial compounds and the routine use of antibiotic drugs in animal feed are believed to have contributed to the rise of antibiotic-resistant bacteria.

## Drugs Used to Treat Fungal or Yeast Infections of the Skin

Fungi and yeast grow in areas that are dark, warm, and moist, such as the feet, perineal area, groin area, underarms, and scalp. Fungus infections include ringworm (tinea capitis, tinea corporis), athlete's foot (tinea pedis), jock itch (tinea cruris), and fungal infections of the nails (onychomycosis). Yeast infections of the skin are caused by *Candida albicans*. Yeast infections most frequently occur in the mouth and vagina, but can also be present on the skin (for example, diaper rash). Fungal and yeast infections can be effectively treated with topical antifungal and antiyeast drugs that alter the cell wall of the fungus or yeast and disrupt its enzyme activity, resulting in cell death. You will notice that some of the same drugs used to treat fungal infections are also used to treat yeast infections. This is because fungi are closely related (biologically) to yeasts.

### Topical Antifungal Drugs

These over-the-counter and prescription antifungal drugs are used to treat superficial fungal infections of the skin or nails.

butenafine (Lotrimin Ultra)

ciclopirox (Loprox, Penlac Nail Lacquer)
(see ■ **FIGURE 17–5**)

clotrimazole (Cruex Cream, Desenex Cream, Lotrimin AF 1%)

econazole (Spectazole)

ketoconazole (Nizoral A-D, Xolegel)
(see ■ **FIGURE 17–6**)

miconazole (Lotrimin AF 2%, Micatin, Ting 2%) (see ■ **FIGURE 17–7**)

naftifine (Naftin)

oxiconazole (Oxistat)

sertaconazole (Ertaczo)

sulconazole (Exelderm)

terbinafine (DesenexMyax, Lamisil AT)

tolnaftate (Aftate, Tinactin, Ting 1%)

triacetin (Fungoid)

undecylenic acid (Cruex, Desenex)

*Note:* The suffix *-conazole* is common to generic antifungal drugs. The *AF* in some trade name drugs stands for *antifungal.*

## Drug Alert!

All of these over-the-counter trade name antifungal drugs are used topically to treat fungal infections. Even though their trade names are very similar, they are actually completely different generic drugs. This can cause confusion on the part of healthcare providers and consumers.

| Trade Name Drug | Generic Name Drug | Drug Form |
|---|---|---|
| Cruex Aerosol/Powder | undecylenic acid | 19% aerosol powder, 10% powder |
| Cruex Cream | clotrimazole | 1% cream |
| | | |
| Desenex Cream | clotrimazole | 1% cream |
| Desenex Powder/Soap | undecylenic acid | 25% powder, soap |
| Desenex, Prescription Strength | miconazole | 2% spray powder |
| DesenexMyax | terbinafine | 1% cream |
| | | |
| Lotrimin AF 1% | clotrimazole | 1% cream, liquid, lotion |
| Lotrimin AF 2% | miconazole | 2% powder, spray |
| Lotrimin Ultra | butenafine | 1% cream |
| | | |
| Ting 1% | tolnaftate | 1% cream |
| Ting 2% | miconazole | 2% spray powder |

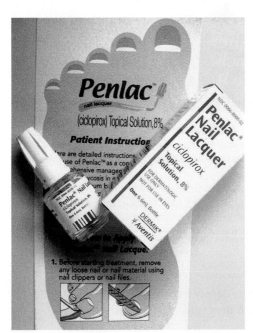

■ **FIGURE 17–5** **Penlac Nail Lacquer.**
The generic antifungal drug ciclopirox comes as a cream or a gel, but it also comes as a topical nail lacquer under the trade name Penlac. This clear nail liquid is applied under the nail, around the cuticle, and on top of the nail plate, as shown in this clever, yet informative, patient information card.

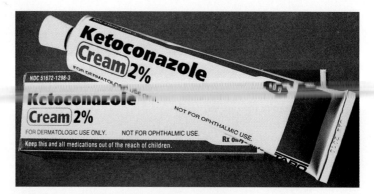

■ **FIGURE 17–6 Tube of ketoconazole.**
Ketoconazole is a topical antifungal drug that is used to treat fungal infections of the skin. This drug form is a 2% cream in a tube. Ketoconzaole is also available in the form of a gel under the trade name Xolegel. No matter which drug form the dermatologist chooses to prescribe after examining a patient with a fungal infection, a generic name drug is always less expensive than a trade name drug.

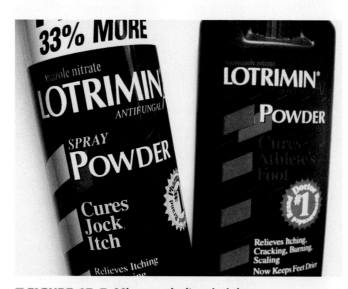

■ **FIGURE 17–7 Miconazole (Lotrimin).**
These two over-the-counter drugs both contain the generic antifungal drug miconazole, and they are both in the form of a powder (aerosol spray or sprinkle powder). However, the Lotrimin on the left advertises that it cures jock itch, while the Lotrimin on the right advertises that it cures athlete's foot. Actually, there is no difference in these drugs or their therapeutic effect because the same fungus (tinea) causes both jock itch (tinea cruris) and athlete's foot (tinea pedis).

## Systemic Antifungal Drugs

When fungal skin infections penetrate deeply into the skin or nails, cover large areas, or are particularly severe, they are treated with drugs that act systemically. These drugs are discussed in Chapter 20.

## Topical Antiyeast Drugs

These over-the-counter and prescription topical drugs are used to treat yeast infections of the skin.

clotrimazole (Cruex Cream, Desenex Cream, Lotrimin AF 1%)

ketoconazole (Nizoral A-D)

miconazole (Lotrimin AF 2%, Micatin, Ting 2%)

nystatin (Mycostatin, Nilstat)

## Systemic Antiyeast Drugs

Severe or widespread yeast infections are treated systemically. These drugs are discussed in Chapter 20.

## Topical Combination Antifungal and Antiyeast Drugs

These combination over-the-counter and prescription drugs contain an antifungal drug (clotrimazole, ketoconazole), antiyeast drug (nystatin), corticosteroid drug (betamethasone, triamcinolone), or a drug that decreases the rate of epithelial cell growth (pyrithione zinc).

Lotrisone (clotrimazole, betamethasone)

Mycolog-II (nystatin, triamcinolone)

Xolegel Duo (ketoconazole, pyrithione zinc)

# Drugs Used to Treat Viral Infections of the Skin

Several different types of viruses cause skin infections. These viruses include herpes simplex virus type 1, which causes cold sores; herpes simplex virus type 2, which causes genital herpes (a sexually transmitted disease); herpes zoster virus, which causes chickenpox and shingles; and the human papilloma virus (HPV), which causes common warts and genital warts.

## Topical Drugs for Herpes Simplex Virus Type 1

Herpes simplex virus type 1 infections only involve the face and mouth and are known as *cold sores*. These drugs interfere with cellular DNA synthesis and keep the herpes virus from reproducing. These are prescription drugs, except for docosanol. The suffix *-vir* is common to generic antiviral drugs.

acyclovir (Zovirax)

docosanol (Abreva)

penciclovir (Denavir)

## Oral Drugs for Herpes Simplex Virus Type 2

Herpes simplex virus type 2 infections are a sexually transmitted disease that is also known as *genital herpes.* These are prescription drugs.

acyclovir (Zovirax)

famciclovir (Famvir)

valacyclovir (Valtrex) (see ■ FIGURE 17–8)

## Topical Drugs for Herpes Zoster Virus

Herpes zoster virus infections or **shingles** are due to a reemergence of the same virus that first caused chickenpox in the patient. After the initial chickenpox infection (as a child), the virus remains dormant in the body until later in life, when stress or illness triggers its emergence. The lesions of herpes zoster (shingles) are particularly painful. The following topical drugs do not treat the viral infection

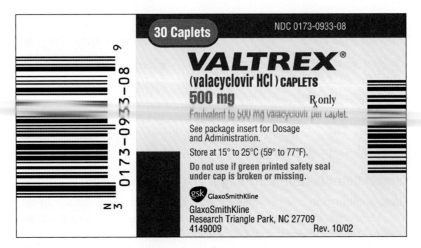

**■ FIGURE 17–8 Drug label for Valtrex.**
The antiviral drug valacyclovir (Valtrex) is used to treat herpes simplex virus type 2 infections, which are also known as *genital herpes*. The suffix *-vir* reminds that this drug is effective against viruses.

but only treat the pain associated with these lesions by exerting a local irritant effect (capsaicin) or anesthetic effect. Capsaicin is an over-the-counter drug; lidocaine is a prescription drug.

capsaicin (Capsin, Zostrix)

lidocaine (Lidoderm Patch)

## *Did You Know?*

The drug capsaicin is a derivative of the habañero chili pepper plant. Some of these chili peppers are so caustic that they will burn your hand if you are not wearing protective gloves. The amount of heat in a chili pepper is measured in Scoville units, which were devised in 1912 by the pharmacist Thomas Scoville. Bhut jolokia chili peppers from India are rated the highest of all peppers—1,041,427 Scoville units. This means that you can still feel the heat when you taste a solution that contains just 1 part Bhut jolokia chili pepper in 1,041,427 parts of a sugar water/alcohol mixture.

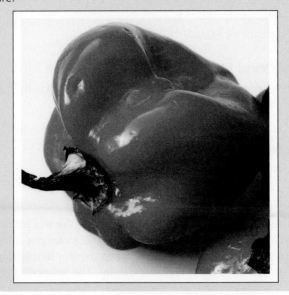

## Oral Drugs for Herpes Zoster Virus

These oral drugs are used to treat herpes zoster infections and shingles. They keep the virus from reproducing by working systemically through the blood and in the deeper tissues of the skin. These are prescription drugs.

acyclovir (Zovirax)

famciclovir (Famvir)

valacyclovir (Valtrex) (see Figure 17–8)

## Drugs to Prevent Herpes Zoster Virus

This drug is a vaccine to prevent herpes zoster infection (shingles). It is given to persons 60 years of age or older who have had chickenpox in childhood and are at risk for developing painful shingles.

Zostavax

## Topical Drugs for Warts

The human papillomavirus causes both common warts (verrucae) and genital warts (condylomata acuminata).

These over-the-counter and prescription keratolytic drugs are applied topically to treat common warts and plantar warts (verrucae). They remove layers of skin, which then removes the wart. They are also used to remove corns, calluses, and the skin plaques associated with psoriasis.

monochloroacetic acid (Mono-Chlor)

salicylic acid (Compound W, Dr. Scholl's) (see ▓ **FIGURE 17–9**)

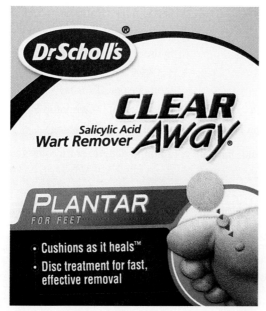

▓ **FIGURE 17–9 Topical wart remover pads.**
These topical pads adhere to the skin. They contain the over-the-counter keratolytic drug salicylic acid to strip away layers of skin, including a plantar wart on the bottom of the foot.

These prescription drugs are applied topically or injected locally to treat genital warts (condylomata acuminata), a sexually transmitted disease caused by the human papillomavirus. These are prescription drugs.

| | |
|---|---|
| fluorouracil (Efudex) | kunecatechins (Veregen) |
| imiquimod (Aldara) | podofilox (Condylox) |
| interferon alfa-2b (Intron A) | podophyllum (Podocon-25) |
| interferon alfa-n3 (Alferon N) | trichloroacetic acid (Tri-Chlor) |

## Did You Know?

Kunecatechins is extracted from green tea leaves. Podofilox is derived from juniper evergreen trees. Podophyllum contains an extract of May apple plant as its active ingredient.

This drug is a vaccine to prevent human papillomavirus (HPV) infection and genital warts. It is given to females ages 9 to 26. It also protects against some strains of HPV that cause cervical cancer.

Gardisil

## Drugs Used to Treat Inflammation and Itching

### Topical Corticosteroid Drugs

Topical corticosteroid drugs, both over-the-counter and prescription, are indicated to treat inflammation and itching caused by contact dermatitis, poison ivy, insect bites, psoriasis, seborrhea, eczema, and yeast or fungal infections. All of these are prescription drugs, except for hydrocortisone, which is available as both a prescription drug and an over-the-counter drug.

| | |
|---|---|
| alclometasone (Aclovate) | fluocinonide (Lidex) |
| amcinonide | flurandrenolide (Cordran) |
| betamethasone (Diprolene, Diprosone, Maxivate) | fluticasone (Cutivate) |
| clobetasol (Temovate) | halcinonide (Halog) |
| clocortolone (Cloderm) | halobetasol (Ultravate) |
| desonide (DesOwen) | hydrocortisone (Dermolate, Westcort) (see ■ FIGURE 17–10) |
| desoximetasone (Topicort) | mometasone (Elocon) |
| dexamethasone (Decadron, Decaspray) | prednicarbate (Dermatop E) |
| diflorasone (Maxiflor, Psorcon E) | triamcinolone (Kenalog) |

*Note:* The suffixes *-sone, -lone,* and *-nide* are common to generic corticosteroid drugs.

## Did You Know?

The topical corticosteroid drug mometasone (Elocon) used to treat skin inflammation is also used to treat asthma under the trade name Asmanex Twisthaler; it is also used intranasally as a spray to treat allergic rhinitis under the heavily advertised trade name Nasonex.

## In Depth

Corticosteroid drugs mimic the action of glucocorticoid hormones secreted by the adrenal gland. Hydrocortisone, introduced in 1952, was the first topical corticosteroid drug. In 1983, hydrocortisone was also the first topical corticosteroid drug to be approved in a nonprescription strength for over-the-counter sales.

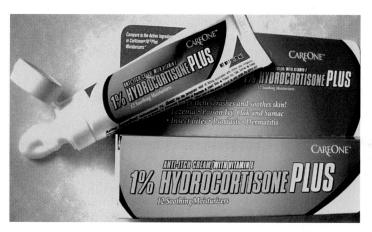

**FIGURE 17–10  Hydrocortisone.**
Over-the-counter generic hydrocortisone is available under many different drug trade names, including Cortizone-5, Dermolate, Cortaid Intensive Therapy, and Lanacort-5, among others. This drug Hydrocortisone Plus contains added vitamin E to soothe the skin.

### Intradermal Corticosteroid Drugs

These corticosteroid drugs are injected directly into individual skin lesions to decrease inflammation.

> betamethasone (Celestone Soluspan)
> methylprednisolone (Depo-Medrol)
> triamcinolone (Aristospan Intralesional)

### Systemic Corticosteroid Drugs

Severe or widespread dermatitis, inflammation, allergic skin conditions, or itching are treated with oral corticosteroid drugs that exert a systemic effect. These are discussed in detail in Chapter 14.

### Topical Antihistamine Drugs

These drugs inhibit inflammation, redness, and itching due to the release of histamine (hence the name *antihistamine),* which is released during an allergic reaction such as contact dermatitis. As a group, these drugs are also known as ***antipruritic drugs*** (*pruritus* is a Latin word that means *itching*). Diphenhydramine is an over-the-counter drug, while doxepin is a prescription drug.

> diphenhydramine (Benadryl)
> doxepin (Zonalon)

*Did You Know?*

The antihistamine drug doxepin is also a tricyclic antidepressant drug that is given orally for depression and marketed under the trade name Sinequan.

### Topical Combination Antihistamine Drugs

These combination drugs contain a topical antihistamine drug (diphenhydramine) to decrease itching, an astringent drug (calamine, zinc oxide) to decrease oozing and exudates, or a topical anesthetic drug (benzocaine) to relieve itching and numb the skin.

> Caladryl (calamine, diphenhydramine)
>
> Calamycin (benzocaine, calamine, zinc oxide)
>
> Ziradryl (diphenhydramine, zinc oxide)

### Oral Antihistamine Drugs

For severe hives, itching, or dermatitis caused by an allergy, these antihistamine drugs are given orally.

> hydroxyzine (Vistaril)
>
> levocetirizine (Xyzal)

### Other Topical Drugs for Inflammation and Itching

These drugs contain vitamins A and D to promote skin healing, oatmeal to decrease itching, or an astringent drug (calamine, zinc oxide). Burow's solution contains the astringent drug aluminum to treat oozing skin inflammations; it was created by Dr. Karl Burow, a German surgeon in the mid-1800s. These are all over-the-counter drugs.

> Burow's solution               vitamins A and D (A and D Medicated)
>
> calamine                            zinc oxide
>
> colloidal oatmeal (Aveeno)

## Drugs Used for Topical Anesthesia

Topical anesthetic drugs provide brief periods of anesthesia to a limited depth in the skin. These drugs block the movement of sodium ions across the cell membrane, part of the process of the transmission of nerve impulses. These over-the-counter and prescription drugs provide temporary symptomatic relief to treat the pain of herpes zoster lesions (shingles) and postherpetic neuralgia. They are also used to treat the pain of abrasions, minor burns, cold sores, rashes, sunburn, eczema, and insect bites.

> benzocaine (Dermoplast)          lidocaine (Lidoderm, Xylocaine, Zingo)
>
> dibucaine (Nupercainal)          pramoxine (Tronothane)

*Note:* The suffix *-caine* is common to topical generic anesthetic drugs.

### Topical Combination Anesthetic Drugs

This combination drug contains a topical anesthetic drug (lidocaine) and an anti-inflammatory drug (hydrocortisone).

> Xyralid (lidocaine, hydrocortisone)

## *Did You Know?*

Zingo is a new formulation and packaging for the anesthetic drug lidocaine. It consists of a single-dose, helium-powered system that delivers powdered lidocaine into the skin. The device is held firmly against the skin while the "start" button is pushed. The powder is propelled with a loud popping sound (a "zing"), similar to that of a balloon popping. Zingo is administered a few minutes prior to starting an intravenous line and is helpful in providing topical anesthesia for pediatric patients, especially those with chronic illness who must frequently have intravenous lines inserted. Its drug advertisement says "Ready. Set. Zingo!"

These combination drugs contain two or three topical anesthetic drugs (benzocaine, butamben, lidocaine, prilocaine, tetracaine). These drugs are used to prevent pain during procedures that involve the skin, such as a biopsy or removal of a skin lesion, or the insertion of an intravenous line. These drugs are prescription drugs. Synera comes in the form of a patch.

Cetacaine (benzocaine, butamben, tetracaine)

EMLA (lidocaine, prilocaine) (see ■ **FIGURE 17–11**)

Synera (lidocaine, tetracaine)

*Note:* Also see the previous section Drugs for Herpes Zoster for a discussion of anesthetic drugs specifically used to treat the pain of shingles.

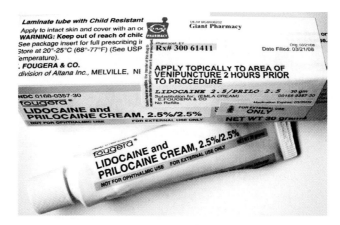

■ **FIGURE 17–11  Combination drug lidocaine with prilocaine.**
This tube contains the combination topical generic anesthetic drugs lidocaine and prilocaine in the form of a cream. This drug was prescribed for a patient who was fearful of having blood drawn. The cream was applied to the skin on the inner aspect of the elbow several hours prior to venipuncture. In the hospital, this topical combination drug is also applied to the skin before starting an intravenous line on a patient. This is the generic version of the combination trade name drug EMLA.

## Drugs Used to Treat Alopecia

Chronic hair loss or alopecia usually begins in middle age in men and women, although inherited tendencies can cause it to occur at an earlier age. In men, lowered testosterone levels and decreased blood flow to the scalp cause the hair follicles to shrink. The hair on the top of the head eventually disappears, leaving a fringe of hair at the back of the head. This is known as male pattern baldness. In women, the onset of menopause causes the level of estradiol produced by the ovaries to be lower than the level of the male hormone androgen (produced by the adrenal cortex) and this hormonal change causes the hair to thin. These drugs are used to treat mild-to-moderate alopecia. They are not effective in all cases, and they must be continued indefinitely to maintain any new hair growth.

These drugs have two different therapeutic effects and are given by two different routes of administration. Healthy hair follicles on the scalp contain a small amount of the substance DHT, while shrinking hair follicles on the balding scalp contain an increased amount of DHT. The oral drug finasteride blocks an enzyme that must be present in order to produce DHT. The topical drug minoxidil dilates the arteries in the scalp to increase blood flow and stimulate hair growth.

> finasteride (Propecia) (see ■ **FIGURE 17–12**)
>
> minoxidil (Rogaine)

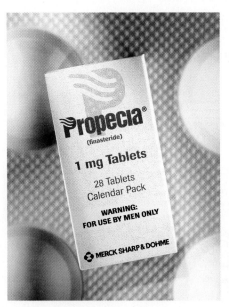

■ FIGURE 17–12  **Finasteride (Propecia).**
This drug is given orally and works systemically to treat male pattern baldness. Interestingly, finasteride, under the trade name Proscar, is given orally to treat benign prostatic hypertrophy in men. The drug blocks an enzyme that is needed to produce another substance that causes the prostate gland to enlarge.

## *Drug Alert!*

The oral drug finasteride (Propecia) is not approved for use in women because of its connection with the male hormone testosterone. Women are advised not to take finasteride. They are also warned not to handle finasteride tablets when they are pregnant because of the risk of birth defects in a male fetus. However, the topical drug minoxidil (Rogaine) is approved to treat both male and female alopecia and does not cause birth defects.

## *Historical Notes*

Minoxidil (Rogaine) was the first drug scientifically shown to stimulate hair growth. For thousands of years, men have smeared smelly stuff on their scalps in a vain attempt to treat baldness. Cleopatra reportedly put a concoction of bear grease, burned mice, deer marrow, and horse teeth on Caesar's bald head. Other baldness remedies have included pigeon droppings, horseradish, and buffalo dung.

Joe Graedon and Teresa Graedon, "People's Pharmacy," *The Baltimore Sun*, April 15, 1997, 3F.

## Drugs Used to Treat Wrinkles

Drugs used to treat wrinkles include topical vitamin A–type drugs, muscle relaxant drugs to relax the muscles that pull the skin into wrinkle lines, or filler drugs to plump up the skin to minimize wrinkle lines. Tretinoin is a topical cream vitamin A–type drug. The other drugs are injected under the skin and their effect lasts several months. Sometimes these drugs are injected together to simultaneously relax the muscle causing the wrinkle while minimizing the wrinkle line. These are prescription drugs.

botulinum toxin type A (Botox) (see ▣ FIGURE 17–13)

human collagen (CosmoDerm, CosmoPlast)

hyaluronic acid (Hylaform, Juvéderm, Restylane)

poly-L-lactic acid (Sculptra)

tretinoin (Renova)

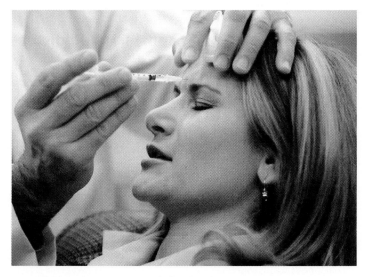

▣ **FIGURE 17–13 Botox injection.**
This woman is receiving the first of three injections to minimize wrinkles on her forehead between the eyebrows. The toxin in Botox relaxes the underlying muscle, and this allows the skin to become smooth.

## Did You Know?

The toxin in Botox that relaxes muscles in the face is the same toxin produced by *Clostridium botulinum*, the bacterium that causes food poisoning. Eating spoiled food that contains this bacterium results in muscle paralysis and eventually death from respiratory arrest. Botox was first used to treat wrinkles by Dr. Carruthers, a Canadian dermatologist. The trade name Botox is made up of the initial letters of **bo**tulinum **tox**in. Botox parties, where many patients gather to receive Botox injections and enjoy food and drinks, are quite popular.

Human collagen is a highly purified product from human sources.

Hyaluronic acid occurs naturally in the skin, but the amount decreases with age. The drug hyaluronic acid used to be manufactured from the combs of chickens, but is now manufactured from nonanimal sources. Hyaluronic acid, under the trade names Hyalgan and Synvisc, is also injected into the joint to improve the thickness and lubricating quality of the synovial fluid in patients with osteoarthritis.

Sculptra is a completely synthetic material. Its antiwrinkle effects last for up to two years.

## Drugs Used to Treat Actinic Keratoses

Actinic keratoses are raised, irregular, rough areas of skin that develop in areas of chronic sun exposure. Topical drugs that are used to treat actinic keratoses include keratolytic drugs (diclofenac), chemotherapy drugs (fluorouracil), and other drugs (aminolevulinic acid, methyl aminolevulinate) used in conjunction with red or blue light photodynamic therapy to cause a chemical reaction in the skin.

aminolevulinic acid (Levulan Kerastick)    fluorouracil (Efudex)

diclofenac (Solaraze)    methyl aminolevulinate (Metvixia)

## Drugs Used to Treat Scabies and Pediculosis

These drugs are used to treat parasites that cause infection in the skin. These parasitic infections, scabies and pediculosis, are treated with scabicide and pediculocide drugs.

### Drugs for Scabies

This skin condition is caused by tiny, barely visible parasites called *mites* that tunnel under the skin and cause itchy lesions. They lay eggs under the skin which then hatch within a week and continue the cycle. The lesions occur on the trunk, pubic area, and in skin folds. The scalp is rarely infected. Scabies can be transmitted to others through contact with furniture, clothing, bedsheets, towels, or close personal contact or sexual intercourse. These topical prescription drugs are used to treat scabies.

crotamiton (Eurax)

lindane

permethrin (Acticin, Elimite)

### Drugs for Pediculosis

This skin condition is caused by an infestation of **lice** and their eggs (nits) that can be found on the scalp, body, and pubic area. Lice feed on human blood, and their bites cause severe itching. Their eggs are attached to body hairs, particularly on the scalp and pubic area. Lice are easily transmitted from one person to another by means of hairbrushes, combs, hats, headphones, towels, clothing, upholstery, carpets, and from close personal contact or sexual intercourse. These topical prescription drugs are used to treat pediculosis.

lindane

malathion (Ovide)

permethrin (Acticin, Elimite)

### Combination Topical Drugs for Treat Pediculosis

These combination over-the-counter drugs contain two pediculocide drugs (pyrethrin, piperonyl) to kill lice.

RID (pyrethrin, piperonyl)

Tisit (pyrethrin, piperonyl)

## Did You Know?

Scabies in humans is caused by the same parasite (*Sarcoptes scabiei*) that causes mange in dogs.

In pediculosis, a single parasite or louse is shaped like a crab, and so laypersons often refer to an infestation of lice as *crabs*. A child who has had lice and has been treated must be examined by a school health aide or nurse before being readmitted to school. Many school districts have a guideline as to how many *nits* (eggs) can be found in the hair before the child must be treated again. The phrase *nit-picking,* which means *to point out tiny details,* comes from the process of picking through the hair looking for lice eggs. A special LiceMeister Comb, a fine-tooth comb, is helpful in removing nits from the hair.

The over-the-counter drug pyrethrin is derived from chrysanthemums. This drug acts on the nervous system of the parasite to paralyze it. Pyrethrin is a common ingredient in flea powder for dogs as well.

## Drug Alert!

The prescription drug lindane is used to treat both scabies and lice, but only if other drugs have been ineffective. Lindane is never the first choice for treatment. In the past, lindane was an agricultural pesticide, but its use was discontinued by the Environmental Protection Agency (EPA) in 2006 because runoff from the fields caused toxic stream pollution. However, despite reports of causing illness and even death, the Food and Drug Administration (FDA) allowed lindane to remain on the market as a drug. Lindane is not prescribed for pregnant women, children under two years of age, or the elderly because of its possible effect on the central nervous system (seizures). This drug is stored in the fat and can be present in breast milk.

## Drugs Used to Treat Burns, Skin Ulcers, and Wounds

Burns, skin ulcers, and deep wounds present unique problems in medical management. They may contain a large amount of necrotic (dead) tissue that must be removed (debrided) before new tissue can form (granulation). In addition, the affected area may produce a large amount of exudate (drainage) that can become infected and must be removed before healing can occur.

## Topical Drugs for Debridement

These topical enzymes dissolve necrotic tissue and scar tissue and allow new tissue to begin to form at the base of a burn, skin ulcer, or wound. These drugs are prescription drugs, except for dextranomer.

anasain/comosain (Vianain)          papain (Accuzyme, Panafil)

collagenase (Santyl)                    trypsin (Granulex)

dextranomer (Debrisan)

### Did You Know?

Vianain contains two enzymes, anasain and comosain, which were originally derived from pineapple. Papain is an enzyme found in papaya fruit; it is also added to meat tenderizer products. Trypsin is an enzyme found in the stomach that digests the proteins in foods.

## Topical Drugs to Absorb Exudate

These over-the-counter topical drugs absorb the tissue fluid that flows from damaged tissues and from wounds.

DuoDerm

IntraSite

Sorbsan

### Did You Know?

Dextranomer (Debrisan) contains tiny polymer beads of dextran that absorb amounts of wound drainage equal to four times their size. Sorbsan contains absorbent calcium fibers.

## Topical Drugs to Stimulate Granulation

This drug stimulates the formation of healthy, new granulation tissue, particularly in skin ulcers in diabetic patients. It is a growth factor derived from human platelets and produced with recombinant DNA technology.

becaplermin (Regranex)

### Did You Know?

Becaplermin (Regranex) was created by taking a gene that produces a certain type of growth factor in cells and, through recombinant DNA technology, inserting it into a yeast cell which was then grown in sufficient quantities to make a drug.

## Topical Anti-Infective Drugs for Burns

These anti-infective drugs are used specifically to treat extensive burns and keep them from becoming infected.

mafenide (Sulfamylon)

nitrofurazone (Furacin)

silver sulfadiazine (Silvadene)

## Did You Know?

The active ingredient in silver sulfadiazine (Silvadene) is actually the chemical element of silver in an ion form.

### Other Topical Drugs for Burns and Wounds

Chlorophyll is an over-the-counter drug that promotes healing and neutralizes the odor from wounds. Manuka honey is taken from actual honey. Metronidazole is a prescription antibacterial and antiprotozoal drug used to treat infected decubitus ulcers.

    chlorophyll derivative (Chloresium)

    manuka honey (Medihoney)

    metronidazole (MetroCream, MetroGel)

## Did You Know?

The Egyptians used honey to treat wounds 4,000 years ago. In 2007, the FDA approved the first honey-impregnated topical sterile absorbent dressing for use on burns, skin ulcers, and wounds. The dressing is made from a seaweed material that absorbs draining fluids, while the honey is manuka honey that comes from Australia and is a strong antibiotic drug that kills bacteria.

## Drugs Used to Treat Vitiligo

Vitiligo is an autoimmune disorder in which melanocytes (pigment cells) in the skin are slowly destroyed, resulting in patchy, slowly spreading areas where there is a complete loss of skin pigmentation. These drugs are used to produce repigmentation of the skin in patients with vitiligo. Dihydroxyacetone and monobenzone are applied topically. Methoxsalen is taken orally and works in conjunction with exposure to ultraviolet light.

    dihydroxyacetone (Chromelin Complexion Blender)

    methoxsalen (Oxsoralen)

    monobenzone (Benoquin)

## Drug Alert!

With their sound-alike pronunciations, be careful not to confuse the trade name drug Chromelin (Complexion Blender), a topical drug used to treat vitiligo, with the generic name drug cromolyn, an inhaled drug used to treat asthma.

# Chapter Review

## Quiz Yourself

1. Explain why some dermatologic diseases can be treated with either topical or systemic drugs.
2. How does the anti-inflammatory and antipruritic effect of a corticosteroid drug differ from that of an antihistamine drug?

3. Explain why vitamin A and vitamin D are used to treat psoriasis.
4. Coal tar preparations and psoralens are prescribed for what dermatologic disease?
5. The drug minoxidil is used to treat both baldness and hypertension. True or false?
6. What type of drug treatment is prescribed when the nails have a severe, embedded fungal infection?
7. What is the difference between acne vulgaris and acne rosacea, and how do the prescribed drug treatments differ?
8. What is the therapeutic effect of these categories of drugs: keratolytic drugs, antipruritic drugs?
9. Salicylic acid is used to treat all of these skin conditions except which one? Warts, acne vulgaris, wrinkles, corns, calluses.
10. Discuss the advantages and disadvantages of the use of triclosan in products and the routine use of antibiotic drugs for patients and in animal feed.
11. List the two uses of the topical drug tretinoin (Retin-A, Renova).
12. What serious adverse effect has been linked to the drug Accutane?
13. Why are some topical antifungal drugs also used to treat yeast infections?
14. Describe the similarities and differences between herpes simplex virus type 1 and herpes simplex virus type 2 infections and the drugs used to treat them.
15. What is a herpes zoster infection and what drugs are used to treat it?
16. Explain what the drug Zingo is and what is unique about how it is administered.
17. What is unusual about the origin of the popular drug Botox?
18. Describe the symptoms of scabies and pediculosis and how they are treated.
19. What condition is Rogaine used to treat and what is its therapeutic effect?
20. To what category of drugs does each of these drugs belong?

a. acyclovir (Zovirax)
b. betamethasone (Maxivate)
c. capsaicin (Capsin, Zostrix)
d. clotrimazole (Lotrimin)
e. collagenase (Santyl)
f. EMLA
g. finasteride (Propecia)
h. halcinonide (Halog)

i. hyaluronic acid (Restylane)
j. isotretinoin (Accutane)
k. Medihoney
l. metronidazole (MetroGel)
m. permethrin (Acticin, Elimite)
n. Sculptra
o. triamcinolone (Kenalog)

## Spelling Tips

| | |
|---|---|
| **alclometasone** | The generic name has an *l* as the second letter, but the trade name drug **Aclovate** does not. |
| **BenzaClin** | Unusual internal capitalization. |
| **benzocaine** | The generic name is spelled with an *o*, but the trade name drug **Benzamycin** is spelled with an *a*. |
| **cortisone** | The generic name is spelled with an *s*, but the trade name drug **Cortizone** is spelled with a *z*. |
| **CosmoDerm** | Unusual internal capitalization. |
| **CosmoPlast** | Unusual internal capitalization. |
| **DesOwen** | Unusual internal capitalization. |
| **DuoDerm** | Unusual internal capitalization. |
| **IntraSite** | Unusual internal capitalization. |
| **MetroGel** | Unusual internal capitalization. |
| **PanOxyl** | Unusual internal capitalization. |
| **Psorcon E** | Silent *p*. |

## Clinical Applications

1. Look at this computer-generated prescription and answer the following questions.
   a. What drug has been prescribed?
   b. To what drug category does this drug belong?
   c. How do you know that this is a topical drug?
   d. What is the strength of the drug?
   e. Translate the entire prescription into plain English.

> *ketoconazole cream 2% apply top BID × 2 weeks*
> *#60g tube #11 RFs*

2. Look at this photograph and answer the following questions.
   a. What is the generic name of this drug?
   b. What dermatologic condition is it used to treat?
   c. What trade name is associated with this generic drug name?

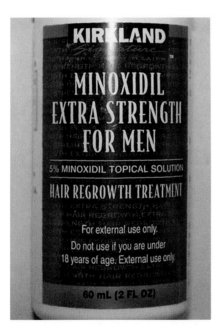

3. Look at this photograph and answer the following questions.
   a. What is the trade name of this drug?
   b. What dermatologic conditions is it used to treat?
   c. What generic name is associated with this trade name drug?

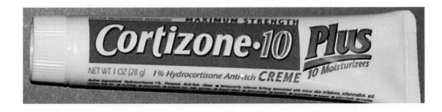

4. Look at this photograph and answer the following questions.
   a. What is the trade name of this drug?
   b. What dermatologic condition is it used to treat?
   c. What generic name is associated with this trade name drug?

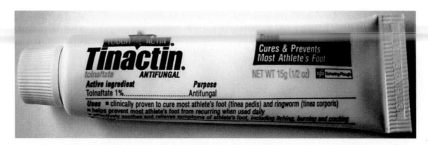

5. Look at this handwritten prescription and answer the following questions.
   a. What drug has been prescribed?
   b. To what drug category does this drug belong?
   c. How do you know that this is a topical drug?
   d. Translate the rest of the prescription into plain English.

℞

EMLA CREAM

Apply topical to area of venopuncture
2 hours prior to procedure

☐ Label     #one tube
Refill 0 - 1 - 2 - 3 - 4 - PRN

## Multimedia Extension Exercises

■ Go to www.pearsonhighered.com/turley and click on the photo of the cover of *Understanding Pharmacology for Health Professionals* to access the interactive Companion Website created for this textbook.

# Ophthalmic Drugs

## Learning Objectives

After you study this chapter, you should be able to

1. Compare and contrast the therapeutic effects of antibiotic drugs, antifungal drugs, antiviral drugs, and anti-inflammatory drugs used to treat the eye.

2. Describe three categories of drugs used to treat eye allergy symptoms and their different therapeutic effects.

3. Describe seven categories of drugs used to treat glaucoma and their different therapeutic effects.

4. Given the generic and trade names of an ophthalmic drug, identify what drug category they belong to, or what disease they are used to treat.

5. Given an ophthalmic drug category, identify several generic and trade name drugs in that category.

Ophthalmic drugs are used to treat diseases of the eye. These diseases include infection or inflammation of the eye, allergy symptoms in the eye, glaucoma, and macular degeneration. Ophthalmic drugs include these topical drugs: antibiotic drugs, corticosteroid drugs, nonsteroidal anti-inflammatory drugs, antihistamine drugs, mast cell stabilizer drugs, decongestant drugs, prostaglandin F drugs, carbonic anhydrase inhibitor drugs, beta-blocker drugs, miotic drugs, cholinesterase inhibitor drugs, monoclonal antibody drugs, topical anesthetic drugs, mydriatic drugs, and other drugs.

## Drugs Used to Treat Eye Infections

Superficial bacterial, fungal, and viral infections can occur in the eye in the areas of the eyelid, cornea, conjunctiva, or tear duct. These infections are treated topically with antibiotic drugs for bacterial infections, sulfonamide drugs for bacterial infections, antifungal drugs for fungal infections, or antiviral drugs for viral infections.

### Topical Antibiotic Drugs for Bacterial Eye Infections

Topical antibiotic drugs disrupt the cell walls of bacteria. Antibiotic drugs are not effective against viral infections. These drugs are used topically to treat bacterial infections of the eyes (see ■ **FIGURE 18–1**).

| | |
|---|---|
| azithromycin (AzaSite) | gentamicin (Garamycin, Gentacidin, Gentak) |
| bacitracin (AK-Tracin) | levofloxacin (Quixin) |
| chloramphenicol (Chloromycetin) | moxifloxacin (Vigamox) |
| ciprofloxacin (Ciloxan) | ofloxacin (Ocuflox) |
| erythromycin (Ilotycin) | polymyxin B |
| gatafloxacin (Zymar) | tobramycin (AK-TOB, Defy, Tobrex) (see ■ FIGURE 18–2) |

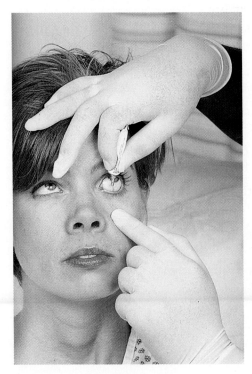

■ **FIGURE 18–1  Ophthalmic ointment.**
The nurse is administering a topical ophthalmic antibiotic ointment to the patient's eye, by pulling down the lower eyelid so that a ribbon of ointment can be laid in the sac between the eye and the lower eyelid. As the patient blinks, the ointment is distributed across the eye. Topical ophthalmic ointment is specially formulated to be nonirritating to the eye; it is not interchangeable with topical ointments used on the skin.

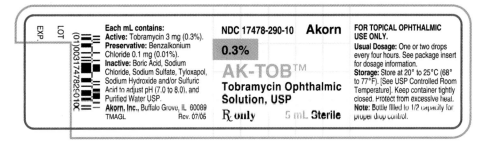

**■ FIGURE 18–2  Drug label for tobramycin (AK-TOB).**
The trade name AK-TOB refers to the drug company Akorn and tobramycin, the generic name of
this drug. The phrase *ophthalmic solution* indicates that this liquid antibiotic drug can only be used
in the eyes.

## Oral Antibiotic Drugs for Severe Bacterial Eye Infections

For severe eye infections, various systemic antibiotic drugs are prescribed. For a discussion of these
drugs, see Chapter 20.

## *Clinical Applications*

If the physician's order is for ophthalmic ointment in the patient's right eye, before you administer
the drug, you have to consciously remember this: as you face the patient, your right-hand side
does not correspond to the patient's right-hand side; it corresponds to the patient's left-hand side.

## Drug Alert!

All topical drugs used in the eye are specially formulated to be physiologically similar to eye
fluids and tears, so as not to damage the delicate tissues of the eye.

Some topical antibiotic drugs for the eye are also available as oral antibiotic drugs.
However, antibiotic drugs can have the same generic drug name, but the names for the
topical eye trade name drug and oral trade name drug are different.

| Generic Antibiotic Drug | Topical Eye Trade Name | Oral Trade Name |
| --- | --- | --- |
| azithromycin | AzaSite | Zithromax |
| ciprofloxacin | Ciloxan | Cipro |
| erythromycin | Ilotycin | Ery-Tab |
| levofloxacin | Quixin | Levaquin |
| moxifloxacin | Vigamox | Avelox |
| ofloxacin | Ocuflox | Floxin |

## Topical Sulfonamide Drugs for Bacterial Eye Infections

This topical anti-infective drug is not categorized as an antibiotic drug, but as an anti-infective drug.
Unlike antibiotic drugs that kill bacteria, this drug only inhibits the growth of bacteria, but it is useful
in treating bacterial infections of the eyelids and eye.

sulfacetamide (Bleph-10, Cetamide, Sulster)

## Focus on Healthcare Issues

Most states either recommend or require a topical anti-infective drug be applied to the eyes of newborn infants to prevent the possibility of infection and possible blindness from gonorrhea (a sexually transmitted disease contracted by the baby as its head moves through the infected birth canal). Anti-Infective drugs used for this purpose include erythromycin (Ilotycin) and silver nitrate. Although silver nitrate has been commonly used for years and is the least expensive of the two drugs, it has several drawbacks. Silver nitrate produces conjunctival irritation/swelling, which may interfere with mother–child bonding, and it is ineffective in preventing eye infections due to *Chlamydia* (another sexually transmitted disease). Erythromycin does not produce irritation and is effective against *Chlamydia*.

### Topical Antifungal Drugs for Fungal Eye Infections

This topical antifungal drug is used to treat fungal infections of the eyelids and eye.

natamycin (Natacyn)

### Topical Antiviral Drugs for Viral Eye Infections

Antiviral drugs are only effective against viruses. They act by inhibiting viral DNA from reproducing. This topical antiviral drug for the eye is specifically effective against herpes simplex virus, type 1 and type 2.

trifluridine (Viroptic)

### Oral Antiviral Drugs for Viral Eye Infections

For antiviral drugs that act systemically against viral infections in the eye, see Chapter 20.

### Other Antiviral Drugs for Viral Eye Infections

These antiviral drugs are effective against cytomegalovirus (CMV) infection of the retina, an infection most often seen in patients with AIDS. This drug is administered as an implant that is placed within the eye in the vitreous humor so that the drug will come in contact with the retina.

ganciclovir (Vitrasert)

## Drugs Used to Treat Eye Inflammation

Inflammation in the eye can be due to injury, trauma, contact with chemicals, allergies, or infection. Topical corticosteroid drugs and nonsteroidal anti-inflammatory drugs are used to treat inflammation in the eye in the areas of the eyelid, cornea, conjunctiva, or tear duct.

### Topical Corticosteroid Drugs for Eye Inflammation

Topical corticosteroid drugs are used topically in the eye to treat inflammation. They suppress the immune system's local inflammatory response.

| | |
|---|---|
| dexamethasone (Maxidex) | loteprednol (Alrex, Lotemax) |
| difluprednate (Durezol) | prednisolone (Econopred Plus, Pred Forte) |
| fluorometholone (Flarex, FML) | rimexolone (Vexol) |

## Other Corticosteroid Drugs for Eye Inflammation

These anti-inflammatory drugs are administered within the eye into the vitreous humor to treat uveitis. Fluocinolone is an implant, while triamcinolone is injected as a solution.

fluocinolone (Retisert)

triamcinolone (Trivaris)

## Topical Nonsteroidal Anti-Inflammatory Drugs for Eye Inflammation

Topical nonsteroidal anti-inflammatory drugs (NSAIDs) are used topically in the eye to treat pain and inflammation. Some of these drugs are used to decrease pain and inflammation after cataract or LASIK surgery on the eye.

| | |
|---|---|
| bromfenac (Xibrom) | ketorolac (Acular) |
| diclofenac (Voltaren) | nepafenac (Nevanac) |

## Oral Anti-Inflammatory Drugs for Eye Inflammation

Anti-inflammatory drugs that act systemically against pain and inflammation in the eye are discussed in Chapter 22.

# Drugs Used to Treat Eye Allergy Symptoms

Allergy symptoms in the eyes occur for the same reason as allergy symptoms in other parts of the body. When a foreign substance, such as pollen, animal dander, or other antigen, enters the body, antibodies from the immune system attach to the antigen and form an antigen-antibody complex that the body can destroy. In the process, histamine is released. Histamine causes vasodilation, and the blood vessels and tissues become swollen, inflamed, and red. Histamine also irritates tissues directly, causing pain and itching. Allergy symptoms in the eyes are treated with topical antihistamine drugs, mast cell stabilizer drugs, and decongestant drugs.

## Topical Antihistamine Drugs for Eye Allergies

These topical antihistamine drugs block the effect of histamine and relieve allergy symptoms in the eyes.

emedastine (Emadine)

olopatadine (Patanol)

## Topical Mast Cell Stabilizer Drugs for Eye Allergies

These topical drugs act as antihistamine drugs, but are also mast cell stabilizer drugs that prevent the cell membranes of mast cells in the eyes from releasing histamine.

| | |
|---|---|
| azelastine (Optivar) | lodoxamide (Alomide) |
| cromolyn (Crolom, Opticrom) | nedocromil (Alocril) |
| epinastine (Elestat) | pemirolast (Alamast) |
| ketotifen (Zaditor) | |

## Topical Decongestant Drugs for Eye Allergies

Topical decongestant drugs constrict the blood vessels in the conjunctiva to reduce redness. These are over-the-counter and prescription drugs.

| | |
|---|---|
| naphazoline (Albalon) | phenylephrine (Mydfrin) |
| oxymetazoline (Visine LR) | tetrahydrozoline (Murine Tears Plus, Visine) |

# Drugs Used to Treat Glaucoma

Glaucoma is a disease whose presenting symptom is increased intraocular pressure. If untreated, it can lead to blindness. Drugs for glaucoma act either by decreasing the amount of aqueous humor circulating in the anterior and posterior chambers (to decrease the intraocular pressure) and/or by constricting the pupil (miosis) to open the angle of contact between the iris and the trabecular meshwork (to allow the aqueous humor to flow freely). Drugs used to treat glaucoma include prostaglandin F agonist drugs, carbonic anhydrase inhibitor drugs, beta-blocker drugs, alpha receptor stimulator drugs, sympathomimetic drugs, miotic drugs, and cholinesterase inhibitor drugs.

## Prostaglandin F Agonist Drugs for Glaucoma

These drugs stimulate prostaglandin F receptors in the eye, which increases the outflow of aqueous humor and decreases the intraocular pressure.

> bimatoprost (Lumigan)
>
> latanoprost (Xalatan)
>
> travoprost (Travatan)

*Note:*  The suffix *-oprost* is common to generic prostaglandin F agonist drugs.

## Carbonic Anhydrase Inhibitor Drugs for Glaucoma

These drugs block the enzyme carbonic anhydrase, which is active in the production of aqueous humor. Acetazolamide and methazolamide are given orally, while the others are topical drugs applied to the eye.

> acetazolamide (Diamox Sequels)          dorzolamide (Trusopt) (see ■ FIGURE 18–3)
>
> brinzolamide (Azopt)                     methazolamide

*Note:*  The suffix *-zolamide* is common to generic carbonic anhydrase inhibitor drugs.

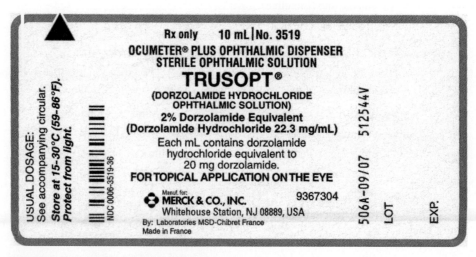

■FIGURE 18–3  Drug label for Trusopt.
Dorzolamide (Trusopt) is a carbonic anhydrase inhibitor drug that treats glaucoma by blocking an enzyme that is needed to make aqueous humor.

## Beta-Blocker Drugs for Glaucoma

These drugs block beta receptors in the eye. This decreases the production of aqueous humor to decrease the intraocular pressure. These drugs have no effect on pupil size and therefore do not cause the blurred vision or night blindness associated with some other glaucoma drugs.

betaxolol (Betoptic) (see ■ FIGURE 18–4)     levobunolol (Betagan Liquifilm)

carteolol (Ocupress)     metipranolol (OptiPranolol)

levobetaxolol (Betaxon)     timolol (Istalol, Timoptic)

*Note:* The suffix *olol* is common to generic beta-blocker drugs.

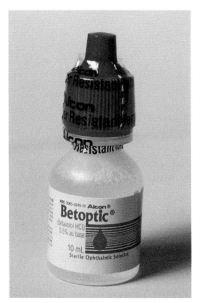

■ FIGURE 18–4 **Drug bottle of betaxolol (Betoptic).** Betoptic is a beta-blocker drug that decreases the production of aqueous humor by blocking beta receptors in the eye. When these receptors are blocked, they cannot be stimulated to make aqueous humor.

## Alpha Receptor Stimulator Drugs for Glaucoma

These drugs stimulate alpha receptors in the eye. This decreases the production of aqueous humor and also increases the outflow of aqueous humor.

apraclonidine (Iopidine)

brimonidine (Alphagan P)

## Sympathomimetic Drugs for Glaucoma

This drug is converted to epinephrine by an enzyme in the eye. Epinephrine is a hormone that acts as part of the sympathetic division of the nervous system. This drug mimics the action of epinephrine by decreasing the production and increasing the outflow of aqueous humor to decrease the intraocular pressure.

dipivefrin (Propine)

## Miotic Drugs for Glaucoma

Miotic drugs have the same effect as acetylcholine, a neurotransmitter for the parasympathetic nervous system. These drugs cause the pupil to constrict, and this increases the outflow of aqueous humor and lowers the intraocular pressure. These were the first drugs to be developed to treat glaucoma.

carbachol (Carboptic, Miostat)

pilocarpine (Pilocar)

### Cholinesterase Inhibitor Drugs for Glaucoma

This drug inhibits cholinesterase, an enzyme that normally destroys acetylcholine. As acetylcholine remains active, it continues to cause the pupil to constrict, and this increases the outflow of aqueous humor and lowers the intraocular pressure.

echothiophate iodide (Phospholine Iodide)

### Combination Drugs for Glaucoma

These combination drugs contain a miotic drug (pilocarpine), epinephrine, a carbonic anhydrase inhibitor drug (dorzolamide), an alpha receptor stimulator drug (brimonidine), and/or a beta-blocker drug (timolol).

Combigan (brimonidine, timolol)

Cosopt (dorzolamide, timolol)

$P_1E_1$, $P_2E_1$ (pilocarpine, epinephrine)

## Drugs Used to Treat Macular Degeneration

Macular degeneration is a chronic, progressive loss of central vision in the area of the macula of the retina. The macula contains the area of the fovea, which is directly opposite from the pupil, and is the area of greatest visual acuity. In age-related macular degeneration, the macula deteriorates with age. This is also called *dry macular degeneration*. In wet macular degeneration, abnormal blood vessels grow under the macula. They are fragile and leak, causing the macula to lift away from the retina with a loss of vision. Pegaptanib (Macugen) blocks vascular endothelial growth factor that causes the new blood vessels to grow. It is injected into the vitreous humor of the eye. Bevacizumab and ranibizumab are monoclonal antibody drugs that also block vascular endothelial growth factor and are administered in the same way. Verteporfin is a phototherapy drug that is given intravenously and then the eye is exposed to a red laser light to activate the drug within the retina.

bevacizumab (Avastin)      ranibizumab (Lucentis)

pegaptanib (Macugen)      verteporfin (Visudyne)

### *Did You Know?*

The monoclonal antibody drugs bevacizumab and ranibizumab are used to treat macular degeneration. Their generic drug names end with the suffix–*mab*, which is an abbreviation for *monoclonal antibody*. Ranibizumab is produced by recombinant DNA technology. It is manufactured by Genentech, which is one of the foremost drug companies producing drugs by recombinant DNA technology. The company's street address is 1 DNA Way.

## Anesthetic Ophthalmic Drugs

Topical anesthetic drugs are used in the eye to facilitate eye examinations and for short surgical procedures, such as foreign body removal or suture removal.

proparacaine (Alcaine, Ophthetic)

tetracaine

# Mydriatic Drugs

These topical drugs are used to dilate the pupil (mydriasis) and paralyze the muscles of accommodation (cycloplegia) in the iris. They block the action of acetylcholine, which normally constricts the pupil. Mydriatic drugs are used to dilate and fix the pupil prior to an eye examination or surgery or to treat inflammatory conditions of the iris and uveal tract of the eye.

| | |
|---|---|
| atropine (Isopto Atropine) | phenylephrine (Mydfrin) |
| cyclopentolate (Cyclogyl, Pentolair) | scopolamine (Isopto Hyoscine) |
| homatropine (Isopto Homatropine) | tropicamide (Mydriacyl) |

## Combination Mydriatic Drugs

These combination drugs contain two mydriatic drugs (cyclopentolate, hydroxyamphetamine, phenylephrine, scopolamine, tropicamide).

Cyclomydril (cyclopentolate, phenylephrine)

Murocoll-2 (scopolamine, phenylephrine)

Paremyd (hydroxyamphetamine, tropicamide)

## *Historical Notes*

The belladonna plant was the original source of the mydriatic drugs atropine and scopolamine. The word *belladonna* means *beautiful lady* in Italian. "Sixteenth century Italian women . . . squeezed the berries of these plants into their eyes to widen and brighten them."

Michael C. Gerald, *Pharmacology: An Introduction to Drugs,* 2d ed., Englewood Cliffs, NJ: Prentice Hall, 1981, p. 149, out of print.

# Combination Ophthalmic Drugs

Combination topical ophthalmic drugs contain one or more antibiotic drugs or an antibiotic drug or sulfonamide drug with a corticosteroid drug. These are all prescription drugs.

These combination topical ophthalmic drugs contain two or three antibiotic drugs (bacitracin, neomycin, polymyxin B).

AK-Poly-Bac Ophthalmic (bacitracin, polymyxin B)

Neosporin Ophthalmic (bacitracin, neomycin, polymyxin B)

Polysporin Ophthalmic (bacitracin, polymyxin B)

These combination topical ophthalmic drugs contain an antibiotic drug (chloramphenicol, gentamicin, neomycin, polymyxin B, tobramycin) and a corticosteroid drug (dexamethasone, ioteprednol, prednisolone).

| | |
|---|---|
| Maxitrol Ophthalmic (dexamethasone, neomycin) | Pred G Ophthalmic (gentamicin, prednisolone) |
| NeoDecadron Ophthalmic (dexamethasone, neomycin) | TobraDex Ophthalmic (dexamethasone, tobramycin) |
| Ophthocort (chloramphenicol, polymyxin B) | Zylet (ioteprednol, tobramycin) |

These combination topical ophthalmic drugs contain a sulfonamide anti-infective drug (sulfacetamide) and a corticosteroid drug (prednisolone).

Blephamide (sulfacetamide, prednisolone)

Metimyd (sulfacetamide, prednisolone)

Vasocidin (sulfacetamide, prednisolone)

These combination topical ophthalmic drugs contain an ophthalmic dye (fluorescein) and an anesthetic drug (benoxinate, proparacaine).

Fluoracaine (fluorescein, proparacaine)

Flurate (fluorescein, benoxinate)

## Drugs Used to Treat Strabismus

Strabismus is a deviation of one or both eyes to the center (cross-eye) or to the side (wall-eye) because of an abnormal shortening of some of the extraocular muscles. This drug is injected to paralyze the muscle fibers and allow them to lengthen. It is also used to treat the related eye muscle disorders of blepharospasm and nystagmus.

botulinum toxin type A (Botox, Dysport)

### Did You Know?

Botulinum toxin type A (Botox) is actually a diluted neurotoxin from the bacterium *Clostridium botulinum* type A that causes food poisoning (botulism) and is present in canned goods that have bulging ends. It is also a popular drug that is injected into the muscles of the face to release deep wrinkles.

## Chapter Review

### Quiz Yourself

1. Why must topical ophthalmic drug forms be different from topical drug forms used on the skin?
2. Discuss the use of silver nitrate versus erythromycin to prevent newborns from developing eye infections due to gonorrhea.
3. Describe how histamine is produced and how it causes redness and inflammation in the eyes.
4. Name three categories of drugs that are used topically to treat allergy symptoms in the eyes.
5. Name seven different categories of drugs used to treat glaucoma and describe the therapeutic effect of each category.
6. What advantage do beta-blocker drugs have over other miotic drugs used to treat glaucoma?
7. What category of ophthalmic drugs is used to dilate the pupil and prepare for an examination of the internal eye?
8. Describe how the therapeutic effect of ophthalmic antihistamine drugs differs from that of ophthalmic mast cell stabilizer drugs.
9. How is the drug botulinum toxin type A used to treat blepharospasm, nystagmus, and strabismus?

**10.** To what category of drugs does each of the following drugs belong and what condition is it used to treat?

a. azithromycin (AzaSite)

b. bevacizumab (Avastin)

c. bimatoprost (Lumigan)

d. brinzolamide (Azopt)

e. dexamethasone (Maxidex)

f. diclofenac (Voltaren)

g. ganciclovir (Vitrasert)

h. ketotifen (Zaditor)

i. levobunolol (Betagan Liquifilm)

j. tetrahydrozoline (Murine Tears Plus, Visine)

k. tobramycin (Defy, Tobrex)

l. triamcinolone (Trivaris)

m. tropicamide (Mydriacyl)

## Spelling Tips

**AzaSite**       Unusual internal capitalization.

gent**a**micin    Generic drug is spelled "mi," but trade name is spelled "my" (Gara**my**cin).

**ophthalmic**    This is correctly pronounced "of-thal-mik." However, because of the pronunciation of optic and optician, which also have to do with the eyes, ophthalmic is commonly mispronounced as "op-thal-mik." This common mispronunciation makes the first *h* silent, and so the word is frequently misspelled with the first *h* omitted.

**OptiPranolol**  Unusual internal capitalization.

## Clinical Applications

**1.** Look at this handwritten prescription and answer the following questions.

a. What drug has been prescribed?

b. To what drug category does this drug belong?

c. What is the therapeutic effect of this drug?

d. What is the strength of this drug?

e. In what drug form does it come?

f. Translate the rest of the prescription into plain English.

---

PAT SMITH, M.D.
27 Oak Leaf Lane
Baltimore, MD  12121
Phone:  322 –7890

Name _____

Address _____

Age _____

$R_X$   *Timoptic 0.25%*
       *Ophthalmic drops*
       *#1*
       *S. gtts ī o.u. BID*

[  ] Contents are labeled
     unless checked

May be refilled 0   1   2   3   4

Signed _____ M.D.

Date _____ 20 ___ DEA No. _____

2. Look at the photograph of this eye drops drug. This drug is listed in Appendix D. Look up "Opcon-A" in Appendix D and answer the following questions.
   a. Is it an over-the-counter or a prescription drug?
   b. What two generic drugs are in this combination drug?
   c. To what category does each of these drugs belong?
   d. What condition is this drug used to treat?

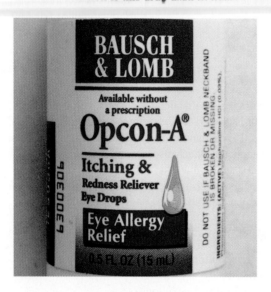

3. Look at the photograph of this eye drops drug and answer the following questions.
   a. What is the name of this drug?
   b. To what category of drugs does it belong?
   c. What condition is this drug used to treat?
   d. In what drug form does this drug come?

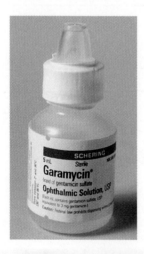

## Multimedia Extension Exercises

■ Go to www.pearsonhighered.com/turley and click on the photo of the cover of *Understanding Pharmacology for Health Professionals* to access the interactive Companion Website created for this textbook.

# Ears, Nose, and Throat Drugs

## Learning Objectives

After you study this chapter, you should be able to

1. Describe the therapeutic effect of decongestant drugs.

2. Describe the role that histamine plays in allergies.

3. Compare and contrast the therapeutic effects of antihistamine drugs and mast cell stabilizer drugs.

4. Describe the therapeutic effect of corticosteroid drugs.

5. Compare and contrast the therapeutic effects of antitussive drugs and expectorant drugs (as discussed in Chapter 10).

6. Compare and contrast the therapeutic effects of antibiotic drugs and antiyeast drugs.

7. Given the generic and trade names of an ENT drug, identify what drug category they belong to or what disease they are used to treat.

8. Given an ENT drug category, identify several generic and trade name drugs in that category.

E ars, nose, and throat (ENT) drugs are used to treat diseases of the ears, nose, or throat. These diseases include swimmer's ear, otitis media, allergic rhinitis, sinus congestion, colds, inflammation, yeast infections in mouth, and coughing. ENT drugs include decongestant drugs, antihistamine drugs, mast cell stabilizer drugs, corticosteroid drugs, antibiotic drugs, antiyeast drugs, and antitussive drugs.

## Decongestant Drugs

Decongestant drugs act as vasoconstrictors to reduce blood flow to edematous mucous membranes in the nose, sinuses, and pharynx. These drugs produce vasoconstriction by stimulating alpha receptors in the smooth muscle around the blood vessels. Decongestant drugs decrease the swelling of mucous membranes, alleviate nasal stuffiness and sinus congestion, allow secretions to drain, and help open up the eustachian tubes to the ears. Decongestant drugs are commonly prescribed for colds and allergies. They can be administered topically as nose drops or nasal sprays, or they can be taken orally. They are over-the-counter drugs as well as prescription decongestant drugs.

naphazoline (Privine)

oxymetazoline (Afrin 12-Hour, Duration)
(see ■ FIGURE 19–1)

phenylephrine (Afrin, Sudafed PE)

pseudoephedrine (Dimetapp, Drixoral, Sudafed, Triaminic)

tetrahydrozoline (Tyzine)

xylometazoline (Otrivin)

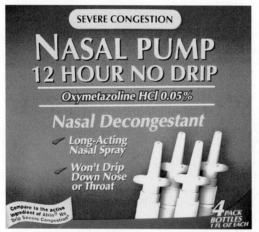

■ FIGURE 19–1 **Oxymetazoline.**
This over-the-counter generic decongestant drug oxymetazoline is also available under the trade names Afrin 12-Hour and Duration. The banner at the bottom left on this box points this out to consumers, advising them to "Compare to the active ingredient of Afrin . . ." Both generic and trade name drugs have the same active ingredient (oxymetazoline), but the generic drug costs less.

## Historical Notes

The drug phenylpropanolamine was included in many popular combination decongestant drugs in the past. Those combination decongestant drugs were withdrawn from the market by the FDA in 2000 when phenylpropanolamine was linked to deaths due to strokes. This change required the reformulation of many combination decongestant drugs. Phenylpropanolamine was also found in many over-the-counter weight loss aids, which were also withdrawn.

## Antihistamine Drugs

Antihistamine drugs exert their therapeutic effect by blocking histamine ($H_1$) receptors in the nose and throat. Histamine is released from mast cells in the tissues when an antibody-antigen complex is created during an allergic reaction. Histamine causes vasodilation, and the blood vessels and mucous membranes become swollen and red. Histamine also irritates these tissues directly, causing pain and itching. Antihistamine drugs block the action of histamine at $H_1$ receptors to dry up secretions, shrink edematous mucous membranes, and decrease itching and redness. A significant side effect of older antihistamine drugs was drowsiness; however, newer antihistamine drugs have a different chemical structure, and they do not produce drowsiness. These are over-the-counter and prescription antihistamine drugs.

azelastine (Astelin) (see ■ **FIGURE 19–2**)

brompheniramine (Lodrane)

carbinoxamine (Histex, Pediatex)

cetirizine (Zyrtec)

chlorpheniramine (Chlor-Trimeton, Efidac)

clemastine (Tavist Allergy)

cyproheptadine

desloratadine (Clarinex)

dexchlorpheniramine

diphenhydramine (Benadryl)

fexofenadine (Allegra)

levocetirizine (Xyzal)

loratadine (Claritin, Tavist) (see ■ **FIGURE 19–3**)

olopatidine (Patanase)

phenindamine (Nolahist)

promethazine (Phenergan)

triprolidine (Zymine)

### In Depth

First-generation antihistamine drugs, such as diphenhydramine (Benadryl), are nonselective in that they bind to both central histamine ($H_1$) receptors in the brain as well as peripheral $H_1$ receptors in body tissues. This drug action in the brain results in drowsiness and impaired performance while driving or operating machinery. Second-generation antihistamine drugs, such as cetirizine (Zyrtec) and loratadine (Claritin), only bind to peripheral $H_1$ receptors in the body tissues; this blocks the action of histamine and relieves the symptoms of redness, inflammation, and itching associated with allergies—without producing drowsiness.

Hydroxyzine (Vistaril) is also a first-generation antihistamine drug. However, it is not used to treat allergies. Instead, its typical side effects of drowsiness and dry mouth are used as therapeutic effects when Vistaril is given as a preoperative drug to calm the patient and decrease oral secretions during endotracheal intubation prior to surgery.

### Did You Know?

Antihistamine drugs are not effective in treating bacteria or viruses that cause the common cold. Although symptoms of allergies and colds are similar, no release of histamine occurs during the common cold. Nevertheless, drug companies combine antihistamine drugs and decongestant drugs in over-the-counter cold remedies because antihistamine drugs have a drying effect on the mucous membranes that is helpful during a cold.

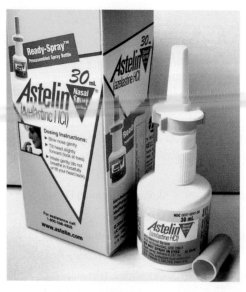

■ **FIGURE 19–2  Azelastine (Astelin).**
This prescription antihistamine drug is administered as a nasal spray. It is used to treat allergic rhinitis, which is characterized by an itchy, runny, stuffy nose.

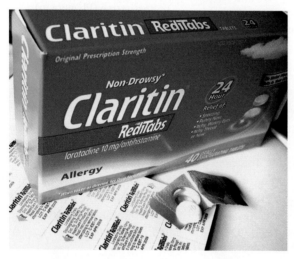

■ **FIGURE 19–3  Loratadine (Claritin).**
This over-the-counter antihistamine drug is used to treat allergy symptoms in the eyes and nose. It is one of the newer antihistamine drugs and does not cause drowsiness. It is advertised in television commercials as helping patients be "Claritin clear," that is, free of the fogginess or drowsiness associated with older antihistamine drugs. The box also reflects this advertising concept by showing a clear sky with just a single cloud. A RediTab is a thin, flat tablet that dissolves quickly in the mouth.

## Drug Alert!

Do not confuse the sound-alike generic name antihistamine drugs desloratadine and loratadine.

You cannot always associate a particular generic drug with a particular trade name. Tavist Allergy contains the generic antihistamine drug clemastine, while Tavist ND (nondrowsy) contains the generic antihistamine drug loratadine. Tavist Allergy/Sinus Headache is a combination drug that contains the antihistamine clemastine plus a decongestant drug and an analgesic drug. Tavist Sinus Maximum Strength is a combination drug that contains a decongestant drug, an analgesic drug, but no antihistamine drug.

## Historical Notes

Terfenadine (Seldane) was introduced in 1985 as the first nonsedating antihistamine drug. This was considered a major breakthrough, as the older antihistamine drugs had the undesirable side effect of causing moderate-to-severe sleepiness. Another nonsedating antihistamine drug astemizole (Hismanal) was also introduced at that time. However, both drugs were taken off the market in 1997 after they were found to cause fatal heart arrhythmias in patients who were also taking erythromycin (an antibiotic drug) or ketoconazole (an antifungal drug), or had liver disease. According to the January/February 2002 issue of the Food and Drug Administration's *FDA Consumer* magazine, the FDA knew of these deaths, but allowed the drugs to continue to be sold until fexofenadine (Allegra), another nonsedating antihistamine drug, became available in 1997. Allegra's chemical structure is just a slightly modified version of the chemical structure of Seldane.

## Mast Cell Stabilizer Drugs

Mast cell stabilizer drugs stabilize the cell membranes of mast cells in the tissues of the nose and prevent them from releasing histamine during the immune system's response to an antigen. This prevents edema of the nasal mucous membranes and sneezing in patients with allergic rhinitis. This is a prescription drug.

> cromolyn (Nasalcrom)

## Corticosteroid Drugs

Corticosteroid drugs act by inhibiting the body's immune response. They decrease inflammation and edema of the mucous membranes. Corticosteroid drugs have no decongestant or antihistamine effect. Corticosteroid drugs are not used to treat the common cold. They are prescription drugs.

### Corticosteroid Drugs for the Nose

These corticosteroid drugs are administered intranasally to treat allergic and nonallergic rhinitis.

> beclomethasone (Beconase)  fluticasone (Flonase, Veramyst)
> budesonide (Rhinocort) (see ■ **FIGURE 19–4**)  mometasone (Nasonex) (see ■ **FIGURE 19–5**)
> ciclesonide (Omnaris)  triamcinolone (Nasacort)
> flunisolide (Nasalide)

## Drug Alert!

These trade name drugs all sound similar to each other, but are not related.

| | |
|---|---|
| Nasacort | (corticosteroid generic drug triamcinolone) |
| Nasalcrom | (mast cell stabilizer generic drug cromolyn) |
| Nasalide | (corticosteroid generic drug flunisolide) |
| Nasonex | (corticosteroid generic drug mometasone) |

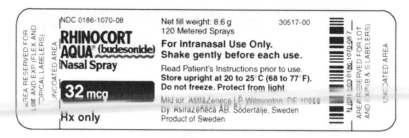

**■ FIGURE 19–4  Drug label for budesonide (Rhinocort).**
Budesonide is a prescription corticosteroid drug that is sprayed into the nose to treat allergy symptoms. The trade name Rhinocort is derived from *rhin/o-* and *-cort. Rhin/o-* is a combining form that means *nose.* Memory tip: It is a rhinoceros that has the large horn on its nose. The suffix *-cort* is an abbreviation for *corticosteroid.*

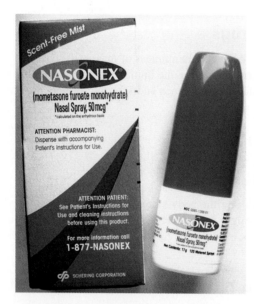

**■ FIGURE 19–5  Mometasone (Nasonex).**
Mometasone (Nasonex) is a corticosteroid drug that is given intranasally to treat allergy symptoms in the nose. All corticosteroid drugs suppress the immune system as they decrease inflammation. However, the nose is an important site where air coming into the lungs is filtered and white blood cells from the immune system normally attack and kill bacteria and viruses. Therefore, a common side effect of intranasal corticosteroid drugs is the development of nasal infections or colds from the suppression of the immune system's activity in the nose.

## Corticosteroid Drugs for the Mouth

This corticosteroid drug is applied topically as a paste to treat mouth ulcers and inflammation.

triamcinolone (Kenalog in Orabase)

## Corticosteroid Drugs for the Ears

This corticosteroid drug is applied topically as a solution in the external ear canal to decrease inflammation associated with allergies or infection.

dexamethasone

# Antibiotic Drugs

Antibiotic drugs are prescribed for colds caused by bacterial infections, particularly streptococci that cause strep throat. Antibiotic drugs are not effective in treating the common cold because it is usually caused by a virus. However, antibiotic drugs may be prescribed preventatively for some patients with viral colds to prevent a subsequent superimposed bacterial infection from developing, although this practice is not recommended as it contributes to the overuse of antibiotic drugs. Antibiotic drugs for colds caused by bacteria are given orally. These drugs are discussed in Chapter 20.

This antibiotic drug is applied topically as a solution in the external ear canal to treat bacterial infections such as swimmer's ear and external otitis, as well as infection of the tympanic membrane (otitis media).

ofloxacin (Floxin Otic)

*Note: Otic* is an adjective that means *pertaining to the ear.*

## Did You Know?

Most people contract two or more colds per year. There are over 120 different viruses, and most colds are caused by viruses. The common cold is considered the single most expensive illness in the United States in terms of time lost from work and school. No drug is currently available to treat viral common colds; available drugs merely provide temporary relief of various symptoms until the cold has run its course.

Sulfonamide drugs are a type of anti-infective drug that inhibits the growth of bacteria. These drugs are given orally to treat an infected tympanic membrane (otitis media) in the ear.

sulfadiazine

sulfisoxazole (Gantrisin Pediatric)

## Antiyeast Drugs

Yeasts, which are one-celled organisms that are closely related to fungi, grow easily in the warm, moist, dark environment of the mouth. This is especially true in patients whose immune systems are compromised by disease. *Candida albicans* yeast infections of the mouth are also known as *oral candidiasis (thrush)* or *monilia*.

These topical antiyeast drugs are used to treat a yeast infection in the mouth (oral candidiasis).

clotrimazole (Mycelex)

nystatin (Mycostatin, Nilstat) (see ■ **FIGURE 19–6**)

Oral antiyeast drugs that act systemically to treat severe yeast infections are discussed in Chapter 20.

## Drug Alert!

Topical antiyeast drugs used to treat oral candidiasis (thrush) are administered in several unique ways. (1) An infant with oral candidiasis is given an oral suspension of the drug. The entire dose is placed in an unattached nipple, and the infant sucks on the nipple until the dose is gone. The drug is not mixed with milk or formula in a bottle because the infant might not drink the entire bottle and would not get the full dose of the drug. Also, the drug should not be diluted with milk or formula because it needs to adhere to the mucous membranes of the oral cavity in order to be effective. (2) An adult with oral candidiasis is told to "swish and swallow" the oral suspension. The swishing action helps to coat all areas of the oral cavity, and swallowing ensures that the drug coats the pharynx and esophagus, which can also be infected. (3) Alternatively, an adult can suck on a troche that contains the antiyeast drug. A troche is an oblong tablet that dissolves in the mouth like a lozenge. *Pastille* is another name for a troche. *Pastille* is a French word that means *little lump of bread.*

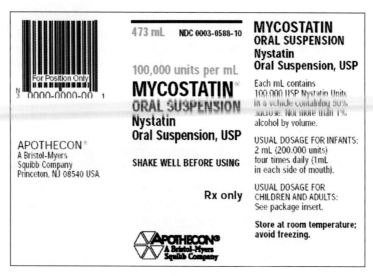

■ **FIGURE 19–6  Drug label for nystatin (Mycostatin).**
Nystatin (Mycostatin) is an antiyeast drug used to treat yeast infections in the mouth. This drug comes in the drug form of an oral suspension. Note the instructions on the label to "Shake well before using." A suspension contains fine, undissolved particles of a drug suspended in a water base. It is important to shake a suspension before measuring the dose so that the drug particles are evenly suspended throughout, rather than settled at the bottom.

## Antitussive Drugs

Antitussive drugs decrease coughing by suppressing the cough center in the brain or by anesthetizing stretch receptors in the respiratory tract. Their main purpose is to control dry, nonproductive coughs. These drugs are not prescribed to treat a productive cough because, when sputum is present, it is important for the patient to cough up this sputum. Benzonatate is a prescripton drug, while dextromethorphan is an over-the-counter drug that is also commonly seen in combination drugs used to treat coughs and colds. The word *antitussive* contains the prefix *anti-* (against), the combining form *tuss/o-* (cough), and the suffix *-ive* (pertaining to); it means *pertaining to against a cough. Dextromethorphan* is abbrevated as *DM* in many trade name antitussive drugs.

   benzonatate (Tessalon)

   dextromethorphan (Robitussin, Vicks 44)

   Some antitussive drugs contain codeine or hydrocodone, which are prescription Schedule III narcotic drugs. These drugs are used to treat severe, nonproductive coughing.

   codeine

   hydrocodone (Hycodan)

## Expectorant Drugs

Expectorant drugs exert an opposite therapeutic effect from that of antitussive drugs. Their therapeutic effect is to help remove sputum from the lungs, and so they are discussed in Chapter 10.

# Combination ENT Drugs

Combination ENT drugs contain various combinations of antihistamine, decongestant, antitussive, and expectorant drugs. They are both prescription and over-the-counter drugs.

## Combination Prescription ENT Drugs

These combination prescription drugs contain an antihistamine drug (cetirizine, chlorpheniramine, desloratadine, fexofenadine, promethazine) and a decongestant drug (phenylephrine, pseudoephedrine).

Allegra-D (fexofenadine, pseudoephedrine)

Clarinex-D (desloratadine, pseudoephedrine)

Phenergan VC (promethazine, phenylephrine)

Rondec (chlorpheniramine, phenylephrine)

Zyrtec-D (cetirizine, pseudoephedrine)

This combination prescription drug contains an antihistamine drug (chlorpheniramine), a decongestant drug (phenylephrine), and a nonnarcotic antitussive drug (dextromethorphan).

Rondec-DM (chlorpheniramine, phenylephrine, dextromethorphan)

These combination prescription drugs contain an antihistamine drug (chlorpheniramine), a decongestant drug (phenylephrine), and a narcotic antitussive drug (dihydrocodeine, hydrocodone). These are Schedule III drugs.

Novahistine (chlorpheniramine, phenylephrine, dihydrocodeine)

Tussionex (chlorpheniramine, hydrocodone)

These combination prescription drugs contain an expectorant drug (guaifenesin) and a narcotic antitussive drug (codeine, hydromorphone). These are Schedule II, III, and IV drugs.

Dilaudid Cough (guaifenesin, hydromorphone)

Hycotuss (guaifenesin, hydromorphone)

Tussi-Organidin (guaifenesin, codeine)

## *Drug Alert!*

Prescription cough syrups that contain a controlled substance are very effective in treating severe coughing, but they also contain a narcotic drug that can be addicting. These narcotic antitussive drugs include codeine (a Schedule IV drug), dihydrocodeine (a Schedule III drug), hydrocodone (a Schedule III drug), and hydromorphone (a Schedule II drug). Schedule drugs cause euphoria (an exaggerated sense of well being and happiness) and slowed muscle movements. The Drug Enforcement Administration (DEA) reports that these prescription cough syrups are easily available to addicts whose drug of abuse is cough syrup from some online pharmacies that do not verify prescriptions sent to them.

The Website for Partnership for a Drug-Free America notes that the nonnarcotic antitussive drug dextromethorphan is also being abused by 1 out of every 10 teenagers. It causes distortions in color and sound, disorientation, hallucinations, and an out-of-body experience, in addition to dizziness, nausea and vomiting, loss of motor control, and a rapid heart rate. Because it is an over-the-counter drug, it is commonly available.

These combination prescription drugs contain a decongestant drug (pseudoephedrine) and an expectorant drug (guaifenesin) to relieve edema and nasal dripping and treat a productive cough.

Entex (guaifenesin, pseudoephedrine)

Guaifenex PSE (guaifenesin, pseudoephedrine) (see ■ FIGURE 19–7)

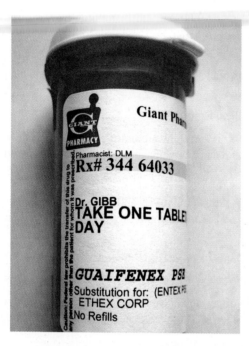

■ **FIGURE 19–7 Prescription bottle of Guaifenex PSE.**
This combination prescription drug contains a decongestant and an expectorant drug to help expel sputum produced from the throat and lungs.

This combination prescription drug contains a nonnarcotic antitussive drug (dextromethorphan) and an expectorant drug (guaifenesin).

Humibid DM (dextromethorphan, guaifenesin)

These combination prescription drugs contain an antibiotic drug (ciprofloxacin, neomycin, polymyxin B) and a corticosteroid drug (dexamethasone, hydrocortisone). They are used topically in the ear to treat infections of the external ear canal (otitis externa) and tympanic membrane (otitis media).

Ciprodex (ciprofloxacin, dexamethasone)

Cipro HC Otic (ciprofloxacin, hydrocortisone)

Coly-Mycin S Otic (hydrocortisone, neomycin)

Cortisporin Otic (hydrocortisone, neomycin, polymyxin B)

Octicair (hydrocortisone, neomycin, polymyxin B)

Otosporin (hydrocortisone, neomycin, polymyxin B)

Pediotic (hydrocortisone, neomycin, polymyxin B)

### Combination Over-the-Counter ENT Drugs

There are hundreds of over-the-counter combination drugs with such common brand names as Claritin-D, Dimetapp, Drixoral, Entex, Excedrin, Mucinex, Pediacare, Polaramine, Primatene, Robitussin, Rondec, Sudafed, Theraflu, Triaminic, and Tylenol. They contain various combinations of an analgesic drug (acetaminophen, ibuprofen, naproxen), a decongestant drug (ephedrine, phenylephrine, pseudoephedrine), an antihistamine drug (brompheniramine, cetirizine, chlorpheniramine, clemastine, dexchlorpheniramine, diphenhydramine, fexofenadine, loratadine, phenyltoloxamine, triprolidine) and an expectorant drug (guaifenesin) or an antitussive drug (dextromethorphan). These over-the-counter drugs are listed in Appendix D.

# Chapter Review

## Quiz Yourself

1. What are the therapeutic effects of decongestant drugs?
2. What is the action of histamine in the body?
3. How do antihistamine drugs exert their therapeutic effect?
4. Why do first-generation antihistamine drugs cause drowsiness as a side effect?
5. Describe the therapeutic effects of antihistamine drugs versus mast cell stabilizer drugs.
6. If there is no release of histamine during a common cold, why are antihistamine drugs included in so many over-the-counter drugs used to treat the common cold?
7. How can you tell from the trade name that the drug Coly-Mycin S Otic is used to treat the ears?
8. Explain why the mouth is a perfect environment for a yeast infection to develop.
9. Describe how the therapeutic effects of antitussive drugs differ from those of expectorant drugs (as discussed in Chapter 10).
10. Describe how an infant with oral candidiasis (thrush) is given an antiyeast drug. Describe two ways in which an adult with this same condition is given an antiyeast drug.
11. To what category of drugs does each of these drugs belong?

    a. cetirizine (Zyrtec)
    b. cromolyn (Nasalcrom)
    c. desloratadine (Clarinex)
    d. dextromethorphan (Robitussin)
    e. fexofenadine (Allegra)

    f. hydrocodone (Hycodan)
    g. mometasone (Nasonex)
    h. nystatin (Mycostatin, Nilstat)
    i. phenylephrine (Afrin)
    j. xylometazoline (Otrivin)

## Spelling Tip

**pseudoephedrine**    In the trade name, the sound for *pseudo-* is spelled *suda-* (Sudafed).

## Clinical Applications

1. Look at this packaged card of individual drug doses and answer the following questions.
   a. What is the trade name of this drug?
   b. What is the generic name of this drug?
   c. To what drug category does this drug belong?
   d. In what form is this drug?
   e. What is the dose contained in each tablet?
   f. Is this an over-the-counter or a prescription drug? How can you tell?

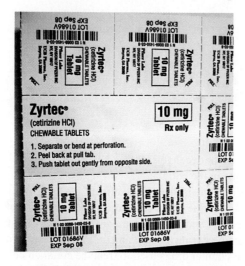

2. Look at this drug package and answer the following questions.
   a. What is the generic name of this drug?
   b. What is the trade name of this drug?
   c. To what drug category does this drug belong?
   d. In what form is this drug?
   e. What is the dose per spray?

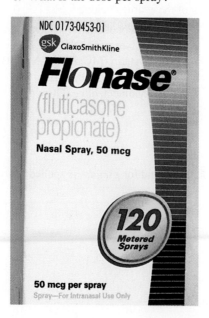

**3.** Look at this drug box and answer the following questions.
   **a.** What is the generic name of this drug?
   **b.** To what drug category does this drug belong?
   **c.** What is the dose strength in each tablet?
   **d.** The box states that the consumer should compare the active ingredient in this drug to what well-known trade name drug?

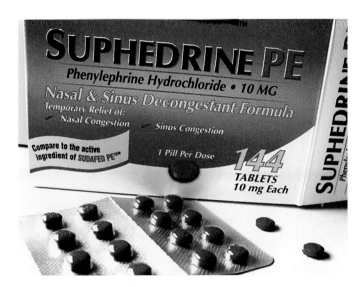

## Multimedia Extension Exercises

■ Go to www.pearsonhighered.com/turley and click on the photo of the cover of *Understanding Pharmacology for Health Professionals* to access the interactive Companion Website created for this textbook.

# Unit Three

# OTHER DRUG CATEGORIES

# 20 Anti-Infective Drugs

## Learning Objectives

After you study this chapter, you should be able to

1. Compare and contrast how different categories of antibiotic drugs kill bacteria.

2. Explain the significance of the beta-lactam ring and penicillinase.

3. Describe the historical milestones in the development of penicillin.

4. Explain how various consumer, medical, and environmental factors produce antibiotic-resistant bacteria.

5. Compare and contrast how different categories of antiviral drugs act to treat HIV and AIDS.

6. Describe the development of drugs used to treat HIV and AIDS.

7. Describe various opportunistic infections associated with HIV and AIDS.

8. Explain why fungal and yeast infections are often treated with the same drugs.

9. Given the generic and trade names of an anti-infective drug, identify what drug category they belong to, or what disease they are used to treat.

10. Given an anti-infective drug category, identify several generic and trade name drugs in that category.

Anti-infective drugs are used to treat systemic (not topical) infections in all parts of the body. These include bacterial infections, viral infections, fungal infections, and yeast infections. Anti-infective drugs include antibiotic drugs (sulfonamides, anti-infectives, penicillins, cephalosporins, aminoglycosides, tetracyclines, and others), antiviral drugs, antifungal drugs, and antiyeast drugs.

## Antibiotic Drugs

### Sulfonamide Anti-Infective Drugs

Sulfonamide anti-infective drugs are a group of drugs that inhibit the growth of bacteria. They are not categorized as antibiotic drugs because they do not actually kill bacteria. Sulfonamide drugs interfere with the growth of some bacteria that must manufacture their own folic acid. Human cells (as well as other types of bacteria) that can utilize folic acid from sources outside their cells are not affected by sulfonamide drugs. Sulfonamide drugs are effective against many gram-negative and gram-positive bacteria. They are commonly used to treat otitis media infections in the ear, urinary tract infections, and meningitis. Sulfonamide drugs are also known as *sulfa drugs.*

> sulfadiazine
>
> sulfisoxazole (Gantrisin Pediatric)

### Historical Notes

In 1934, a German researcher was screening chemicals for possible medicinal use. A red dye used to color cloth was tested. It seemed to cure streptococcal infections in mice. The researcher's own daughter was dying of streptococcal septicemia (blood poisoning) from pricking her finger. In desperation, he injected her with the dye and she recovered. The red dye was converted in the body into the anti-infective sulfa drug sulfanilamide. For this discovery, he won the Nobel Prize. Until the introduction of penicillin, sulfa drugs were the only anti-infective drugs available to treat bacterial infections.

### Penicillin Antibiotic Drugs

Penicillin antibiotic drugs are a group of drugs that kill bacteria. These drugs share the common molecular structure of a **beta-lactam ring** (see ■ FIGURE 20–1). All penicillin drugs interfere with the cell wall that surrounds a bacterium, disrupting the intracellular contents and causing cell death. Human cells have a cell membrane rather than a cell wall, and so they are not affected by penicillin drugs. Penicillin drugs are used to treat a wide variety of gram-positive, gram-negative, and anaerobic bacterial infections and are used to treat the sexually transmitted diseases of gonorrhea and syphilis. Antibiotic drugs, such as the penicillin drug amoxicillin, that are able to kill a variety of different types of bacteria are known as *broad spectrum antibiotic drugs.*

| | |
|---|---|
| amoxicillin (Amoxil, Moxatag) | penicillin G benzathine (Bicillin L-A, Permapen) |
| ampicillin (Principen) | penicillin G procaine |
| dicloxacillin | penicillin V (Penicillin VK, Veetids) |
| nafcillin | piperacillin |
| oxacillin | ticarcillin (Ticar) |
| penicillin G (Pfizerpen) (see ■ FIGURE 20–2) | |

*Note:* The suffix *-cillin* is common to generic penicillin antibiotic drugs.

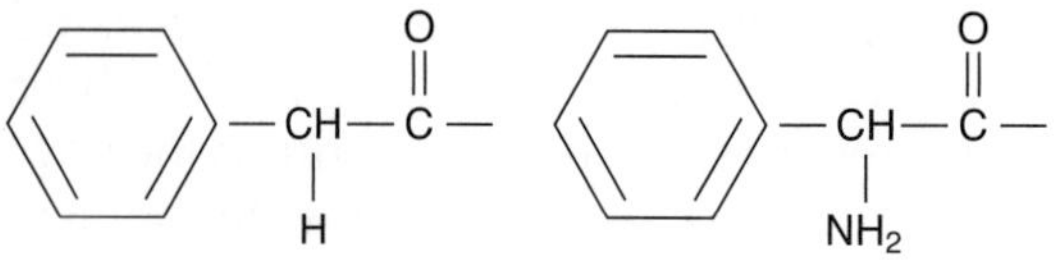

penicillin G          ampicillin

**■ FIGURE 20–1 Chemical structures.**
These are the chemical structures of penicillin G and
ampicillin, showing the beta-lactam ring that is common
to all drugs in the penicillin category of antibiotic drugs.

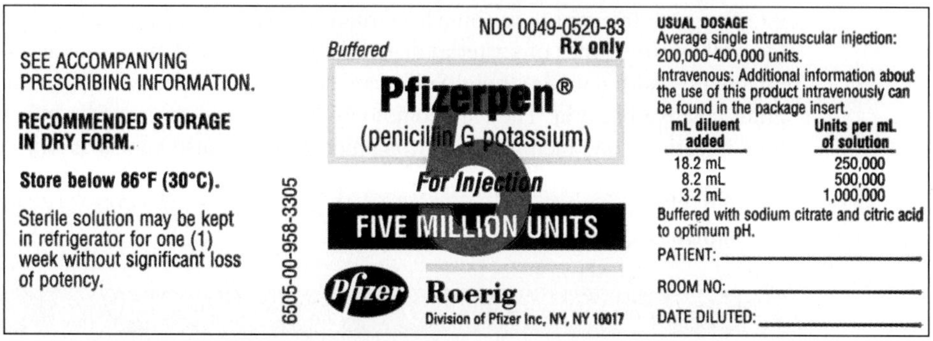

**■ FIGURE 20–2 Drug label for penicillin G potassium (Pfizerpen).**
This drug belongs to the penicillin category of antibiotic drugs. Note that the drug label shows that
the dose of Pfizerpen is measured in units, not in milligrams. The unusual spelling of the trade name
Pfizerpen reflects the drug company's name Pfizer plus the suffix *-pen* for *penicillin*.

Drugs in the penicillin category differ from each other in the following ways:

- Some are inactivated by gastric acid and cannot be given orally (penicillin G drugs).
- Most are inactivated by **penicillinase** (all penicillin drugs, except dicloxacillin, nafcillin, and oxacillin). The enzyme penicillinase is produced by penicillin-resistant bacteria and is also known as *beta lactamase* because it inactivates penicillin drugs by breaking their chemical structure at the site of the beta-lactam ring.
- Most have little antibiotic activity against gram-negative bacteria (all penicillin drugs, except piperacillin and ticarcillin).

## *Historical Notes*

In 1928, the Scottish bacteriologist, Alexander Fleming, was looking for drugs that would
inhibit the growth of the bacterium staphylococcus. He concluded his experiments and went
on vacation, after instructing an assistant to wash the culture plates that were soaking in the
sink. When Fleming returned from vacation, the plates had not been washed. One culture
plate had remained above the water and on it had grown a blue-green mold with a ring
around it where the staphylococcus bacteria had been killed. Fleming identified this mold as

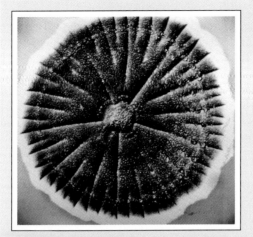

*Penicillium notatum;* however, he was unable to extract a drug from this. (The mold itself contained only 1 part penicillin per 2 million parts mold.) He wrote a paper about his finding, but it remained generally unknown to the scientific world.

Later, during World War II, work on penicillin resumed. Two researchers in England were afraid all of the drug would be destroyed in the bombing of London. Therefore, they smeared some of the mold inside their coat jackets and brought it to the United States, where penicillin could be produced.

A 43-year-old policeman was the first person to be injected with penicillin. He was dying of septicemia, which had begun as an abscess when a rose thorn scratched his face. Penicillin was in such short supply that his urine was saved each day and the penicillin in it was extracted to provide the next day's dose. He was given the world's entire supply of penicillin. He responded well to the treatment, but on the fifth day the supply of penicillin ran out, and he relapsed and died.

Because the mold *Penicillium notatum* only grew on the surface of a culture medium, it had to be produced in many shallow bottles and the yield was very small. Later, researchers found the strain *Penicillium chrysogenum* on a moldy cantaloupe in Peoria, Illinois. It was approximately 20 times more potent than the original mold and could be grown in larger quantities. When the United States entered World War II in December 1941, the government took immediate control of the supplies and production of penicillin and advised the Committee on Medical Research to distribute the drug carefully for medical investigation. The first small amounts of commercially produced penicillin became available in 1942. By the end of that year, 100 patients had been treated with it.

On Wednesday, July 28, 1943, the *Pittsburgh Press* ran an article entitled, "Penicillin Drug Hailed as Boon to Mankind." The article noted that penicillin took its place alongside the sulfonamide drugs as a deadly enemy of infection and disease. By 1945, *penicillin* had become a household word, and the word *antibiotic* was coined as well.

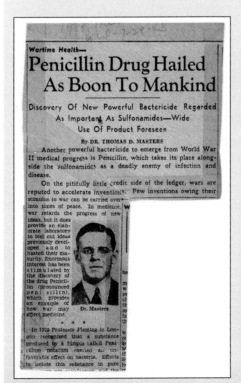

## Cephalosporin Antibiotic Drugs

Cephalosporin antibiotic drugs are a group of drugs that kill bacteria. They interfere with the cell wall that surrounds each bacterium, causing disruption of the intracellular contents and cell death. This group of antibiotic drugs is further divided into first-generation, second-generation, and third generation cephalosporin drugs. This designation has nothing to do with when these antibiotic drugs were discovered or first marketed, but instead divides them according to their therapeutic antibiotic properties. Cephalosporin drugs are used to treat a wide variety of gram-negative and anaerobic bacterial infections, some gram-positive bacterial infections, and are used to treat the sexually transmitted disease of gonorrhea.

## *Drug Alert!*

Cephalosporin drugs and penicillin drugs are structurally similar, and patients who are allergic to penicillin drugs may have an allergic reaction if given cephalosporin antibiotic drugs.

First-generation cephalosporin drugs have a fairly broad spectrum of effectiveness against various bacteria, but are not very effective against bacteria that produce penicillinase.

cefadroxil (Duricef)

cefazolin

cephalexin (Keflex)

Second-generation cephalosporin drugs are more effective than first-generation cephalosporin drugs against bacteria that produce penicillinase. They are also effective against more gram-positive bacteria.

| | |
|---|---|
| cefaclor (Ceclor) | cefoxitin (Mefoxin) |
| cefditoren (Spectracef) | cefprozil (Cefzil) |
| cefotetan (Cefotan) | cefuroxime (Ceftin, Zinacef) |

Third-generation cephalosporin drugs are the most effective of all the cephalosporin drugs against bacteria that produce penicillinase. Third-generation cephalosporin drugs also show the greatest effectiveness against gram-negative and gram-positive bacteria. These drugs can also pass through the blood–brain barrier and are useful for treating meningitis. The cost of third-generation cephalosporin drugs is higher than that of other cephalosporin drugs.

| | |
|---|---|
| cefdinir (Omnicef) (see ■ FIGURE 20–3) | cefpodoxime (Vantin) |
| cefepime (Maxipime) | ceftazidime (Ceptaz, Fortaz) |
| cefixime (Suprax) | ceftibuten (Cedax) |
| cefoperazone (Cefobid) | ceftizoxime (Cefizox) |
| cefotaxime (Claforan) | ceftriaxone (Rocephin) |

*Note:* Generic cephalosporin antibiotic drugs begin with *cef-, cefa-, cefe-, cefi-, cefo-,* or *cepha-.*

## *Historical Notes*

The fungus *Cephalosporium,* from which the first cephalosporin drugs were produced, was discovered in a sewer outlet near Sardinia (an island off the coast of Italy) in 1948.

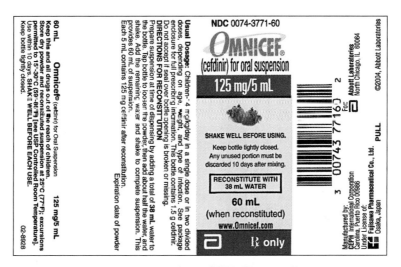

**■ FIGURE 20–3 Drug label for cefdinir (Omnicef).**
This cephalosporin drug comes in the drug form of an oral suspension that
contains tiny, undissolved particles of the drug suspended in a liquid. Note the
label instruction that says to "Shake well before using," so that the drug
particles can be evenly distributed throughout the liquid before the dose is
measured.

## Drug Alert!

Most bacteria have developed resistant strains that are immune to certain antibiotic drugs.
This has happened because antibiotic drugs have been so widely prescribed and are often
prescribed for conditions that do not warrant antibiotic drug use. Many parents do not know
that a viral infection cannot be treated with an antibiotic drug, and so they incorrectly
pressure the physician to prescribe an antibiotic drug; sometimes the physician gives in to this
pressure. A study conducted by the University of Tennessee found that pediatricians
incorrectly prescribe antibiotic drugs 42 percent of the time. According to the Centers for
Disease Control and Prevention (CDCP), pediatricians will prescribe antibiotic drugs more
often if they perceive the parents expect their child to be given an antibiotic drug. The
American Academy of Pediatrics guidelines state that educating parents is the single most
important issue in reducing the overuse of antibiotic drugs. Many physicians now give
parents pamphlets describing how antibiotic drugs are overused in order to convey the idea
that just because they are not prescribing an antibiotic drug does not mean that they are
giving incomplete medical care. Also, antibiotic drugs are given to animals so that they can
be housed in crowded conditions that would normally cause disease. The meat from these
animals contains traces of antibiotic drugs. The nonprofit Union of Concerned Scientists
reported that 16 million pounds of antibiotic drugs were given to animals annually in the
1980s, and this increased to 25 million pounds in 2001. In addition to that, patients take
about 3 million pounds of antibiotic drugs each year. Antibiotic drugs are the fourth most
commonly prescribed drug category, and the CDCP estimates that 50 percent of all prescriptions for antibiotic drugs are not necessary. Each year, about 14,000 Americans die because
of infections caused by antibiotic-resistant bacteria.

### Aminoglycoside Antibiotic Drugs

Aminoglycoside antibiotic drugs are a group of drugs that kill bacteria. They interfere with the synthesis of protein in the bacterial wall. This disrupts the intracellular contents and causes the bacterium to die. Aminoglycoside drugs are primarily effective against gram-negative bacteria. Some aminoglycoside drugs (kanamycin, neomycin) are not absorbed from the intestine into the blood, and so they are given orally as a bowel prep to inhibit intestinal bacteria prior to abdominal surgery. Aminoglycoside drugs are used to treat a wide variety of gram-negative and some gram-positive bacterial infections.

| | |
|---|---|
| amikacin (Amikin) | neomycin |
| gentamicin | paromomycin (Humatin) |
| kanamycin (Kantrex) | tobramycin (TOBI, Tobrex) |

*Note:* The suffix *-micin* or *-mycin* is common to generic aminoglycoside antibiotic drugs.

## Drug Alert!

All aminoglycoside antibiotic drugs have the potential to cause toxic effects to the auditory nerve (**ototoxicity**) or to the kidneys (**nephrotoxicity**). Patients receiving aminoglycoside antibiotic drugs are carefully monitored with hearing tests (audiograms) and blood tests (BUN and creatinine) for kidney function.

## In Depth

How does a physician know which category of antibiotic drugs to prescribe for a particular patient? The physician gives the patient a prescription for an antibiotic drug that seems appropriate for the patient's symptoms. While the patient is still in the office (before taking the first dose of the antibiotic drug), the physician collects a specimen of the infected area and sends it to a laboratory for a culture and sensitivity test. In the laboratory, the specimen (urine, blood, mucus, pus, saliva, etc.) is swabbed onto a Petri dish (see ■ **FIGURE 20–4a**). The dish is allowed to incubate and grow colonies of the bacterium. The results show the bacterial colonies, and these are used to identify what bacterium (or different kinds of bacteria) is causing the infection. The bacterium is then swabbed onto another Petri dish, and disks with specific concentrations of different antibiotic drugs are added. The Petri dish is incubated. The antibiotic drugs that are effective against that bacterium will have a large zone of inhibition (clear ring) around their disk where the bacterium was not able to grow (see ■ **FIGURE 20–4b**). The result of the laboratory test is sent to the physician. The physician then checks to see that the preliminary antibiotic drug that was prescribed is one that is effective in treating the type of bacterium causing the patient's infection. If it is not, the physician will write a prescription for a different antibiotic drug.

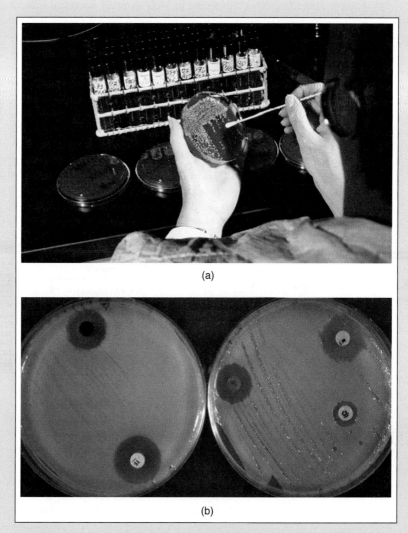

(a)

(b)

■ **FIGURE 20–4  Culture and sensitivity testing.**
(a) This laboratory technician has a cotton swab containing mucus from a patient's throat and is streaking it across the surface of a Petri dish. This Petri dish contains blood agar, a medium that is particularly good for growing streptococcus, a bacterium that causes strep throat. (b) These Petri dishes show small or large rings of inhibition (clear zones of no bacterial growth) around different antibiotic disks. A large ring of inhibition signifies that the antibiotic drug in that disk is very effective in killing the bacterium.

## Tetracycline Antibiotic Drugs

Tetracycline antibiotic drugs inhibit the growth of bacteria by inhibiting protein synthesis in the cell wall of the bacterium. Tetracycline drugs are used to treat a wide variety of gram-negative and gram-positive bacterial infections, as well as other bacterial infections, and are used to treat the sexually transmitted diseases of gonorrhea and syphilis.

demeclocycline (Declomycin)                    minocycline (Dynacin, Minocin)

doxycycline (Vibramycin, Vibra-Tabs)        tetracycline (Sumycin)

(see ■ FIGURE 20–5)

*Note:*  The suffix *-cycline* is common to generic tetracycline antibiotic drugs.

## Drug Alert!

Tetracycline drugs can cause permanent discoloration of the teeth; therefore, they are not prescribed for pregnant women (to protect the fetus's developing teeth) or for children under age 8 (whose permanent teeth are still developing).

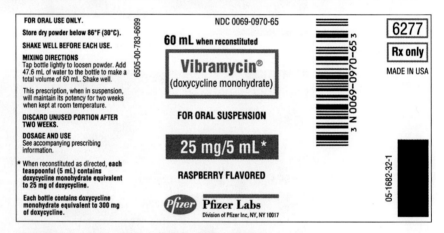

**■ FIGURE 20–5  Drug label for Vibramycin.**
Doxycycline (Vibramycin) is used to treat a wide variety of gram-negative and gram-positive bacterial infections. It also has special uses in treating the infections of Lyme disease, malaria, and anthrax from bioterrorism.

## Carbapenem Antibiotic Drugs

Carbapenem antibiotic drugs are a group of drugs that kill bacteria. These drugs interfere with the structure of the cell wall of the bacterium and cause cell death. Carbapenem antibiotic drugs are effective against some gram-negative and gram-positive bacteria.

doripenem (Doribax)

ertapenem (Invanz)

meropenem (Merrem I.V.)

## Monobactam Antibiotic Drugs

Monobactam antibiotic drugs are a group of drugs that kill bacteria. These drugs interfere with the structure of the cell wall of the bacterium and cause cell death. Monobactam antibiotic drugs are effective against gram-negative bacteria.

aztreonam (Azactam)

## Quinolone Antibiotic Drugs

Quinolone antibiotic drugs are a group of drugs that kill bacteria. These drugs interfere with the bacterium's DNA and cause cell death. Quinolone antibiotic drugs are effective against gram-negative bacteria.

cinoxacin

nalidixic acid (NegGram)

## Fluoroquinolone Antibiotic Drugs

Fluoroquinolone antibiotic drugs are a group of drugs that kill bacteria. These drugs inhibit an enzyme that is essential to bacterial DNA replication and this causes cell death. Fluoroquinolone antibiotic drugs are effective against gram-negative bacteria, some gram-positive bacteria, and other types of bacteria and are used to treat the sexually transmitted disease of gonorrhea.

ciprofloxacin (Cipro) (see ■ FIGURE 20–6)  moxifloxacin (Avelox)

gemifloxacin (Factive)  norfloxacin (Noroxin)

levofloxacin (Levaquin) (see ■ FIGURE 20–7)  ofloxacin (Floxin)

lomefloxacin (Maxaquin)

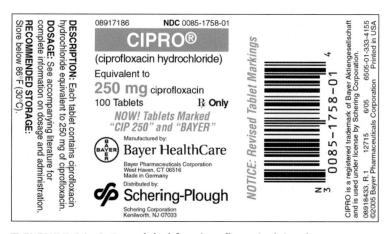

■ **FIGURE 20–6 Drug label for ciprofloxacin (Cipro).**
The fluoroquinolone antibiotic drug ciprofloxacin (Cipro) is effective against a wide variety of bacterial infections and is a commonly prescribed antibiotic drug.

## Macrolide Antibiotic Drugs

Macrolide antibiotic drugs are a group of drugs that either inhibit or kill bacteria by interfering with RNA and protein synthesis within the bacteria. Macrolide antibiotic drugs are effective against some gram-negative bacteria, some gram-positive bacteria, anaerobic bacteria, and other types of bacteria and are used to treat the sexually transmitted diseases of gonorrhea and syphilis. Clarithromycin is used in combination with other drugs to treat gastric ulcers caused by *H. pylori* infection. Azithromycin and clarithromycin are used to prevent *Mycobacterium avium-intracellulare* infection in AIDS patients.

azithromycin (Zithromax) (see ■ FIGURE 20–8)

clarithromycin (Biaxin)

erythromycin (Eryc, Ery-Tab) (see ■ FIGURE 20–9)

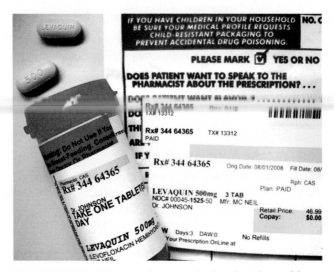

■ **FIGURE 20–7  Levaquin prescription bottle and bag.**
Levaquin is the trade name for the generic drug levofloxacin, an
antibiotic drug that belongs to the fluoroquinolone category. This
prescription is for a 3-day supply to treat a mild urinary tract
infection prior to a surgical procedure. Although most antibiotic
drugs have plain and unlabeled tablets, the Levaquin tablet is not
only labeled with the drug name on one side of the tablet, but the
reverse side of the tablet has the tablet strength of 500 (for
500 mg). Notice the red warning label on the prescription bottle that
says "Do not use if you are breastfeeding." Notice the blue notice on
the prescription bag that requests child-resistant packaging.

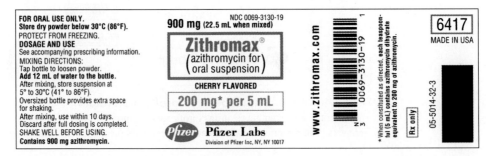

■ **FIGURE 20–8  Drug label for Zithromax.**
The macrolide antibiotic drug azithromycin (Zithromax) has a half life of 68 hours. That means it
takes 68 hours for the body to excrete one half of a single dose of Zithromax. This extended
therapeutic effect is good because it makes it possible to take Zithromax just once a day for five days
to complete treatment, while most other antibiotic drugs have a shorter half life and have to be taken
two or three times a day for seven days or more. Also, the patient is less likely to forget to take a
dose of once-a-day Zithromax. However, if the patient has an allergic reaction to Zithromax, that
reaction will last longer and could be more severe.

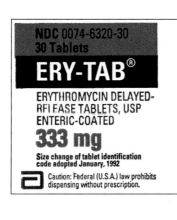

NDC 0074-6320-30
30 Tablets

**ERY-TAB®**

ERYTHROMYCIN DELAYED-
RELEASE TABLETS, USP
ENTERIC-COATED

**333 mg**

Size change of tablet identification
code adopted January, 1992

Caution: Federal (U.S.A.) law prohibits
dispensing without prescription.

Do not accept if break-away
ring on cap is broken or
missing. Keep tightly closed.
Each tablet contains:
Erythromycin ............. 333 mg
Usual adult dose: One tablet
every eight hours.
See enclosure for full
prescribing information.
DOSAGE MAY BE
ADMINISTERED WITHOUT
REGARD TO MEALS.
Each white tablet bears
the a and Abbo-Code EH for
product identification.
U.S. Pat. No. 4,340,582
©Abbott
Abbott Laboratories
North Chicago, IL60064, U.S.A.

**■ FIGURE 20-9  Drug label for ery-thromycin (Ery-Tab).**
The trade name of the drug Ery-Tab makes it easy
to remember that the generic name for this drug is
erythromycin and that it comes in the drug form of
a tablet.

## Other Antibiotic Drugs

These are other antibiotic drugs that are used to treat gram-positive bacterial infections. Vancomycin is used to treat serious infections, particularly methicillin-resistant staphylococcal infections.

clindamycin (Cleocin)

telithromycin (Ketek)

vancomycin (Vancocin)

## *Focus on Healthcare Issues*

*Staphylococcus aureus* is a gram-positive bacterium. For years, this bacterium could be killed by the penicillin category of drugs. Then it developed strains that were resistant to the penicillin drugs and to methicillin, the most common drug in the penicillin category at that time (methicillin is no longer on the market). This resistant strain of bacteria was named methicillin-resistant *Staphylococcus aureus* (MRSA) (pronounced "MER-sah"). MRSA causes serious and sometimes fatal infections in hospitalized patients, and now has been found in patients who are in other healthcare facilities and even at home. MRSA exists in the noses of some healthcare providers who are not ill, but inadvertently pass it to hospitalized patients whose immune systems are unable to combat it. Nonsymptomatic healthcare providers with MRSA colonies in the nose are treated with topical mupirocin (Bactroban), and infected hospitalized patients are treated with intravenous vancomycin or linezolid. Unfortunately, some strains of MRSA have now also become resistant to vancomycin. Drug companies are racing to create new antibiotic drugs that can take the place of vancomycin in combating these resistant bacteria.

### Combination Antibiotic Drugs

This combination drug contains two different penicillin drugs.

> Bicillin C-R (penicillin G benzathine, penicillin G procaine)

These combination drugs contain an antibiotic drug (erythromycin, trimethoprim) and a sulfonamide anti-infective drug (sulfamethoxazole, sulfisoxazole).

> Bactrim (trimethoprim, sulfamethoxazole)
>
> Pediazole (erythromycin, sulfisoxazole)
>
> Septra (trimethoprim, sulfamethoxazole)

This combination drug contains a carbapenem antibiotic drug (impenem) and a drug (cilastin) that inhibits an enzyme in the kidneys that normally breaks down carbapenem.

> Primaxin (imipenem, cilastatin)

This combination drug contains two antibiotic drugs that do not belong to any particular category of drugs but are chemically related to each other. It is used to treat some methicillin-resistant and vancomycin-resistant bacterial infections.

> Synercid (dalfopristin, quinupristin)

These combination drugs contain a penicillin antibiotic drug (ampicillin, amoxicillin, piperacillin, ticarcillin) that is inactivated by penicillinase from resistant bacteria and another drug (clavulanic acid, sulbactam, tazobactam) that inactivates bacterial penicillinase. These drugs are used to treat infections caused by penicillin-resistant bacteria.

> Augmentin (amoxicillin, clavulanic acid)
>
> Timentin (ticarcillin, clavulanic acid)

> Unasyn (ampicillin, sulbactam) (see ■ **FIGURE 20–10**)
>
> Zosyn (piperacillin, tazobactam)

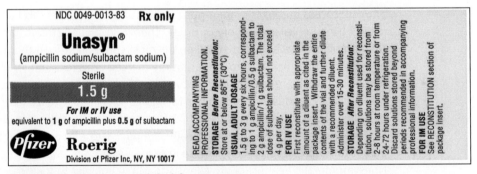

■ **FIGURE 20–10 Drug label for Unasyn.**
The two generic drugs (ampicillin and sulbactam) in the combination drug Unasyn are clearly marked on the drug label. This drug is only given by the intramuscular (IM) or intravenous (IV) route of administration, as noted on the label.

## Drugs Used to Treat HIV and AIDS

Acquired immunodeficiency syndrome (AIDS) is an eventually fatal disease in which the human immunodeficiency virus (HIV) attaches to CD4 receptors on helper T lymphocytes (a specific type of white blood cell in the immune system) and directs the lymphocyte to produce more HIV using the lymphocyte's own DNA. As the newly produced viruses are released, the lymphocyte is destroyed. The viruses then infect more helper T lymphocytes and further weaken the immune system. As large numbers of helper T cells are destroyed, the action of suppressor T cells (CD8 lymphocytes) is unopposed, and this further suppresses the immune response. Although the body produces antibodies against HIV, the immune system is never able to eradicate the virus. HIV is transmitted through contact with an infected individual, contaminated blood, or used needles, or when an infected mother transmits the virus to the fetus or a breastfeeding infant.

## Historical Notes

Azidothymidine (AZT, zidovudine, Retrovir) was originally synthesized in 1974. It was tested as a treatment for cancer but was not effective. Other uses for it were not investigated and it was simply shelved.

The word **retrovirus** was coined in 1977 and is a shortened form of the phrase *reverse transcriptase* plus the word *virus.* The human immunodeficiency virus (HIV) is a retrovirus because it contains reverse transcriptase, an enzyme that transcribes or encodes RNA (instead of the usual DNA) for its genetic information.

In 1984, although there were only 3,000 reported cases of AIDS in the United States, researchers at the National Cancer Institute, including the codiscoverer of the AIDS virus, Dr. Robert Gallo, approached Burroughs Wellcome drug company to develop a drug to treat AIDS. Although other drug companies were also approached, their concern about working with the deadly virus, as well as the apparently limited use for the drug at that time, resulted in unenthusiastic responses. Burroughs Wellcome, however, responded to the request and tested many different drugs, one of which was AZT.

In 1986, clinical testing of AZT was begun using a double-blind study in which severely ill AIDS patients were divided into two groups: One group received AZT while the control group received a placebo. Shortly after the study was begun, it was stopped when it was found that those in the control group had a 40 percent mortality rate while those receiving AZT had only a 6 percent mortality rate. In March 1988, just four months after a new drug application was filed, the FDA approved AZT.

Burroughs Wellcome chose the generic name zidovudine for this new AIDS drug and the trade name Retrovir. The trade name refers to the fact that the AIDS virus belongs to a category of viruses known as *retroviruses.*

Zidovudine was used extensively by itself to treat HIV infection for many years, but can no longer be given alone because HIV has developed resistance to it.

A person infected with HIV usually remains without symptoms for four to five years but, with the progressive decrease in the number of T lymphocytes, symptoms of fever, night sweats, weakness, diarrhea, weight loss, fatigue, and swollen glands begin. The dividing line between a diagnosis of HIV infection and a diagnosis of AIDS is determined by the presence or absence of the following indicators.

CD4 lymphocyte count below 200 cells/mm$^3$

Presence of opportunistic infections/diseases

Drug therapy for AIDS focuses on drugs to suppress the virus, as well as drugs to treat any secondary opportunistic infections that develop. Drugs used to treat HIV inhibit the growth of the retrovirus but are unable to kill it. They are, however, able to decrease the **viral load** (total number of viruses in the blood and lymphocytes) and delay the onset of AIDS and clinical complications from opportunistic infections. The goal of drug therapy is to suppress HIV replication as much as possible for as long as possible.

These antiviral drugs are used to treat HIV and AIDS: protease inhibitor drugs, nucleoside reverse transcriptase inhibitor drugs, nonnucleoside reverse transcriptase inhibitor drugs, nucleotide analog reverse transcriptase inhibitor drugs, fusion inhibitor drugs, and integrase inhibitor drugs.

### Protease Inhibitor Drugs for HIV and AIDS

Protease inhibitor drugs inhibit the viral enzyme protease. This enzyme breaks down certain proteins in the virus, an important last step that must happen before the virus can reproduce. Without the action of the enzyme, the virus dies.

atazanavir (Reyataz)

darunavir (Prezista)

fosamprenavir (Lexiva)

indinavir (Crixivan) (see ■ **FIGURE 20–11**)

nelfinavir (Viracept)

ritonavir (Norvir)

saquinavir (Fortovase, Invirase)

tipranavir (Aptivus)

*Note:* The suffix *-navir* is common to generic protease inhibitor drugs.

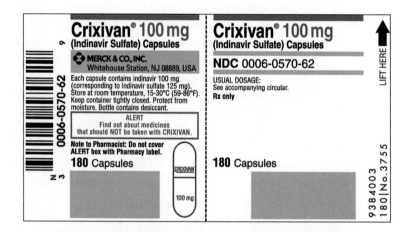

■ **FIGURE 20–11  Drug label for indinavir (Crixivan).**
Indinavir (Crixivan), other protease inhibitor drugs, and other drugs used to treat HIV/AIDS are given orally in the form of a capsule, tablet, or oral liquid. The exception to this is the category of fusion inhibitor drugs, which must be given by subcutaneous injection.

### Nucleoside Reverse Transcriptase Inhibitor Drugs for HIV and AIDS

These drugs inhibit reverse transcriptase, an enzyme that the virus needs to reproduce itself. These drugs also become part of the viral DNA chain, which causes it to break, and the virus dies.

abacavir (Ziagen)

didanosine (Videx)

emtricitabine (Emtriva)

lamivudine (Epivir) (see ■ **FIGURE 20–12**)

stavudine (Zerit)

zalcitabine (Hivid)

zidovudine (Retrovir) (see ■ **FIGURE 20–13**)

*Note:* The suffix *–vir* in the trade name drugs Epivir and Retrovir shows that they are antiviral drugs. The spelling of the trade name drug Hivid references HIV, the infection it is used to treat.

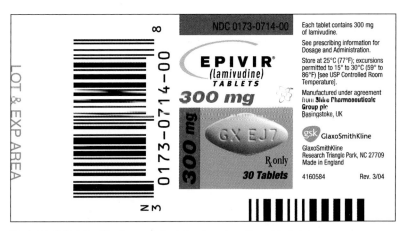

■ **FIGURE 20–12  Drug label for lamivudine (Epivir).**
This interesting diamond-shaped tablet is the nucleoside reverse transcriptase
inhibitor drug lamivudine (Epivir), used to treat HIV and AIDS.

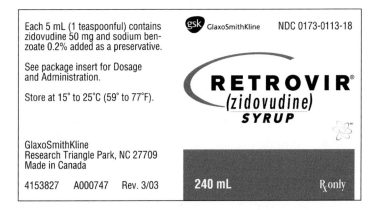

■ **FIGURE 20–13  Drug label for zidovudine (Retrovir).**
The trade name Retrovir is a direct link to its therapeutic effect against the
retrovirus HIV and AIDS.

## *Drug Alert!*

The antipsychotic drug lithium (Lithobid), which is used to treat the mania of bipolar disorder, has a known side effect of causing the white blood cell count to increase. This side effect becomes the therapeutic effect when treating AIDS patients who have a low white blood cell count from being treated with zidovudine.

### Nonnucleoside Reverse Transcriptase Inhibitor Drugs for HIV and AIDS

These drugs bind directly to reverse transcriptase, an enzyme needed to reproduce viral DNA, and disrupt its activity, causing the virus to die.

delavirdine (Rescriptor)        etravirine (Intelence)

efavirenz (Sustiva)             nevirapine (Viramune)

### Nucleotide Analog Reverse Transcriptase Inhibitor Drugs for HIV and AIDS

These drugs inhibit reverse transcriptase, an enzyme that the virus needs to reproduce itself. These drugs also become part of the viral DNA chain, which causes it to break, causing the virus to die. Nucleotide reverse transcriptase inhibitor drugs act in the same way as nucleoside reverse transcriptase inhibitor drugs, except they are preactivated and act more quickly in the body.

> tenofovir (Viread)

### Fusion Inhibitor Drugs for HIV and AIDS

Fusion inhibitor drugs block HIV when it tries to fuse its viral membrane with the cell membrane of the CD4 lymphocyte. Because the virus cannot fuse with the lymphocyte, it is unable to reproduce itself. This drug can only be given by the subcutaneous route of administration and must be injected twice a day.

> enfuvirtide (Fuzeon)

### Integrase Inhibitor Drugs for HIV and AIDS

Integrase inhibitor drugs block integrase, an enzyme used by HIV to insert its genetic material into a CD4 lymphocyte. Without this enzyme, HIV is unable to reproduce itself.

> raltegravir (Isentress)

## Combination Drugs for HIV and AIDS

These combination drugs contain a protease inhibitor drug (lopinavir, ritonavir), a nonnucleoside reverse transcriptase inhibitor drug (efavirenz), a nucleoside reverse transcriptase inhibitor drug (abacavir, emtricitabine, lamivudine, zidovudine), and/or a nucleotide analog reverse transcriptase inhibitor drug (tenofovir).

*Note:* The protease inhibitor drug lopinavir is not available as an individual drug.

Aptripla (efavirenz, emtricitabine, tenofovir)

Combivir (lamivudine, zidovudine)

Epzicom (abacavir, lamivudine)

Kaletra (lopinavir, ritonavir) (see ■ FIGURE 20–14)

Trizivir (abacavir, lamivudine, zidovudine)

Truvada (emtricitabine, tenofovir)

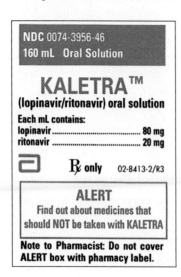

■ **FIGURE 20–14** Drug label for Kaletra.
Kaletra is a combination drug that contains two protease inhibitor drugs to treat HIV and AIDS. Note the red box warning on the label. This drug can cause life-threatening reactions if taken with these drugs: rifampin (for tuberculosis), St. John's wort (herbal antidepressant), Zocor (for a high cholesterol level), Halcion (for insomnia), phenobarbital (for seizures), or dexamethasone (corticosteroid drug for inflammation).

## Historical Notes

Originally, HIV-positive patients were not begun on drug therapy until they began to exhibit symptoms. Later, the standard treatment was to treat patients with one antiviral drug as soon as a diagnosis of HIV was made. The first study of combined therapy showed that using two or more antiviral drugs increased the CD4 cell count so significantly that combination therapy (the so-called "AIDS cocktail") became the standard treatment in 1996. Current drug therapy uses two or three antiviral drugs in combination; this is more effective than one drug and also decreases the risk of developing resistant strains of HIV. Several individual antiviral drugs are given at the same time, or the physician can prescribe a single tablet that contains two different antiviral drugs. In 2006, the FDA approved the first combination drug to contain three different AIDS drugs: Atripla.

### Other Drugs for HIV and AIDS

These drugs are only used to treat a specific strain of HIV or they are orphan drugs that have been approved by the FDA to treat HIV and AIDS. Receptin is made by recombinant DNA technology in which the protein from a CD4 receptor (on a lymphocyte) is inserted into bacteria and reproduced in sufficient quantities to make a drug. This drug binds to the part of HIV that would normally combine with the CD4 lymphocyte. VaxSyn HIV-1 contains an antigen to HIV.

| | |
|---|---|
| carbovir | interferon beta-1a (Rebif) |
| dextran sulfate | interferon beta-1b (Betaseron) |
| dideoxyinosine | lithium (Lithobid) |
| diethyldithiocarbamate (Imuthiol) | maraviroc (Selzentry) |
| HIV immune globulin (Hivig) | recombinant human soluble CD4 (Receptin) |
| HIV neutralizing antibodies (Immupath) | tumor necrosis factor-binding protein |
| human immune globulin (Gamimune N) | VaxSyn HIV-1 |

### Vaccine for HIV and AIDS

In 1988, the National Institutes of Health began efforts to develop an AIDS vaccine. A vaccine, which consists of purified protein genetic material from the human immunodeficiency virus (HIV), is reproduced using recombinant DNA technology. The purpose of the vaccine is to stimulate the body to produce antibodies against HIV. Because the vaccine only contains pieces of the virus, it cannot cause AIDS. However, because HIV continues to mutate, no vaccine has yet been approved by the FDA, although many are in the clinical trials phase.

## Drugs Used to Treat Conditions Related to HIV and AIDS

The immune system of a patient with an HIV infection is also unable to defend against **opportunistic infections,** such as candidiasis, coccidioidomycosis, CMV retinitis, histoplasmosis, toxoplasmosis, *Salmonella, Mycobacterium avium-intracellulare* infection, and *Pneumocystis carinii* pneumonia. These uncommon diseases have an unusual opportunity to attack the compromised immune systems of patients with HIV, and so they are known as *opportunistic infections.* Also, HIV patients are prone to develop the rare cancers of Kaposi's sarcoma and Burkitt's lymphoma. AIDS wasting syndrome is characterized by extreme weight loss and loss of muscle mass.

### AIDS Wasting Syndrome Drugs

These drugs are used to stimulate the appetite of AIDS patients, build muscle mass, and treat extreme weight loss. Some of these are orphan drugs whose only indication is treating AIDS wasting syndrome.

Others are prescription hormone, growth hormone, or anabolic steroid drugs. Dronabinol is a Schedule III drug derived from marijuana.

| | |
|---|---|
| Cachexon | oxymetholone (Anadrol-50) |
| dihydrotestosterone (Androgel-DHT) | sermorelin (Geref) |
| dronabinol (Marinol) | somatropin (BioTropin, Serostim) |
| megestrol (Megace) | testosterone (AndroGel) |
| oxandrolone (Oxandrin) | thalidomide (Synovir) |

## Did You Know?

After the drug thalidomide was used to treat morning sickness in pregnant women in Europe and caused the severe birth defect of phocomelia ("seal limbs") in their babies, it was withdrawn from the market. It would have become an obscure footnote in medical history but, in 1997, it was discovered to be useful in treating cancer, AIDS, and leprosy. The potential side effects of this drug are so great that it is only considered as a viable treatment option for life-threatening diseases. The FDA regulates the use of thalidomide in two ways: (1) by limiting the number of physicians who can prescribe it, and (2) by requiring women taking the drug not to have sex or to use two forms of birth control if they do have sex (so that there is virtually no risk of the woman giving birth to a child with phocomelia). Thalidomide is now an official prescription drug used to treat multiple myeloma, leprosy, graft-versus-host disease, and several types of cancers. It is also officially recognized as an orphan drug to treat Crohn's disease and AIDS wasting syndrome.

### AIDS-Related Diarrhea Drugs

These orphan drugs slow intestinal transit time and are used to treat AIDS-related diarrhea that is not responsive to regular prescription antidiarrheal drugs.

bovine colostrum

lactobin

octreotide (Sandostatin)

### *Pneumocystis carinii* Pneumonia Drugs

*Pneumocystis carinii* pneumonia (PCP) is the most common serious infection and complication of AIDS and eventually affects about three-fourths of all AIDS patients. *Pneumocystis carinii* is a protozoan that seldom causes symptoms in healthy individuals, but it is a life-threatening infection in AIDS patients. These anti-infective drugs are specifically used to treat this infection.

| | |
|---|---|
| atovaquone (Mepron) | piritrexim |
| dapsone | primaquine |
| eflornithine (Ornidyl) | trimetrexate (Neutrexin) |
| pentamidine (NebuPent, Pentam 300) | |

These combination drugs contain an antibiotic drug (trimethoprim) and a sulfonamide anti-infective drug (sulfamethoxazole) for treating *Pneumocystis carinii* pneumonia in AIDS patents.

Bactrim (sulfamethoxazole, trimethoprim)

Septra (sulfamethoxazole, trimethoprim)

### *Mycobacterium avium-intracellulare* Complex Infection Drugs

*Mycobacterium avium-intracellulare* complex (MAC) infection is a common, late-stage complication of AIDS that occurs in about 40 percent of AIDS patients. It is caused by two related bacteria, *Mycobacterium avium* and *Mycobacterium intracellulare,* whose names are often combined. MAC infection affects the intestines and other organs in the body. Drugs used to treat a MAC infection include antituberculosis drugs, macrolide antibiotic drugs, fluoroquinolone antibiotic drugs, aminoglycoside antibiotic drugs, and orphan drugs. At least two of these drugs are used together to treat a MAC infection.

| | |
|---|---|
| amikacin (Amikin) | gentamicin liposomal (Maitec) |
| aminosidine (Gabbromicina) | piritrexim |
| azithromycin (Zithromax) | rifabutin (Mycobutin) |
| ciprofloxacin (Cipro) | rifampin (Rifadin, Rimactane) |
| clarithromycin (Biaxin) | rifapentine (Priftin) |
| ethambutol (Myambutol) | |

## *Did You Know?*

*Mycobacterium tuberculosis,* the bacterium that causes tuberculosis, has a waxy bacterial cell wall that makes it difficult to kill. *Mycobacterium avium* and *Mycobacterium intracellulare* belong to this same category of bacteria. The drug rifabutin, used to treat a MAC infection, is structurally related to the drugs used to treat tuberculosis. Many antituberculosis drugs are used as one of the two drugs needed simultaneously to treat a MAC infection. The drug action of rifabutin against Mycobacterium is reflected in the trade name drug Mycobutin.

## Drugs Used to Treat Other Viral Infections

Antiviral drugs are used to treat infections caused by herpes simplex virus, human papillomavirus, cytomegalovirus, influenza virus, and respiratory syncytial virus.

Topical and oral drugs used to treat herpes simplex virus type 1 (cold sores), herpes simplex virus type 2 (genital herpes), herpes zoster, and the human papillomavirus that causes common warts (verrucae) and genital warts (condylomata acuminata) are discussed in Chapter 17.

### Drugs for Cytomegalovirus Infection

These antiviral drugs are used to prevent cytomegalovirus (CMV) infection in AIDS patients and organ transplant patients. These are immunoglobulin drugs and antiviral drugs.

cytomegalovirus immunoglobulin (CytoGam)

ganciclovir (Cytovene)

valganciclovir (Valcyte)

Drugs used to treat CMV infections of the retina are discussed in Chapter 18.

### Drugs for Influenza Virus Infection

These antiviral drugs are used to prevent or treat influenza A or influenza B infections (the "flu").

| | |
|---|---|
| amantadine (Symmetrel) | rimantadine (Flumadine) |
| influenza virus vaccine (Fluarix, FluMist) | zanamivir (Relenza) |
| oseltamivir (Tamiflu) | |

*Focus on Healthcare Issues*

Flu shots are given prophylactically to prevent influenza. They use either the whole virus, a part of the virus, or a surface antigen from the virus to provoke the body's immune response and create temporary immunity. Annual revaccination is necessary to provide protection against the most current strains of the two most common and dangerous flu families: influenza A and influenza B viruses. Each February, the Centers for Disease Control and Prevention (CDCP) selects those stains of influenza that are most prevalent in Asia and other parts of the world to include in the flu vaccine that will be offered in the United States the following fall before the start of flu season. Flu viruses mutate constantly and create many new subtypes, and so the influenza vaccine must be reformulated every year. Persons who get flu shots can still get the flu from other strains of the influenza virus not included in the flu vaccine.

### Drugs for Respiratory Syncytial Virus Infection

These antiviral drugs are used to prevent and treat respiratory syncytial virus (RSV) infection in hospitalized pediatric patients or those with lung disease.

palivizumab (Synagis)

respiratory syncytial virus immunoglobulin (Hypermune RSV, RespiGam)

ribavirin (Virazole)

## Drugs Used to Treat Fungal and Yeast Infections

Fungi can cause disease topically or systemically. Fungi are related to yeasts and both of these organisms are treated with many of the same antifungal (or antiyeast) drugs. Antifungal drugs act by binding to a specific receptor on the cell membrane of the fungus or yeast, changing the permeability of the membrane, and causing the cellular contents to leak out. Fungi and yeasts are opportunistic organisms that grow most successfully when the patient's immune system is already compromised and under stress. In immunocompromised patients, such as patients with cancer or AIDS or in those who are undergoing bone marrow transplantation, fungal and yeast infections can become widespread and extremely serious.

### Topical Drugs for Fungal Infections

Topical fungal infections of the skin include ringworm, athlete's foot, and jock itch, all of which are caused by the fungus *Tinea*. A fungal infection of the nails (onychomycosis) can be treated topically if the infection has not reached the nailbed. Topical antifungal drugs used to treat these fungal infections are discussed in Chapter 17.

### Oral and Intravenous Drugs for Fungal Infections

When a fungal infection becomes embedded in the nailbed and the nail becomes misshapen, thickened, and discolored, then it must be treated with oral antifungal drugs that act systemically through the blood to reach the tissues around the nail. These oral and intravenous antifungal drugs also act systemically to treat severe fungal infections in other parts of the body, such as aspergellosis, blastomycosis, cryptococcus, and histoplasmosis.

amphotericin B (Fungizone)

caspofungin (Cancidas)

fluconazole (Diflucan) (see ■ FIGURE 20–15)

flucytosine (Ancobon)

griseofulvin (Grifulvin)

itraconazole (Sporanox)

ketoconazole (Nizoral)

posaconazole (Noxafil)

terbinafine (Lamisil)

voriconazole (Vfend)

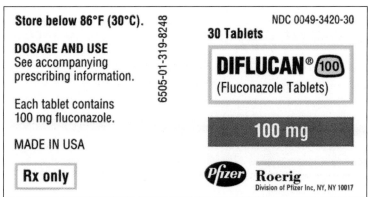

■ **FIGURE 20–15** **Drug label for fluconazole (Diflucan).**
The antifungal drug fluconazole (Diflucan) is given orally (this drug label is for the 100 mg tablet of Diflucan), as well as intravenously to treat severe or even life-threatening fungal infections.

### Drugs for Yeast Infections

Topical yeast infections caused by *Candida* can occur in the mouth. Topical antiyeast drugs used to treat these infections are discussed in Chapter 19.

These antiyeast drugs are given orally and intravenously, and they act systemically to treat severe yeast infections (candidiasis) in the mouth that extend into the esophagus and stomach or are in other parts of the body. Many of the antifungal drugs listed previously are also used to treat systemic yeast infections.

amphotericin B (Fungizone)

anidulafungin (Eraxis)

caspofungin (Cancidas)

fluconazole (Diflucan)

flucytosine (Ancobon)

itraconazole (Sporanox)

ketoconazole (Nizoral)

micafungin (Mycamine)

nystatin (Mycostatin, Nilstat)

posaconazole (Noxafil)

voriconazole (Vfend)

## Drugs Used to Treat Eye Infections

Topical antibiotic drugs used to treat bacterial eye infections are discussed in Chapter 18.

## Drugs Used to Treat Kaposi's Sarcoma

Kaposi's sarcoma is a rare, cancerous condition that affects the skin and other organs in AIDS patients. Drugs used to treat Kaposi's sarcoma are discussed in Chapter 21.

## Drugs Used to Treat Skin Infections

Topical drugs used to treat bacterial, viral, and fungal skin infections are discussed in Chapter 17.

## Drugs Used to Treat Tuberculosis

Drugs used to treat tuberculosis are discussed in Chapter 10.

## Drugs Used to Treat Urinary Tract Infections

Drugs used to treat urinary tract infections are discussed in Chapter 7.

## Drugs Used to Treat Vaginal Yeast Infections

Drugs used to treat vaginal yeast infections are discussed in Chapter 13.

# *Chapter Review*

## Quiz Yourself

1. Describe how sulfonamide drugs exert their therapeutic effect.
2. Describe how some penicillin-resistant bacteria inactivate penicillin.
3. Name at least four different categories of antibiotic drugs.
4. Describe the historical milestones in the development of penicillin.
5. Why are tetracycline antibiotic drugs not given to pregnant women or children under eight years of age?
6. What are two potentially toxic effects of aminoglycoside drugs?
7. Define each of these phrases: *broad spectrum antibiotic, retrovirus, opportunistic infection.*
8. If a patient is allergic to amoxicillin, what other category of antibiotic drugs could also cause an allergic reaction?
9. What is the difference between the three generations of cephalosporin drugs?
10. Why can the antibiotic drug Zithromax be taken just once a day, when other antibiotic drugs need to be taken two or three times a day?
11. What is the consequence of the overprescription of antibiotic drugs and the use of antibiotic drugs in animal feed?
12. Define these abbreviations: *AIDS, HIV, CDCP, MRSA.*
13. How does the HIV virus reproduce in the body?
14. Describe the development of drugs used to treat HIV and AIDS.
15. When does a patient's diagnosis change from HIV to AIDS?
16. Describe several ways antiviral drugs kill or block the human immunodeficiency virus.
17. Why is an AIDS vaccine difficult to develop?
18. Name three opportunistic infections that affect AIDS patients.
19. Describe the relationship between drugs used to treat MAC infection in AIDS patients and antitubercular drugs.
20. What two distinct and very different medical uses does the drug lithium have?
21. What is the history of the drug thalidomide?
22. How and why does the CDCP reformulate the flu vaccine each year?
23. Why are some antifungal drugs also useful in treating yeast infections?

**24.** To what category of drugs does each of these drugs belong?

**a.** amoxicillin (Amoxil, Moxatag)
**b.** azithromycin (Zithromax)
**c.** cefoxitin (Mefoxin)
**d.** ceftriaxone (Rocephin)
**e.** ciprofloxacin (Cipro)
**f.** doxycycline (Vibramycin, Vibra-Tabs)
**g.** efavirenz (Sustiva)
**h.** erythromycin (Eryc, Ery-Tab)

**i.** ketoconazole (Nizoral)
**j.** nalidixic acid (NegGram)
**k.** nelfinavir (Viracept)
**l.** oseltamivir (Tamiflu)
**m.** pentamidine (NebuPent)
**n.** stavudine (Zerit)
**o.** tobramycin (TOBI)
**p.** zidovudine (Retrovir)

## Spelling Tips

| | |
|---|---|
| **BioTropin** | Unusual internal capitalization. |
| **CytoGam** | Unusual internal capitalization. |
| **FluMist** | Unusual internal capitalization. |
| **Gamimune N** | This immunoglobulin drug (spelled with two *m's*) has just one *m*. |
| **NebuPent** | Unusual internal capitalization. |
| **NegGram** | Unusual internal capitalization. |
| **Pfizerpen** | Unusual spelling based on the drug company's name Pfizer. |
| **RespiGam** | Unusual internal capitalization. |
| **TOBI** | Unusual for all capital letters. |
| **VaxSyn** | Unusual internal capitalization. |

## Clinical Applications

**1.** Look at this prescription bag and drug label and answer the following questions.
   **a.** What two antibiotic drugs are included in this one prescription combination drug?
   **b.** If this prescription had been filled with the trade name drug, what would its name be?

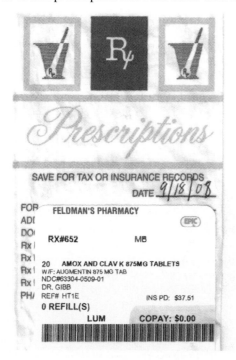

2. Look at these two drug labels and answer the following questions.
   a. To what category of antibiotic drugs do both of these drugs belong?
   b. Besides the difference in the color of the drug labels, name three main differences between these two drugs as seen on these drug labels.

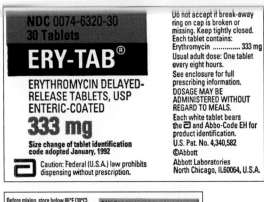

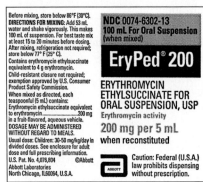

3. Look at these two handwritten prescriptions and give the name of the drug and the dose prescribed for each one.

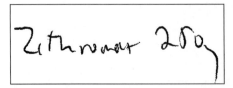

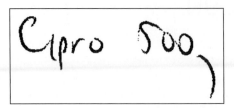

**4.** Look at this drug label and answer the following questions.
    **a.** What is the name of this generic drug?
    **b.** What is the trade name associated with it?
    **c.** To what category of drugs does it belong?
    **d.** In what drug form and dose strength does it come?

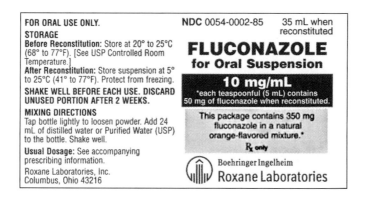

FOR ORAL USE ONLY.
**STORAGE**
**Before Reconstitution:** Store at 20° to 25°C (68° to 77°F). [See USP Controlled Room Temperature.]
**After Reconstitution:** Store suspension at 5° to 25°C (41° to 77°F). Protect from freezing.
**SHAKE WELL BEFORE EACH USE. DISCARD UNUSED PORTION AFTER 2 WEEKS.**
**MIXING DIRECTIONS**
Tap bottle lightly to loosen powder. Add 24 mL of distilled water or Purified Water (USP) to the bottle. Shake well.
**Usual Dosage:** See accompanying prescribing information.
Roxane Laboratories, Inc.
Columbus, Ohio 43216

NDC 0054-0002-85    35 mL when reconstituted
**FLUCONAZOLE**
**for Oral Suspension**
**10 mg/mL**
*each teaspoonful (5 mL) contains 50 mg of fluconazole when reconstituted.
This package contains 350 mg fluconazole in a natural orange-flavored mixture.*
R̠ only
Boehringer Ingelheim
**Roxane Laboratories**

**5.** Look at this handwritten prescription and answer the following questions.
    **a.** What is the name of the prescribed drug?
    **b.** Is this a generic name or a trade name?
    **c.** To what category of drugs does this drug belong?
    **d.** What dose and what drug form are prescribed?
    **e.** Translate the rest of the prescription into English words.

**PAT SMITH, M.D.**
27 Oak Leaf Lane
Baltimore, MD  12121
Phone:  322 –7890

Name *Donna Bell*
Address *27 Windsor Place*
*Balto, MD. 12121*  Age  *26*

**R**x

*Ampicillin 250 mg Caps*
*Disp. #30*
*Sig: + cap QID for*
*urinary infection*

721723
11/28/01

[  ] Contents are labeled
    unless checked

May be refilled 0 ① 2  3  4

Signed *T. Smith*  M.D.

Date  *11 / 27*  20 *01* DEA No. *AS1522209*

**6.** Look at this drug label and answer the following questions.
   **a.** What is the generic name of this drug?
   **b.** What is the trade name of this drug?
   **c.** To what category of drugs does it belong?
   **d.** What disease is it used to treat?
   **e.** What is the drug form and the dose strength?

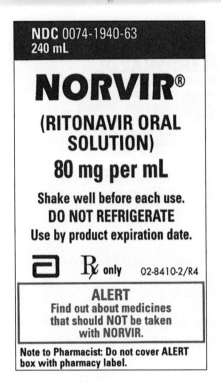

**NDC** 0074-1940-63
240 mL

# NORVIR®

## (RITONAVIR ORAL SOLUTION)

## 80 mg per mL

Shake well before each use.
**DO NOT REFRIGERATE**
Use by product expiration date.

℞ only    02-8410-2/R4

**ALERT**
Find out about medicines
that should **NOT** be taken
with **NORVIR**.

**Note to Pharmacist: Do not cover ALERT
box with pharmacy label.**

## Multimedia Extension Exercises

■ Go to www.pearsonhighered.com/turley and click on the photo of the cover of *Understanding Pharmacology for Health Professionals* to access the interactive Companion Website created for this textbook.

# Chemotherapy Drugs

## CHAPTER CONTENTS

## Learning Objectives

After you study this chapter, you should be able to

1. Name several main categories of chemotherapy drugs.

2. Compare and contrast the therapeutic effects of antimetabolite chemotherapy drugs, alkylating chemotherapy drugs, and demethylating chemotherapy drugs.

3. Describe how the therapeutic effect of antibiotic chemotherapy drugs differs from that of regular antibiotic drugs.

4. Explain why hormonal chemotherapy drugs are only used to treat certain types of cancer.

5. Compare and contrast the therapeutic effects of mitosis inhibitor chemotherapy drugs, platinum chemotherapy drugs, chemotherapy enzyme drugs, and retinoid chemotherapy drugs.

6. Compare and contrast the therapeutic effects of interleukin, interferon, monoclonal antibody chemotherapy drugs, and immunomodulator chemotherapy drugs.

7. Explain the role that corticosteroid drugs play in treating cancer.

8. Explain how cancer is treated with a vaccine.

9. Describe the advantages of using a chemotherapy protocol to treat cancer.

10. Describe the types of drugs used to treat the side effects and toxicity of chemotherapy drugs.

11. Given the generic and trade names of a chemotherapy drug, identify the drug category to which they belong.

12. Given a chemotherapy drug category, identify several generic and trade name drugs in that category.

A **neoplasm** is a new growth of cells that may be benign or malignant. All malignant neoplasms are classified as **cancer**, a Latin word meaning *crab,* because cancer metastasizes or spreads outward from the original site like the legs of a crab. Uncontrolled cell division and metastasis to other parts of the body are identifying characteristics of cancer cells. As cancerous cells invade tissues and organs, normal function is compromised and sometimes impaired to the point of death, unless treatment with surgery, radiation, or chemotherapy drugs is begun.

## Did You Know?

Cancer cells are the anarchists of the body, for they know no law, pay no regard for the commonwealth, serve no useful function, and cause disharmony and death in their surrounds.

Michael Gerald, *Pharmacology: An Introduction to Drugs,* 2nd ed. Englewood Cliffs, NJ: Prentice Hall, 1981, p. 574, out of print.

To properly treat any type of cancer, the physician must determine two things: the type of cancer and the stage of the cancer. To determine the type of cancer, a biopsy is taken from the tumor site or a blood specimen is drawn to examine blood cells. The extent of cancer progression is referred to as the **stage**. The stage indicates whether or not the cancer has spread beyond the original or primary site and metastasized to secondary sites, such as regional lymph nodes or other parts of the body. The selection of appropriate chemotherapy drugs is based on the type of cancer and the stage of the cancer. A treatment that is appropriate for one type of cancer is usually not appropriate for a different type of cancer and may not even be appropriate for the same cancer that has progressed to a more advanced stage. Only when the type of cancer and its stage has been determined can the physician select an appropriate chemotherapy drug treatment regimen.

Drugs used to treat cancers or malignant neoplasms are known as *chemotherapy drugs* or *antineoplastic drugs.* Chemotherapy drugs are most effective when initiated during the early stages of cancer when there are fewer cancer cells present in the body. Most chemotherapy drugs exert their effect against rapidly dividing cancer cells.

However, some normal cells in the body also divide rapidly—cells lining the GI tract, hair cells, and blood cells. These normal cells are greatly affected by chemotherapy, with resulting inflammation of the mouth and GI tract, loss of hair, and decreased numbers of RBCs and WBCs. Other chemotherapy drugs—targeted chemotherapy—target their effects against gene mutations that are only found in cancer cells.

**Adjuvant therapy** refers to chemotherapy (or radiation therapy) that is given to cancer patients after they have had surgery to remove a tumor. The purpose of adjuvant therapy is to aid in eradicating any remaining tumor cells. The word *adjuvant* is taken from a Latin word meaning *aiding.*

A **remission** occurs when cancerous cells stop actively reproducing. Some cancer patients experience a complete remission following chemotherapy, others have a partial remission, but some patients actually experience tumor growth while being treated with chemotherapy. When the tumor size increases or new metastatic lesions appear despite chemotherapy, the patient is said to have failed chemotherapy. A new combination of chemotherapy drugs may then be tried.

## Did You Know?

At the time of diagnosis of acute leukemia, 1 trillion cancer cells are generally present and widely distributed throughout the body of the patient. If an antileukemic drug were able to kill 99.9 percent of those cells, the patient would show symptomatic improvement even though he or she would still harbor 1 billion cancer cells.

Michael Gerald, *Pharmacology: An Introduction to Drugs,* 2nd ed. Englewood Cliffs, NJ: Prentice Hall, 1981, p. 574, out of print.

Chemotherapy drugs include antimetabolite chemotherapy drugs, alkylating chemotherapy drugs, demethylating chemotherapy drugs, chemotherapy antibiotic drugs, hormonal chemotherapy drugs, mitosis inhibitor chemotherapy drugs, platinum chemotherapy drugs, chemotherapy enzyme drugs, retinoid chemotherapy drugs, interleukin chemotherapy drugs, interferon chemotherapy drugs, monoclonal antibody drugs, as well as many chemotherapy drugs that do not fit into specific categories.

## Antimetabolite Chemotherapy Drugs

Antimetabolite chemotherapy drugs act against metabolites, important byproducts produced from other substances in the cell during the process of metabolism. These metabolites are active in the production of cellular DNA. Antimetabolite chemotherapy drugs work during cell division in one of two ways: They take the place of an important metabolite, or they block an enzyme that produces an important metabolite. This disrupts cell metabolism and the cancer cell dies. Antimetabolite chemotherapy drugs target rapidly dividing cells, such as cancer cells, that have a high rate of metabolism. The category of antimetabolite chemotherapy drugs includes purine analog chemotherapy drugs, pyrimidine analog chemotherapy drugs, and folic acid blocker chemotherapy drugs.

### Purine Analog Chemotherapy Drugs

Purine is a molecule that forms the base upon which adenine and guanine are built. These two substances are important components of the DNA molecule in each cell. An **analog** is a drug that is created by slightly modifying the molecular structure of another substance (in this case, a purine). Purine analog chemotherapy drugs take the place of the purine base structure, and so the normal metabolites (adenine, guanine) cannot be built, DNA cannot be produced, and the cancer cell cannot divide. These drugs are used to treat different types of leukemia.

cladribine (Leustatin)          mercaptopurine (Purinethol)

clofarabine (Clolar)            pentostatin (Nipent)

fludarabine (Fludara)           thioguanine (Tabloid)

### Pyrimidine Analog Chemotherapy Drugs

Pyrimidine is a molecule that forms the base upon which cytosine, thymine, and uracil are built. These three substances are important components of the DNA molecule. Pyrimidine analog chemotherapy drugs take the place of the pyrimidine base structure, and so the normal metabolites (cytosine, thymine, uracil) cannot be built, DNA cannot be produced, and the cancer cell cannot divide. These drugs are used to treat many different types of cancer.

capecitabine (Xeloda)           fluorouracil (Adrucil)
  (see ■ FIGURE 21–1)        gemcitabine (Gemzar)

cytarabine (DepoCyt, Tarabine)  troxacitabine (Troxatyl)

floxuridine (FUDR)

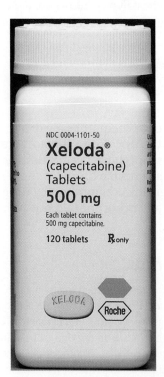

■ **FIGURE 21–1 Capecitabine (Xeloda).**
This pyrimidine analog chemotherapy drug is used to treat cancer of the breast, colon, and rectum.

## Did You Know?

The pyrimidine analog chemotherapy drug cytarabine was developed from a substance found in Caribbean sea sponges.

# Drug Alert!

Although fluorouracil is used to treat many types of cancers, it is also used topically under the trade name Efudex to treat some noncancerous conditions of the skin. When you see that a patient is on topical fluorouracil, do not automatically conclude that the patient has a cancerous skin condition. Fluorouracil is not used topically to treat skin cancer; it is used to treat actinic keratoses (roughened areas of skin due to chronic exposure to the sun) and condylomata acuminata (genital warts).

## Folic Acid Blocker Chemotherapy Drugs

Folic acid is a B vitamin whose metabolite is important in DNA production in the cell. Folic acid blocker chemotherapy drugs act as antagonists in that they compete with folic acid for the same enzyme. This enzyme normally changes folic acid into the metabolite that carries purine to a forming DNA molecule. Without the folic acid metabolite, purine is not available, DNA cannot be produced, and the cancer cell cannot divide. These drugs are used to treat many different types of cancer.

methotrexate (Trexall) (see ▣ **FIGURE 21–2**)

pemetrexed (Alimta)

trimetrexate (Neutrexin)

*Note:* The suffixes -*trexate* and -*trexed* are common to generic folic acid blocker chemotherapy drugs.

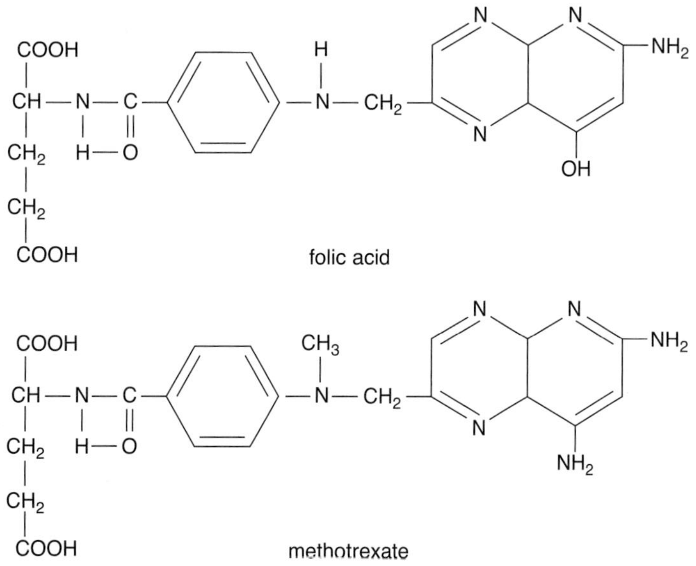

▣ **FIGURE 21–2 Chemical structures of folic acid and methotrexate.**
Folic acid blocker chemotherapy drugs, such as methotrexate, are very similar in chemical structure to folic acid, the B vitamin whose action they block.

## Alkylating Chemotherapy Drugs

Alkylating chemotherapy drugs cause alkylation, a chemical reaction in which an alkyl group from the chemotherapy drug is substituted for a hydrogen molecule in DNA and/or RNA. This causes abnormal cross-linking in the DNA strands, and the cancer cell cannot divide. The category of alkylating chemotherapy drugs includes nitrogen mustard chemotherapy drugs, nitrosourea chemotherapy drugs, and other alkylating chemotherapy drugs.

### Nitrogen Mustard Chemotherapy Drugs

Nitrogen mustard chemotherapy drugs insert an alkyl group into the DNA. This causes cross-linking to occur in the strands of DNA, DNA cannot be produced, and the cancer cell cannot divide. These drugs are used to treat many different types of cancer.

bendamustine (Treanda)

chlorambucil (Leukeran)

cyclophosphamide (Cytoxan, Neosar)

estramustine (Emcyt)

ifosfamide (Ifex)

mechlorethamine (Mustargen)

melphalan (Alkeran)

### *Historical Notes*

In the early 1900s, the only treatments available for cancer were surgical excision and radiation therapy. The discovery of the first chemotherapy drug, nitrogen mustard, came about serendipitously. During the 1940s, researchers who were reviewing medical records from World War I noticed that Allied soldiers who were exposed to the chemical weapon nitrogen mustard gas had a decreased level of WBCs. It was thought that this adverse effect could be used as a therapeutic effect in patients with leukemia whose WBC counts were abnormally elevated. Nitrogen mustard (the drug mechlorethamine) and its derivative drugs are still used to treat leukemia today.

### Nitrosourea Chemotherapy Drugs

Nitrosourea chemotherapy drugs insert an alkyl group into both DNA and RNA. DNA and RNA cannot be produced and the cancer cell cannot divide. These drugs also inhibit enzymes within the cell. These drugs are used to treat many different types of cancer.

carmustine (BiCNU, Gliadel)

lomustine (CeeNU)

Sarmustine

streptozocin (Zanosar)

### Other Alklyating Chemotherapy Drugs

These alkylating chemotherapy drugs insert an alkyl group into the DNA, but they also have other effects as well that prevent the cancer cell from dividing. These drugs are used to treat many different types of cancer.

altretamine (Hexalen)

busulfan (Myleran)

dacarbazine (DTIC-Dome)

procarbazine (Matulane)

temozolomide (Temodar)

thiotepa (Thioplex)

## Demethylating Chemotherapy Drugs

Demethylating chemotherapy drugs inhibit the enzyme methyltransferase. This enzyme normally transfers a methyl group and inserts it into DNA (a process known as methylation) during cell division. Demethylating chemotherapy drugs inhibit this enzyme. Because the DNA lacks a methyl group, the cell cannot divide and this particularly affects rapidly dividing cancer cells. These drugs also have a direct cytotoxic effect on abnormal blood cells in the bone marrow. These drugs are used to treat leukemia or lymphoma.

azacitidine (Vidaza)

decitabine (Dacogen)

nelarabine (Arranon)

*Note:* The suffixes *-bine* and *-dine* are common to demethylating chemotherapy drugs.

## Chemotherapy Antibiotic Drugs

Chemotherapy antibiotic drugs are not interchangeable with regular antibiotic drugs. Regular antibiotic drugs that are used to treat infection act on the cell walls of bacteria. Human cells, which do not have a cell wall (they only have a cell membrane), are not affected by antibiotic drugs that treat bacterial infections. However, unlike regular antibiotic drugs, chemotherapy antibiotic drugs do affect human cells. Chemotherapy antibiotic drugs inhibit the production of DNA, RNA, and some cellular proteins. Some of these drugs block the enzyme that normally splits each DNA strand into two strands prior to cell division. Chemotherapy antibiotic drugs are used to treat many different types of cancer.

| | |
|---|---|
| bleomycin (Blenoxane) | epirubicin (Ellence) |
| dactinomycin (Cosmegen) | idarubicin (Idamycin) |
| daunorubicin (Cerubidine) | mitomycin (Mutamycin) |
| doxorubicin (Adriamycin)<br>(see ■ FIGURE 21–3) | valrubicin (Valstar) |

*Note:* The suffixes *-rubicin* and *-mycin* are common to generic chemotherapy antibiotic drugs.

## *Historical Notes*

In the 1950s, Italian researchers extracted the drug doxorubicin from a fungus-like bacterium found in the soil near an ancient castle in Italy. This bacterium produces a bright red pigment. French researchers discovered it at the same time. Together, both groups decided on a name for the drug: daunorubicin, which was taken from *Dauni* (an ancient people that lived in that region of Italy) and *rubis* (the French word for *ruby*). Italian researchers then modified the original molecular structure and created the new generic drug doxorubicin, and assigned it the trade name Adriamycin (named for the Adriatic Sea off the coast of Italy).

## *Drug Alert!*

Some chemotherapy drugs have older drug names that were used during clinical trials before the generic and trade name drugs were marketed. Such is the case for dactinomycin (which was formerly known as *actinomycin D*), cisplatin (which was formerly known as *cis-platinum*), and for many other chemotherapy drugs.

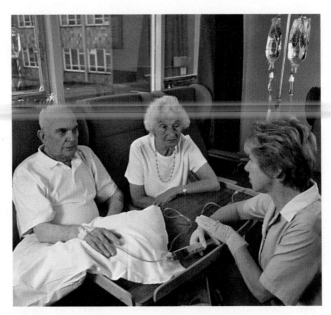

**▧ FIGURE 21–3 Intravenous administration of doxorubicin (Adriamycin).**
This elderly man is receiving an intravenous dose of doxorubicin (Adriamycin). He already has a continuously running intravenous line in place (see intravenous bags in the upper right hand corner). The nurse is administering this drug according to the drug instructions which say that the drug is not to be inserted into the intravenous bag (because the dose would be diluted and it would take several hours for the drug to reach the patient), but is to be given directly into the intravenous tubing, slowly, as a single dose over about 5 minutes. Most intravenous drugs are clear, but doxorubicin has a unique red color. Doxorubicin is used to treat many different types of cancer.

## Hormonal Chemotherapy Drugs

Certain cancers need hormones to grow, particularly cancers that arise from tissues that are influenced by the male sex hormone testosterone or by the female sex hormones estradiol and progesterone. These cancers have receptors on the surface of their cells for those hormones, and the growth of these cancers is stimulated by those hormones. Chemotherapy drugs used to treat these cancers block the effect of those hormones or surround the cancer cells with a hormone that has the opposite hormonal effect. The category of hormonal chemotherapy drugs includes androgen hormonal chemotherapy drugs, antiandrogen hormonal chemotherapy drugs, estrogen hormonal chemotherapy drugs, antiestrogen hormonal chemotherapy drugs, progestin hormonal chemotherapy drugs, gonadotropin-releasing hormone chemotherapy drugs, aromatase inhibitor hormonal chemotherapy drugs, and other hormonal chemotherapy drugs.

### Androgen Hormonal Chemotherapy Drugs

Androgen hormonal chemotherapy drugs act in a similar way to that of the main male (androgen) hormone testosterone, which is produced by the testicles. Androgen hormonal chemotherapy drugs are used to treat breast cancer in females because they create a male hormone environment, which is the opposite from what the breast cancer cells need to grow. These are Schedule III drugs.

fluoxymesterone (Androxy)

methyltestosterone (Testred, Virilon)

testosterone (Delatestryl)

*Note:* The suffix *-terone* is common to generic androgen hormonal chemotherapy drugs.

### Antiandrogen Hormonal Chemotherapy Drugs

Antiandrogen hormonal chemotherapy drugs bind to and block receptors in prostate gland tissue that are normally stimulated by testosterone. With the effect of testosterone blocked, the prostate gland cancer cannot grow.

bicalutamide (Casodex)

flutamide

nilutamide (Nilandron)

*Note:* The suffix *-lutamide* is common to generic antiandrogen hormonal chemotherapy drugs.

### Estrogen Hormonal Chemotherapy Drugs

Estrogen hormonal chemotherapy drugs act in a similar way to that of the main female hormone estradiol, which is produced by follicles of the ovary. Estrogen hormonal chemotherapy drugs are used to provide **palliative treatment** for advanced breast cancer and/or advanced prostate cancer. Palliative treatment provides relief from symptoms but is not intended to cure.

conjugated estrogens (Premarin)      estradiol (Delestrogen, Estrace)

esterified estrogens (Menest)      raloxifene (Evista)

## *Focus on Healthcare Issues*

Raloxifene (Evista) is advertised on the television as the only drug that is able to prevent and treat osteoporosis and, at the same time, prevent breast cancer in postmenopausal women who are at high risk for developing breast cancer. Research studies show that this drug decreased the risk of breast cancer by 44 percent; however, it increased the risk of a fatal stroke from a blood clot by 49 percent, according to the July 13, 2006, issue of *The New England Journal of Medicine*.

### Antiestrogen Hormonal Chemotherapy Drugs

Antiestrogen hormonal chemotherapy drugs bind to and block receptors in breast tissue that are normally stimulated by estradiol. With the effect of estradiol blocked, the breast cancer cannot grow.

fulvestrant (Faslodex)

tamoxifen (Soltamox)

toremifene (Fareston)

## *Did You Know?*

Tamoxifen is also given prophylactically to women who are at high risk for developing breast cancer before they develop breast cancer.

## Progestin Hormonal Chemotherapy Drugs

Progestin hormonal chemotherapy drugs act in a similar way to that of the female hormone progesterone, which is produced by the corpus luteum of the ovary. Progestin hormonal chemotherapy drugs are used to treat breast cancer in females because they contain a different female hormone than the estradiol that the breast cancer needs to grow.

medroxyprogesterone (Depo-Provera, Provera) (see ■ **FIGURE 21–4**)

megestrol (Megace)

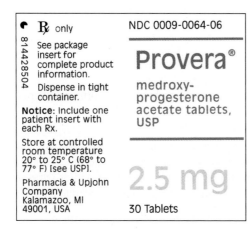

■ **FIGURE 21–4  Drug label for medroxyprogesterone (Provera).**
This progestin hormonal chemotherapy drug is used to treat breast cancer, but it is also used to treat abnormal uterine bleeding in women who do not have cancer.

## Gonadotropin-Releasing Hormone Chemotherapy Drugs

These drugs are a synthetic reproduction (analog) of the body's own gonadotropin-releasing hormone (GnRH). Normally, GnRH is produced by the hypothalamus, and its action causes the anterior pituitary gland to secrete luteinizing hormone. Luteinizing hormone then stimulates the testes in men to produce testosterone and the ovaries in women to produce estradiol and progesterone. Gonadotropin-releasing hormone chemotherapy drugs compete with GnRH and block GnRH receptors on the anterior pituitary gland, so that the anterior pituitary gland is not stimulated to secrete luteinizing hormone. Without luteinizing hormone, the testes do not produce testosterone and the ovaries do not produce estradiol or progesterone. Without testosterone, prostate gland cancer cannot grow. Without estradiol, breast and ovarian cancers cannot grow.

| | |
|---|---|
| abarelix (Plenaxis) | leuprolide (Eligard, Lupron) |
| goserelin (Zoladex) | triptorelin (Trelstar) |
| histrelin (Vantas) | |

*Note:* The suffixes *-lide, -relin,* and *-relix* are common to these generic chemotherapy drugs.

## Aromatase Inhibitor Hormonal Chemotherapy Drugs

During menopause, the level of estradiol secreted by the ovaries declines. The main source of estradiol in postmenopausal women is androgens from the adrenal glands which are converted by the enzyme aromatase to estrone and then to estradiol. Aromatase inhibitor chemotherapy drugs bind to the enzyme aromatase and hinder its action, and so estradiol is not produced. Without estradiol, the breast cancer cells cannot grow. Some, but not all, of these drugs are also used to treat cancer of the prostate gland in men, because they produce the opposite hormonal environment from what the prostate gland cancer needs to grow.

anastrozole (Arimidex)    letrozole (Femara)

exemestane (Aromasin)    testolactone

### Other Hormonal Chemotherapy Drugs

These drugs inhibit other hormones normally produced by the body. Mitotane inhibits corticosteroid hormones secreted by the adrenal gland and is used to treat cancer of the cortex of the adrenal gland. Thyrotropin alfa is derived from thyroid-stimulating hormone (which is produced by the anterior pituitary gland). Thyrotropin alfa is used to treat thyroid cancer.

mitotane (Lysodren)

thyrotropin alfa (Thyrogen)

## Mitosis Inhibitor Chemotherapy Drugs

Mitosis inhibitor chemotherapy drugs act at very specific times during the early stages of **mitosis** (the process of cell division). Mitosis inhibitor drugs affect dividing cells and keep them from completing the process of cell division. These drugs have their greatest effect on cells that divide often, so their effect is felt more on cancer cells than on normal cells. The category of mitosis inhibitor chemotherapy drugs includes podophyllotoxin chemotherapy drugs, topoisomerase chemotherapy drugs, taxane chemotherapy drugs, vinca alkaloid chemotherapy drugs, and other mitosis inhibitor chemotherapy drugs.

### Podophyllotoxin Chemotherapy Drugs

Podophyllotoxin chemotherapy drugs are semisynthetic drugs created from a toxin found in the fleshy root of the Mayapple, whose scientific name is *Podophyllum peltatum*. During cell division, these drugs keep new DNA from being formed, break strands of DNA, or cause DNA strands to abnormally cross-link to each other so the cancer cell cannot divide. Etoposide is used to treat many different types of cancer, but teniposide is only used to treat leukemia and non-Hodgkin's lymphoma.

etoposide (Etopophos, VePesid)

teniposide (Vumon)

*Note:* The suffix *-poside* is common to generic podophyllotoxin chemotherapy drugs.

### Topoisomerase Inhibitor Chemotherapy Drugs

Topoisomerase inhibitor chemotherapy drugs affect the enzyme topoisomerase. This enzyme normally relieves the twisting stress on the spiral strands of DNA by creating a break in a single strand so that the strands can separate and be copied during cell division. This break is repaired later in the process. Topoisomerase inhibitor chemotherapy drugs bind to the enzyme topoisomerase and prevent the enzyme from creating the initial break in the DNA strand, and so the cancer cell cannot divide. These drugs are used to treat many different types of cancer.

irinotecan (Camptosar)

mitoxantrone (Novantrone)

topotecan (Hycamtin)

### Taxane Chemotherapy Drugs

Taxane chemotherapy drugs disrupt the microtubular network in the cytoplasm of the cell during cell division. As a cell divides, centrioles migrate to either end of the cell and microtubules form spindle fibers that radiate from the centrioles and connect the chromosomes. Taxane chemotherapy drugs allow the microtubules to form, but the microtubules do not function properly, and the cancer cell cannot divide. These drugs are used to treat many different types of cancer.

docetaxel (Taxotere)

paclitaxel (Taxol) (see ■ **FIGURE 21–5**)

*Note:* The suffix -*taxel* is common to generic taxane chemotherapy drugs.

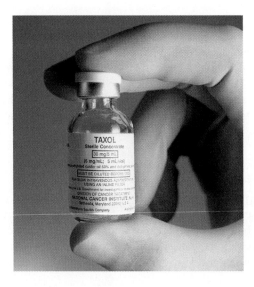

■ **FIGURE 21–5  Vial of paclitaxel (Taxol).**
This vial contains the liquid chemotherapy drug paclitaxel (Taxol). This drug is given intravenously. The healthcare professional will insert a needle into the rubber-stopper top of the vial and use a syringe to remove the prescribed dose of this chemotherapy drug.

## Did You Know?

The taxane chemotherapy drugs are so named because they were originally derived from an extract of the bark of the Pacific yew tree whose scientific name is *Taxus brevifolia*. Paclitaxel was the first of the taxane chemotherapy drugs. This yew tree, which only grows in the Pacific Northwest, is small and grows slowly, and collection of the bark kills the tree. Now, the needles of European and Himalayan yews are used because they contain 10 times more paclitaxel and harvesting of the needles does not kill the trees.

### Vinca Alkaloid Chemotherapy Drugs

Vinca alkaloid chemotherapy drugs interfere with the production of DNA and RNA and also interfere with cellular metabolism and the production of the energy need to complete cell division. They also bind to tubulin in the microtubules, and the cancer cell cannot divide. These drugs are used to treat many different types of cancer.

vinblastine (Velban)

vincristine (Vincasar)

vinorelbine (Navelbine)

*Note:* The suffixes *-bine* and *-tine* are common to generic vinca alkaloid chemotherapy drugs.

## Did You Know?

Vinblastine and vincristine are extracted from the Madagascar rosy periwinkle plant. The scientific name for this common evergreen ground-cover plant is *Vinca rosea*. It takes over 6 tons of periwinkle leaves to produce 1 ounce of drug.

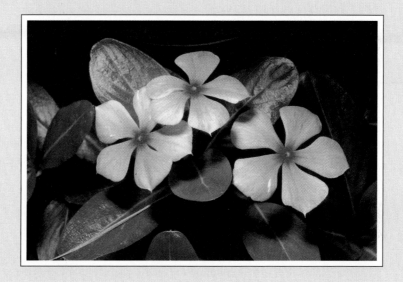

### Other Mitosis Inhibitor Chemotherapy Drugs

This drug ixabepilone belongs to the group of epothilone mitosis inhibitor chemotherapy drugs. Ixabepilone is the only drug in this group. This drug is used to treat breast cancer.

ixabepilone (Ixempra)

## Platinum Chemotherapy Drugs

Platinum chemotherapy drugs contain the precious metal platinum. Platinum chemotherapy drugs create cross-links in DNA strands, and the cancer cell cannot divide. These drugs are used to treat many different types of cancers.

carboplatin (Paraplatin)

cisplatin

oxaliplatin (Eloxatin)

*Note:* The suffix *-platin* is common to generic platinum chemotherapy drugs.

## Did You Know?

Platinum is a precious metal that is mostly mined in South Africa. It takes 10 tons of ore to produce 1 ounce of platinum. Cisplatin was the first of the platinum chemotherapy drugs. It was discovered when a researcher at Michigan State University was studying whether bacteria could multiply in an electrical field. He placed platinum electrodes that would conduct electricity into a solution of bacteria. When the electrical field was turned on, the bacteria did not multiply, but they also did not multiply when the electrical field was turned off. He found that it was the platinum in the electrodes that was toxic to the bacteria. This ability to stop a cell from dividing was later applied to the treatment of cancer. The generic drug name cisplatin was approved by the FDA in 1978. The drug was originally known as *cis-platinum* because it was in the *cis* isomer form of the platinum molecule. (When specific functional groups of a molecule are both located on the same side of the molecule, this is a *cis* isomer, but when those groups are located on opposite sides of the molecule, that is the *trans* isomer.).

## Chemotherapy Enzyme Drugs

Chemotherapy enzymes drugs are enzymes that break down the amino acid asparagine. Human cells can synthesize their own supply of asparagine, and so asparagine is not one of the eight essential amino acids that the body needs to produce protein. Leukemia cells, however, cannot synthesize their own asparagine. By breaking down asparagine, the chemotheraphy drug deprives the cancer cell of asparagine, and the cell cannot build protein or divide. These chemotherapy drugs are used to treat leukemia.

> asparaginase (Elspar)
>
> erwinia L-asparaginase (Erwinase)
>
> pegaspargase (Oncaspar)

*Note:* The suffix *-ase* is common to generic chemotherapy enzyme drugs (and to all enzymes).

## Did You Know?

Asparaginase is derived from the common intestinal bacterium *Escherichia coli* (*E. coli*) that causes most urinary tract infections. Cancer patients who are hypersensitive to asparaginase can be treated with pegaspargase, a modified form of asparaginase that contains polyethylene glycol (PEG).

## Retinoid Chemotherapy Drugs

Retinoid chemotherapy drugs are structurally related to vitamin A (retinoic acid). Normally, vitamin A regulates cell differentiation and growth, particularly in the skin. Retinoid chemotherapy drugs bind to vitamin A receptors on cancer cells and help them become more normal in their cell differentiation and growth. Alitretinoin is used topically to treat the cancerous skin lesions of T-cell lymphoma and Kaposi's sarcoma. Bexarotene comes as both a topical and oral drug and is used to treat the cancerous skin lesions of T-cell lymphoma. Tretinoin is given orally; it helps white blood cells to mature and is used to maintain a remission in patients who have already been treated for leukemia.

alitretinoin (Panretin)

bexarotene (Targretin)

tretinoin (Vesanoid)

## *Did You Know?*

The generic drug tretinoin is also available as a topical drug. As the trade name drug Retin-A, it is used topically to treat acne vulgaris. As the trade name drug Renova, it is used topically to treat skin wrinkles.

In 2005, *ABC World News Tonight* reported that researchers had found that 1,000 mg of vitamin D per day could prevent cancer of the breast, ovaries, and uterus in women and cancer of the prostate gland in men. In 2007, the same television show reported that a vitamin D deficiency allowed cancer cells to grow. Vitamin D deficiency is widespread because people spend less time in the sun and, when they do, they wear sunscreen, which prevents the rays of the sun from generating vitamin D in the skin.

## Interleukin Chemotherapy Drugs

Interleukins are proteins that are secreted by white blood cells when they encounter bacteria or antigens. Interleukins act as a signal that tells the immune system to produce more white blood cells to combat the infection or inflammation. (The prefix *inter-* means *between,* the combining form *leuk/o-* means *white,* and the suffix *-in* means *substance* because interleukins are a substance that communicates between white blood cells in the blood and those being formed in the bone marrow). This interleukin chemotherapy drug is used to treat many different types of cancer.

aldesleukin (Proleukin, Teceleukin)

## Interferon Chemotherapy Drugs

Interferon is an immunomodulator chemical that is released by a cell when it is invaded by a virus. Interferon stimulates the surrounding cells to produce certain proteins that prevent the virus from spreading. Interferon chemotherapy drugs are manufactured by recombinant DNA technology and are used to treat many different types of viral diseases and cancer.

interferon alfa-1b

interferon alfa-2b (Intron A)

interferon beta-1a (Avonex, Rebif)

interferon gamma-1b (Actimmune)

peginterferon alfa-2a (Pegasys)

peginterferon alfa-2b (PEG-Intron)

## Monoclonal Antibody Drugs

Monoclonal antibody (MAb) drugs are created using recombinant DNA technology. This process takes human antibodies and modifies them so that they selectively bind to specific antigens on the surface of cancer cells. As the monoclonal antibody combines with the antigen, it destroys the cancer cell. These drugs are used to treat many different types of cancer.

| | |
|---|---|
| alemtuzumab (Campath) | nimotuzumab |
| bevacizumab (Avastin) | Ovarex |
| catumaxomab (Removab) | panitumumab (Vectibix) |
| Cea-Cide | Panorex |
| cetuximab (Erbitux) | rituximab (Rituxan) |
| oprutuzumab (LymphoCIDE) | siplizumab |
| gemtuzumab (Mylotarg) | Theragyn |
| lintuzumab (Zamyl) | trastuzumab (Herceptin) |
| Melimmune | |

*Note:* The suffix *-mab* is common to generic monoclonal antibody drugs and represents the abbreviation for *monoclonal antibody* (MAb).

### Combination Monoclonal Antibody Drugs

These combination drugs contain a monoclonal antibody drug (ibritumomab, murine MAb Lym-1, tositumomab) and the same monoclonal antibody drug labeled with a radioactive isotope (indium-111, iodine-131, yttrium-90). The monoclonal antibody drug binds to specific antigens on the surface of a cancer cell and kills the cell. The radioactive monoclonal antibody drug has the same effect, but brings with it a lethal dose of radiation to kill the cancer cell. These drugs are only used to treat non-Hodgkin's lymphoma.

Bexxar (tositumomab, iodine-131)
Oncolym (murine monoclonal antibody Lym-1, iodine-131)
Zevalin (ibritumomab, indium-111, yttrium-90)

## Immunomodulator Chemotherapy Drugs

Immunomodulator chemotherapy drugs modulate or regulate the immune system. They are active against cancer cells, but also inhibit inflammation and the formation of new blood vessels. These drugs are used to treat multiple myeloma. Thalidomide is also used to treat other types of cancer.

lenalidomide (Revlimid)
thalidomide (Thalomid)

### Did You Know?

After the drug thalidomide was used to treat morning sickness in pregnant women in Europe and caused the severe birth defect of phocomelia ("seal limbs") in their babies, it was withdrawn from the market. It would have become an obscure footnote in medical history but, in 1997, it was discovered to be useful in treating cancer, AIDS, and leprosy. Thalidomide is also used to treat graft-versus-host disease after bone marrow transplantation in patients with leukemia.

Other immunomodulator drugs are commonly used to treat noncancerous diseases in which the immune system is attacking the body's own cells (diseases such as rheumatoid arthritis, multiple sclerosis, psoriasis, and Crohn's disease).

## Protein-Tyrosine Kinase Inhibitor Chemotherapy Drugs

Protein-tyrosine kinase inhibitor chemotherapy drugs block the enzyme protein-tyrosine kinase and other kinases that play a role in cell growth. An abnormal version of the tyrosine kinase enzyme was found to be produced by the Philadelphia chromosome (see the In Depth feature) in patients with a certain type of leukemia. Protein-tyrosine kinase inhibitor chemotherapy drugs block this enzyme, and the cancer cell cannot divide. Dasatinib and imatinib are used to treat leukemia. Sunitinib is used to treat stomach and kidney cancer. Sorafenib inhibits protein-tyrosine kinase as well as other types of kinases and is categorized as a multikinase inhibitor chemotherapy drug. It is used to treat cancer of the liver and kidney. Tipifarnib and vandetanib inhibit several different kinases. Tipifarnib is used to treat leukemia. Vandetanib is used to treat thyroid gland cancer. Vandetanib also inhibits epidermal growth factor receptors, as described in the next section.

dasatinib (Sprycel)

imatinib (Gleevec)
  (see ■ **FIGURE 21–6**)

nilotinib (Tasigna)

sorafenib (Nexavar)

sunitinib (Sutent)

temsirolimus (Torisel)

tipifarnib (Zarnestra)

vandetanib (Zactima)

*Note:* The suffix *-nib* is common to these generic chemotherapy drugs.

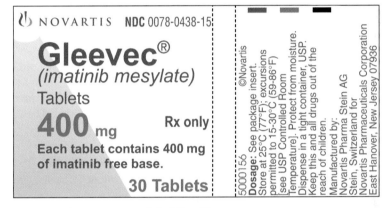

■ **FIGURE 21–6 Drug label for Gleevec.**
Imatinib (Gleevec) is a chemotherapy drug that is used to treat leukemia. It inhibits the abnormal enzyme protein-tyrosine kinase that is present in leukemia cells.

## *In Depth*

There are many types of leukemia. Until 2001, chronic myeloid leukemia (CML) had no treatment available except bone marrow transplantation. This type of leukemia occurs during the division of cells in the bone marrow when genetic material is mistakenly transferred between chromosomes 9 and 22, creating an abnormal chromosome known as the *Philadelphia chromosome.* This abnormal chromosome then produces an abnormal version of an enzyme (Ber-Abl). Normally, this enzyme directs the body to replace the number of WBCs that die each day. However, the abnormal version of the enzyme directs the body to continually produce too many WBCs, which is the main symptom of leukemia.

Imatinib (Gleevec) binds with the abnormal enzyme so that it cannot use ATP, a cellular energy source. Without energy, the enzyme ceases to function. A patient with leukemia must take this drug for life. Now, some forms of chronic myeloid leukemia have become resistant to imatinib and must be treated with dasatinib.

## Epidermal Growth Factor Receptor Inhibitor Chemotherapy Drugs

Epidermal growth factor stimulates cells to grow. Receptors for epidermal growth factor are found on the cell surfaces of normal cells, but more receptors are found on cancer cells, which is why they grow rapidly. Epidermal growth factor receptor inhibitor chemotherapy drugs insert a phosphate molecule into the normal epidermal growth factor molecule; this hinders its action so that it cannot bind with the receptor on the cancer cell. Without epidermal growth factor stimulating the receptor, the cancer cell cannot grow. (See the In Depth feature box, opposite.) These drugs are used to treat many different types of cancer.

erlotinib (Tarceva)

gefitinib (Iressa)

lapatinib (Tykerb)

*Note:* The suffix *-tinib* is common to these generic chemotherapy drugs.

## Corticosteroid Drugs

Corticosteroid drugs are derived from the anti-inflammatory hormone cortisol, which is secreted by the cortex of the adrenal gland. Corticosteroid drugs are given to decrease the tissue inflammation caused by chemotherapy drugs. Corticosteroid drugs also act directly to suppress the production of excessive WBCs in patients with leukemia or lymphoma. They are also used to treat the anemia caused by chemotherapy drugs.

dexamethasone (Decadron)

methylprednisolone

oxymetholone (Anadrol-50)

prednisone (Deltasone, Meticorten) (see ■ FIGURE 21–7)

triamcinolone (Kenalog)

*Note:* The suffixes *-lone* and *-sone* are common to generic corticosteroid drugs.

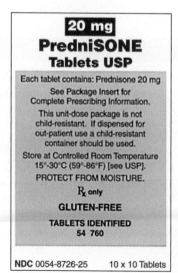

**20 mg**

**PredniSONE**

**Tablets USP**

Each tablet contains: Prednisone 20 mg

See Package Insert for
Complete Prescribing Information.

This unit-dose package is not
child-resistant. If dispensed for
out-patient use a child-resistant
container should be used.

Store at Controlled Room Temperature
15°-30°C (59°-86°F) [see USP].

PROTECT FROM MOISTURE.

℞ only

**GLUTEN-FREE**

TABLETS IDENTIFIED
54 760

NDC 0054-8726-25     10 x 10 Tablets

■ **FIGURE 21–7 Drug label for prednisone.**
Corticosteroid drugs, such as prednisone, can be given alone or given in a fixed combination with chemotherapy drugs in a chemotherapy protocol.

## *In Depth*

Protein-tyrosine kinase inhibitor chemotherapy drugs and epidermal growth factor receptor inhibitor chemotherapy drugs are known as **targeted chemotherapy.** These drugs do not kill rapidly dividing cells as most chemotherapy drugs do. Instead, they attack specific abnormalities (abnormal enzymes and genes, increased numbers of receptors) that are only found in cancer cells. In that way, they "target" only cancer cells.

## Other Chemotherapy Drugs

These chemotherapy drugs exert a therapeutic effect through various mechanisms, or their effect is not well understood. Many are orphan drugs that are only used to treat a specific type of cancer.

| | |
|---|---|
| Actimid | beta alethine (Betathine) |
| adenosine | Borocell |
| Advexin | bortezomib (Velcade) |
| Allovectin-7 | Cavatak |
| Ampligen | cilengitide |
| amsacrine (Amsidyl) | cinacalcet (Sensipar) |
| arsenic trioxide (Trisenox) | cloretazine |
| augmerosen (Genasense) | coumarin (Onkolox) |

## *Drug Alert!*

Do not confuse the chemotherapy drug coumarin, which is an orphan drug used to treat kidney cancer, with the sound-alike drug Coumadin, which is a common trade name anticoagulant drug used to prevent blood clots.

| | |
|---|---|
| Cytoimplant | fenretinide |
| decitabine (Dacogen) | Gimatecan |
| denileukin (Ontak) | Hepacid |
| depsipeptide | herpes simplex virus gene |
| diaziquone | histamine (Maxamine) |
| edotreotide (OctreoTher) | homoharringtonine |
| efaproxiral | HuMax-CD4 |
| eniluracil | hydroxyurea (Droxia, Hydrea) |
| enzastaurin | hypericin |

iboctadekin                    ImmTher

idoxuridine                    Immurait

imexon (Amplimexon)            Imuvert

## Did You Know?

Imuvert is an orphan drug that is an extract of *Serratia marcescens,* a gram-negative bacterium that causes urinary tract infections and wound infections.

IntraDose                      Neovastat

lestaurtinib                   PAN-Cide

Leuvectin                      Panzem

Melanocid                      Pentacea

mitoguazone (Apep)             phenylbutyrate

mitolactol                     porfimer (Photofrin)

Mylovenge

## Did You Know?

Porfimer (Photofrin) is a photosensitizing drug that is used to treat superficial cancers of the skin and of the mucous membranes that line the esophagus and bladder. The drug is injected intravenously and then laser treatment using intense light directed locally at the cancer causes the release of free radicals to kill the cancer cells that have been sensitized by the drug.

porfiromycin (Promycin)        Taxoprexin

Remitogen                      temoporfin (Foscan)

Revlimid                       thymalfasin (Zadaxin)

Rexin-G                        tiazofurin

sodium iodide-131 (Iodotope)   tirapazamine

sodium phosphate-32            TransMID

suramin (Metaret)

## Did You Know?

TransMID is an orphan drug that contains a modified diphtheria toxin, the toxin produced by the bacterium that children are vaccinated against to prevent diphtheria. This drug is used to treat glioblastoma, a type of brain cancer. The drug is delivered through a catheter placed in the brain, in small doses (so as not to put too much fluid pressure on the brain) over four to five days.

treosulfan (Ovastat)              vorinostat (Zolinza)

trimetrexate (Neutrexin)          Xomazyme-791

triptorelin (Trelstar)

## Cancer Vaccines

Unlike flu vaccines that are given prior to the flu season to prevent patients from getting influenza, cancer vaccines are given after the patient has cancer. Cancer vaccines stimulate the immune system to attack cancer cells. The vaccine targets a specific type of cancer by including in the vaccine a fragment of protein that is unique to that type of cancer. BCG is used to treat bladder cancer. Melacine, Canvaxin, and M-Vax are used to treat malignant melanoma. O-Vax is used to treat ovarian cancer. Oncophage is used to treat kidney cancer and malignant melanoma.

BCG (TheraCys)                    M-Vax

DCVax-Brain                       O-Vax

Melacine                          Oncophage

melanoma cell vaccine (Canvaxin)

### Did You Know?

BCG is a vaccine used to treat bladder cancer. It is a specially prepared weakened, but live strain (**b**acille **C**almette-**G**uérin) of the bacterium that causes tuberculosis in cows (*Mycobacterium bovis*). In third-world countries where human tuberculosis is common, BCG is given as a vaccine to stimulate the body to make antibodies against the similar human tuberculosis bacterium (*Mycobacterium tuberculosis*).

## Chemotherapy Protocols

Chemotherapy protocols were introduced in the late 1960s in order to combine the effectiveness of several chemotherapy drugs and direct them against one specific type of cancer. Prior to this, only single-agent chemotherapy drugs were used. In selecting drugs for a chemotherapy protocol, the success of each drug in treating that type of cancer is compared with that of other drugs. The most successful drugs are combined into one protocol. The different therapeutic effects of the various chemotherapy drugs maximize the effectiveness of therapy, while minimizing the side effects that would be caused by a large dose of just one drug. Today, chemotherapy protocols are used to treat nearly every type of cancer. Protocols are designated by acronyms that combine the first letters of the generic name drug or trade name drug or an abbreviation of that drug name in the name of the protocol.

| Protocol Name | Chemotherapy Drug |
|---|---|
| MACC | **m**ethotrexate |
| | **A**driamycin (doxorubicin) |
| | **c**ycylophosphamide (Cytoxan) |
| | **C**eeNU (lomustine) |

*Note:* You can find a comprehensive list of the abbreviations of chemotherapy protocols and the chemotherapy drugs they contain in Appendix C.

## Drug Alert!

Well-known chemotherapy protocols CHOP and MOPP include the chemotherapy drug vincristine, which is represented by the "O" in the protocol abbreviations. The "O" stands for Oncovin, a former trade name of vincristine. Even though Oncovin has been discontinued and is no longer available, these chemotherapy protocols have kept their original abbreviation that includes the "O." Healthcare professionals are expected to know that the "O" stands for "Oncovin" (even though that trade name drug is no longer on the market) and that the generic drug vincristine is part of the chemotherapy protocol.

## *Focus on Healthcare Issues*

In preparing chemotherapy drugs, pharmacists must maintain sterile technique to protect the immunocompromised cancer patient from infection and also to protect themselves from the toxic effects of exposure to the chemotherapy drug. Working under a laminar flow hood maintains a sterile work environment, as chemotherapy drugs are injected into bags of intravenous fluids. A laminar flow hood constantly takes in the surrounding air, passes it through a HEPA filter to remove all bacteria, and then blows the purified air throughout the work space. This pharmacist is wearing gloves and a gown to maintain a sterile environment, but also to protect her skin and clothing from exposure to the chemotherapy drug. Chemotherapy drugs are included on lists of known human carcinogens. The Occupational Safety and Health Administration (OSHA), a federal government agency, issues guidelines for minimizing exposure to all types of hazardous substances, including chemotherapy drugs.

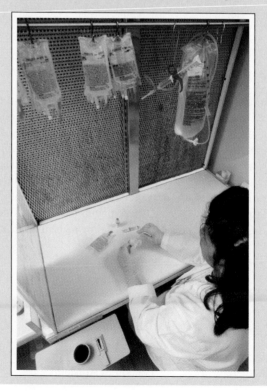

## Drugs Used to Treat Specific Cancers

Because cancer is a life-threatening disease, old as well as new chemotherapy drugs are constantly being evaluated for their effectiveness against specific types of cancer. A complete list of chemotherapy drugs, vaccines, and orphan drugs currently used to treat specific types of cancer is available on the Website for this textbook.

## Drugs Used to Protect Against Chemotherapy Toxicity

Chemotherapy drugs target rapidly dividing cancer cells. However, their effects are also felt in other areas where cells normally divide rapidly, such as in the mucous membranes lining the mouth and intestines and in the bone marrow.

These drugs are used to treat oral mucositis and dry mouth caused by chemotherapy drugs or radiation therapy.

| | |
|---|---|
| amifostine (Ethyol) | palifermin (Kepivance) |
| benzydamine (Tantum) | pilocarpine (Salagen) |
| chlorhexidine (Peridex) | sucralfate (Carafate) |

Granulocyte colony-stimulating factor (G-CSF) is a substance that normally is produced by the body to stimulate the production of neutrophils, the white blood cells that kill bacteria and fight infection. Granulocyte colony-stimulating factor drugs are used to treat decreased levels of neutrophils that occur after chemotherapy or after bone marrow transplantation. Neutrophils belong to the category of white blood cells known as granulocytes, because their cellular cytoplasm shows large purple granules when stained and viewed under the microscope. These drugs are produced by recombinant DNA technology by inserting the human gene that produces G-CSF into rapidly dividing bacteria or yeast cells.

filgrastim (Neupogen) (see ■ **FIGURE 21–8**)

pegfilgrastim (Neulasta)

sargramostim (Leukine)

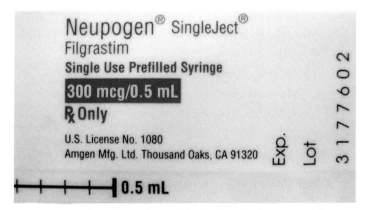

■ **FIGURE 21–8  Drug label for filgrastim (Neupogen).**
The generic name filgrastim reflects the therapeutic effect of this drug, which is **gra**nulocyte **stim**ulation. Filgrastim (Neupogen) was the first of the granulocyte colony-stimulating factor drugs to be introduced. It, like all of the granulocyte colony-stimulating factor drugs, is created using recombinant DNA technology.

Some chemotherapy drugs are known to be toxic to particular organs of the body, such as the bladder, kidneys, or heart. When a patient receives a chemotherapy drug that is known to be toxic to a particular organ, the patient is also given a drug to protect that organ from toxicity. These drugs exert a cytoprotective effect that protects the cells of that organ against the toxic side effects of a specific chemotherapy drug. Amifostine protects the kidneys from toxicity due to cisplatin and cyclophosphamide. Dexrazoxane protects the heart from toxicity due to doxorubicin and epirubicin. Mesna protects the bladder from toxicity due to ifosfamide. Sodium thiosulfate protects the kidneys from toxicity due to platinum chemotherapy drugs. Other chemotherapy drugs are known to be toxic in general, and these drugs are used when those chemotherapy drugs are given. Ethiofos protects against toxicity due to cisplatin and cyclophosphamide. Glucarpidase protects against toxicity due to methotrexate. Leucovorin, L-leucovorin, and levoleucovorin protect against toxicity due to methotrexate or fluorouracil.

| | |
|---|---|
| amifostine (Ethyol) | L-leucovorin (Isovorin) |
| dexrazoxane (Zinecard) | levoleucovorin (Fusilev) |
| ethiofos | mesna (Mesnex) |
| glucarpidase (Voraxaze) | sodium thiosulfate |
| leucovorin (Wellcovorin) | |

## Did You Know?

Leucovorin is a derivative of the B vitamin folic acid. Administration of leucovorin after methotrexate chemotherapy is known as **leucovorin rescue** because the drug rescues the patient from the toxic effects of methotrexate. Leucovorin is also known as *citrovorum factor* and *folinic acid.*

This drug is used to stimulate red blood cell production to treat anemia caused by the cancer itself or by the treatment of chemotherapy drugs or radiation therapy (see ■ **FIGURE 21–9**).

epoetin alfa (Epogen, Procrit)

These bone resorption inhibitor drugs are used to treat an elevated level of calcium caused by cancer and bone metastases, in which bone is broken down and releases calcium into the blood.

etidronate (Didronel)

gallium nitrate (Ganite)

zoledronic acid (Zometa)

## Antiemetic Drugs Used with Chemotherapy

Chemotherapy drugs kill rapidly dividing cancer cells, but they also affect the rapidly dividing cells in the mucous membrane of the GI tract, causing irritation. These drugs also directly stimulate the vomiting center in the brain. In addition, some chemotherapy drugs cause the release of serotonin in the small intestine, which stimulates the vomiting reflex. The nausea and vomiting that occur as a result of chemotherapy can be so severe and prolonged that, without antiemetic

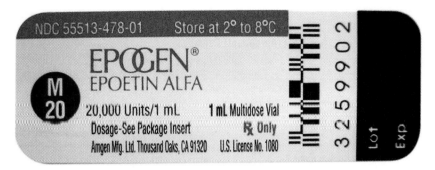

**■ FIGURE 21–9 Drug label for epoetin alfa (Epogen).**
Epoetin alfa (Epogen) has a therapeutic effect that is similar to that of erythropoietin. Erythropoietin is a hormone secreted by the kidneys in response to anemia (low levels of red blood cells). Erythropoietin increases the rate at which red blood cells are produced in the bone marrow. In cancer patients, an abnormality of cytokines decreases the effect of natural erythropoietin. Also, chemotherapy drugs and radiation therapy can diminish the ability of the bone marrow to produce red blood cells. So the drug epoetin alfa is given to act in the place of natural erythropoietin to increase the rate of red blood cell production in cancer patients who have anemia.

drugs, the patient might elect to discontinue life-saving chemotherapy. Therefore, antiemetic drugs are often given prophylactically prior to beginning chemotherapy. These drugs, many of which block serotonin, are used specifically to treat the nausea and vomiting associated with chemotherapy.

aprepitant (Emend)
  (see ■ **FIGURE 21–10**)

dolasetron (Anzemet)

dronabinol (Marinol)

droperidol (Inapsine)

granisetron (Kytril)

nabilone (Cesamet)

ondansetron (Zofran)

palonosetron (Aloxi)

## *Did You Know?*

The antiemetic drug dronabinol (Marinol) is derived from the marijuana plant. The Latin name for the marijuana plant is *Cannabis sativa,* and the active components in marijuana that produce physical and psychological effects are known as *cannabinoids.* The drug dronabinol (Marinol) is a cannabinoid, and it is also known by its chemical name delta-9-tetrahydrocannabinol, abbreviated delta-9-THC, or just THC. In addition to its use as an antiemetic drug, dronabinol (Marinol) is also used as an appetite stimulant for patients with AIDS. Nabilone is a synthetic cannabinoid drug.

  See Focus on Healthcare Issues in Chapter 1 for an overview of the debate to legalize other forms of marijuana.

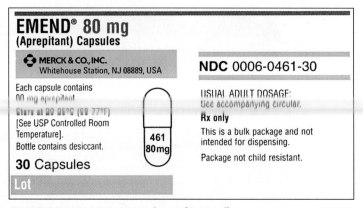

**■ FIGURE 21–10 Aprepitant (Emend).**
Aprepitant (Emend) has a unique effect that differs from that of other
antiemetic drugs given to treat chemotherapy-induced nausea and
vomiting. Emend crosses the blood–brain barrier and blocks neurokinin-1
(NK-1) receptors in the brain. When these receptors are stimulated by
substance P, they cause nausea and vomiting. Other antiemetic drugs
block serotonin or dopamine receptors. Emend is often given with other
antiemetic drugs to increase synergistically the total therapeutic effect of
preventing nausea and vomiting.

# *Chapter Review*

## Quiz Yourself

1. What two steps does the physician need to take before selecting an appropriate chemotherapy
   drug treatment regimen for a particular patient?
2. Define these words and phrases: *neoplasm, stage, adjuvant therapy, remission, analog, mitosis, chemotherapy protocol, leucovorin rescue.*
3. What is the etymology (word origin) of the word *cancer?*
4. In what way are purine analog chemotherapy drugs and pyrimidine analog chemotherapy
   drugs the same, and in what way are they different?
5. The molecular structure of methotrexate is very similar to the molecular structure of
   which B vitamin?
6. How did the chemical weapons of war used in World War I lead to the development of a
   chemotherapy drug?
7. Only chemotherapy antibiotic drugs, not regular antibiotic drugs, are used to treat cancer.
   Explain why this is true.

8. How do hormonal chemotherapy drugs treat breast cancer?
9. How were the platinum chemotherapy drugs discovered?
10. Explain the therapeutic effect of chemotherapy enzyme drugs with respect to the amino acid asparagine.
11. Which two chemotherapy drugs are each given to women who are at high risk of developing breast cancer to prevent them from developing it?
12. Explain the therapeutic effect of retinoid chemotherapy drugs with respect to vitamin A.
13. Interleukins are a signaling protein in the body. What do they signal?
14. Why do many chemotherapy drugs cause a side effect of nausea and vomiting?
15. What organs of the body are particularly affected by the toxicity of these chemotherapy drugs: doxorubicin, ifosfamide, cisplatin?
16. To what category of drugs does each of these drugs belong?

| | |
|---|---|
| **a.** asparaginase (Elspar) | **o.** timatinib (Gleevec) |
| **b.** bexarotene (Targretin) | **p.** irinotecan (Camptosar) |
| **c.** bleomycin (Blenoxane) | **q.** lapatinib (Tykerb) |
| **d.** busulfan (Myleran) | **r.** lomustine (CeeNU) |
| **e.** chlorambucil (Leukeran) | **s.** methotrexate (Trexall) |
| **f.** cisplatin | **t.** raloxifene (Evista) |
| **g.** cyclophosphamide (Cytoxan, Neosar) | **u.** tamoxifen (Soltamox) |
| **h.** doxorubicin (Adriamycin) | **v.** teniposide (Vumon) |
| **i.** exemestane (Aromasin) | **w.** thalidomide (Thalomid) |
| **j.** filgrastim (Neupogen) | **x.** topotecan (Hycamtim) |
| **k.** fludarabine (Fludara) | **y.** trastuzumab (Herceptin) |
| **l.** fluorouracil (Adrucil) | **z.** valrubicin (Valstar) |
| **m.** gemtuzumab (Mylotarg) | **aa.** vinblastine (Velban) |
| **n.** goserelin (Zoladex) | |

## Spelling Tips

| | |
|---|---|
| **Bexxar** | Unusual double *x*. |
| **BiCNU** | Unusual internal capitalization. |
| **CeeNU** | Unusual internal capitalization. |
| **DepoCyt** | Unusual internal capitalization. |
| **DTIC-Dome** | Unusual internal capitalization. |
| **epoetin alfa** | Unusual spelling of the Greek letter *alpha*. |
| **FUDR** | All capital letters. |
| **interferon alfa** | Unusual spelling of the Greek letter *alpha*. |
| **LymphCIDE** | Unusual internal capitalization. |
| **paclitaxel** | Spelled with an "e" versus the trade name **Taxol,** which is spelled with an "o." |
| **PEG-Intron** | Unusual internal capitalization. |
| **TheraCys** | Unusual internal capitalization. |
| **thyrotropin alfa** | Unusual spelling of the Greek letter *alpha*. |
| **VePesid** | Unusual internal capitalization. |

## Clinical Applications

1. Look at this vial of a chemotherapy drug and answer the following questions.
   a. What is the generic name of this drug?
   b. What is the trade name of this drug?
   c. To what category of drugs does this drug belong?
   d. What is the therapeutic effect of this drug?
   e. What parts of this photograph give you a clue that this chemotherapy drug is given intravenously?
   f. What is the natural source that was used to develop this drug?
   g. Name three other natural sources that were used to develop chemotherapy drugs.

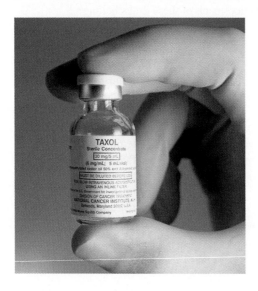

2. If you saw a nurse using a syringe to inject a chemotherapy drug directly into the intravenous tubing near the needle in the patient's arm and the chemotherapy drug in the syringe was red, what chemotherapy drug do you think was being given?

3. Look at this drug label and answer the following questions.
   a. What is the trade name of this drug?
   b. What is the generic name of this drug?
   c. How is the dose of this drug measured?
   d. How is this drug used to treat cancer patients? What is its therapeutic effect?

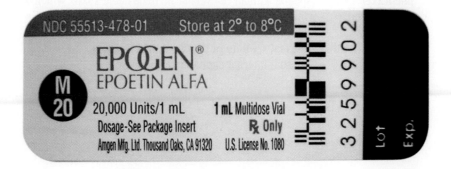

**4.** Look at this drug label and answer the following questions.
   **a.** What is the trade name of this drug?
   **b.** What is the generic name of this drug?
   **c.** What is the dose strength?
   **d.** What is the route of administration?
   **e.** What is the therapeutic effect of this drug in cancer patients?

Do not mix with calcium-containing infusion solutions.

Store at 25°C (77°F); excursions permitted to 15°C-30°C (59°F-86°F).

85054701

Rx only

484180

**NDC** 0078-0387-25

**Zometa**®
(zoledronic acid) Injection
Concentrate for
Intravenous Infusion
**4 mg/5 mL**
US

Manufactured by
Novartis Pharma Stein AG
Stein, Switzerland for
Novartis Pharm. Corp.
E. Hanover, NJ 07936

484185

EXP./LOT

## Multimedia Extension Exercises

■ Go to www.pearsonhighered.com/turley and click on the photo of the cover of *Understanding Pharmacology for Health Professionals* to access the interactive Companion Website created for this textbook.

# 22

# Analgesic Drugs

## CHAPTER CONTENTS

## Learning Objectives

After you study this chapter, you should be able to

1. Compare and contrast the therapeutic effects of various nonnarcotic analgesic drug categories.

2. Describe the four therapeutic effects of aspirin.

3. Explain what types of analgesic drugs are controlled substances and schedule drugs.

4. Describe the therapeutic effects of narcotic analgesic drugs.

5. Discuss the common side effects of narcotic drugs and give two examples of how those side effects can be used as therapeutic effects.

6. Give two reasons why nonnarcotic and narcotic drugs are often used together in combination drugs.

7. Compare and contrast the therapeutic effects of various drug categories used to treat migraine headaches.

8. Given the generic and trade names of an analgesic drug, identify what drug category they belong to.

9. Given an analgesic drug category, identify several generic and trade name drugs in that category.

Pain is a common component of most disease processes. Pain can be mild and chronic, or severe and acute. The ideal analgesic drug would (1) provide maximum pain relief, (2) produce no side effects, and (3) cause no dependence or addiction. Unfortunately, the ideal analgesic drug does not exist. Nonnarcotic analgesic drugs are only effective for mild-to-moderate pain, while drugs that effectively relieve severe pain are usually addictive (narcotic analgesic drugs). Nonnarcotic analgesic drugs are the first step in pain control, and their advantages are that they are nonaddicting, inexpensive, and many of them are over-the-counter drugs that can be purchased without a prescription. Narcotic analgesic drugs, on the other hand, are able to relieve or control severe pain that cannot be treated by other analgesic drugs. Drugs used to treat pain include nonnarcotic analgesic drugs (salicylate analgesic drugs, nonsalicylate analgesic drugs, nonsteroidal anti-inflammatory drugs) and narcotic analgesic drugs.

## Salicylate Analgesic Drugs

Salicylate analgesic drugs are in a general category that includes aspirin and other chemically related drugs. Salicylate analgesic drugs have three distinct therapeutic effects.

- **Analgesic.** Provide relief from mild-to-moderate pain by inhibiting the release of prostaglandins from damaged tissue.
- **Anti-inflammatory.** Decrease inflammation, also by inhibiting the release of prostaglandins from damaged tissue.
- **Antipyretic.** Reduce fever by acting on the hypothalamus to cause vasodilation and sweating. This increases heat loss from the skin and lowers an elevated body temperature.

The salicylate drug aspirin has a fourth therapeutic effect that is unique and not shared by any of the other salicylate drugs.

- **Anticoagulant.** Aspirin prolongs the clotting time of the blood by inhibiting thromboxane, a substance in the blood that normally causes platelets to aggregate and form a clot.

| | |
|---|---|
| aspirin (Bayer Aspirin, Ecotrin, Empirin) (see ■ FIGURE 22–1) | magnesium salicylate (Doan's) (see ■ FIGURE 22–2) |
| diflunisal (Dolobid) | salsalate (Salsitab) |

### *Did You Know?*

In the 1950s, so many doctors relied on aspirin to treat so many conditions that the physician's phrase "Take two aspirins and call me in the morning" became a part of popular culture.

### *Historical Notes*

Aspirin was first introduced in 1899, although for many years prior to that it was used for pain relief in its natural form from willow bark. The drug aspirin is also known by its chemical name and abbreviation *acetylsalicylic acid* (ASA), which was derived from *salix,* a Latin word that means *willow.* The drug category name *salicylate* was derived from acetylsalicylic acid, the first drug in that category.

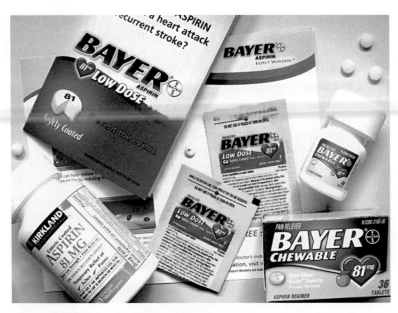

■ **FIGURE 22–1  Low-dose aspirin.**
Because regular aspirin was such a popular and well-used analgesic drug at a dose of 325 mg, the phrase "low-dose aspirin" was coined when it was discovered that a daily 81 mg dose of aspirin could prevent heart attacks and strokes. This Bayer brochure states this fact with the catchy phrase "Prevent the event." The brochure has a cut-away illustration showing the "safety coated" tablet, which has an outer enteric coating that makes it dissolve in the small intestine to prevent gastric upset, a common side effect of aspirin. Notice the "81" imprinted on it. Another low-dose Bayer aspirin tablet product is based on the familiar orange-flavored baby aspirin taken by children, as seen in the orange/pink tablets and box at the right of the photograph. Many other drug manufacturers also make low-dose 81 mg tablets.

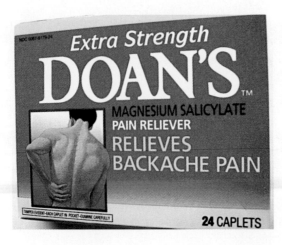

■ **FIGURE 22–2  Doan's drug box.**
Doan's is a popular, over-the-counter analgesic trade name drug. It belongs to the salicylate category of analgesic drugs and contains the generic drug magnesium salicylate. This analgesic drug is commonly used to treat muscle pain and stiffness, particularly in the back.

## *Focus on Healthcare Issues*

One low-dose (81 mg) tablet of aspirin daily—at a cost of only pennies a day—has been found to decrease the risk of a heart attack or stroke in patients with coronary artery disease or those who have had bypass surgery or an angioplasty. WebMD recommends that, if you think you are having a heart attack, you should call 911 and take a full-strength dose of aspirin (325 mg) while you wait for the ambulance to arrive.

In addition, according to Dr. Isadore Rosenfeld (*Parade* magazine, January 1, 2006, p. 8), the regular use of aspirin has also been shown to decrease the risk of cancer of the esophagus, stomach, intestines, and prostate gland.

The regular use of aspirin, however, has a down side. Because aspirin is an acid (acetylsalicylic acid) and is irritating to the stomach, long-term use may cause stomach ulcers. To reduce stomach irritation, aspirin is available as an enteric-coated tablet (trade name Ecotrin) that dissolves only in the higher pH environment of the duodenum. Aspirin is also combined with antacid drugs (aluminum, calcium, or magnesium) to protect the stomach. This combination is known as *buffered aspirin.*

## *Drug Alert!*

Aspirin used regularly for longer than 10 years has been linked to the development of cataracts in the eyes. Also, the use of aspirin to treat the aches and pains of a viral illness has been linked to the occurrence of Reye's syndrome. Reye's syndrome causes liver damage, an increased serum level of ammonia, and encephalitis. Therefore, treating the symptoms of a viral illness (cold, flu, chickenpox) with aspirin is no longer recommended. Instead, acetaminophen (Tylenol) is used.

## *Did You Know?*

Prostaglandins, which are present throughout the body and exert various effects, were so named because they were originally isolated from the prostate gland.

## Nonsalicylate Analgesic Drugs

Nonsalicylate analgesic drugs include acetaminophen and other drugs that have a different therapeutic effect from that of acetaminophen.

### Acetaminophen

Acetaminophen is a nonsalicylate analgesic drug that is not related to aspirin or any of the previously described salicylate drugs. Acetaminophen has two distinct therapeutic effects.

- **Analgesic.**    The mechanism by which acetaminophen relieves pain is unclear.
- **Antipyretic.**    Acetaminophen reduces fever by acting on the hypothalamus to cause vasodilation and sweating. This increases heat loss from the skin and lowers an elevated body temperature. (This is the same mechanism of action as that of aspirin).

Acetaminophen does not have the anti-inflammatory properties that aspirin has, and so acetaminophen cannot be used to treat inflammation. Acetaminophen does not have the anticoagulant effect that aspirin has, and so acetaminophen cannot be used to prevent a heart attack or stroke. On the other hand, acetaminophen does not cause the stomach irritation that aspirin does, and so patients who cannot take aspirin because of stomach upset can take acetaminophen.

acetaminophen (Panadol, Tylenol) (see ■ FIGURE 22–3)

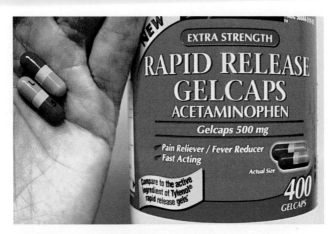

■ **FIGURE 22–3 Acetaminophen.**
The over-the-counter generic drug acetaminophen comes
in many forms and strengths. Each of these colorful gelcaps
contains 500 mg of acetaminophen. A normal adult dose is two
gelcaps (1000 mg) every four to six hours as needed for pain.
Be careful when you read a drug label: This bottle contains
400 gelcaps, but the dose of each gelcap is 500 mg.
Acetaminophen also comes as a suppository, a drug form
that is given to patients who are vomiting and cannot take a drug
orally.

## Historical Notes

Within just a few days of each other in 1982, seven people in the Chicago area died after having taken Extra Strength Tylenol capsules laced with cyanide. The first death was that of a 12-year-old girl who had taken the drug for cold symptoms. Several other deaths were in a single family who shared the same contaminated bottle of Tylenol capsules. Each capsule contained 10,000 times the amount of cyanide needed to kill a person. Chicago police drove through the neighborhoods with loudspeakers, and television network broadcasts warned consumers not to take Tylenol. Tylenol's drug company, Johnson & Johnson, immediately removed 31 million bottles of Tylenol capsules from store shelves and offered to replace already-purchased Tylenol capsules with Tylenol tablets. In response to this tragedy, the FDA set a deadline for all drug companies to convert to tamper-resistant packaging. The legacy of the Tylenol murders is still with us today in the form of tamper-resistant packaging (see ■ FIGURE 22–4). No one has ever been charged with the Tylenol murders.

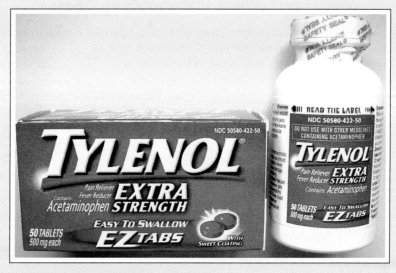

**■ FIGURE 22–4 Tylenol.**

Tylenol was the first drug to have a plastic safety seal on the top of each drug container to prevent tampering with the drug prior to purchase by the consumer. After the plastic seal is removed, the container also has a childproof safety cap that prevents children from accessing the drug. Tylenol is still the most well-known trade name of the generic drug acetaminophen. Tylenol comes in many drug forms: tablet, chewable tablet, caplet, melt-away (dispersible) tablet, gelcap, capsule, liquid elixir and oral infant drops. This box of Tylenol contains small, rounded tablets that the drug company has chosen to name EZ tabs because they are easy to swallow.

## Other Nonsalicylate Analgesic Drugs

These nonsalicylate analgesic drugs are used to treat moderate-to-severe pain. Tramadol inhibits the neurotransmitters norepinephrine and serotonin. It also activates narcotic receptors in the brain and spinal cord to relieve pain, although it does not have the potential for addiction that narcotic drugs have. Ziconotide is used to treat chronic pain.

> clonidine (Duraclon)
> tramadol (Ultram)
> ziconotide (Prialt)

### *Did You Know?*

Clonidine (Duraclon) is an orphan drug that is given continuously via the epidural route to treat severe pain in patients with cancer. It blocks pain receptors in the spinal cord and prevents pain signals from reaching the brain. However, clonidine is best known as the antihypertensive drug (trade name Catapres). It blocks alpha receptors in the brain, decreases the release of norepinephrine, and allows the blood vessels to dilate to lower the blood pressure.

Ziconotide (Prialt) is derived from the venom of a cone snail that lives in the coral reefs around the Phillipines. The FDA said that this is the first time it has approved a drug that is the exact chemical duplicate of a substance found in the ocean. Any substance secreted by a sea creature must be very concentrated because it is diluted immediately with sea water. The drug ziconotide is 1,000 times stronger than morphine. It can only be given through a catheter placed within the membranes around the spinal cord.

## Nonsteroidal Anti-Inflammatory Drugs

Nonsteroidal anti-inflammatory drugs (NSAIDs) have an analgesic effect because they inhibit the production of prostaglandins. These drugs have less of a tendency than salicylate drugs to cause stomach irritation and ulcers. NSAIDs are structurally similar enough to aspirin that patients who are allergic to aspirin should not take NSAIDs. These drugs are used to treat mild-to-moderate pain and inflammation, particularly from osteoarthritis, rheumatoid arthritis, bursitis, tendinitis, gout, migraine headaches, dysmenorrhea, and other painful conditions.

celecoxib (Celebrex) (see ■ **FIGURE 22–5**)

diclofenac (Cataflam, Flector, Voltaren)

etodolac

fenoprofen (Nalfon)

flurbiprofen (Ansaid)

ibuprofen (Advil, Motrin) (see ■ **FIGURE 22–6**)

indomethacin (Indocin)

ketoprofen

ketorolac

meclofenamate

mefenamic acid (Ponstel)

meloxicam (Mobic)

nabumetone

naproxen (Aleve, Naprosyn)

oxaprozin (Daypro)

piroxicam (Feldene)

sulindac (Clinoril)

tolmetin

*Note:* The suffix *-profen* is common to generic nonsteroidal anti-inflammatory drugs.

## *Did You Know?*

All nonsteroidal anti-inflammatory drugs can be given orally as a capsule or tablet. However, only diclofenac can be given in all of these drug forms and routes of administration: orally as a tablet (Cataflam, Voltaren), topically as a gel (Voltaren Emugel), or topically as a transdermal patch (Flector).

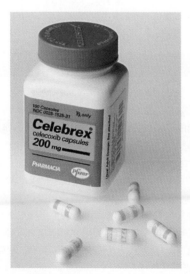

■ **FIGURE 22–5  Celecoxib (Celebrex).**
Celecoxib (Celebrex) is a COX-2 inhibitor drug. Celecoxib was the first drug in this drug category when it was introduced in 1998 as a new way to treat the pain and inflammation of osteoarthritis. The drugs rofecoxib (Vioxx) and valdecoxib (Bextra) were later added to the COX-2 inhibitor drug category. However, Vioxx was taken off the market in 2004 and Bextra in 2005 because of an increased risk of heart attack and stroke. At the current time, there is only one drug—Celebrex—in the category of COX-2 inhibitor drugs.

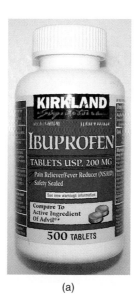

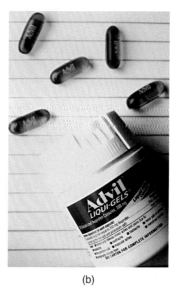

(a)                              (b)

■ **FIGURE 22–6  Ibuprofen (Advil).**
Ibuprofen belongs to the analgesic drug category known as
nonsteroidal anti-inflammatory drugs or NSAIDs. (a) This bottle
contains the generic name drug ibuprofen in a solid tablet form.
Notice that its label calls attention to the fact that this generic
drug has the same active ingredient (and therefore the same
pain-relieving effect) as the familiar, but more expensive, trade
name drug Advil. (b) This bottle contains the trade name drug
Advil in the form of a Liqui-Gel, a fast-dissolving gelatin
capsule. The drug inside is in a liquid form that is rapidly
absorbed through the stomach and into the blood to provide
the fastest possible pain relief. Ibuprofen is also available as
the over-the-counter trade name drug Motrin IB and as the
prescription trade name drug Motrin.

## *In Depth*

When body tissue is damaged, the fluid within the cells is released, and the enzyme
cyclooxygenase (COX) converts this fluid to prostaglandins. The prostaglandins then stimulate
pain receptors in the area. The greater the amount of tissue damage, the more prostaglandins
that are produced and the greater the pain that is felt.

There are two types of the cyclooxygenase (COX) enzyme: COX-1 and COX-2. The
COX-1 enzyme produces prostaglandins that cause pain, but it is also active in platelet
aggregation, in regulating blood flow, and in protecting the mucous membranes of the
stomach from the irritating effect of gastric acid. The COX-2 enzyme's only action is to
produce prostaglandins that cause pain.

Analgesic drugs, such as aspirin and NSAIDs, inhibit the COX-1 enzyme. This blocks the
production of the prostaglandins that cause pain, but it also disrupts the protective action
that prostaglandins have on the stomach. That is why aspirin and NSAIDs can cause stomach
upset and peptic ulcers. The COX-2 inhibitor drugs selectively inhibit only the COX-2 enzyme
and so control pain without any adverse effects on the stomach.

# Drug Alert!

The nonsteroidal anti-inflammatory drug diclofenac (Voltaren) is now available as a topical gel to treat the pain of osteoarthritis. It is the first prescription topical skin gel approved by the FDA for treating the pain of osteoarthritis.

The nonsteroidal anti-inflammatory drug indomethacin (Indocin) is used to treat the pain of osteoarthritis, rheumatoid arthritis, and gout, but it has another unusual use: It is given intravenously to newborn infants to close a persistent patent ductus arteriosus, a part of the fetal circulation that should normally close soon after birth.

## Focus on Healthcare Issues

Studies have shown that elderly people who regularly take an NSAID or aspirin are 55 percent less likely to develop Alzheimer's disease.

## Combination Nonnarcotic Analgesic Drugs

These over-the-counter combination drugs contain a salicylate drug (aspirin) and a stimulant drug (caffeine).

Anacin, Anacin Maximum Strength (aspirin, caffeine)

Bayer Extra Strength Back & Body Pain (aspirin, caffeine)

These over-the-counter combination drugs contain a salicylate drug (aspirin) and an antacid drug (aluminum, calcium, magnesium, sodium bicarbonate) to minimize stomach irritation.

Alka-Seltzer with Aspirin (aspirin, sodium bicarbonate)

Ascriptin (aspirin, aluminum, calcium, magnesium)

Bayer Buffered Aspirin (aspirin, aluminum, calcium, magnesium)

Bayer Plus Extra Strength (aspirin, calcium)

Bufferin (aspirin, calcium, magnesium)

This over-the-counter combination drug contains a salicylate drug (magnesium salicylate) and a sedative drug (phenyltoloxamine).

Mobigesic (magnesium salicylate, phenyltoloxamine)

These over-the-counter combination drugs contain a salicylate analgesic drug (aspirin), a nonsalicylate analgesic drug (acetaminophen), and a stimulant drug (caffeine).

Excedrin Migraine (aspirin, acetaminophen, caffeine)

Excedrin Extra Strength (aspirin, acetaminophen, caffeine)

Vanquish (aspirin, acetaminophen, caffeine)

These over-the-counter combination drugs contain a nonsalicylate analgesic drug (acetaminophen) and a stimulant drug (caffeine).

Excedrin Aspirin Free (acetaminophen, caffeine)

Excedrin Tension Headache (acetaminophen, caffeine)

This prescription combination drug contains a nonsalicylate analgesic drug (acetaminophen) and a nonsteroidal anti-inflammatory drug (tramadol).

Ultracet (acetaminophen, tramadol)

These prescription combination drugs contain a salicylate analgesic drug (aspirin) or a nonsalicylate analgesic drug (acetaminophen), a stimulant drug (caffeine), and a barbiturate sedative drug (butalbital).

Fioricet (acetaminophen, caffeine, butalbital)

Fiorinal (aspirin, caffeine, butalbital)

This prescription combination drug contains a nonsteroidal anti-inflammatory analgesic drug (diclofenac) and a GI protectant drug (misoprostol)

Arthrotec (diclofenac, misoprostol)

## *Did You Know?*

The combination drugs Fioricet and Ultracet give a clue in their trade names as to what generic analgesic drug they contain. Their trade drug names both end in the suffix *-cet,* which stands for *acetaminophen.*

## Narcotic Analgesic Drugs

Narcotic drugs are used to treat moderate-to-severe pain, and they also produce sedation and a sense of well-being (euphoria). Narcotic drugs relieve pain by binding to opiate receptor sites in the brain, thus blocking pain impulses coming to the brain from nerves in the body. There are several different types of opiate receptors, and this explains why some narcotic drugs have a stronger potential for addiction than other narcotic drugs. This difference in the potential for addiction led to the creation of different categories of schedule drugs (see ■ **FIGURE 22–7**). All narcotic drugs are schedule drugs (Schedules II to IV). Interestingly, however, the narcotic drug nalbuphine is not a schedule drug (although it can only be obtained with a prescription).

buprenorphine (Buprenex)

butorphanol (Stadol)

codeine

fentanyl (Actiq, Duragesic, Ionsys)

hydromorphone (Dilaudid) (see ■ **FIGURE 22–8**)

levorphanol (Levo-Dromoran)

meperidine (Demerol)

methadone (Dolophine, Methadose) (see ■ **FIGURE 22–9**)

morphine (MS Contin, Roxanol)

nalbuphine (Nubain)

oxycodone (OxyContin, Roxicodone) (see ■ **FIGURE 22–10**)

oxymorphone (Numorphan, Opana)

pentazocine (Talwin)

propoxyphene (Darvon, Darvon-N)

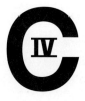

■ **FIGURE 22–7  Symbol for a schedule drug.**
All drugs that have the potential to cause addiction are classified as schedule drugs. This symbol *C* indicates that the drug is a controlled substance and therefore a schedule drug, This symbol must always appear on the drug label. The Roman numeral inside of it (II, III, or IV) indicates the assigned level of the schedule drug and corresponds to how addicting the drug is. Schedule II drugs are highly addictive. This symbol for a Schedule IV drug indicates that the drug is mildly addictive. See Chapter 1 for an in-depth discussion of schedule drugs.

## Drug Alert!

Do not confuse the narcotic analgesic drug Duragesic (generic name fentanyl), which is a Schedule II drug used to treat severe pain, with the nonnarcotic prescription analgesic drug Duraclon (generic name clonidine), which is used to treat moderate-to-severe pain in cancer patients but is also used to treat hypertension, atrial fibrillation, postoperative shivering, restless legs syndrome, and many other conditions that are unrelated to pain control.

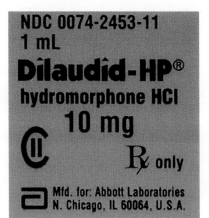

**NDC 0074-2453-11**
**1 mL**
**Dîlaudîd-HP®**
**hydromorphone HCl**
**10 mg**
Ⓒ II      ℞ only
Mfd. for: Abbott Laboratories
N. Chicago, IL 60064, U.S.A.

■ **FIGURE 22–8  Drug label for hydromorphone (Dilaudid).**
Hydromorphone (Dilaudid) is a very effective narcotic drug that is used to treat severe pain. It is a Schedule II drug, and therefore it has the greatest potential to cause addiction of any narcotic drug.

## Drug Alert!

The narcotic drug fentanyl is available in several different drug forms: tablet, lozenge on a stick, and transdermal patch. Fentanyl (Actiq), which is used to treat breakthrough pain in cancer patients, comes as a lozenge on a stick. Informally, the drug is known as the *Actiq lollipop.* Fentanyl comes in two different transdermal patch forms: Duragesic and Ionsys. Duragesic comes in several different strengths of transdermal patches, each of which delivers a set dose of fentanyl each hour. The patch is applied to the skin and left in place to deliver continuous pain relief for 72 hours. The Duragesic patch is used by many patients with chronic, severe pain who are at home or in a skilled nursing facility or hospice. The Ionsys transdermal patch comes with a recessed button. Before dispensing this patch, the pharmacist pushes the button in and releases it twice (double click) and then waits to hear an audible beep that confirms that the patch is activated. The nurse then applies the transdermal patch to the patient's skin. If the patch does not have good contact with the skin, it will beep. The Ionsys patch releases 80 individual doses of fentanyl over 24 hours. This transdermal patch is only used in the hospital, and patients are not discharged home on this transdermal patch.

## Did You Know?

The narcotic drug morphine is more accurately known as *morphine sulfate.* The trade name drug MS Contin reflects the abbreviation for morphine sulfate (MS) and the fact that the drug provides continuous pain relief (Contin), as a controlled-release tablet.

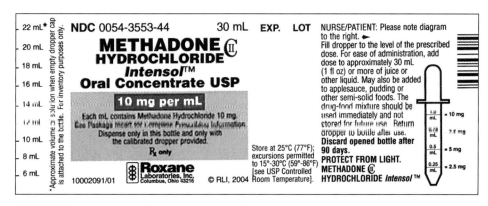

■ **FIGURE 22-9** **Drug label for methadone.**

Methadone is well known for its use in treating recovering narcotic drug addicts. It is a Schedule II narcotic drug that is able to treat severe pain but, because it does not produce the high degree of euphoria that other narcotic drugs do, it is not generally a drug of abuse. When it is given to recovering narcotic drug addicts, in the setting of a methadone outpatient clinic, it prevents the addict from experiencing narcotic withdrawal symptoms while it slowly decreases the addict's physical and psychological dependence on narcotic drugs.

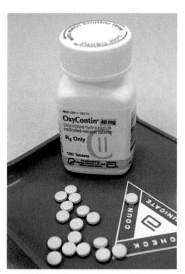

■ **FIGURE 22-10** **Oxycodone (OxyContin).**

Oxycodone (OxyContin) is used to treat severe pain. Because it is a Schedule II drug—see the symbol on the label—it has a high potential for addiction. The drug bottle is sitting on a blue pill-counting tray in the pharmacy. This tray helps the pharmacist count out the exact number of tablets specified in the patient's prescription. The logo in the center of the tray reminds the pharmacist to "Check, Counsel, Communicate." Oxycodone is also a popular drug of abuse that is sold on the street and now can be more easily obtained through unscrupulous on-line Internet pharmacies.

## *Focus on Healthcare Issues*

OxyContin was introduced in 1995 as a Schedule II drug for treating moderate-to-severe pain. Today, OxyContin is the best selling narcotic drug in the United States. Physicians wrote almost 7 million prescriptions for OxyContin in 2001. Oxycodone (OxyContin) has launched an epidemic of drug abuse that some law enforcement officials compare to the crack cocaine epidemic of the 1980s. One U.S. detoxification treatment clinic reported that 75 percent of its patients were recovering OxyContin addicts. Pharmacies that carry OxyContin have been the target of armed robberies, and this drug can be obtained more easily than illegal drugs by writing forged prescriptions or stealing from hospital supplies.

*(continued)*

## *Focus on Healthcare Issues* (continued)

Oxycodone is available under several other trade names besides OxyContin, but addicts use OxyContin because it is a time-release formula that contains up to 10 times more narcotic than other forms of oxycodone. The time-release formula is meant to control pain for 12 hours; however, addicts crush the tablet and then snort the powder or dissolve the tablet and then inject the liquid intravenously so that the full narcotic dose takes effect immediately and produces a "high." The drug company that makes OxyContin, in cooperation with the FDA, has put new warning labels on the drug; however, it is the illegal sale and use of the drug that has been responsible for multiple deaths and an epidemic of addiction.

In 2008, the Maryland Society of Addiction Medicine reported that buprenorphine has become a new drug of abuse on a national scale. From 2006 to 2007, arrests in Baltimore for selling oxycodone were up 7 percent, but arrests for selling buprenorphine were up 215 percent.

(D. Donovan and F. Schulte, "'Bupe' seizures rise," *The Baltimore Sun,* April 18, 2008, p. 16A).

## *Did You Know?*

The word *narcotic* is derived from the Greek word *narke,* which means *numbness.* Natural opiate-like substances in the body known as **endorphins** were designed to occupy specific receptor sites in the body and produce a natural feeling of pain relief without the use of drugs. Narcotic drugs activate these same receptor sites.

The existence of different opiate receptors also accounts for the different types of side effects that are seen with narcotic drugs. Common side effects of narcotic drugs include constipation, respiratory depression, sedation, and euphoria. It is the presence of significant euphoria that causes some narcotic drugs to be more psychologically addicting than others. Another common narcotic side effect, suppression of the cough center (antitussive effect), is used as a therapeutic effect by using a narcotic drug as a prescription cough syrup (e.g., Hycodan). For a discussion of antitussive drugs, see Chapter 19. For narcotic drugs that use the side effect of constipation as a therapeutic effect to treat diarrhea, see Chapter 8.

## *Historical Notes*

Opium is obtained from the dried seeds of the poppy flower. The receptors in the body that are stimulated by opium and other narcotic drugs are known as *opiate receptors.* Morphine was first isolated from opium in 1815. Because it could cause unconsciousness, morphine was named for Morpheus (the Greek god of dreams, who was the son of Hypnos, the Greek god of sleep). Morphine was used extensively during the Civil War to treat the pain of battle wounds, resulting in a very high rate of addiction among veterans. Heroin, a semisynthetic narcotic drug, was introduced in 1898 and was thought to be a nonaddicting substitute for morphine. However, it proved to be more addicting than morphine. At present, heroin is classified as a Schedule I drug with no medical uses because of its high potential for physical and psychological addiction. In 1939, meperidine (Demerol), the first synthetic narcotic drug, was introduced. Today, narcotic drugs can be derived from opium or synthetically manufactured. The original drug opium is still on the market. It can be found in the combination analgesic drug B&O Supprettes (a Schedule II drug), but it can also be found as tincture of opium in the Schedule III drug paregoric, which is only used to treat diarrhea. Because a common side effect of all narcotic drugs is constipation, paregoric uses this side effect as a therapeutic effect to treat diarrhea.

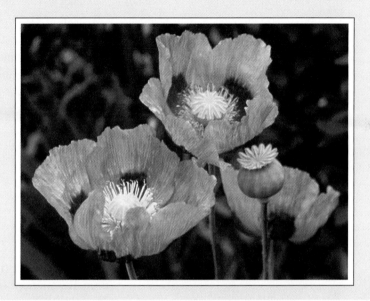

## Combination Nonnarcotic and Narcotic Analgesic Drugs

Nonnarcotic and narcotic drugs are often given in combination with each other for two reasons.

1. The nonnarcotic drug provides a foundation of pain relief upon which the narcotic drug can build; therefore, less narcotic drug is needed to effectively control the pain.
2. The therapeutic effects of this combination of drugs treat the two components of pain—pain from the stimulation of nerve endings and pain that is heightened by anxiety.

These combination drugs contain a salicylate analgesic drug (aspirin) and a narcotic analgesic drug (codeine, dihydrocodeine, hydrocodone, oxycodone, pentozocine). They may also contain a barbiturate sedative drug (butalbital) and a stimulant drug (caffeine). These drugs are Schedule II and III drugs.

Empirin w/ Codeine No. 3 (aspirin, codeine)

Empirin w/ Codeine No. 4 (aspirin, codeine)

Fiorinal w/ Codeine (aspirin, codeine, butalbital, caffeine)

Lortab ASA (aspirin, hydrocodone)

Percodan (aspirin, oxycodone)

Roxiprin (aspirin, oxycodone)

Synalgos-DC (aspirin, dihydrocodeine)

Talwin Compound (aspirin, pentozocine)

These combination drugs contain a nonsalicylate analgesic drug (acetaminophen) and a narcotic analgesic drug (codeine, hydrocodone, oxycodone, pentazocine, propoxyphene). They may also contain a barbiturate sedative drug (butalbital) and a stimulant drug (caffeine). These drugs are Schedule III, IV, or V drugs (see ▇ **FIGURE 22–11**).

Darvocet-N (acetaminophen, propoxyphene)

Fioricet w/ Codeine (acetaminophen, codeine, butalbital, caffeine)

Lorcet (acetaminophen. hydrocodone)

Lortab (acetaminophen, hydrocodone)

Percocet (acetaminophen, oxycodone)

Roxicet (acetaminophen, oxycodone)

Roxilox (acetaminophen, oxycodone)

Talacen (acetaminophen, pentazocine)

Tylenol w/ Codeine (acetaminophen, codeine)

Tylenol w/ Codeine No. 2 (acetaminophen, codeine)

Tylenol w/ Codeine No. 3 (acetaminophen, codeine)

Tylenol w/ Codeine No. 4 (acetaminophen, codeine)

Tylox (acetaminophen, oxycodone)

Vicodin (acetaminophen, hydrocodone)

Zydone (acetaminophen, hydrocodone)

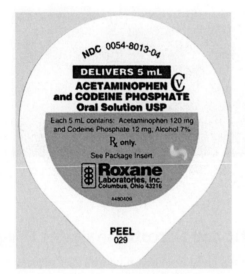

▇ **FIGURE 22–11 Drug label for the combination drug acetaminophen with codeine.**
This Schedule V combination analgesic drug contains the nonsalicylate drug acetaminophen and the narcotic drug codeine. This is not a trade name drug, and so both generic drug names are given on the label. This label is the peel-off top on a small plastic container that holds the liquid form (oral solution) of this combination Schedule V drug that is used to treat mild-to-moderate pain.

These combination drugs contain a nonsteroidal anti-inflammatory analgesic drug (ibuprofen) and a narcotic analgesic drug (hydrocodone). These are Schedule III drugs.

Ibudone (ibuprofen, hydrocodone)

Vicoprofen (ibuprofen, hydrocodone)

This combination drug contains a narcotic analgesic drug (opium) and an antispasmodic drug (belladonna). This is a Schedule II drug.

B&O Supprettes (opium, belladonna)

This combination drug contains a narcotic drug (pentazocine) and a narcotic antagonist drug (naloxone). This is a Schedule IV drug.

Talwin NX (naloxone, pentazocine)

# *Drug Alert!*

The sound-alike combination drugs Fioricet and Fiorinol as well as Percocet and Percodan can easily be confused. These drugs contain acetaminophen (Fioricet, Percocet), and these drugs contain aspirin as the nonnarcotic analgesic drug (Fiorinol, Percodan). You can remember which drugs are which by associating **acet**aminophen with Fiori**cet** and Perco**cet**.

In the combination drug Tylenol w/ Codeine, the *w/* stands for *with.* Tylenol w/ Codeine comes in several strengths. Tylenol w/ Codeine is the first strength, and it contains 12 mg of codeine. Tylenol w/ Codeine No. 2 is the second strength, and it contains 15 mg of codeine. Tylenol w/ Codeine No. 3 is the third strength and it contains 30 mg of codeine. Tylenol w/ Codeine No. 4 is the fourth strength and it contains 60 mg of codeine. It is important to note that Tylenol w/ Codeine (with 12 mg of codeine) is a Schedule V drug, but all of the other drugs are Schedule III drugs because of the larger dose of codeine.

Empirin w/ Codeine No. 3 contains 30 mg of codeine, and Empirin w/ Codeine No. 4 contains 60 mg of codeine (which corresponds to the numbering and amount of codeine in Tylenol w/ Codeine No. 3 and Tylenol w/ Codeine No. 4).

*Note:* There is no such drug name as Tylenol w/ Codeine No. 1, Empirin w/ Codeine No. 1, or Empirin w/ Codeine No. 2.

## Drugs Used to Treat Migraine Headaches

A migraine headache is a specific type of headache that has a sudden onset with severe, throbbing pain, often on just one side of the head. It is often accompanied by nausea and vomiting, and sensitivity to light. The pain of a migraine headache is caused by a constriction of the arteries in the brain followed by a sudden dilation, accompanied by the release of neuropeptides by the trigeminal nerve (a nerve that travels from deep within the skull outward to the jaw, cheeks, eyes, and forehead). The dilation of the arteries causes pain, and the neuropeptides cause inflammation. Drugs used to treat migraine headaches include serotonin receptor agonist drugs, ergotamine drugs, beta-blocker drugs, calcium channel blocker drugs, antidepressant drugs, and other drugs.

### Serotonin Receptor Agonist Drugs for Migraine Headaches

Serotonin is a neurotransmitter that normally constricts the arteries in the brain. Prior to the occurrence of a migraine, there are elevated levels of serotonin. The serotonin levels then suddenly decrease, and this causes rebound dilation of the arteries in the brain and throbbing pain. These drugs stimulate serotonin receptor sites on the arteries and cause them to constrict again. These drugs also stimulate serotonin receptors on the trigeminal nerve to treat the pain of migraine headaches. Serotonin receptor agonist drugs are used to treat migraine headaches once they have occurred.

| | |
|---|---|
| almotriptan (Axert) | rizatriptan (Maxalt) |
| eletriptan (Relpax) | sumatriptan (Imitrex) (see ■ **FIGURE 22–12**) |
| frovatriptan (Frova) | valproic acid (Stavzor) |
| naratriptan (Amerge) | zolmitriptan (Zomig) |

*Note:* The suffix *-triptan* is common to generic serotonin receptor agonist drugs.

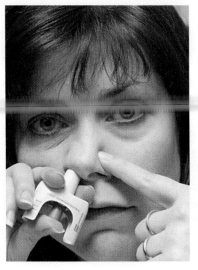

**■ FIGURE 22–12  Sumatriptan (Imitrex) nasal spray.**
While most serotonin receptor agonist drugs used to treat migraine headaches come in a tablet form, sumatriptan is unique in that it comes as a tablet that is taken orally, as a liquid that is injected subcutaneously, and as a liquid that is sprayed into the nose. The nasal spray liquid drug begins to exert a therapeutic effect more rapidly than a tablet because it does not have to disintegrate before it can be absorbed.

### Ergotamine Drugs for Migraine Headaches

Ergotamine drugs constrict the arteries in the brain without significantly reducing blood flow. They stimulate serotonin receptors, but also act on receptors for norepinephrine and dopamine. Ergotamine drugs are used to prevent or treat migraine headaches.

> dihydroergotamine (Migranal)
>
> ergotamine (Ergomar)

## Did You Know?

Ergotamine is derived from ergot, a fungus that affects rye and other grasses.

### Beta-Blocker Drugs for Migraine Headaches

Beta-blocker drugs keep the arteries dilated to prevent the initial vasoconstriction that is the beginning of a migraine headache. These drugs are used to prevent migraine headaches.

> atenolol (Tenormin)                     propranolol (Inderal)
>
> metoprolol (Lopressor, Toprol-XL)        timolol (Blocadren)
>
> nadolol (Corgard)

### Calcium Channel Blocker Drugs for Migraine Headaches

Calcium channel blocker drugs slow the movement of calcium ions through calcium channels and into the smooth muscle around the arteries in the brain. With less calcium available within the cells, the smooth muscles relax, and the arteries remain dilated. These drugs are used to prevent migraine headaches.

> diltiazem (Cardizem)
>
> verapamil (Calan, Covera-HS)

## Antidepressant Drugs for Migraine Headaches

Antidepressant drugs treat depression and depression associated with anxiety, but also have been found to be helpful in treating migraine and tension headaches.

amitriptyline

amoxapine

desipramine (Norpramin)

doxepin (Sinequan)

imipramine (Tofranil)

nortriptyline (Aventyl, Pamelor)

protriptyline (Vivactil)

## Other Drugs for Migraine Headaches

Other drugs treat migraine headaches in a variety of different ways. Baclofen is a muscle relaxant drug. Chlorpromazine and prochlorperazine are antipsychotic drugs that are also indicated for the treatment of migraine headaches. Gabapentin, levetiracetam, and topiramate are antiseizure drugs that are also indicated for the treatment of migraine headaches. Lithium is best known for its ability to treat the manic phase of bipolar disorder, but it is also used to treat cluster headaches, a type of migraine headache.

baclofen (Lioresal)

chlorpromazine (Thorazine)

gabapentin (Neurotin)

levetiracetam (Keppra)

lithium (Lithobid)

prochlorperazine (Compazine)

topiramate (Topamax)

## Drug Alert!

Topiramate is best known as an antiseizure drug and is used to treat both generalized tonic-clonic seizures as well as simple partial seizures. However, it has many other indications as well, and is used to treat bipolar disorder, binge eating and bulimia nervosa, alcohol and cocaine dependence, as well as migraine headaches. *Monthly Prescribing Reference* for physicians and pharmacists stated in 2008 that Topamax is the number one prescribed drug for migraine headaches.

## Combination Drugs for Migraine Headaches

This combination drug contains a serotonin receptor agonist drug (sumatriptan) and a nonsteroidal anti-inflammatory drug (naproxen).

Treximet (sumatriptan, naproxen)

These combination drugs contain a vasoconstrictor drug (ergotamine, isometheptene), an analgesic drug (acetaminophen), a stimulant drug (caffeine), and/or a sedative drug (dichloralphenazone).

Cafergot (ergotamine, caffeine)

Duradrin (isometheptene, acetaminophen, dichloralphenazone)

Midrin (isometheptene, acetaminophen, dichloralphenazone)

## Drugs Used to Treat Narcotic Drug Addiction

Drugs used to treat narcotic drug addiction are discussed in Chapter 16.

## Drugs Used to Treat Analgesic or Narcotic Drug Overdose

Drugs used to treat analgesic drug or narcotic drug overdoses are discussed in Chapter 24.

## Analgesic Drugs Used to Treat Dysmenorrhea

Analgesic drugs used to treat painful menstrual cramps (dysmenorrhea) are discussed in Chapter 13.

## Analgesic Drugs Used to Treat the Skin

Topical analgesic drugs used to treat painful skin conditions are discussed in Chapter 17.

 *Chapter Review*

### Quiz Yourself

1. Describe the four therapeutic effects of aspirin.
2. Describe the two therapeutic effects of acetaminophen.
3. What is one advantage and one disadvantage that nonnarcotic analgesic drugs have when compared to narcotic analgesic drugs?
4. What is the therapeutic effect of buffered aspirin?
5. Explain why nonnarcotic and narcotic analgesic drugs are often given in combination with each other.
6. Why do aspirin and NSAIDs cause stomach upset and ulcers?
7. Why shouldn't aspirin be given to those who have the aches and pains of a viral illnesss?
8. Describe what the enzyme COX does and describe the therapeutic effect of the COX-2 inhibitor drug celecoxib (Celebrex).
9. What unique use does the NSAID indomethacin (Indocin) have?
10. Why do some narcotic drugs have a stronger potential for causing addiction than other narcotic drugs?
11. Describe the role of endorphins in the body.
12. Name five categories of drugs used to treat migraine headaches, and describe the therapeutic effect of each category.
13. To what category of drugs does each of these drugs belong, or what is its therapeutic effect?

    a. celecoxib (Celebrex)          g. oxycodone (OxyContin)
    b. fentanyl (Actiq, Duragesic, Ionsys)    h. propoxyphene (Darvon)
    c. hydromorphone (Dilaudid)       i. sumatriptan (Imitrex)
    d. meperidine (Demerol)          j. topiramate (Topamax)
    e. naproxen (Aleve, Naprosyn)     k. tramadol (Ultram)
    f. oxaprozin (Daypro)

## Spelling Tips

**Ansaid** versus **NSAID**
Trade name of a nonsteroidal anti-inflammatory drug sounds like the pronounced abbreviation for the drug category.

**MS Contin**
Unusual double capital.

**OxyContin**
Unusual internal capitalization.

## Clinical Applications

**1.** Look at this handwritten prescription and answer the following questions.
   **a.** What is the name of the drug that is prescribed here?
   **b.** Is this a generic name drug or a trade name drug?
   **c.** To what drug category does this drug belong?
   **d.** What strength of the drug is being prescribed?
   **e.** In what drug form is this drug manufactured?
   **f.** Translate the rest of the prescription into English.

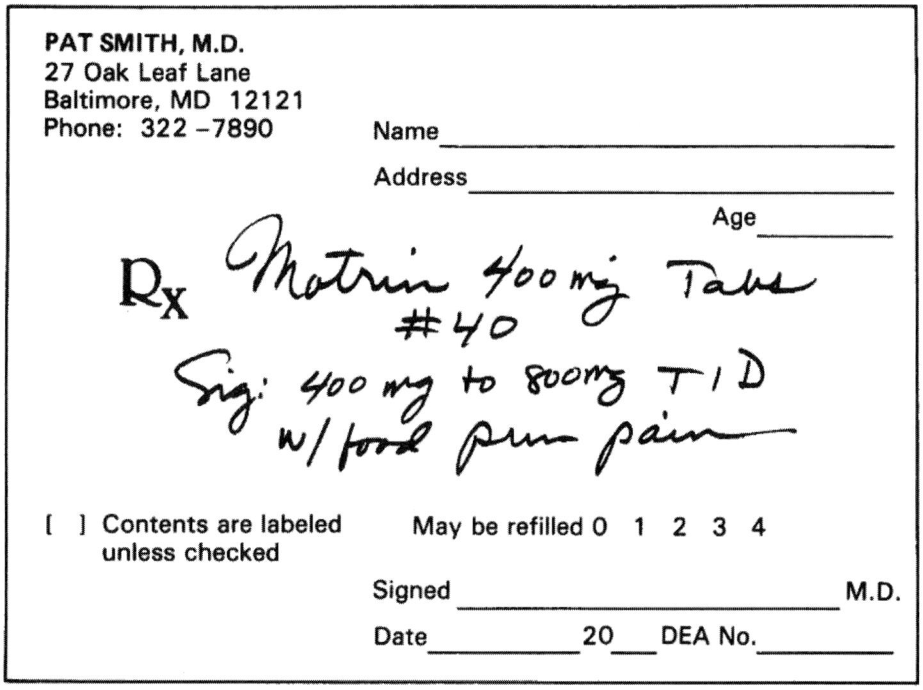

```
PAT SMITH, M.D.
27 Oak Leaf Lane
Baltimore, MD  12121
Phone:  322 –7890        Name_____

                         Address_____

                                               Age_____

Rx   Motrin  400 mg  Tabs
           #40
     Sig: 400 mg to 800mg  TID
          w/ food  prn  pain


[  ] Contents are labeled      May be refilled  0  1  2  3  4
     unless checked

                         Signed _____ M.D.

                         Date_____ 20___ DEA No._____
```

# 23 Anesthetic Drugs

## CHAPTER CONTENTS

## Learning Objectives

After you study this chapter, you should be able to

1. Describe some historical milestones in the discovery of anesthetic drugs.

2. Compare and contrast how local, regional, spinal, and epidural anesthetic drugs are given.

3. Explain the significance of *MPF* in the trade names of some anesthetic drugs.

4. Describe various categories of drugs that are given preoperatively and their therapeutic effects.

5. Compare and contrast how barbiturate drugs versus narcotic drugs versus inhaled anesthetic gases produce general anesthesia.

6. Given the generic and trade names of an anesthetic drug, identify what drug category they belong to.

7. Given an anesthetic drug category, identify several generic and trade name drugs in that category.

Anesthesia is defined as the absence of feeling, sensation, or pain. Anesthesia can be obtained on the skin (by topical application of anesthetic drugs), in the skin and deeper tissues (by subcutaneous local injection), in one body part (by regional nerve block), in the trunk and lower extremities (by epidural or spinal anesthesia), or in the entire body (by general anesthesia that produces unconsciousness).

Topical, local, regional, epidural, or spinal anesthesia is obtained when an anesthetic drug blocks the flow of sodium ions across the membranes of nerve cells, thereby blocking the production of nerve impulses that convey the message of pain.

General anesthesia, on the other hand, involves a loss of pain sensation through deep sedation of the central nervous system and unconsciousness. This results in the total body anesthesia that is needed for many surgical procedures.

The word *anesthetic* contains the prefix *an-* (without; not), the combining form *esthet/o-* (sensation; feeling) and the suffix *-ic* (pertaining to); the word means *pertaining to without sensation* or *pertaining to not feeling*.

## Topical Anesthetic Drugs for the Skin, Nose, and Mouth

Anesthetic drugs in the form of creams, gels, ointments, and sprays are applied to the skin to produce topical anesthesia. These drugs are discussed in Chapter 17. Anesthetic drugs in the form of gels and liquids are used to produce topical anesthesia in the nose and mouth. These drugs are discussed in Chapter 19.

## Local, Regional, Spinal, and Epidural Anesthetic Drugs

Anesthesia may be produced locally, regionally, or throughout a larger region via the spine (spinal and epidural).

For **local anesthesia,** an anesthetic drug is given by subcutaneous injection into the skin to anesthetize a small area of skin and adjacent tissues (see ▨ **FIGURE 23–1**). Local anesthesia is used during minor surgical procedures, such as biopsies, or during dental surgery.

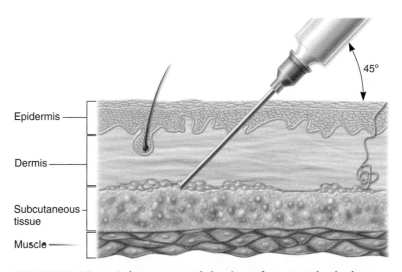

Epidermis

Dermis

Subcutaneous tissue

Muscle

45°

▨ **FIGURE 23–1 Subcutaneous injection of an anesthetic drug.**
To achieve local anesthesia, the needle is inserted at a 45-degree angle, and the anesthetic drug is injected into the fatty subcutaneous tissue, but not into the muscle layer.

For **regional anesthesia,** an anesthetic drug is given by subcutaneous injection near a nerve plexus (group of nerves) and its branches. Regional anesthesia is used during surgery on an extremity to provide anesthesia for just that region. This is also known as *nerve block anesthesia.*

For **spinal anesthesia,** an anesthetic drug is given by injection into the subarachnoid space between the vertebrae of the lumbar region of the back.

For **epidural anesthesia,** an anesthetic drug is given by injection into the epidural space (a space filled with fatty tissue and blood vessels that is located between the dura matter of the spinal cord and the vertebrae); the drug then moves into the subarachnoid space to produce anesthesia.

These anesthetic drugs are used to produce local, regional, spinal, and/or epidural anesthesia.

bupivacaine (Marcaine, Sensorcaine)          procaine (Novocain)

chloroprocaine (Nesacaine)                    ropivacaine (Naropin) (see ■ FIGURE 23–3)

lidocaine (Xylocaine) (see ■ FIGURE 23–2)    tetracaine (Pontocaine)

mepivacaine (Carbocaine, Polocaine)

*Note:* The suffix *-caine* is common to generic and trade name anesthetic drugs used to produce local, regional, spinal, or epidural anesthesia.

## Historical Notes

Lidocaine (Xylocaine), the most widely used topical, local, regional, and spinal anesthetic drug, was introduced in 1948.

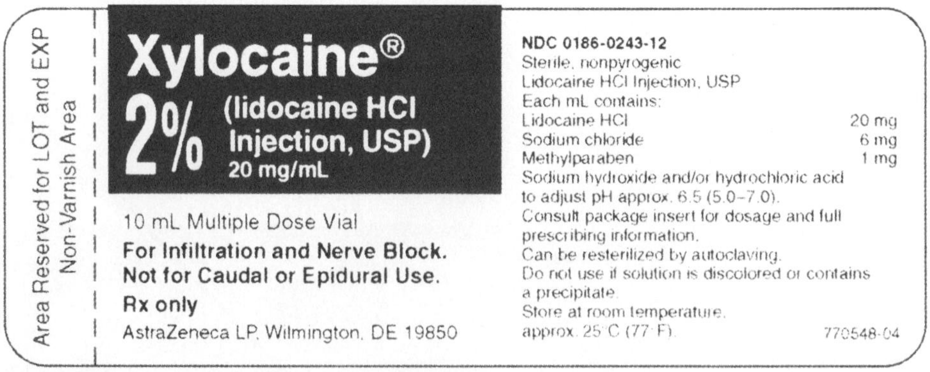

**Xylocaine®**
**2%** (lidocaine HCl Injection, USP)
**20 mg/mL**

Area Reserved for LOT and EXP Non-Varnish Area

10 mL Multiple Dose Vial
**For Infiltration and Nerve Block.**
**Not for Caudal or Epidural Use.**
**Rx only**
AstraZeneca LP, Wilmington, DE 19850

NDC 0186-0243-12
Sterile, nonpyrogenic
Lidocaine HCl Injection, USP
Each mL contains:
Lidocaine HCl                          20 mg
Sodium chloride                         6 mg
Methylparaben                           1 mg
Sodium hydroxide and/or hydrochloric acid
to adjust pH approx. 6.5 (5.0–7.0).
Consult package insert for dosage and full
prescribing information.
Can be resterilized by autoclaving.
Do not use if solution is discolored or contains
a precipitate.
Store at room temperature.
approx. 25°C (77°F).                 770548-04

■ **FIGURE 23–2  Drug label for Xylocaine.**
This form of lidocaine (Xylocaine) is only used for local (i.e., infiltration) and regional (i.e., nerve block) anesthesia. Other forms of Xylocaine are used for topical, spinal, or epidural anesthesia.

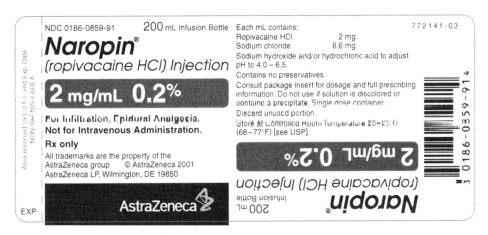

**■ FIGURE 23–3 Drug label for ropivacaine (Naropin).**
Ropivacaine (Naropin) is an anesthetic drug that is injected to produce local or epidural anesthesia. Notice that the label says "For infiltration, epidural anesthesia." Infiltration anesthesia is another name for local anesthesia. The drug label clearly indicates that this drug is not to be given intravenously.

## Combination Anesthetic Drugs

This combination drug contains two anesthetic drugs (bupivacaine, lidocaine). It is used to provide local or regional anesthesia.

Duocaine (bupivacaine, lidocaine)

## *Focus on Healthcare Issues*

Some trade name anesthetic drugs (Nesacaine MPF, Sensorcaine MPF, Xylocaine MPF, etc.) contain the abbreviation *MPF*, which stands for *methylparaben free*. Methylparaben, a preservative with antibiotic and antifungal effects, is often present in liquid anesthetic drugs that are in vials or ampules. Some patients have an immediate and severe allergic reaction to methylparaben, and so it has been eliminated from some anesthetic drugs. Those anesthetic drugs that do not contain methylparaben are labeled *MPF*.

The local anesthetic drugs bupivacaine and lidocaine are available with or without epinephrine in the solution. Epinephrine (Adrenalin) is a powerful vasoconstrictor that decreases blood flow to the tissue where it is injected. This therapeutic effect prolongs the anesthetic action of the drug. The use of epinephrine is contraindicated in certain areas of the body, such as the tip of the nose, and the fingers, toes, and ears, because the blood supply there is limited and excessive local vasoconstriction could lead to necrosis and skin sloughing. In those areas, an anesthetic drug without epinephrine is used for local anesthesia.

*Historical Notes*

For centuries, the South American Indians chewed the leaves of the coca bush for their euphoric effect. Cocaine, which is derived from these leaves, was recognized as a topical anesthetic drug in 1880 and is still used as a topical anesthetic and vasoconstrictor drug for ENT procedures. For many years, synthetic substitutes for cocaine were sought. This led to the discovery of procaine (Novocain), the prototype of local anesthetic drugs.

## Drugs Used During the Preoperative Period

Various categories of drugs are given preoperatively. These include antihistamine drugs, anticholinergic drugs, antianxiety drugs, narcotic drugs, barbiturate drugs, and antipsychotic drugs.

These antihistamine drugs are given preoperatively to provide sedation as well as to dry up oral secretions to facilitate endotracheal intubation.

hydroxyzine (Vistaril)

promethazine (Phenergan)

These anticholinergic drugs are given preoperatively to block the action of acetylcholine and decrease oral secretions to facilitate endotracheal intubation.

atropine

glycopyrrolate (Robinul)

These benzodiazepine antianxiety drugs are given preoperatively to relieve anxiety and provide sedation. A larger dose of diazepam will produce amnesia during minor surgical/dental procedures and endoscopic procedures; the patient is able to respond to commands to facilitate the procedure, but has little memory of events upon awakening. They are Schedule IV drugs.

diazepam (Valium)

lorazepam (Ativan)

midazolam

These narcotic drugs are given preoperatively to relieve pain and provide sedation. They are Schedule II drugs, except for pentazocine, which is a Schedule IV drug.

levorphanol (Levo-Dromoran)          oxymorphone (Numorphan, Opana)

meperidine (Demerol)                 pentazocine (Talwin)

morphine (Duramorph)

These barbiturate drugs are given preoperatively to produce sedation. They are Schedule II drugs.

pentobarbital

secobarbital (Seconal)

This antipsychotic drug is give preoperatively to decrease anxiety. It is not a schedule drug.

chlorpromazine (Thorazine)

## Drugs Used to Obtain General Anesthesia

General anesthesia involves the loss of consciousness as a means of producing a generalized anesthesia throughout the body, a technique that distinguishes it from all other types of anesthesia. In the operating room, the patient is first given a drug to induce general anesthesia. Once the patient is unconscious and intubated with an endotracheal tube, other anesthetic drugs are given to maintain general anesthesia throughout the surgical procedure. Drugs for the **induction of anesthesia** are generally given intravenously; drugs used to maintain general anesthesia may be given intravenously or by inhalation.

## Historical Notes

In 1874, Dr. Oré of France demonstrated the first use of intravenous anesthetic drugs during surgery. In 1920, the technique of endotracheal intubation was perfected. This allowed greater control of patient ventilation and anesthetic administration during surgical procedures.

### Intravenous Drugs for the Induction and Maintenance of General Anesthesia

Intravenous drugs provide a rapid loss of consciousness. This helps the anesthesiologist to initiate anesthesia quickly while minimizing patient anxiety. These intravenous drugs include ultrashort-acting barbiturate drugs, narcotic drugs, sedative drugs, and antianxiety drugs. Some of these drugs are used by themselves to provide light sedation during short procedures, such as endoscopies. Usually, one (or more) of these drugs is used in combination with an anesthetic gas to provide a balanced and sustained level of general anesthesia. These intravenous drugs are classified as Schedule II, III, or IV drugs, but the short duration of their use during surgery eliminates the possibility of addiction.

These ultrashort-acting barbiturate drugs are used to induce general anesthesia or are used in combination with other drugs to help maintain general anesthesia. Barbiturate drugs depress the central nervous system and produce sedation. In higher doses, they produce unconsciousness, but they have no analgesic effect. They are Schedule III or Schedule IV drugs.

methohexital (Brevital)

thiopental (Pentothal)

## Historical Notes

In 1935, thiopental (Pentothal), a barbiturate drug, was found to rapidly induce general anesthesic drug administration when given intravenously. It is still used today.

These narcotic drugs are used to induce general anesthesia or are used in combination with other drugs to help maintain general anesthesia. Narcotic drugs bind with opiate receptors in the brain to block pain. In higher doses, they produce unconsciousness. They are Schedule II drugs, except for pentazocine, which is a Schedule IV drug.

alfentanil (Alfenta)                oxymorphone (Numorphan, Opana)

fentanyl (Sublimaze)                pentazocine (Talwin)

meperidine (Demerol)                remifentanil (Ultiva)

morphine (Duramorph)                sufentanil (Sufenta)

These sedative and benzodiazepine antianxiety drugs are used to induce general anesthesia or are used in combination with other drugs to maintain general anesthesia. Etomidate and propofol are sedative drugs, but are not schedule drugs. Ketamine is a Schedule III drug. Lorazepam and midazolam are benzodiazepine antianxiety drugs and are Schedule IV drugs.

etomidate (Amidate)            midazolam

ketamine (Ketalar)             propofol (Diprivan)

lorazepam (Ativan)

## Inhaled General Anesthetic Drugs

These anesthetic drugs are in the form of a gas that is inhaled to induce or maintain general anesthesia (see ■ FIGURE 23–4). These drugs are used in conjunction with one or more of the intravenous anesthetic drugs described previously. They are not schedule drugs.

desflurane (Suprane)           isoflurane (Forane)

enflurane (Ethrane)            sevoflurane (Ultane)

halothane

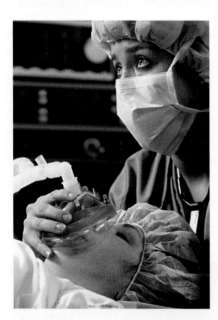

■ **FIGURE 23–4  Inhaled general anesthetic drug.**
This anesthesiologist is administering an inhaled anesthetic drug in the form of a gas to induce and maintain general anesthesia in this patient, who is about to undergo a surgical procedure.

## *Historical Notes*

The first mention of general anesthesia is in the book of Genesis when God caused a deep sleep to fall on Adam prior to removing a rib from his side to create Eve.

For many centuries, the only pain relief available during surgical procedures was from the use of alcohol or opium. These drugs failed to produce complete anesthesia, and surgeries were performed as quickly as possible, with assistants holding down the patient.

In 1772, nitrous oxide ($N_2O$) was discovered. Rather than being utilized as an anesthetic drug, it was inhaled at social parties to produce euphoria and was commonly known as *laughing gas*. Nitrous oxide was not recognized an inhaled drug that could produce general anesthesia until the 1860s.

During the first half of the 1800s, surgery was performed without the benefit of general anesthesia. In the PBS television series *Treasure Houses of Great Britain*, the story was told of the Marquis de Angelcy, whose leg was destroyed by cannon shot during the battle of Waterloo (1815). His leg was sawed off without the benefit of general anesthesia. The surgeon wrote afterward that he was amazed that the patient's pulse did not vary during the operation. The Marquis' only recorded comment was, "I do not think the saw was very sharp."

In 1846, William Morton, a Boston dentist, recognized that inhaled ether could produce general anesthesia. He gave the first public demonstration of surgery performed under ether anesthesia at Massachusetts General Hospital. The word *anesthesia* was coined at that time to describe the effects of ether. A monument at Morton's grave reads:

*Inventor and Revealer of Anaesthetic Inhalation.*
*Before Whom, in All Time, Surgery was Agony.*
*By Whom, Pain in Surgery Was Averted and Annulled.*
*Since Whom, Science Has Control of Pain.*

Alfred Gilman, Louis Goodman, et al., *The Pharmacologic Basis of Therapeutics*, 7th ed. New York: Macmillan Publishing Company, 1985, p. 261.

From its first use in 1846, ether enjoyed great popularity as an inhaled general anesthetic drug. However, it had an extremely unpleasant odor, was highly explosive, and frequently produced severe postoperative vomiting. Its use was discontinued in the 1960s.

At approximately the same time that ether was discovered, the Scottish obstetrician James Simpson introduced the general anesthetic gas chloroform. Chloroform had two advantages over ether: It had a more pleasant odor, and it was not explosive. However, it was much more toxic, and its use was associated with a higher mortality rate. Its use was discontinued after World War I.

Thus, within the scope of 17 years, the first three inhaled general anesthetic drugs—ether, chloroform, and nitrous oxide—were introduced. None of these remain on the market today, although nitrous oxide was only recently discontinued.

In 1929, the fourth general anesthetic drug, cyclopropane, was discovered by accident during research on another chemical. Cyclopropane was used widely until the late 1950s, when its use was curtailed due to the danger of explosion in operating rooms that then contained more and more electrical equipment.

No further advances were made in inhaled general anesthetic drugs until 1956, when halothane was developed from research with fluorine (conducted during World War II to produce the atomic bomb). Halothane marked the beginning of a new category of inhaled general anesthetic drugs that are still used today.

## Neuromuscular Blocker Drugs Used During General Anesthesia

Neuromuscular blocker drugs are given intravenously to block nerve transmissions throughout the body, to reduce resistance to endotracheal intubation, and to produce skeletal muscle relaxation. This last effect is particularly important during abdominal surgery when the muscles of the abdominal wall must relax in order to allow adequate visualization of the operative field within the abdominal cavity.

atracurium (Tracrium)                    rocuronium (Zemuron)

cisatracurium (Nimbex)                   succinylcholine (Anectine, Quelicin)

mivacurium (Mivacron)                    vecuronium (Norcuron)

pancuronium

*Note:* The suffixes *-curium* and *-curonium* are common to generic neuromuscular blocker drugs.

These drugs are used to reverse the effects of neuromuscular blocker drugs used during general anesthesia.

edrophonium (Reversol, Tensilon)

Enlon-Plus

## Drugs Used During the Postoperative Period

Nausea and vomiting can often occur in the postoperative period. Surgery, particularly abdominal surgery, can temporarily stop peristalsis. Then, as fluids accumulate in the GI tract, they cause distension and trigger postoperative nausea and vomiting. Drugs used to treat postoperative nausea and vomiting are discussed in Chapter 8.

## *Historical Notes*

For centuries, the South American Indians used arrows dipped in curare for hunting animals and in battle. This drug caused death by muscle paralysis. It was unknown to the rest of the world until 1595, when Sir Walter Raleigh brought it to England. Not until the 1940s, however, was curare introduced as the first neuromuscular blocker drug to be used during general anesthesia. Until that time, abdominal surgery presented a challenge to both the surgeon and the anesthesiologist because the abdominal muscles remained taut and unyielding except with the deepest level of general anesthesia. With curare, the anesthesiologist could maintain a lighter level of general anesthesia, while still obtaining complete abdominal wall relaxation.

## *Chapter Review*

### Quiz Yourself

1. Describe some historical milestones in the discovery of anesthetic drugs.
2. Define these words and phrases: *anesthesia, epidural anesthesia, general anesthesia, induction of anesthesia, regional anesthesia.*
3. What is the significance of the abbreviation *MPF* when seen in the trade name of some anesthetic drugs?
4. Why is epinephrine not added to the anesthetic drug lidocaine for anesthesia during procedures on the fingers?
5. Describe the five categories of drugs that are given preoperatively and their therapeutic effects.

6. If a Schedule II narcotic drug is used to induce general anesthesia, why does the patient not become addicted?
7. Describe the difference in the therapeutic effects of these drugs given to produce general anesthesia: ultrashort-acting barbiturate drugs, narcotic drugs.
8. Name several inhaled gases that are used to maintain general anesthesia.
9. What is the therapeutic effect of neuromuscular blocker drugs?
10. To what category of drugs does each of these drugs belong?

a. desflurane (Suprane)
b. fentanyl (Sublimaze)
c. halothane
d. hydroxyzine (Vistaril)
e. lidocaine (Xylocaine)

f. meperidine (Demerol)
g. methohexital (Brevital)
h. sufentanil (Sufenta)
i. vecuronium (Norcuron)

## Spelling Tips

**fentanyl**    Spelled with a *y*, but remifentan**i**l is spelled with an *i*.
**Novocain**    Does not have a final *e*, unlike other anesthetic trade name drugs.

## Multimedia Extension Exercises

■ Go to www.pearsonhighered.com/turley and click on the photo of the cover of *Understanding Pharmacology for Health Professionals* to access the interactive Companion Website created for this textbook.

CHAPTER

# 24 Emergency Drugs, Intravenous Fluids, and Blood Products

## Learning Objectives

After you study this chapter, you should be able to

1. Describe several routes for administering emergency drugs.

2. Describe the various types of drugs given during emergency resuscitation
   and their therapeutic effects.

3. Compare and contrast the site of action and therapeutic effect of various drugs
   used to treat drug overdose, suicide attempt, or accidental poisoning.

4. Describe the physiology of anaphylaxis and how drugs are used to treat it.

5. Describe the various ways in which intravenous fluids are administered.

6. Name several types of intravenous fluids.

7. Name several types of blood and blood products.

8. Compare and contrast the therapeutic effect of blood and blood products with
   that of plasma and plasma products.

There are several types of life-threatening emergencies that require prompt intervention with drugs: cardiac or respiratory arrest, shock from trauma or infection, anaphylaxis, or drug overdose. Unless these problems can be corrected within a matter of minutes, oxygen levels in the blood decrease, carbon dioxide and lactic acid levels in the blood increase, the blood pH becomes acidic, cellular metabolism in the vital organs slowly comes to a halt, and the patient dies.

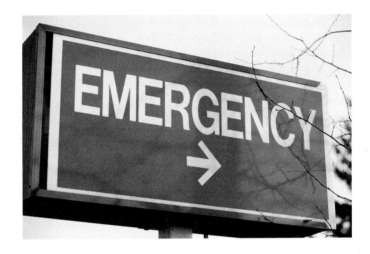

Basic life support measures, as performed in **cardiopulmonary resuscitation (CPR)**, involve mechanically circulating the blood and inflating the lungs with air. **Advanced cardiac life support (ACLS)** includes the use of drug therapy. A **crash cart** containing all necessary emergency drugs and resuscitative equipment is available in every patient area in the hospital, in physicians' offices and clinics, and in other healthcare facilities.

## Routes of Administration for Emergency Drugs

Most of the routes used to administer emergency drugs are different from the routes normally used to administer drugs. This is because of the need to have the drugs take immediate effect throughout the body. In an emergency, most routes of administration result in too slow an absorption rate for the drug to produce a therapeutic effect before the patient dies.

### Intravenous Route

Drugs are injected into an intravenous (I.V.) line or given by I.V. push or bolus to produce a maximum drug effect in the shortest period of time. Following successful resuscitation, continuous I.V. drip infusion is used. The I.V. route is by far the most common route for administering emergency drugs.

### Endotracheal Route

Drugs are administered by placing them into an endotracheal tube. As the lungs are mechanically ventilated, the drug solution is propelled into the lungs, where it is absorbed by the lung tissue and rapidly enters the blood. Therapeutic systemic drug levels can be achieved, but only certain drugs can be administered by this route.

# Drug Alert!

Healthcare professionals use the acronym NAVEL, as given in the *Advanced Cardiac Life Support (ACLS) Guidelines,* to help them remember which emergency drugs are appropriate to give via an endotracheal tube.

N    naloxone (Narcan)
A    atropine
V    vasopressin*
E    epinephrine (Adrenalin)
L    lidocaine (Xylocaine)

*Other sources also include Valium and Ventolin.

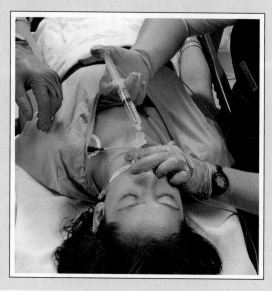

### Intracardiac Route

Intracardiac injection is not used frequently, but can be valuable when other routes have failed to produce a therapeutic effect. This route carries with it the risk of pneumothorax, cardiac tamponade, or coronary artery laceration if the injection is not properly placed within the left ventricle. Only the drugs calcium chloride and epinephrine (Adrenalin) can be given by the intracardiac route of administration.

## Drugs for Emergency Resuscitation

Emergency drugs are used to correct a life-threatening cardiac arrhythmia in which the heart is beating extremely fast, extremely slow, or has stopped completely (asystole). Emergency drugs are also used to increase an extremely low blood pressure.

### Drugs for Life-Threatening Cardiac Arrhythmias and Asystole

Lidocaine is indicated for the management of life-threatening ventricular fibrillation and is the drug of choice in resuscitative efforts for patients with this problem. It inhibits the flow of sodium into the myocardial cell; this slows the electrical impulse that causes the heart to fibrillate. This drug has no therapeutic effect if the heart is already in asystole.

lidocaine (Xylocaine)

Atropine blocks the action of acetylcholine released from the vagus nerve. The vagus nerve is part of the parasympathetic division of the nervous system that innervates the heart. When acetylcholine is released, the heart rate slows. Atropine blocks this action and is used specifically to treat severe bradycardia and bradyarrhythmias such as heart block (see ▇ **FIGURE 24-1**).

atropine

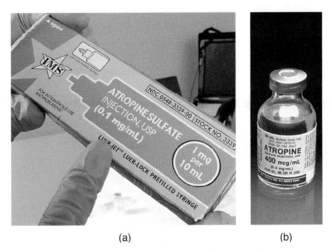

(a)          (b)

▇ **FIGURE 24-1 Drug packaging for atropine.**
Atropine is used to treat severe bradycardia and is given via the intravenous route of administration. Atropine is also given via the endotracheal route of administration to decrease bronchial secretions during resuscitation or surgery. (a) This package contains a prefilled syringe of atropine. (b) Atropine also comes in vials (shown) and ampules.

The hormone epinephrine is secreted by the adrenal medulla and acts as a neurotransmitter in the sympathetic division of the nervous system in response to pain, danger, or stress. Epinephrine prepares the body to respond with either "flight or fight" by

- stimulating alpha receptors to constrict the peripheral blood vessels and raise the blood pressure
- stimulating beta$_1$ receptors in the heart and blood vessels to increase the heart rate and cardiac output and raise the blood pressure
- stimulating beta$_2$ receptors in the lungs to relax bronchial smooth muscle, dilate the bronchi, and increase air flow to the lungs.

The drug epinephrine (Adrenalin) has these same actions (see ▇ **FIGURE 24-2**). Epinephrine makes the myocardium more responsive to the use of a defibrillator that can restore a normal rhythm. If the heart has stopped beating completely (asystole), epinephrine can actually stimulate contractions of the myocardium. As epinephrine stimulates the heart to beat, it also helps to maintain blood pressure and blood flow to the heart and brain to improve the chances of a successful resuscitative effort.

epinephrine (Adrenalin)

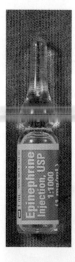

■ **FIGURE 24–2  Ampule of epinephrine.**
The drug epinephrine has the same effects as epinephrine secreted by the medulla of the adrenal gland. An ampule is a slender glass container with a main body and an elongated top. An alcohol swab is placed around the neck (narrow indentation) of the ampule, and the ampule is quickly snapped into two pieces. A syringe is used to withdraw the drug solution from the body of the broken ampule. An ampule can be used only once and the remaining, unused drug must be discarded because it contains no preservative.

## Drug Alert

The medulla of the adrenal gland secretes the hormone epinephrine, which is also known as *adrenaline* (a combination of the combining form *adrenal/o-* (adrenal gland) and the suffix *-ine* (substance pertaining to). As a drug, epinephrine is the generic name drug, but Adrenalin (without a final *e*) is the trade name drug. The slang form for the drug epinephrine is *epi.*

Calcium chloride is used to stimulate the myocardium to contract more forcefully and may even stimulate a contraction when the heart is in asystole and has failed to respond to epinephrine.

    calcium chloride

### Vasopressor Drugs

These drugs stimulate beta$_1$ receptors to increase the heart rate; they also stimulate alpha receptors in the blood vessels to produce vasoconstriction and raise the blood pressure. Vasopressor drugs also have the desirable effect of maintaining blood flow to the kidneys so that kidney ischemia does not later result in renal failure, which would complicate an otherwise successful resuscitative effort.

    dopamine                          norepinephrine (Levophed)

    epinephrine (Adrenalin)           phenylephrine (Neo-Synephrine)

    isoproterenol (Isuprel)

### Drugs for Metabolic Acidosis

During cardiac and respiratory arrest, the pH of the blood decreases rapidly as carbon dioxide and waste products accumulate in the blood. In this environment of severe acidosis, the effectiveness of any emergency drug is greatly diminished. These drugs correct acidosis by buffering excess hydrogen ions and returning the blood pH to within a normal range. There is controversy as to the true effectiveness of sodium bicarbonate. It may actually increase acidosis through a chemical reaction that releases more $CO_2$ into the blood. The American Heart Association guidelines recommend using it only after other measures have failed.

    sodium bicarbonate

    tromethamine (Tham)

## Did You Know?

Sodium bicarbonate is combined with aspirin or acetaminophen in the over-the-counter trade name drugs Alka-Seltzer and Bromo Seltzer and is given orally as an antacid to neutralize excess acid in the stomach and treat an upset stomach and heartburn.

## Drugs Used to Treat a Drug Overdose, Suicide Attempt, or an Accidental Poisoning

Any drug or substance, when ingested in large amounts, can be toxic and fatal. Treatment consists of removing the drug from the stomach (emetic drugs), binding the ingested drug to another substance to make it inert (absorbent drugs), and/or inactivating the drug in the blood (antagonist drugs).

### Emetic Drugs

Drugs that induce vomiting are useful only if the patient is conscious and will not aspirate vomited stomach contents. Emetic drugs are not helpful if the overdosed drug has already been absorbed from the stomach into the blood.

ipecac syrup

## Focus on Healthcare Issues

Bulimia is a psychiatric disease in which patients eat excessive amounts of food (binge) and then try to rid themselves of the food (purge) by using ipecac syrup to induce vomiting or laxative drugs to have increased bowel movements. Some patients with bulimia take two or more doses of ipecac syrup each day. This is an abuse of the drug and can have adverse effects on the heart, causing arrhythmias and heart damage.

### Absorbent Drugs

Absorbent drugs bind to overdosed drugs or toxic substances so that they cannot be absorbed from the stomach into the blood. They are administered orally to patients who are conscious or via a nasogastric tube to patients who are unconscious. This treatment is not effective if the overdosed drug or toxic substance has already been absorbed from the stomach into the blood.

activated charcoal

### Narcotic Antagonist Drugs

An overdose of a narcotic drug can be reversed by giving a narcotic antagonist or blocker drug intravenously. Narcotic antagonist drugs compete for the same receptor sites as the narcotic drug, block those receptors, and decrease the narcotic drug's effects of unconsciousness, respiratory depression, and hypotension. (See Chapter 22 for a list of generic and trade name narcotic drugs.)

nalmefene (Revex)

naloxone (Narcan) (see ■ FIGURE 24–3)

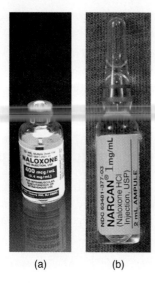

(a)          (b)

■ **FIGURE 24–3  Naloxone (Narcan).**
(a) This vial contains the generic drug naloxone. A vial has a rubber stopper
in its top so that multiple doses of the drug can be withdrawn at different
times. (b) This ampule contains the trade name drug Narcan. The generic
name naxolone is printed beneath in parentheses.

## Tranquilizer Antagonist Drugs

An overdose of a benzodiazepine-type antianxiety drug can be reversed by giving this antagonist or
blocker drug intravenously. It competes for the same receptor sites as the tranquilizer drug, blocks
those receptors, and decreases the tranquilizer drug's effects. (See Chapter 16 for a list of generic
and trade name benzodiazepine drugs.)

> flumazenil (Romazicon)

## Antidepressant Antagonist Drugs

An overdose of a tricyclic-type antidepressant drug can be reversed by giving this antagonist or
blocker drug intravenously. It competes for the same receptor sites as the antidepressant drug,
blocks those receptors, and decreases the antidepressant drug's effects. (See Chapter 16 for a list of
generic and trade name tricyclic antidepressant drugs.)

> physostigmine (Antilirium)

## Other Drugs for Overdose

This drug is used to treat an overdose of the cardiac drug digoxin. Because of digoxin's low therapeutic index (narrow margin between the therapeutic dose and a toxic dose) and its long half-life, it
is not uncommon for elderly patients to experience digoxin toxicity. (See Chapter 11 for a list of
digoxin drugs.)

> digoxin immune Fab (Digibind, Digidote)

This drug is used to treat acetaminophen overdose. It protects the liver, the main site of symptoms
from acetaminophen overdose. The exact mechanism of its action is not known.

> acetylcysteine (Acetadote, Mucomyst)

This drug is used to treat ethylene glycol and methanol poisoning. Ethylene glycol (antifreeze)
abused recreationally or swallowed accidentally can result in central nervous system damage, blindness,
or death. Methanol (wood alcohol) is found in commercial solvents and paints.

> fomepizole (Antizol)

## Did You Know?

Digoxin immune Fab is an antigen-binding fragment obtained from sheep that have been treated to produce antibodies against the drug molecule of digoxin. The word *Fab* in the generic name stands for *fragment, antibody binding.* The trade name Digidote comes from *digi-* for *digitalis* and *-dote* for *antidote.*

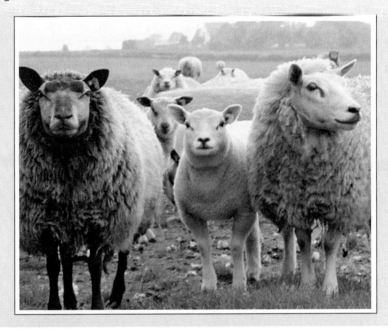

These drugs are used used to treat cyanide poisoning or pesticide (organophosphate) poisoning or an overdose of anticholinesterase drugs used to treat myasthenia gravis.

hydroxocobalamin (Cyanokit)          sodium nitrite

methylene blue (Urolene Blue)        sodium thiosulfate

pralidoxime (Protopam)

## Did You Know?

Sometimes, an alcoholic patient will drink methanol instead of ethanol (liquor). In the body, methanol is metabolized into formaldehyde, a toxic chemical that is used by pathologists to preserve biopsied tissue specimens.

Methylene blue is a dye that is used to stain tissue samples (Gram's stain, Wright's stain). It is used during surgery to stain tissue that is abnormal so that it can be excised. It is also an antiseptic drug that is included in many combination drugs to treat urinary tract infections (hence its trade name Urolene Blue).

These drugs are used to treat lead, mercury, arsenic, gold, iron, or aluminum toxicity and poisoning.

deferasirox (Exjade)                    edetate calcium disodium (Calcium Disodium Versenate)

deferoxamine (Desferal)                 succimer (Chemet)

dimercaprol (BAL In Oil)

## Drugs Used to Treat Anaphylaxis

Any allergic reaction involves the release of histamine. However, in anaphylaxis, massive amounts of histamine are released. This causes two life-threatening conditions: severe vasodilation (which causes an extreme drop in blood pressure and shock) and bronchoconstriction (which severely limits air flow in and out of the lungs). This drug constricts the blood vessels to restore a normal blood pressure and relaxes bronchial smooth muscle to allow adequate air flow.

epinephrine (Adrenalin, EpiPen) (see ■ FIGURE 24–4)

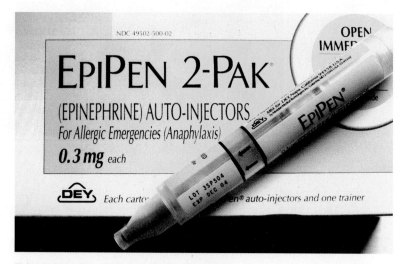

■ **FIGURE 24–4  Epinephrine (EpiPen).**
Patients with severe allergies to foods or insect bites often keep an EpiPen with them at all times in case of an unexpected severe allergic reaction. Note that the box says that it is for allergic emergencies/anaphylaxis. The EpiPen is a prefilled syringe (auto-injector) that the patient can quickly use to inject epinephrine into the thigh muscle.

## Intravenous Fluid Administration

Intravenous (I.V.) fluids may be prescribed and administered for any of these reasons:

- ■ To correct decreased levels of body fluid volume
- ■ To correct decreased levels of electrolytes or glucose
- ■ To provide nutritional support to patients who are NPO or who are temporarily unable to take in sufficient nutrients or fluids
- ■ To administer drugs
- ■ To administer blood or plasma products
- ■ To maintain venous access between drug doses.

### Types of Intravenous Fluid Administration

Intravenous (I.V.) fluid therapy and drugs to be given intravenously are administered in various ways.

1. **Continuous Infusion.**   In continuous infusion, the intravenous fluid flows continuously at a predetermined rate through an intravenous line and into a vein. The rate is ordered by the physician (e.g., 100 cc/hr) and is calculated on the basis of the patient's weight, fluid volume needs, and heart/kidney function. An intravenous (I.V.) line includes a bag containing I.V. fluid, connecting tubing, and a needle or flexible catheter inserted in the vein. Additional equipment can include an infusion pump that automatically infuses a set amount of fluid. This method is known as *intravenous drip*. A drug can be injected into the I.V. bag and administered continuously over several hours along with the I.V. fluid, at the same rate of flow prescribed for the I.V. fluid. A label stating the name of the drug, the dose, and the date and time is placed on the I.V. bag.

2. **I.V. Piggyback.**   A drug can be added to the intravenous fluids in a very small I.V. bag whose tubing is connected into the main I.V. tubing. Because the drug is mixed with a smaller amount of I.V. fluid, it is administered in an hour or less, even as the main I.V. continues at the prescribed rate of flow.

3. **I.V. Push.**   When the therapeutic effect of a drug needs to take effect almost immediately, the drug is injected all at one time (a **bolus**) through a **port** (rubber stopper) into the end of the I.V. tubing closest to the patient.

4. **Keep the Vein Open (KVO).**   If the patient does not need a large volume of I.V. fluid, but does need to have access maintained via the I.V. route, the physician can order the I.V. fluid to infuse at a very slow rate to just keep the vein open (KVO) and patent.

5. **Saline or Heparin Lock.**   This special device allows I.V. access without the need for continuously infusing I.V. fluids. It provides a convenient way to administer intravenous drugs on an intermittent basis. It contains a small reservoir that holds saline or heparin and keeps the vein free of clots. Because heparin can cause hemorrhaging, saline is more commonly used.

## Intravenous Fluids

The most commonly used intravenous (I.V.) fluids contain dextrose, electrolytes, or a combination of both.

### In Depth

Glucose, a simple sugar, is the only form of carbohydrate that cells can use as a source of energy. Intravenous fluids contain a glucose-type sugar known as *dextrose.* Dextrose has the same chemical structure as glucose, but the molecule is an isomer that is rotated in a right-hand direction (*dextr/o-* means *right*) when compared to the glucose molecule. However, the action of dextrose in the body is identical to that of glucose.

### Dextrose Intravenous Fluids

There are many different concentrations of dextrose and water intravenous fluids.

dextrose 2.5% in water

dextrose 5% in water (D5W)

dextrose 10% in water (D10W)

Dextrose also comes in concentrations of 20%, 25%, 30%, 40%, 50%, 60%, and 70%. These more concentrated intravenous fluids have a special use. They are administered as a bolus injection through an existing I.V. line to patients who have severely low blood sugar levels, including diabetic patients and premature infants.

## Sodium Intravenous Fluids

If a patient does not need dextrose, an intravenous fluid consisting of just sodium ($Na^+$), chloride ($Cl^-$), and water can be administered. Sodium is an important electrolyte in both the intracellular and extracellular fluids in the body. The intravenous fluid contains these electrolytes in proportions that parallel those in tissue fluids. This concentration is known as a *physiologic salt solution* or **normal saline (NS)**. Sometimes an intravenous fluid of **half normal saline** is ordered. This is written as 0.45% NaCl.

normal saline (NS) (0.9% NaCl) (see ■ **FIGURE 24–5**)

half normal saline (0.45% NaCl) (see Figure 24–5)

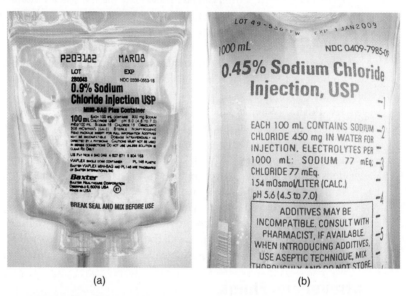

(a)                                              (b)

■ **FIGURE 24–5  Bags of normal saline and half normal saline intravenous fluids.**
(a) Normal saline is an intravenous fluid of 0.9% sodium chloride and water. It contains the electrolytes sodium ($Na^+$) and chloride ($Cl^-$) in the same proportions as in tissue fluids. (b) Half normal saline also contains the electrolytes sodium and chloride, but at half the concentration of normal saline. Half normal saline is written as 0.45% (not 0.5%), because 0.45% is one half of 0.9%.

## Combination Intravenous Fluids

Dextrose in varying concentrations and normal saline or half normal saline can be combined into a single intravenous fluid.

dextrose 5%, normal saline
   (D5/0.9% NaCl)

dextrose 5%, half normal saline
   (D5/0.45% NaCl)

dextrose 10%, normal saline
   (D10/0.9% NaCl)

dextrose 10%, half normal saline
   (D10/0.45% NaCl)

This combination intravenous fluid contains fixed amounts of dextrose and water with sodium, potassium, calcium, chloride, and lactate. The added electrolytes and lactate are known as **lactated Ringer's (LR)** or **Ringer's lactate (RL)**, named for the English physiologist, Sidney Ringer. *Crystalloid* is the name of a general category that refers to any intravenous fluid that provides dextrose and sodium chloride alone or in combination with other electrolytes.

dextrose 5% in lactated Ringer's (D5/LR)

## Total Parenteral Nutrition

Dextrose and electrolyte intravenous fluids are used to maintain fluid and electrolyte balance and supply calories, but they are unable to completely meet long-term nutritional needs. Specifically, they lack protein, fat, and vitamins. Patients whose nutritional needs cannot be met with dextrose and electrolyte fluids can be given a specially prepared intravenous fluid known as *total parenteral nutrition (TPN)*. It contains specific amounts of essential amino acids (proteins), as well as electrolytes, vitamins, and minerals, individually tailored to the patient's needs according to the physician's orders (see **FIGURE 24–6**). TPN is also known as ***hyperalimentation solution***. TPN, as

**TPN ORDER FORM**
**TOTAL PARENTERAL NUTRITION**

**ORDERING GUIDELINES:** To order standard TPN solution, check appropriate box(s). To change a standard additive in a TPN solution, re-write ALL additives in the OTHER column. Electrolytes are ordered per LITER and drug additives are ordered per KILOGRAM.

FOR INFORMATIONAL PURPOSES ONLY:

Electrolytes

Ca = ______
Phos = ______
Mg = ______

| | | | |
|---|---|---|---|
| Fluid Limit ______ mL / kg / day | | Cal ______ kcal / kg / day | |
| TPN ______ mL / kg / day | | Pro ______ g / kg / day | |
| Lipid ______ mL / kg / day | | Lipid ______ g / kg / day | |
| Other ______ mL / kg / day | | Na ______ mEq / kg / day | |
| Other ______ mL / kg / day | | K ______ mEq / kg / day | |

Comments ______

Weight ______ kg    Chronological age ______ months ______ yr.
TPN Solution ______ mL / kg / day    Diagnosis ______
Rate ______ mL / hour over ______ hours    Bag number ______

☐ **PERIPHERAL SOLUTION**

| * AMINO ACID | DEXTROSE |
|---|---|
| ☐ 1% | ☐ 10% |
| ☐ 2% | ☐ 12.5% |
| ☐ 2.5% | ☐ ____% |
| ☐ ____% | |

☐ **CENTRAL SOLUTION**

| * AMINO ACID | DEXTROSE |
|---|---|
| ☐ 1% | ☐ 15% |
| ☐ 2% | ☐ 20% |
| ☐ 2.5% | ☐ ____% |
| ☐ 3% | |
| ☐ 5% | |
| ☐ ____% | |

**ADDITIVE PROFILE**
Check appropriate box. To change standard, re-write all additives in OTHER column.

| ADDITIVE | ☐ STANDARD per liter | ☐ OTHER per liter |
|---|---|---|
| Sodium chloride | 15 mEq | mEq |
| Sodium acetate | 15 mEq | mEq |
| Sodium phosphate | None | mEq |
| Potassium chloride | 5 mEq | mEq |
| Potassium phosphate | 15 mEq (10.2 mMol) | mEq |
| Potassium acetate | None | mEq |
| Calcium gluconate | 20 mEq > 2.5 kg<br>30 mEq ≤ 2.5 kg | mEq |
| Magnesium sulfate | 4 mEq | mEq |
| Heparin | 500 units | units |
| Standard multivitamins | Standard | |
| † Standard trace elements | Standard | |
| | | |
| | | |
| | | |

**INTRAVENOUS LIPIDS 20%**
Total volume of______mL over______hours at______mL / hour. Infuse over 22–24 hours.
Maximum infusion rate for 20% lipid is 0.8 mL/ kg / hour for infants ≤ 33 wks gestation.

*** AMINO ACIDS**
Children ≤ 1 year receive Trophamine® + 40 mg L-cysteine / g protein delivered.
Children > 1 year receive standard amino acids.
**OTHER**
† Infants ≤ 2.5 kg. will receive a total of 400 μg / kg / day zinc.

Physician's Signature______ Date / Time Written______

**FIGURE 24–6 Total parenteral nutrition (TPN) order form.**
This preprinted physician order form allows the physician to customize the amounts of amino acids, electrolytes, vitamins, and minerals in a patient's TPN fluids. TPN is prepared in the hospital pharmacy.

well as intravenous lipids (described later), must be administered through a special long-term intravenous (Broviac or Hickman) catheter that is inserted into the subclavian vein or superior vena cava.

## Intravenous Lipids

To meet a patient's dietary fat requirements, a separate intravenous solution of lipids may be ordered. This solution is in the form of soybean or sunflower oil, along with water, glycerin, and egg yolk. Lipids (fats) are a more concentrated source of calories than dextrose (fats contain about 30% more calories per gram than dextrose), and lipids also contain essential fatty acids. Intravenous lipids are only given to patients who are unable to take oral feedings for an extended period of time.

Intralipid

Liposyn

## Intravenous Multivitamins

These drugs are a specially formulated combination of 12 vitamins for intravenous administration. They contain 9 water-soluble vitamins and 3 fat-soluble vitamins. (There are actually 4 fat-soluble vitamins that can be given as drugs but the fourth one—vitamin K—cannot be given intravenously.)

Berocca Parenteral Nutrition          Infuvite

Cernevit-12                           M.V.I.-12

## *Did You Know?*

A unit of whole blood contains 500 mL. The common phrase "a pint of blood" is fairly accurate and easy for laypersons to remember. One pint is equivalent to 473.17 mL, or nearly 1 unit of blood. Each year, Americans donate 15 million units of blood. Whole blood can be divided into its component parts (red blood cells, platelets, and plasma), and each part given to a different patient, as needed. About 8 million Americans receive transfusions of blood or blood products each year.

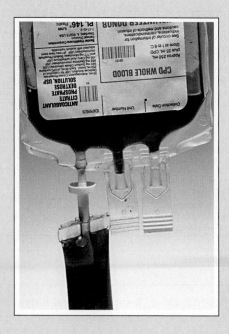

## Blood and Blood Products

Blood for transfusion is available as units of whole blood, packed red blood cells, and platelets.

### Whole Blood, Citrated

Whole blood contains all of the cellular components (red blood cells, white blood cells, and platelets), as well as plasma and its constituents (albumin, globulins, clotting factors, and electrolytes). *Citrated* refers to the anticoagulant (citrate) that is commonly used to preserve whole blood and prolong its refrigerated shelf life. Whole blood provides complete correction of blood loss by supplying both blood cells and plasma in the correct proportions. It provides the red blood cells needed to carry oxygen and carbon dioxide until the patient's own body is able to produce replacement red blood cells. Before whole blood can be given as a transfusion, the patient and the unit of blood must both be typed (for blood type) and crossmatched (to each other) to assure compatibility and avoid a transfusion reaction (hemolysis of red blood cells due to incompatibility of blood types).

### Packed Red Blood Cells

Packed red blood cells (PRBCs) are a concentrated preparation of RBCs in a small amount of plasma. PRBCs have an advantage over whole blood in that they can be given without causing fluid overload. This is of special importance in patients with congestive heart failure and in premature infants, who need the benefits of whole blood but cannot tolerate the increased blood volume. However, PRBCs do not contain the plasma proteins and clotting factors that are needed by some patients. PRBCs must be typed and crossmatched before being given to a patient.

---

### *Historical Notes*

Dr. Karl Landsteiner, a Viennese pathologist, categorized blood into four types: A, B, AB, and O. He won a Nobel Prize for this in 1930. In 1937, the first blood bank opened at Cook County Hospital in Chicago. In 1940, Dr. Landsteiner also discovered the Rh factor. Both the blood type and the presence or absence of the Rh factor determine which patients can receive that blood in a blood transfusion. The most common blood type is O positive, and the least common is AB negative. Blood type O negative is known as *the universal donor* because all patients can be given O negative blood without it causing a transfusion reaction.

---

### Platelets

Platelets are extracted from whole blood and suspended in a small amount of plasma. Platelets are crossmatched for best results, but in an emergency (and because platelets have a shelf life of only five days and supplies are limited) unmatched platelets may be given. Unmatched platelets do not provoke a transfusion reaction, but the body's antibodies quickly destroy them and they are less effective than matched platelets. Platelets are given to patients with thrombocytopenia or leukemia or to patients whose bone marrow is depressed after radiation or chemotherapy.

## Plasma and Plasma Volume Expanders

Plasma and plasma volume expanders do not contain blood cells. Plasma is derived from whole blood that has undergone plasmapheresis to remove the blood cells. Plasma has an advantage over blood in that it does not need to be typed and crossmatched. Plasma is given to hemophiliac patients who need clotting factors and to restore blood volume and electrolytes to normal levels in patients with severe burns, but it cannot raise the patient's hematocrit or contribute to the oxygen-carrying capacity of the blood.

## Focus on Healthcare Issues

Whole blood and red blood cells have a refrigerated shelf life of 42 days, according to the American Red Cross. However, a 2008 study reported in the *New England Journal of Medicine* found that patients undergoing heart surgery were more likely to die or have complications if they were given blood transfusions with blood that was more than two weeks old.

Patients preparing to have surgery can donate a unit of their own blood in advance so they can receive it during surgery. This is known as *an autologous blood transfusion*.

### Fresh Frozen Plasma

Fresh frozen plasma (FFP) consists of plasma that contains all of the plasma proteins and clotting factors. It is frozen to prolong its shelf life and then thawed to room temperature before being administered intravenously.

### Plasma Protein Fraction

Plasma protein fraction (PPF) is derived from plasma. It contains 5% plasma proteins (the most abundant of which is albumin) mixed with normal saline. It contains no clotting factors.

Plasmanate

Plasma-Plex

Protenate

### Albumin

This solution, derived from plasma, contains only the plasma protein albumin and no clotting factors. It is prepared in 5% and 25% solutions; the 5% solution approximates the concentration of normal blood plasma.

Albuminar

Albutein

Plasbumin

### Cryoprecipitate

This is a plasma extract prepared by freezing and then slowly thawing plasma. It contains concentrated amounts of factor VIII, von Willebrand's factor, and fibrinogen. It is used to treat hemophiliacs and patients with von Willebrand's disease.

## Historical Notes

In 1964, while watching a bag of plasma thaw, Dr. Judith Pool, a Stanford University researcher, noticed stringy flakes settling to the bottom; these subsequently turned out to be factor VIII and other clotting factors. Dr. Pool developed a method for separating the clotting factors from frozen plasma. The product was named *cryoprecipitate*. *Cryo-* is a combining form that means *frozen,* and *precipitate* means *something that separates out from a solution.*

## *Focus on Healthcare Issues*

Each lot of clotting factor is made from the pooled plasma of 15,000 to 60,000 donors. There are never enough volunteer donors, so companies pay plasma donors. The process of blood donation, separation of blood cells from plasma, and return of the blood cells to the donor is known as **plasmapheresis**.

Plasma, albumin, and cryoprecipitate are all prepared from pooled units of donor plasma. These are tested for hepatitis and HIV and heat-treated for 10 hours to reduce the risk of transmitting these diseases. However, these precautions are not totally effective in eliminating the viruses, particularly HIV. Because of this, many hemophiliacs who were repeatedly treated with clotting factors in the past developed hepatitis and AIDS.

All donated blood is tested for syphilis, hepatitis, and HIV according to guidelines established by the Food and Drug Administration (FDA), the federal organization that is responsible for the safety of blood and blood products in the United States. The FDA has banned blood donated by people who have lived in or visited Europe for a certain length of time because of the possibility of contamination with the microorganism that causes mad cow disease and a fatal neurological disease in humans. Although the United States has the safest blood supply in the world, there is still a small risk of transfused blood being contaminated with an infectious disease.

Elaine DePrince, *Cry Bloody Murder: A Tail of Tainted Blood.* New York: Random House, 1997, p. 27, 31, 37.

### Plasma Volume Expanders

Plasma volume expanders are manufactured from complex carbohydrates and normal saline. They do not need to be refrigerated, and they retain their potency for many months. Plasma volume expanders have an advantage over blood products in that they do not need to be typed or crossmatched. Plasma volume expanders are given intravenously to restore blood volume to normal levels.

dextran (Macrodex, Rheomacrodex)

hetastarch (Hespan)

hydroethyl starch (Voluven)

## *Did You Know?*

Dextran consists of synthetic complex carbohydrates with repeating three-dimensional structural units. Normal saline is able to enter these three-dimensional structures to form a viscous fluid that can be used as a substitute for plasma.

The combination of the bacteria *Streptococcus mutans* (present in the mouth) and sucrose (table sugar) produces dextran. The viscous and sticky dextran biofilm absorbs lactic acid produced by other bacteria in the mouth and holds it in contact with the teeth, producing tooth decay.

Hetastarch is derived from a waxy starch commonly found in potatoes, wheat, and corn. When hetastarch is mixed with normal saline and administered intravenously, it forms a solution similar in viscosity to normal plasma.

# Chapter Review

## Quiz Yourself

1. List five emergency drugs that can be given via an endotracheal tube. What is the acronym that helps you remember these drugs?
2. Describe the potential hazards involved in administering an emergency drug via the intracardiac route.
3. Name the drug of choice for resuscitating patients with ventricular arrhythmias.
4. What emergency drug is given to treat bradycardia?
5. Why is a drug sometimes needed to treat metabolic acidosis during cardiac and respiratory arrest?
6. What is the effect of ipecac syrup and how is it abused by some patients?
7. What is the therapeutic effect of activated charcoal? What are its limitations?
8. Why do patients taking digoxin often develop a drug toxicity?
9. What is something unique about the drug digoxin immune Fab?
10. What drug is used to treat anaphylaxis and what are its two therapeutic effects?
11. Define these words and phrases: *I.V. push, bolus, I.V. piggyback, I.V. drip, saline or heparin lock.*
12. Describe the contents and use of total parenteral nutrition (TPN).
13. What is lacking in intravenous dextrose and saline fluids?
14. Name three types of blood and blood cellular products.
15. What advantage does whole blood or PRBCs have over plasma?
16. Name three plasma volume expanders.
17. What federal agency is responsible for the safety of blood products in the United States?

## Spelling Tips

**intravenous**      Often misspelled and mispronounced as *intervenous.*
**parenteral**       Often misspelled as *parental.*

## Clinical Applications

1. Look at this photograph and answer the following questions.
    a. What is the name of the drug in the back row on the left?
    b. Is this a generic or trade name?
    c. What are the therapeutic effects of this drug?
    d. What is the name of the drug in the back row in the middle?
    e. Is this a generic or trade name?
    f. What is this drug used to treat?
    g. What is the name of the drug in the back row on the right?
    h. Is this a generic or trade name?
    i. What is this drug used to treat?
    j. What is the name of the drug in the front row?

**k.** Is this a generic or trade name?

**l.** What is this drug used to treat?

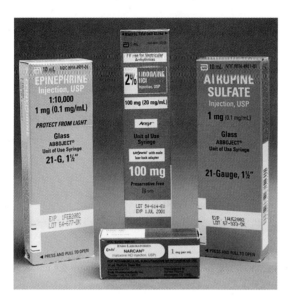

**2.** Look at this photograph and answer the following questions.

**a.** Besides water, what other ingredients are in this intravenous fluid?

**b.** Which of these ingredients are electrolytes and which is a sugar?

**c.** Another name for this intravenous fluid is 5% dextrose and half normal saline. If ½ is written as 0.5%, why is "half normal saline" written as 0.45%?

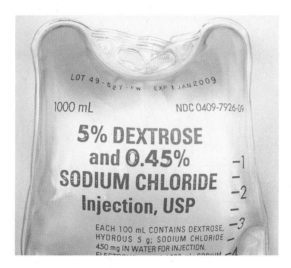

## Multimedia Extension Exercises

■ Go to www.pearsonhighered.com/turley and click on the photo of the cover of *Understanding Pharmacology for Health Professionals* to access the interactive Companion Website created for this textbook.

# Appendix A
# Sound-Alike Drug Names

There are many, many drugs on the market, some of which have very similar-sounding names. These sound-alike drugs can be the source of great confusion to students and healthcare professionals and often are the cause of medication errors.

The Institute for Safe Medication Practices (ISMP) receives 1,200 to 1,500 reports of deaths or serious injuries each year due to drug errors, and 25 percent of these errors are caused by sound-alike drug names. The *United States Pharmacopoeia* (USP) Medication Errors Reporting Program found that 15 percent of all reported errors involved sound-alike drugs. The Joint Commission on Accreditation of Healthcare Organizations (JCAHO) requires that all accredited healthcare facilities maintain a list of sound-alike drugs.

This is a list of sound-alike drugs gathered from many different sources.

| | | | |
|---|---|---|---|
| Accupril | Accutane | carboplatin | cisplatin |
| Accutane | Accuzyme | Celebrex | Cerebyx |
| AcipHex | Aricept | Celexa | Zyprexa |
| Actonel | Actos | codeine | Cardene |
| Adderall | Inderal | Coumadin | coumarin |
| Advicor | Advil | cycloserine | cyclosporine |
| alfentanil | fentanyl | Cytomel | Symmetrel |
| Aldara | Alora | dactinomycin | daptomycin |
| Alkeran | Leukeran | Denavir | indinavir |
| Allegra | Viagra | Depo-Medrol | Solu-Medrol |
| Anbesol | Anusol | desloratadine | loratadine |
| Ansaid | NSAID | DiaBeta | Zebeta |
| Antivert | Axert | dihydrocodeine | hydrocodone |
| Anzemet | Avandamet | Diovan | Zyban |
| arformoterol | formoterol | Diprivan | Ditropan |
| Aricept | AcipHex | dobutamine | dopamine |
| Asmalix | Asmanex | docetaxel | Taxol |
| atracurium | cisatracurium | Elmiron | Imuran |
| Avinza | Evista | enalapril | Enalaprilat |
| azithromycin | erythromycin | erythromycin | azithromycin |
| Baridium | barium | Evista | Avinza |
| Baridium | Pyridium | fentanyl | sufentanil |
| Benadryl | Benylin | Flomax | Flonase |
| calciferol | calcipotriene | Flonase | Flomax |

| | | | |
|---|---|---|---|
| folic acid | folinic acid | pentosan | pentostatin |
| foscarnet | Foscavir | Perdiem | permethrin |
| Hivid | Hivig | Perdiem | Prodium |
| Humalog | Humulin | Pitocin | Pitressin |
| hydralazine | hydroxyzine | Plavix | Plax |
| hydrocodone | hydromorphone | Prilosec | Prozac |
| hydrocortisone | hydrocodone | Procort | Procrit |
| hydromorphone | morphine | Protonix | Protopic |
| Inderal | Adderall | Pyridium | Baridium |
| indinavir | Denavir | Remifemin | remifentanil |
| isotretinoin | tretinoin | salicylic acid | salicylsalicyclic acid |
| K-Dur | K-Lor | Sarafem | Serophene |
| Lamictal | Lamisil | Seasonale | Seasonique |
| Lamictal | Lomotil | Serophene | Serostim |
| Lasix | Luvox | Solu-Cortef | Solu-Medrol |
| leucovorin | Leukeran | Solu-Medrol | Depo-Medrol |
| leucovorin | L-leucovorin | sufentanil | fentanyl |
| leucovorin | levoleucovorin | Taxol | docetaxel |
| Leukeran | Alkeran | Taxol | Paxil |
| Lexapro | Loxitane | Teladar | Temodar |
| Librium | Valium | Tiazac | Ziac |
| loratadine | desloratadine | TobraDex | Tobrex |
| Lotrimin | Lotrisone | tretinoin | isotretinoin |
| Luvox | Lasix | Tronolane | Tronothane |
| Luxiq | Luxor | Ultrace | Ultratrace |
| Maxzide | Microzide | valacyclovir | valganciclovir |
| melphalan | Myleran | Valium | Librium |
| MiraLax | Mirapex | Viagra | Allegra |
| MS Contin | OxyContin | Xanax | Zantac |
| Neosar | Neosol | Zantac | Xanax |
| Neurontin | Noroxin | Zebeta | DiaBeta |
| nitroglycerin | nitroprusside | Ziac | Tiazac |
| Norflex | norfloxacin | Zyban | Diovan |
| oxycodone | OxyContin | Zinacef | Zithromax |
| paclitaxel | Taxol | Zyprexa | Celexa |
| paclitaxel | Paxil | Zyrtec | Zantac |
| Paxil | Taxol | Zyvox | Zovirax |

# *Appendix B*

# Glossary of Key Words with Definitions

**absorption**   The first step in the drug cycle. Absorption involves the movement of a drug from the site of administration through tissues and into the blood. For most drug forms, absorption involves three steps: disintegrating, dissolving, and absorption. Only drugs given intravenously entirely bypass the step of absorption.

**acetylcholine**   Neurotransmitter that is released in the synapse between a motor neuron and a voluntary skeletal muscle cell. It is also released in the synapse between a neuron of the parasympathetic division of the nervous system and a smooth muscle cell, a cardiac muscle cell, or a gland. Acetylcholine activates cholinergic receptors on the cell. Its effect is blocked by anticholinergic drugs.

**addiction**   An acquired physical and/or psychological dependence on a substance. This substance can be a readily available item such as alcohol (beer, wine, liquor, ETOH, rubbing alcohol, wood alcohol), nicotine (cigarettes, cigars, chewing tobacco), inhalants (fumes and propellants), or an over-the-counter drug. This substance can also be a prescription drug (amphetamines, opioids, sedatives, or tranquilizers) or an illegal street drug (marijuana, cocaine, LSD, PCP). Addiction is characterized by the habitual use of the drug, increasing tolerance to the effects of the drug, the tendency to increase the drug dose in order to experience a greater effect, and the appearance of withdrawal symptoms when deprived of the drug. Legal drugs that have some potential to cause addiction are classified by law as controlled substances and are known as *schedule drugs*.

**adjuvant therapy**   The use of an additional, supporting type of treatment or therapy after the initial treatment or therapy for a disease has been completed.

> Example: The administration of chemotherapy drugs after another type of therapy (surgery or radiation therapy) has already been used as the primary treatment for the cancer.

**adrenergic drugs**   Categories of drugs that stimulate adrenergic receptors of the sympathetic division of the nervous system and produce changes in the body characteristic of the "fight-or-flight response" caused by the neurotransmitter epinephrine. These changes include increasing the heart rate, constricting smooth muscles around the arteries to raise the blood pressure, relaxing smooth muscles around the bronchi to increase air flow to the lungs, dilating the pupils for better vision, constricting arteries in the nasal mucosa to open up the nasal airways, causing skeletal muscles and the liver to release stored glycogen to provide more energy, causing the beta cells of the pancreas to release more insulin to metabolize glucose, and relaxing the smooth muscles of the stomach and intestines to decrease peristalisis and digestion. Also known as *sympathomimetic drugs* because they mimic the effect of the neurotransmitter epinephrine from the sympathetic division of the nervous system.

**adrenergic receptors**   Cell membrane structures that respond to the neurotransmitters epinephrine and norepinephrine from the sympathetic division of the nervous system, as well as to adrenergic drugs. Adrenergic receptors include $alpha_1$, $alpha_2$, as well as $beta_1$, and $beta_2$ receptors. Alpha$_1$ and alpha$_2$ receptors (also known as $\alpha$-adrenergic receptors) respond to norepinephrine and drugs that act in a similar way. Beta$_1$ and beta$_2$ receptors (also known as $\beta$-adrenergic receptors) respond to epinephrine and drugs that act in a similar way. (The Greek letters $\alpha$ and $\beta$ mean *alpha* and *beta*.)

**adverse effect**   A drug effect that is a severe side effect. Adverse effects are not as common as side effects, and so some adverse effects of a drug become apparent only after the drug has been taken by a large number of patients.

**afterload**   The blood pressure in the main arteries, against which the left ventricle must push when it contracts to pump blood out of the heart. The higher the afterload, the greater the chance of eventual heart failure. Antihypertensive drugs decrease the cardiac afterload.

**agonist drugs**   Categories of drugs that take the place of an important chemical in the body or stimulate a specific receptor on the cell membrane normally activated by that chemical, "unlock" the receptor, and activate a response. The response is like that of the chemical that normally activates that receptor. Agonist drugs have a drug effect that is opposite that of antagonist drugs.

**albumin**   The major protein in the plasma (liquid portion) of the blood. It is a large molecule that exerts osmotic pressure. It binds with drugs and keeps them from being excreted by the kidneys.

**allergic reaction**   Local or systemic reaction of the body to a foreign substance (e.g., pollen, animal dander, venom, or drug) in which histamine is released. An allergic reaction can be mild with localized itching, redness, and swelling, or it can be systemic with bronchoconstriction, hypotension, and shock.

**alpha receptor**   See *adrenergic receptor*.

**ampule**   A small, slender, glass container with a main body and a narrow, elongated neck. An ampule contains certain liquid drugs used only for injection or intravenous administration (see ■ **FIGURE B–1**.) An ampule is broken open by placing an alcohol swab around the neck (narrowest part) and briskly snapping both ends of the ampule apart. A syringe is used to withdraw the liquid drug from the body of the broken ampule. An ampule contains enough drug for one dose. Once an ampule is opened, the drug inside it is not saved or reused because it does not contain any preservative. Ampules often contain drugs used in emergency resuscitation, such as epinephrine (Adrenalin), calcium chloride, or 50% dextrose (D50). The word *ampule* has no proper abbreviation and should always be written in full, although it may be dictated as "amp."

Sample dictation: The patient was given an amp of D50 with relief of her hypoglycemic symptoms.

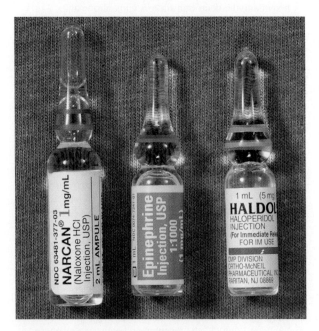

■ **FIGURE B–1  Three ampules.**
These ampules contain the emergency drugs Narcan (to treat an overdose of a narcotic drug), epinephrine (to stimulate the heart), and Haldol (an antipsychotic drug).

**analgesic drug**   A drug that selectively suppresses pain without producing sedation.

**analog**   A drug obtained by slightly modifying the molecular structure of another drug. Analogs are created for the purpose of changing the original drug's characteristics in order to produce a new, improved drug with fewer side effects or a stronger therapeutic effect.

**anaphylactic shock**   The most severe form of an allergic reaction. The release of massive amounts of histamine causes bronchospasm, shock, and even death. Also known as *anaphylaxis*.

**anesthetic drug**   A drug that eliminates pain. A local anesthetic drug eliminates pain in a limited area because of its local effect on sensory nerves. A general anesthetic drug eliminates pain as well as voluntary muscle control by inducing unconsciousness.

**antacid drug**   A drug that neutralizes excessive acid in the stomach.

**antagonism**   Condition in which two drugs taken together combine to produce an effect that is less than the intended effect for either drug.

**antagonist drugs**   Categories of drugs that bind to specific receptors on the cell membrane and block the substance in the body that normally activates that receptor. Antagonist drugs can also block another drug from activating that receptor. Antagonist drugs have a drug effect that is opposite that of agonist drugs.

**antiarrhythmic drug**   A drug that corrects a cardiac arrhythmia, such as an abnormally slow, abnormally fast, or irregular heart rate.

**antibiotic drug**   A drug used to treat infection by killing (bactericidal) or inhibiting the growth (bacteriostatic) of disease-causing (pathogenic) bacteria.

**antibody**   Substance released by the immune system in response to the presence of a foreign substance or drug. See also *antigen*.

**anticholinergic drugs**   Categories of drugs that block the effect of the neurotransmitter acetylcholine at the site of cholinergic receptors. Anticholinergic drugs have the opposite effect of cholingic drugs. Anticholinergic drugs exert a predictable set of side effects known as *anticholinergic side effects*. The ABCs of anticholinergic side effects: A, anticholinergic; B, blurred vision, bladder retention; C, constipation; D, dry mouth.

**anticoagulant drug**   A drug that prevents the clotting of blood.

**anticonvulsant drug**   A drug that prevents or treats epileptic seizures.

**antidepressant drug**   A psychotherapeutic drug that produces mood elevation and relieves depression.

**antidiabetic drug**   A drug used to treat diabetes mellitus. Antidiabetic drugs can be insulin that is injected when the pancreas does not produce insulin, or they can be drugs that are given orally that stimulate the pancreas to secrete more insulin.

**antidiarrheal drug**   A drug that treats diarrhea.

**antiemetic drug**   A drug that prevents or relieves nausea and vomiting. (The combining form *emet/o-* means *vomiting*.)

**antifungal drug**   An anti-infective drug that can kill fungi and is used to treat fungal infections.

**antigen**    Any foreign substance in the body that the immune system recognizes as foreign and sends antibodies against. An antigen can be pollen, a drug, an implanted device, or even red blood cells in a blood donation from another person.

**antihistamine drug**    A drug used to decrease the symptoms of inflammation, redness, edema, and itching caused by the release of histamine during an allergic reaction.

**antihypertensive drug**    A drug that lowers high blood pressure (hypertension).

**anti-inflammatory drug**    A drug used to decrease symptoms of inflammation by inhibiting the release of prostaglandins.

**antineoplastic drug**    A drug that is selectively toxic to rapidly dividing cells, such as malignant cells, and is used to treat cancer. The word *neoplasm* means *new growth*. Also known as a ***chemotherapy drug***.

**antipruritic drug**    A drug that prevents or relieves itching. (*Pruritus* means *itching*.)

**antipyretic drug**    A drug that decreases the body temperature in a patient with a fever.

**antiseptic drug**    A drug that inhibits the growth of bacteria, but does not destroy them. Antiseptic drugs are used topically, not internally.

**antispasmodic drug**    A drug used to stop the spasm of voluntary or involuntary muscles.

**antitussive drug**    A drug that suppresses coughing. (The combining form *tuss/o*-means *cough*.)

**antiviral drug**    An anti-infective drug that can kill or inhibit the growth of viruses and is used to treat viral infections.

**apothecary system**    Old system of drug measurement that originally came from England. It included drug doses such as the minim, grain, scruple, and dram. These have been discontinued, except for the grain, which is still used to measure some drugs, although the drug label shows the measurement of grains (gr) and the more common equivalent measurement of milligrams (metric system of measurement).

**bactericidal drug**    An anti-infective drug that kills bacteria. Most antibiotic drugs are bactericidal.

**bacteriostatic drug**    An anti-infective drug that inhibits the growth of bacteria but does not kill them. Some antibiotic drugs are bacteriostatic.

**beta receptor**    See *adrenergic receptor*.

**beta-lactam ring**    Molecular ring structure within the penicillin molecule.

**beta-lactamase**    Enzyme produced by penicillin-resistant bacteria. It inactivates penicillin by breaking the penicillin molecule at the site of the beta-lactam ring.

**bioavailability**    Extent to which a drug is able to reach cellular receptors and make its effect felt in the body. That portion of the total drug dose that, after absorption, is actually available to interact with receptors and produce a therapeutic effect. Bioavailability is determined by a number of factors influencing absorption, including drug composition (inert fillers and buffers), drug particle size, and stomach pH. Bioavailability can be tested by obtaining blood levels of the drug at various intervals after administration.

**biotransformation**    See *metabolism*.

**blood–brain barrier**    Network that exists between the capillary walls of blood vessels in the brain and the surrounding brain tissues. Many drugs are able to pass through the blood–brain barrier and exert an effect, but some are not.

**bolus**    The whole amount of a liquid drug injected in a short period of time through a port (rubber stopper) in the I.V. tubing by gently pushing on the plunger of the syringe. This is often referred to as ***I.V. push***.

**bore of a needle**    The diameter of the internal hole that runs the length of a needle. The word *bore* is synonymous with *gauge*, but the bore of a needle is never assigned a number during the manufacturing process. The bore of a needle is simply designated as either small or large. See also *gauge*.

   Sample dictation: A large-bore I.V. was inserted and normal saline allowed to run in.

**brand name**    See *trade name*.

**bronchodilator drug**    A drug that relaxes the smooth muscles that surround the bronchi. This allows them to dilate, which increases air flow into the lungs.

**buccal route**    Route of administration in which the drug (usually in a tablet form) is placed between the cheek and the lower teeth and is allowed to disintegrate slowly and dissolve in the saliva.

**butterfly needle**    Specially designed needle that is of a very short length and high gauge. It has distinctive color-coded tabs of plastic on each side (see ■ **FIGURE B–2**). These tabs help control the needle when it is inserted into a vein. The tabs also help hold the needle in place when it is taped

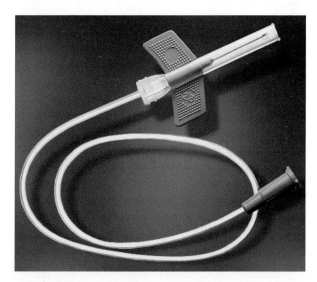

■ **FIGURE B–2** Butterfly needle with extension tubing.

down. The tabs make the needle appear like the wings of a butterfly. Butterfly needles are most often used to draw blood or start intravenous lines on premature infants or on elderly patients with fragile veins.

**caplet**   Tablet form of a drug in which the tablet is coated and in the form of an elongated capsule.

**capsule**   Drug form that comes in two varieties. The first is a soft, one-piece gelatin shell with the liquid drug inside. The second type of capsule is a hard shell manufactured in two pieces that fit together and hold the powdered or granular drug inside (see ■ **FIGURE B–3**). Hard capsules come in a variety of colors. In written prescriptions, *capsule* is sometimes abbreviated as *cap* or *caps*.

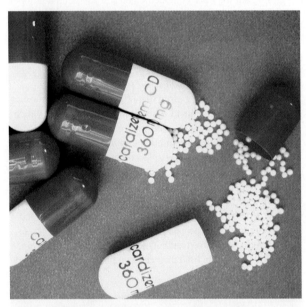

**■ FIGURE B–3 Capsule.**
These are two-piece capsules, and they are filled with granules of drug rather than powdered drug.

**chemical name of a drug**   Name that is assigned by the International Union of Pure and Applied Chemistry (IUPAC). The chemical name accurately describes the molecular structure. The chemical name is commonly used by drug companies and researchers, but is too lengthy and complicated for everyday use by healthcare professionals.

**chemotherapy drug**   See *antineoplastic drug*.

**cholinergic drugs**   Categories of drugs that stimulate cholinergic receptors of the parasympathetic division of the nervous system and produce changes in the body characteristic of the "rest-and-digest" response. These changes include decreasing the heart rate, relaxing smooth muscles around the arteries to lower the blood pressure, and constricting smooth muscles around the stomach and intestines to increase peristalsis and digestion.

**cholinergic receptors**   Cell membrane structures that respond to the neurotransmitter acetylcholine from the parasympathetic division of the nervous system, as well as to cholinergic drugs. The adjective *cholinergic* is derived from the noun *acetylcholine*. There are two types of cholinergic receptors: muscarinic and nicotinic.

**chronotherapy**   Method of drug therapy that attempts to coordinate the administration and metabolism of a drug to the body's own biological rhythms.

**control group**   Group of patients during clinical drug trials that receives a placebo rather than the actual drug being tested. However, neither the patients nor the physician-investigators know which patients are receiving the drug and which patients are in the control group.

**controlled substances**   See *schedule drugs*.

**corticosteroid drug**   A drug that suppresses the response of the immune system and is used to treat severe inflammation.

**cream**   Drug form that is a semisolid emulsion of oil (lanolin or petroleum) and water, the main ingredient being water. Emulsifying agents are added to keep the oil and water mixed together. Creams are applied topically and exert a topical or local effect.

**cubic centimeter**   Unit of measurement of volume from the metric system for liquid drug doses. It is equivalent to a milliliter. *Cubic centimeter* is abbreviated as *cc*.

**decongestant drug**   A drug that decreases congestion of the mucous membranes of the sinuses and nose.

**dependence**   A physical or psychological need for a drug. Physical dependence consists of physical changes that occur in the body in response to the presence of the drug. These can include pleasant physical sensations, such as relaxation or stimulation. Psychological dependence consists of psychological changes that occur in the body in response to the presence of the drug. These can include euphoria or sedation. When the drug is withheld, the body exhibits withdrawal symptoms: physical signs of sweating, nausea, cramps, etc., and psychological signs, such as a compelling desire to obtain more drug.

**dextrorotary**   The structure of a drug molecule which, when light is passed through it, bends the light to the right. The combining form *dextr/o-* means *right*. The generic name of some drugs indicates that they are dextrorotary molecules (e.g., dextromethorphan, dextroamphetamine). Also see *isomer*.

**diluent**   An agent such as sterile normal saline or sterile water that is used to reconstitute the powdered form of a drug to prepare it for injection (e.g., bacteriostatic diluent that has a preservative in it to retard bacterial growth). The word *diluent* is frequently misspelled and mispronounced as *dilutent* because of its association with the word *dilute*.

**disinfectant**   An agent (not used as a drug) that kills microorganisms. It is used to sterilize instruments and surfaces.

**distribution**   The second step in the drug cycle. Once a drug has been absorbed from body tissues and into the blood, it is distributed throughout the body via the circulatory system.

**diuretic drug**    A drug used to treat edema and hypertension by causing the kidneys to excrete more sodium and water and therefore more urine.

**dopamine**    Neurotransmitter that is released in the synapse between neurons of the central nervous system within the cerebral cortex, hypothalamus, limbic system, and the midbrain.

**dose**    See *loading dose, maintenance dose, therapeutic dose, toxic dose*.

**dram**    See *apothecary system*.

**drug cycle**    See *absorption, distribution, metabolism*, and *excretion*.

**drug holiday**    Discontinuation of a drug for a few days. This is done in patients with Parkinson's disease who need larger and larger doses of a drug over time, but then the side effects of that drug become intolerable.

**drug idiosyncrasy**    Type of drug reaction that is not a side effect, adverse reaction, or allergic reaction. It is an individual's unique reaction to a drug, based on the person's genetic makeup.

**drug of choice**    A drug that has been shown to be of particular clinical value in treating a specific disease. It is preferred above all other similar drugs because of its superior therapeutic effect. The drug of choice can change when a new drug is introduced for treating a specific disease and is found to be superior to the older drug.

**effervescent tablet**    Tablet form of a drug that is dissolved in a glass of water before being swallowed.

**efficacy**    How effective a drug is at producing a desired result.

**elixir**    Drug form that is a liquid and contains the drug in a water and alcohol base with added sugar and flavoring.

**emulsion**    Drug form that is a liquid that contains fat globules dispersed uniformly throughout a water base.

**endorphins**    Neurotransmitter released in the synapse between neurons in the hypothalamus, thalamus, and brainstem. Endorphins are one of several natural pain relievers produced by the brain. The word *endorphins* is a combination of the words *endogenous* (produced within) and *morphine* (a strong, pain-relieving drug).

**enteric-coated tablet**    Tablet form of a drug that is covered with a special coating that resists stomach acid but dissolves in the alkaline environment of the small intestine to avoid irritating the stomach.

**epinephrine**    Hormone secreted by the adrenal medulla. It is released into the blood and acts as a neurotransmitter that activates many receptors in the sympathetic division of the nervous system. It is secreted during times of exercise, stress, or danger and initiates the automatic "fight or flight" response of the body by increasing the heart rate, constricting the arteries to increase the blood pressure, dilating the pupils, and dilating the bronchi to increase air flow to the lungs.

**excretion**    The fourth and final step in the drug cycle. Excretion of a drug takes place through the kidneys (urine) and also in smaller amounts through the skin, saliva, tears, and breast milk.

**expectorant drug**    A drug that thins mucus in the respiratory tract to make it easier to cough up and out of the chest.

**first-pass effect**    Initial metabolism of a drug by liver enzymes when the drug is given by the oral route. The drug is absorbed from the intestines into the portal vein to the liver. The drug must first pass through the liver before it can enter the general circulation. For some drugs, the first-pass effect is so extensive that most of the drug dose is immediately metabolized, and the drug must be given by a different route of administration in order to be therapeutic.

**frequency distribution curve**    Mathematical representation that shows the numbers of people who respond or do not respond to a particular drug and at what doses. This is calculated during the clinical trials of a drug before it is approved for marketing.

**gauge of needle**    The diameter of the internal hole that runs the length a needle. The lower the gauge number, the larger the diameter of the hole will be. For example, a 15-gauge needle has a large hole that allows blood to flow freely without clotting during a blood donation. An 18- to 22-gauge needle is used for intramuscular injections in adults. A 27-gauge needle is a very fine needle that is used for an intravenous line in a premature baby with tiny veins. Gauge is abbreviated as G (e.g., 27G needle). See also *bore*.

**gene splicing**    See *recombinant DNA technology*.

**generic name of drug**    Name given to a chemical substance by the drug company together with the United States Adopted Names (USAN) Council. There is always only one generic drug name related to a specific chemical name.

**genetic engineering**    See *recombinant DNA technology*.

**grain**    See *apothecary system*.

**gram**    Measurement of the metric system. One gram equals 1,000 milligrams. The abbreviation for *gram* is g.

**half-life**    The time required for drug levels in the serum to decrease from 100 percent to 50 percent. The half-life of a drug can be significantly prolonged when liver or kidney disease results in decreased metabolism or excretion of a drug. The shorter a drug's half-life, the more frequently it must be administered to sustain therapeutic levels.

**heparin or saline lock**    A special type of device that allows for permanent intravenous access when the patient does not need I.V. fluids. It consists of a flexible catheter inserted in the vein and an outer rubber port for access that contains a small reservoir of heparin that keeps the vein free of clots. It is a convenient way to administer I.V. drugs on an intermittent basis. Because heparin can cause hemorrhaging and is incompatible with some drugs, saline is more commonly used.

**histamine**    Substance released when an antibody from the immune system combines with an antigen (foreign substance or drug) in an allergic reaction. Histamine produces mild-to-severe allergic symptoms, depending on the amount released: itching, swelling, redness, sneezing, wheezing, bronchospasm, shock, and even death. See *anaphylactic shock*.

**hypodermic**    General word for an injection administered under the skin. It includes subcutaneous injections as well as intramuscular injections.

**inhalation**    Route of administration that involves inhaling a drug that is in a gas, liquid, or powder form. The drug is absorbed through the alveoli of the lungs.

**inhaler**    See *metered-dose inhaler*.

**insulin syringe**    A syringe designed to measure and administer only insulin (see ■ **FIGURE B–4**). It is calibrated in units, not in milliliters (or cubic centimeters), as are all other syringes. The attached needle is the appropriate length for a subcutaneous injection, which is the route of administration by which injected insulin is given.

structural relationship to each other. Dextrorotary and levorotary drugs are isomers with identical chemical structures. See also *dextrorotary* and *levorotary*.

**laxative drug**    A drug used to relieve constipation by promoting a bowel movement by stimulating peristalsis in the large intestine or by softening the stool.

**levorotary**    The structure of a drug molecule which, when light is passed through it, bends the light to the left. The combining form *levo-* means *left*. The generic name of some drugs indicates that they are levorotary molecules (e.g., levodopa). Also, *levorotary* can be abbreviated as *L*, as in the drugs L-dopa and L-asparaginase. See also *isomer*.

**loading dose**    Drug dose that is given if the therapeutic effect of a drug is needed immediately. The loading dose is generally twice the maintenance dose. Digoxin (Lanoxin) is often given in a loading dose to patients in acute congestive heart failure. The loading dose is given only once; then the maintenance dose is used for subsequent treatment. See also *maintenance dose*.

**lozenge**    Tablet form of a drug formed from a hardened base of sugar and water containing the drug and other flavorings.

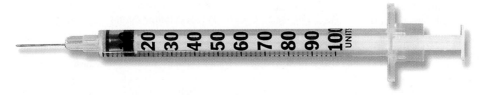

■ **FIGURE B–4**  **Insulin syringe.**

**intra-arterial route**    Route of administration in which a liquid drug is injected into an artery.

**intra-articular route**    Route of administration in which a liquid drug is injected into a joint.

**intracardiac route**    Route of administration in which a liquid drug is injected directly into the heart during emergency resuscitation following cardiac arrest.

**intradermal route**    Route of administration in which a liquid drug is injected into the dermis, the layer of skin just below the epidermis.

**intramuscular route**    Route of administration in which a liquid drug is injected into a muscle.

**intravenous route**    Route of administration in which a liquid drug is injected directly into a vein.

***in vitro* testing**    Testing of a drug that is done in a laboratory in test tubes (*in vitro* is Latin for *in glass*).

***in vivo* testing**    Testing of a drug that is carried out in animals or humans (*in vivo* is Latin for *in living*).

**isomer**    A drug that has the same chemical formula (the same types and numbers of atoms in its molecule) as another drug, but has those atoms arranged in a different way—either with different chemical bonds or in a different

Lozenges are never swallowed, but are allowed to dissolve slowly into a liquid to release the drug topically in the mouth and throat.

**maintenance dose**    Drug dose that is the standard dose prescribed by the physician. See also *loading dose*.

**median effective dose ($ED_{50}$)**    The dose at which 50 percent of animals show a therapeutic response to a drug during testing.

**median toxicity dose ($TD_{50}$)**    The dose at which 50 percent of animals have toxic levels of the drug during testing.

**metabolism**    The third step in the drug cycle. Metabolism gradually transforms or metabolizes the drug from its original active form to a less active, or even inactive, form. This process is accomplished in the liver, the principal organ or metabolism, by the action of liver enzymes. Also known as *biotransformation*.

**metabolite**    The inactive form of a drug after metabolism. It is a waste product that must be removed from the body. However, some drugs are actually administered in an inactive form and remain inactive until they are metabolized by the liver. Then this metabolite form of the drug becomes the active form. See also *prodrug*.

**metered-dose inhaler**    Drug dispenser with a mouthpiece and aerosol canister. The canister is filled with a bronchodilator drug in a liquid, aerosol, or powder form. When the canister is pushed down, the drug is dispensed through the mouthpiece as a puff, and the patient inhales the drug.

**microgram**    Unit of measurement from the metric system for drug doses. One thousand micrograms equals one milligram. Abbreviated as *mcg*.

**milliequivalent**    Unit of measurement from the metric system for drug doses. An equivalent is the molecular weight of an ion divided by the number of hydrogen ions it reacts with. Doses of potassium are measured in milliequivalents. Abbreviated as *mEq*.

**milligram**    Unit of measurement from the metric system for drug doses. One thousand milligrams equals one gram. Abbreviated as *mg*.

**milliliter**    Unit of measurement of volume from the metric system for liquid drug doses. One thousand milliliters equals one liter. Abbreviated as *mL*. It is the equivalent of a cubic centimeter.

**molecular pharmacology**    The study of the chemical structures of drugs and the effect of drugs at the molecular level within cells.

**mydriatic drug**    A drug that dilates the pupil of the eye to facilitate an eye examination.

**nasogastric route**    Route of administration in which a liquid drug is given through a nasogastric tube that is passed from the nose through the esophagus to the stomach. This route is used to administer drugs to patients who cannot take oral drugs.

**needle**    Very narrow and long metal cylinder with an internal hole. It is attached to a syringe or to intravenous tubing. Needles are classified according to gauge and length. The **gauge** is the diameter of the internal hole that runs the length of a needle. The length of the needle varies from ½ inch for the needle on an insulin syringe, ⅝ inch for the needle on a tuberculin syringe, and 1½ inches for the needle used for an intramuscular injection. See also *bore, butterfly needle,* and *gauge*.

**norepinephrine**    Hormone secreted by the adrenal medulla. It is released into the blood and acts as a neurotransmitter that activates receptors in the sympathetic division of the nervous system. It is secreted during sleep and throughout the day.

**ointment**    Drug form that is a semisolid emulsion of oil (lanolin or petroleum) and water, the main ingredient being oil. Ointments are applied topically and usually exert a topical or local effect.

**over-the-counter drug**    Drug that can be purchased without a prescription and is generally considered safe for consumers to use if the label's directions are followed carefully and all warnings are heeded.

**parenteral route**    Phrase that theoretically includes all routes of administration other than the oral route; but in clinical usage, parenteral administration commonly includes these routes: intradermal, subcutaneous, intramuscular, and intravenous.

**pastille**    See *troche*.

**pathogen**    An agent (e.g., bacteria, virus, fungus, prion, etc.) that causes disease.

**peak level**    The highest serum level achieved following a single dose of a drug, as determined by a blood test. If the peak level is too high, the patient can develop toxicity. If the peak level is too low, the drug will not have a therapeutic effect.

**pharmacodynamics**    The mechanism of action by which drugs produce their effects (desired or undesired) based on time and dose. It includes determining the frequency distributions, median effective dose, median toxicity dose (in animals), half-life, and therapeutic index.

**pharmacogenetics**    How the genetic makeup of different people affects their response to certain drugs.

**pharmacogenomics**    Using genome technology to discover new drugs.

**pharmacokinetics**    Description of how drugs move through the body in the processes of absorption, distribution, metabolism, and excretion. See also *drug cycle*.

**pharmacotherapy**    Using drugs to affect the body therapeutically to prevent disease, to diagnose disease, or to treat disease.

**placebo**    A drug form that exerts no pharmacologic effect, no therapeutic effect, and no side effects when administered. Placebos are used in double-blind research studies in which neither the researcher nor the patient knows whether the medication given was the drug being tested or was a placebo. Placebos are commonly sugar pills or injections of sterile normal saline solution. Interestingly, while it is physiologically impossible for a placebo to exert any pharmacologic effect, patients often report a decrease in certain types of symptoms and can even experience "side effects" when given a placebo. These effects are quite real and demonstrate that, in some situations, the power of suggestion can produce changes within the body that closely mimic the pharmacologic effect of an actual drug. The word *placebo* means *I will please* in Latin.

**plasma proteins**    See *albumin*.

**polypharmacy**    The practice of taking many different prescription and over-the-counter drugs, often without the knowledge of the physician.

**port**    A self-sealing rubber stopper in the I.V. tubing. It can be used again and again. Liquid drugs are injected through it into an intravenous line or a needle is inserted into it through which to administer a piggyback I.V. bag. A heparin lock also contains a port.

**potency**    Amount of therapeutic effect a drug can produce at a specific dose. A more potent drug will produce a therapeutic effect at a lower dose compared to another drug.

**prescription drug**   A drug that is not safe to use except under professional medical supervision. Prescription drugs can only be obtained with a written prescription or voice order from the physician, dentist, nurse practitioner, or other healthcare provider whose license permits this. Prescription drugs are also known as *legend drugs* because the drug company or pharmacist adds one of these two legend ends (inscriptions) to the drug package or to the filled prescription bottle: "Caution: Federal law prohibits dispensing without a prescription" or "Rx only."

**prodrug**   A drug that becomes active only after it is metabolized by the liver. The prefix *pro-* means *before,* and *prodrug* refers to the drug that is administered before the active drug is produced.

**prophylaxis**   Prevention of a disease or a condition. A drug given prophylactically is administered before the onset of a disease or other condition in order to prevent its occurrence (e.g., birth control pills, flu shots, and vaccines; an antibiotic drug is given prophylactically to patients with a history of rheumatic heart disease prior to undergoing surgery or a tooth extraction). This word is from the Greek, meaning *to keep guard before.*

**proprietary drug**   Another name for a trade name or brand name drug. The trade name for a drug is selected by the drug company that owns the right to use that particular trade name. *Proprietary* is a legal word that expresses that ownership.

**protocol**   A standardized, written plan of treatment for a particular type of disease. Protocols are based on medical research and findings that have shown what types of treatment have been successful in the past. A protocol details what types of treatments should be given, including what drugs should be given and in what doses.

> Examples: A chemotherapy protocol details which chemotherapy drugs should be given, in what order they should be given, and in what doses to treat a particular type of cancer. Protocols for the emergency treatment of chest pain include what signs and symptoms to look for during the initial history and physical examination, what laboratory tests to order, and what drugs to administer and their doses.

> Protocols can be developed by any group: national healthcare organizations, individual hospitals, individual care units within a hospital, physicians' offices, community emergency medical teams, and so forth. Protocols are reviewed periodically and revised as new, more effective treatments become available.

**prototype**   The original drug from which all other drugs in that same category were developed or to which their therapeutic effects are compared. For example, chlorpromazine (Thorazine) is the prototype of all phenothiazine derivative drugs used to treat psychosis. The prototype drug does not always remain the drug of choice for treatment. It may be replaced by newer drugs. Do not confuse *prototype* with *prodrug*. See also *drug of choice*.

**racemic**   Descriptive word for a drug that is composed of equal amounts of dextrorotary and levorotary isomers. See also *isomer*.

> Sample dictation: The patient was treated with racemic epinephrine.

**receptor**   Structure on the cell membrane that binds to substances in the body (neurotransmitters, hormones, antigens, and so forth) or to substances introduced into the body (drugs, chemicals, and so forth). Binding to a substance causes the receptor to be stimulated or to be blocked so that other substances cannot bind to it.

**recombinant DNA technology**   Drug design and production technology that uses enzymes in a test tube (*in vitro*) to cut apart a segment of a DNA molecule from a human cell. This segment specifically directs the production of a particular substance in the body. The technique of gene cloning allows the production of a large supply of this DNA segment. The DNA segments are then spliced (recombined) with the DNA in a bacterial cell. As the bacterium multiplies, it carries the new DNA with it, and it becomes part of the genetic makeup of all subsequent generations of bacteria. The bacteria are now preprogrammed to make supplies of that particular substance that can be used as a drug. In huge vats, these bacteria can produce unlimited quantities of drugs. Also known as *gene splicing* or *genetic engineering*.

**schedule drugs**   Drugs with the potential for abuse and dependence (addiction). They are regulated by the Drug Enforcement Administration (DEA). Schedule drugs are divided into five categories or schedules based on their potential for physical or psychological dependence. These drugs are known as *controlled substances*.

**scored tablet**   Tablet form of a drug that has an indented line running across it, so that it can be easily broken into equal pieces to produce an accurate but reduced dose.

**sedative drugs**   Categories of drugs that include tranquilizer drugs, as well as the less frequently used barbiturate drugs, to decrease agitation and anxiety.

**serotonin**   Neurotransmitter released in the synapses between neurons in the limbic system, hypothalamus, cerebellum, and spinal cord.

**side effect**   A drug effect other than the intended therapeutic effect. Side effects can be mild and temporary, moderate and annoying, or severe enough that the drug must be discontinued.

**slow-release tablet**   Tablet form of a drug that provides a continuous, sustained release of the drug. The drug trade name often includes the abbreviation *CR* (controlled release), *SR* (slow release), *LA* (long acting), or *XL* (extended length).

**solution**   Drug form that is a liquid and contains the drug in a sterile water, saline, and/or alcohol base. Solutions can be aqueous or viscous. Solutions never need to be mixed as the drug concentration is always the same in every part of the solution, even after prolonged standing.

**subcutaneous route**   Route of administration in which a liquid drug is injected into the fatty layer beneath the dermis. This route is used to administer insulin injections and allergy shots.

**sublingual route**   Route of administration in which the drug (usually in a tablet form) is placed under the tongue and allowed to disintegrate slowly and dissolve in saliva.

**suppository**   Drug form that is composed of a solid base of glycerin or cocoa butter containing the drug. Suppositories are manufactured in appropriate sizes for rectal or vaginal insertion and also come in adult and pediatric sizes.

**suspension**   Drug form that is a liquid that contains fine, undissolved particles of a drug suspended in a water or oil base. After prolonged standing, these fine particles gradually settle to the bottom of the container (due to the action of gravity). Drugs that come as a suspension must always be shaken before administration.

**sympathomimetic drugs**   See *adrenergic drugs*.

**synergism**   Condition in which two drugs taken together combine to produce an effect that is greater than the independent effect of each drug. Synergism can be either beneficial or detrimental.

**syringe**   A long plastic cylinder with a plunger that fits inside it. It is used with a needle to inject liquid drugs. See also *insulin syringe* and *tuberculin (TB) syringe*.

**syrup**   Drug form that is a liquid and contains the drug in a thickened water base with added sugar and flavorings, but no alcohol. Syrups are sweeter and more viscous (thicker) than elixirs.

**tablet**   Drug form that is solid and contains active drug (as a dried powder) plus inert ingredients (binders and fillers) to provide bulk and ensure a standardized tablet size. Tablets come in many colors and shapes.

**target organ**   The specific organ (e.g., heart or lungs) that the therapeutic effect of a drug is directed toward. With antibiotic drugs, the target organ is not an organ but a pathogenic organism (e.g., a bacterium).

**TB syringe**   See *tuberculin syringe*.

**therapeutic dose**   Drug dose that is in the correct amount to produce a therapeutic effect, not a subtherapeutic effect, and not a toxic effect.

**therapeutic effect**   Drug effect that is the intended effect to prevent, control, improve, or cure symptoms, conditions, or diseases of a physiological or psychological nature. The drug's main effect for which it was prescribed.

**therapeutic index**   The therapeutic index is calculated during animal testing of a new drug. It reflects the relative margin of safety between the dose needed to produce a therapeutic effect and the dose that produces a toxic effect in animals.

The higher the therapeutic index number, the more desirable, because it indicates that the drug has a wide margin of safety. For example, penicillin has a therapeutic index of greater than 100. The therapeutic index of digoxin (Lanoxin) is less than 2, however, and it is not uncommon for patients being given a therapeutic dose to begin to exhibit symptoms of toxicity.

**tincture**   Drug form that is a liquid and contains the drug in a water and alcohol base (e.g., topical iodine tincture to disinfect the skin). Tinctures are never taken internally.

**titrate**   To determine the smallest dose that will produce the desired therapeutic effect for a particular individual.

**tolerance**   A decreased susceptibility to the effects of an abused drug because of continued use. See also *addiction*.

**topical route**   Route of administration in which the drug is applied directly to the mucous membranes, skin, eyes, or ears. The therapeutic effect of the drug only extends to the local area.

**toxic effect**   Drug effect that occurs when serum levels of a drug rise above the therapeutic level and the drug becomes a poison to the body. Also known as *toxicity*.

**toxicology**   The study of the toxic or poisonous effects of chemicals or drugs on humans, animals, and the environment.

**trade name**   Drug name selected by the drug company when the FDA gives final approval for marketing. The trade name is specifically designed to be easy to remember and, if possible, to suggest how the drug is used. Also known as the *brand name*.

**tranquilizer drugs**   Category of drugs that includes minor tranquilizer drugs that are used to treat anxiety and neurosis and major tranquilizer drugs that are used to treat psychosis.

**transdermal patch**   Drug form that is a patch that is applied to the skin. The patch releases a small amount of drug over a long period of time, usually for one to two days. The drug in a transdermal patch is designed to exert a systemic effect in the body, not a topical effect on the skin.

**troche**   Drug form that is in an oblong-shaped tablet and has a base of sugar. The troche dissolves into a paste to release the drug topically in the mouth. *Pastille*, a French word that means *little lump of bread*, is another name for a *troche*.

**trough level**   The lowest serum level of a drug that occurs just before the next dose is to be given, as determined by blood tests. If the trough level is too low, this indicates that the drug is being given at a subtherapeutic level and the drug dose needs to be increased.

**tuberculin (TB) syringe**   A small syringe often manufactured with an attached 25-gauge needle, the tuberculin syringe only holds a total of 1 mL of liquid drug (see ■ FIGURE B–5). It is calibrated to measure liquid drug doses as small as 0.01 mL. It is used to administer the intradermal Mantoux test that shows prior exposure to tuberculosis; hence its name. It is also used for pediatric injections and allergy injections.

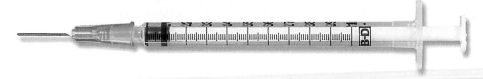

■ **FIGURE B–6** **Tuberculin syringe.**
A tuberculin syringe is calibrated to measure liquid drug doses to 0.01 milliliter (mL).

**umbilical artery/vein route**   Route of drug administration in which a liquid drug is injected into the umbilical artery or vein in the umbilical cord of a newborn infant.

**unit**   Unit of measurement used to measure doses of insulin and some other drugs like penicillins and some vitamins.

**vasodilator drug**   A drug that relaxes smooth muscles in the walls of arteries to dilate the arteries, to increase blood flow, and to decrease the blood pressure.

**vasopressor drug**   A drug that constricts smooth muscles in the walls of arteries to constrict the arteries and increase the blood pressure.

**vial**   A small glass bottle containing a liquid or powder for injection (see ■ **FIGURE B–6**). The top is an aluminum cap to protect a rubber stopper beneath until the vial is opened. The self-sealing rubber stopper in the cap allows a liquid (diluent) to be injected for reconstitution of a powder drug. The rubber stopper also allows repeated doses of the drug to be drawn from the same vial. To withdraw the drug from a vial, the vial is turned upside down, a syringe is inserted through the rubber stopper, air is injected into the vial, and the drug dose is withdrawn. A vial can be used multiple times. The rubber stopper is cleansed with alcohol before each dose is withdrawn.

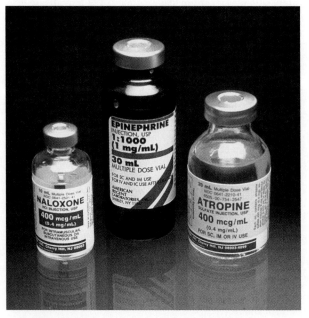

■ **FIGURE B–6** **Vial.**
These vials contain the drugs naloxone (Narcan) (to treat an overdose of a narcotic drug), epinephrine (to stimulate the heart), and atropine (to treat an abnormally slow heart rate).

# Glossary of Abbreviations, Short Forms, Symbols, and their Meanings

Abbreviations, short forms and symbols are commonly used in all types of medical documents. However, they can mean different things to different people and their meanings can be misinterpreted.

This glossary includes abbreviations, short forms, symbols, and their meanings that are

- in printed or handwritten drug prescriptions
- preprinted or handwritten on physician's order sheets
- in the generic name or trade name of a drug
- drug routes of administration
- drug units of measurement
- diseases and conditions commonly treated with drugs
- healthcare professionals who prescribe, dispense, or administer drugs
- professional health organizations
- healthcare locations where drugs are administered
- the names of drug companies
- commonly associated with drugs
- not recommended for use by JCAHO* and ISMP.■

\* An asterisk beside an abbreviation means it is included (or may be included in the future) on a list compiled by the Joint Commission on Accreditation of Healthcare Organizations (JCAHO). The JCAHO list contains abbreviations that have been the cause of drug errors. These abbreviations should not be used, and the JCAHO's National Safety Goal states that these abbreviations also must appear on a facility's "Do Not Use" list. This is a short list because it is the minimum required by JCAHO to obtain facility accreditation. However, because these abbreviations are still used by some healthcare providers, they are included here.

■ A square beside an abbreviation means it is from a more comprehensive list of abbreviations that should not be used, as compiled by the Institute for Safe Medication Practices (ISMP). The ISMP list is derived from the *United States Pharmacopoeia* Medication Error Reporting Program.

## Abbreviations or Short Forms with Their Meanings

**AACP**   American Association of Colleges of Pharmacy
**AAMT**   (see *AHDI*)
**AARP**   American Association of Retired Persons
**ABC**   abacavir
**ABD** or **abd**   abdomen
**ABV**   Adriamycin, bleomycin, vinblastine (chemotherapy protocol)
**ABVD**   Adriamycin, bleomycin, vinblastine, dacarbazine (chemotherapy protocol)
**a.c.**   before meals (Latin, *ante cibum*)

**ACE**   angiotensin-converting enzyme
Adriamycin, Cytoxan, etoposide (chemotherapy protocol)
**ACEI**   angiotensin-converting enzyme inhibitor
**ACS**   acute coronary syndrome
**ACT**   activated cell therapy
actinomycin D (older name for dactinomycin)
**ACTH**   adrenocorticotropic hormone
**AC-TH**   Adriamycin, cyclophosphamide, Taxotere, Herceptin (chemotherapy protocol)
**A.D.** or **AD**■   right ear (Latin, *auris dextra*)

**A-D**  antidiarrheal or antidandruff (in the trade name of a drug)

**ADD**  attention deficit disorder

**ADE**  adverse drug event

**ADEK**  fat-soluble vitamins A, D, E, and K

**ADH**  antidiuretic hormone

**ADHD**  attention-deficit/hyperactivity disorder

**ad lib.**  as needed or as desired (Latin, *ad libitum*)

**ADR**  adverse drug reaction

**aer.**  aerosol

**AF**  antifungal (in the trade name of a drug)
    atrial fibrillation

**A fib**  atrial fibrillation

**AgNO₃**  silver nitrate

**AHA**  acetohydroxamic acid
    American Hospital Association

**AHDI**  Association for Healthcare Documentation Integrity

**AHF**  antihemophilic factor

**AHIMA**  American Health Information Management Association

**AIDS**  acquired immunodeficiency syndrome

**AK**  Akorn (drug company)

**ALL**  acute lymphocytic leukemia

**ALS**  amyotrophic lateral sclerosis

**AM, A.M.** or **A.M.**  morning, between midnight and noon (Latin, *ante meridiem*)

**AMA**  against medical advice
    American Medical Association

**AMI**  acute myocardial infarction

**AML**  acute myelogenous leukemia

**Amp**  ampule

**ANDA**  abbreviated new drug application

**APAP**  acetaminophen (N-acetyl-P-aminophenol)

**APhA**  American Pharmaceutical Association

**APV**  amprenivir

**aq.** or **AQ**  aqueous, water based (Latin, *aqua*)

**AR**  antireflux (in the trade name of a drug)

**Ara-A** or **ARA A■**  vidarabine (chemotherapy drug)

**Ara-C**  cytarabine (chemotherapy drug)

**ARAC-DNR**  Ara-C, daunorubicin (chemotherapy protocol)

**ARB**  angiotensin II receptor blocker

**ARC**  AIDS-related complex

**ARDS**  adult respiratory distress syndrome
    acute respiratory distress syndrome

**ARF**  acute renal failure

**ARMD**  age-related macular degeneration

**A.S.** or **AS■**  left ear (Latin, *auris sinister*)

**ASA**  acetylsalicylic acid
    aminosalicylic acid

**ASAP**  as soon as possible

**ASC**  ambulatory surgery center

**ASCVD**  arteriosclerotic cardiovascular disease

**ASHD**  arteriosclerotic heart disease

**ATG**  antithymocyte globulin

**ATZ**  atazanavir

**A.U.** or **AU■**  both ears (Latin, *auris unitas*)
    each ear (Latin, *auris uterque*)

**AV** or **A-V**  atrioventricular

**AZDU**  3'-azido-2',3' dideoxyuridine (drug for HIV)

**AZT■**  azidothymidine (zidovudine)

**BBB**  blood–brain barrier

**B-CAVe**  bleomycin, CeeNu, Adriamycin, vinblastine (chemotherapy protocol)

**BCG**  bacillus of Calmete and Guérin (vaccine)

**BCNU**  carmustine (chemotherapy drug)

**BCVPP**  BiCNU, Cytoxan, vinblastine, procarbazine, prednisone (chemotherapy protocol)

**B-D** or **BD**  Becton-Dickinson (medical supply manufacturer)

**BEP**  bleomycin, etoposide, cisplatin (Platinol) (chemotherapy protocol)

**BiCNU**  carmustine (chemotherapy drug)

**B.I.D., b.i.d.,** or **bid**  twice a day (Latin, *bis in die*)

**BIG**  botulism immune globulin

**BIP**  bleomycin, ifosfamide, cisplatin (Platinol) (chemotherapy protocol)

**BLM**  bleomycin

**BMS**  Bristol-Myers Squibb (drug company)

**BOM**  bilateral otitis media

**BP**  blood pressure

**BPH**  benign prostatic hypertrophy

**BRCA**  breast cancer (gene)

**BSS**  balanced salt solution
    bismuth subsalicylate

**BT■**  bedtime

**Bx**  biopsy

**Ca** or **Ca⁺⁺**  calcium

**CA** or **Ca**  cancer, carcinoma

**CaCl**  calcium chloride

**CAD**  coronary artery disease

**CAF**  Cytoxan, Adriamycin, fluorouracil (chemotherapy protocol)

**CAMP**  Cytoxan, Adriamycin, methotrexate, procarbazine (chemotherapy protocol)

**cap** or **caps**  capsule(s)

**CAP**  Cytoxan, Adriamycin, cisplatin (Platinol) (chemotherapy protocol)

**CAVE**  Cytoxan, Adriamycin, vincristine, etoposide (chemotherapy protocol)

**C&S**  culture and sensitivity

**CBC**  complete blood count

**cc*,■**  cubic centimeter

**CC**  chief complaint
    calcium channel (in the trade name of a drug)

**CCB**  calcium channel blocker

**CCNU**  lomustine (chemotheraphy drug)

**CCU**  coronary care unit

**CD**  controlled dose

**CDB**   cisplatin, dacarbazine, BiCNU (chemotherapy protocol)

**CDCP**   Centers for Disease Control and Prevention

**CD4**   receptor on helper T lymphocyte

**CDDP**   cisplatin (chemotherapy drug)

**CDE**   Cytoxan, doxorubicin, etoposide (chemotherapy protocol)

**CEA**   carcinoembryonic antigen

**CEF**   Cytoxan, epirubicin, fluorouracil (chemotherapy protocol)

**CEV**   Cytoxan, etoposide, vincristine (chemotherapy protocol)

**CF**   cystic fibrosis

**CHAP**   Cytoxan, Hexalen, Adriamycin, cisplatin (Platinol) (chemotherapy protocol)

**chemo**   chemotherapy

**CHF**   congestive heart failure

**CIS**   carcinoma *in situ*

**CISCA**   cisplatin, Cytoxan, Adriamycin (chemotherapy protocol)

**Cl** or **Cl⁻**   chloride

**CLL**   chronic lymphocytic leukemia

**CMA**   certified medical assistant

**CMF**   Cytoxan, methotrexate, fluorouracil (chemotherapy protocol)

**CMFP**   Cytoxan, methotrexate, fluorouracil, prednisone (chemotherapy protocol)

**CMFVP**   Cytoxan, methotrexate, fluorouracil, vincristine, prednisone (chemotherapy protocol)

**CML**   chronic myelogenous leukemia

**CMT**   certified medical transcriptionist

**CMV**   cytomegalovirus
cisplatin, methotrexate, vinblastine (chemotherapy protocol)

**CNF**   Cytoxan, Novantrone, fluorouracil (chemotherapy protocol)

**CNM**   certified nurse midwife

**CNS**   central nervous system

**comp.**   compound

**COMT**   catecholamine-o-methyl transferase

**COPD**   chronic obstructive pulmonary disease

**COX**   cyclooxygenase

**CP**   cerebral palsy

**CPhT**   certified pharmacy technician

**CPR**   cardiopulmonary resuscitation
computerized patient record

**CPZ■**   Compazine

**CQ**   cigarette quit (in the trade name of a drug)

**CQI**   continuous quality improvement

**CR** or **C-R**   controlled release (in the trade name of a drug)

**CRF**   chronic renal failure

**CRNA**   certified registered nurse anesthetist

**CT**   chewable tablet

**CV**   cardiovascular

**CVA**   cerebrovascular accident

**CVD**   cisplatin, vinblastine, dacarbazine (chemotherapy protocol)

**CVI**   carboplatin, VePesid, ifosfamide (chemotherapy protocol)

**CVP**   Cytoxan, vincristine, prednisone (chemotherapy protocol)

**CVPP**   CeeNu, vinblastine, procarbazine, prednisone (chemotherapy protocol)

**D**   decongestant (in the trade name of a drug)

**d** or **D**   right (Latin, *dextra*); day; daily

**DAW**   dispense as written

**D.C.**   Doctor of Chiropractic

**D/C■**   discontinue
discharge

**DCF**   2'-deoxycoformycin (pentostatin)

**DCT**   daunorubicin, cytarabine, thioguanine (chemotherapy protocol)

**DDAVP**   1-desamino[8-D-arginine]vasopressin (desmopressin)

**ddC**   zalcitabine (chemotherapy drug)

**ddI**   didanosine (chemotherapy drug)

**D.D.S.**   Doctor of Dental Surgery

**DEA**   Drug Enforcement Administration

**DF**   diarrhea formula (in the trade name of an infant formula)

**DFC**   *Drug Facts and Comparisons*

**D5NS**   dextrose 5% in normal saline (intravenous fluid)

**D5W**   dextrose 5% in water (intravenous fluid)

**d4T**   stavudine

**D.H.E.**   dihydroergotamine (in the trade name of a drug)

**DHEA**   dehydroepiandrosterone

**DHHS**   Department of Health and Human Services

**DHPG**   ganciclovir

**DHT**   dihydrotachysterol

**DI**   diabetes insipidus

**DIC**   disseminated intravascular coagulation

**dig**   digoxin

**Disp.**   dispense

**DJD**   degenerative joint disease

**DKA**   diabetic ketoacidosis

**DLV**   delavirdine

**DM**   dextromethorphan (in the trade name of a drug)

**DMSA**   succimer

**DMSO**   dimethyl sulfoxide

**DNA**   deoxyribonucleic acid

**DNR**   do not resuscitate (patient status)
daunorubicin (chemotherapy drug)

**D.O.**   Doctor of Osteopathy

**DOT**   directly observed therapy

**D.P.M.**   Doctor of Podiatric Medicine

**DPT■**   Demerol, Phenergan, Thorazine
diphtheria, tetanus, pertussis

**DR**   drug resistant

**Dr.**   doctor

**DRC**   delayed-release capsule

**DRG**   diagnosis-related groups

**D.S. or DS**   double strength (in the trade name of a drug) discharge summary; dextromethorphan and pseudoephedrine (in the trade name of a drug)

**DT**   delirium tremens

**DTaP**   diphtheria, tetanus, and pertussis (vaccine)

**DTC**   direct to consumer (advertising)

**DTIC**   dacarbazine (chemotherapy drug)

**DVI**   double viral inactivation (in the trade name of a drug)

**DVP**   daunorubicin, vincristine, prednisone (chemotherapy protocol)

**DVT**   deep venous thrombosis

**DX**   dextromethorphan

**Dx**   diagnosis

**EAP**   etoposide, Adriamycin, cisplatin (Platinol) (chemotherapy protocol)

**EBV**   Epstein-Barr virus

**EC**   enterocolitis (in the trade name of a drug)

**ED**   emergency department erectile dysfunction

**ED₅₀**   $ED_{50}$   median effective dose for 50 percent of animals tested

**EDTA**   edentate

**EENT**   eyes, ears, nose, and throat

**E.E.S.**   erythromycin ethynil succinate

**EFP**   etoposide, fluorouracil, cisplatin (Platinol) (chemotherapy protocol)

**EFV**   efavirenz

**EHR**   electronic health record

**ELF**   etoposide, leucovorin, fluorouracil (chemotherapy protocol)

**elix.**   elixir

**EMLA**   eutectic mixture of lidocaine (and prilocaine) (topical anesthetic drug)

**EMMA**   Electronic Medication Management Assistant

**EMR**   electronic medical record

**EPR**   electronic patient record

**ENT**   ears, nose, and throat

**epi**   epinephrine

**EPO**   erythropoietin

**ER**   extended release (in the trade name of a drug) estrogen receptor emergency room

**ERYC**   trade name for erythromycin

**ES**   extra strength (in the trade name of a drug)

**ET**   effervescent tablet (in the trade name of a drug) endotracheal

**ETOH**   ethyl alcohol (ethanol, grain alcohol)

**ETT**   endotracheal tube

**EVA**   etoposide, vinblastine, Adriamycin (chemotherapy protocol)

**EX**   extended (action) (in the trade name of a drug)

**FA**   folic acid (in the trade name of a drug)

**Fab or F(ab)**   fragment (of antibody that contains) antigen binding (sites)

**FAC**   fluorouracil, Adriamycin, Cytoxan (chemotherapy protocol)

**FAM**   fluorouracil, Adriamycin, mitomycin (chemotherapy protocol)

**FAMTX**   fluorouracil, Adriamycin, methotrexate (chemotherapy protocol)

**FAP**   fluorouracil, Adriamycin, cisplatin (Platinol) (chemotherapy protocol)

**FDA**   Food and Drug Administration

**Fe**   iron

**FEC**   fluorouracil, epirubicin, Cytoxan (chemotherapy protocol)

**FeSO₄**   ferrous sulfate

**FFP**   fresh frozen plasma

**5-FU**   5-fluorouracil (fluorouracil) (chemotherapy drug)

**5-HT**   serotonin

**fl. oz.**   fluid ounce

**4-ASA**   4-aminosalicylic acid

**FML**   fluorometholone

**FS**   formulated with sucrose (in the trade name of a drug)

**FSH**   follicle-stimulating hormone

**FUDR**   fluorodeoxyuridine (floxuridine) (chemotherapy drug)

**FUO**   fever of unknown origin

**Fx**   fracture

**g**   gram

**GC**   gonococcus gonorrhea

**G-CSF**   granulocyte colony-stimulating factor

**GDF**   growth and development factor

**GERD**   gastroesophageal reflux disease

**GH**   growth hormone

**GHB**   gamma hydroxybutyrate (street drug, a "date rape drug")

**GI**   gastrointestinal

**gm**   an incorrect abbreviation for *gram*

**GM-CSF**   granulocyte-macrophage colony-stimulating factor

**GnRH**   gonadotropin-releasing hormone

**GP**   guaifenesin and phenylephrine (in the trade name of a drug)

**gr.**   grain

**GSK**   GlaxoSmithKline (drug company)

**gt.**   drop (Latin, *gutta*)

**gtt.**   drops (Latin, *guttae*)

**GU**   genitourinary

**GVHD**   graft-versus-host disease

**GYN**   gynecology

**h.**   hour (Latin, *hora*)

**H₁**   $H_1$   histamine type 1 (receptor)

**H₂** histamine type 2 (receptor)

**H&P** history and physical (examination)

**HAV** hepatitis A virus

**HBIG** hepatitis B immune globulin

**HBr** hydrobromide

**HBV** hepatitis B virus

**HC** hydrocortisone
Huntington's chorea
hydrocodone and chlorpheniramine (in the trade name of a drug)

**HCA** hydrocortisone acetate

**HCG** or **hCG** human chorionic gonadotropin

**HCl■** hydrochloride
hydrochloric acid

**HCT■** hydrochlorothiazide
hydrocortisone
hematocrit

**HCTZ** hydrochlorothiazide

**HCV** hepatitis C virus

**HD** high dose (in the trade name of a drug)
Huntington's disease
hydrocodone with decongestant (in the trade name of a drug)

**HDL** high-density lipoprotein

**HDMTX** high-dose methotrexate

**HFA** hydrofluoroalkane (propellant in aerosol drugs)

**HGC** hard gel capsule

**HIB** or **Hib** *Hemophilus influenzae* type b (vaccine)

**HIV** human immunodeficiency virus

**HLA** human leukocyte antigen

**HMD** hyaline membrane disease

**HMG-CoA** 3-hydroxy-3-methylglutaryl-coenzyme A (reductase)

**HMO** health maintenance organization

**HN** high nitrogen (in the trade name of an enteral feeding solution)

**HO** or **H.O.** house officer

**HP** high potency (in the trade name of a drug)

**HPD** hydrocodone, phenylephrine, and diphenhydramine (in the trade name of a drug)

**HPI** history of present illness

**HPV** human papillomavirus

**hr** hour

**HRT** hormone replacement therapy

**HS■** half strength
hydrocodone and pseudoephedrine (in the trade name of a drug)

**h.s.■** bedtime, hour of sleep (Latin, *hora somni*)

**HSV** herpes simplex virus

**HTN** hypertension

**Hx** history

**I&O** intake and output

**IB** ibuprofen

**IBD** inflammatory bowel disease

**IBS** irritable bowel syndrome

**ICD** International Classification of Diseases

**ICE** ifosfamide, carboplatin, etoposide (chemotherapy protocol)

**ICE-T** ifosfamide, carboplatin, etoposide, Taxol (chemotherapy protocol)

**ICU** intensive care unit

**ID** intradermal

**IDDM** insulin-dependent diabetes mellitus

**IDV** indinivir

**IFN** interferon

**IFRS** intraoral fluoride-releasing system

**IgA** immunoglobulin A

**IgD** immunoglobulin D

**IgE** immunoglobulin E

**IgG** immunoglobulin G

**IGIM** immune globulin intramuscular (injection)

**IGIV** immune globulin intravenous

**IgM** immunoglobulin M

**IJ■** injection

**IL** interleukin

**I.M.** or **IM** intramuscular

**IN■** intranasal

**IND** Investigational New Drug

**INH** isoniazid (isonicotinic acid hydrazide)

**inj** or **INJ** injection

**IOM** Institute of Medicine

**IOP** intraocular pressure

**IPA** ifosfamide, cisplatin (Platinol), Adriamycin (chemotherapy protocol)

**IPV** inactivated poliovirus (vaccine)

**IRS** insulin resistance syndrome

**ISMO** isosorbide mononitrate

**ISMP** Institute for Safe Medication Practices

**IU***,■ International Unit

**IUPAC** International Union of Pure and Applied Chemistry

**I.V.** or **IV** intravenous

**IVP** intravenous push
intravenous pyelography

**IVPB** intravenous piggyback

**JCAHO** Joint Commission for Accreditation of Healthcare Organizations

**K** or **K⁺** potassium

**KCl** potassium chloride

**kg** kilogram

**KI** potassium iodide

**KT** ketoprofen

**KVO** keep the vein open

**l** or **L** left (Latin, *levo*)
liter

**LA** or **L.A.** or **L-A** long acting (in the trade name of a drug)

**LAIV**   live attenuated influenza vaccine
**lb.**   pound
**LDL**   low-density lipoprotein
**LHRH**   luteinizing hormone-releasing hormone
**LIG**   lymphocyte immune globulin
**liq.**   liquid
**LMWH**   low molecular weight heparin
**LP**   low potency
**L-PAM**   melphalan (chemotherapy drug)
**LPN**   licensed practical nurse
**LPV**   lopinavir and ritonavir
**LR**   lactated Ringer's (intravenous fluid)
**LSD**   lysergic acid diethylamide (street drug)

**MAb**   monoclonal antibody
**MAC**   methotrexate, actinomycin D, Cytoxan (chemotherapy protocol)
**MACC**   methotrexate, Adriamycin, Cytoxan, CeeNu (chemotherapy protocol)
**MAID**   mesna, Adriamycin, ifosfamide, dacarbazine (chemotherapy protocol)
**MAO**   monoamine oxidase
**MAOI**   monoamine oxidase inhibitor
**MBC**   methotrexate, bleomycin, cisplatin (chemotherapy protocol)
**mcg**   microgram
**MCT**   medium-chain triglycerides
**MCV4**   meningococcal vaccine
**MD**   muscular dystrophy
**M.D.**   Doctor of Medicine
**MDI**   metered-dose inhaler
**MDR**   multidrug resistant
    minimum daily requirement
**MDRTB**   multidrug-resistant tuberculosis
**mEq.**   milliequivalent
**mets**   metastases
**mg**   milligram
**mg/kg/day**   milligrams (of drug) per kilograms (of body weight) per day
**mg/m²**   milligrams (of drug) per meter squared (of body surface area)
**MgSO₄***,■   magnesium sulfate
**MHC**   major histocompatibility complex
**MI**   myocardial infarction
**MICE**   mesna, ifosfamide, carboplatin, etoposide (chemotherapy protocol)
**μg***,■   microgram (Greek μ, *micro*)
**MIH**   procarbazine (chemotherapy drug)
**MINE**   mesna, ifosfamide, Novantrone, etoposide (chemotherapy protocol)
**mL**   milliliter
**mmHg**   millimeters of mercury (Hg)
**MMR**   measles, mumps, and rubella (vaccine)
**MN**   midnight

**M.O.M.** or **MOM**   milk of magnesia
**MPF**   methylparaben free
**MPH**   methylphenidate
**MPSV4**   meningococcal polysaccharide vaccine
**MR#**   medical record number
**mRNA**   messenger ribonucleic acid
**MRSA**   methicillin-resistant *Staphylococcus aureus*
**MS***,■   magnesium sulfate
    morphine sulfate
    multiple sclerosis
**MSIR**   trade name for morphine sulfate immediate release
**MSO₄***   morphine sulfate
**MST**   magnesium salicylate tablet
**MTC**   mitomycin-C (mitomycin) (chemotherapy drug)
    magnetic targeted carrier
**MTC-DOX**   magnetic targeted carrier-doxorubicin
**MTX**■   methotrexate
**M-VAC**   methotrexate, vinblastine, Adriamycin, cisplatin (chemotherapy protocol)
**M.V.I.-12**   multivitamins intravenous, 12 (different vitamins)
**MVP**   mitomycin, vinblastine, cisplatin (chemotherapy protocol)
**MVPP**   Mustargen, vinblastine, procarbazine, prednisone (chemotherapy protocol)

**Na** or **Na⁺**   sodium
**NaCl**   sodium chloride
**N&V**   nausea and vomiting
**NAVEL**   Narcan, atropine, vasopressin (or Valium or Ventolin), epinephrine, and lidocaine
**NCD**   nanocrystal colloidal dispersion
**NCPA**   National Association of Community Pharmacists
**ND**   nondrowsy (in the trade name of a drug)
**NDA**   New Drug Application
**NDC**   National Drug Code
**NF**   *National Formulary*
**NFL**   Novantrone, fluorouracil, leucovorin (chemotherapy protocol)
**NFV**   nelfinavir
**NG**   nasogastric (tube)
**NICU**   neurologic intensive care unit
    newborn intensive care unit
**NIDDM**   non–insulin-dependent diabetes mellitus
**NIH**   National Institutes of Health
**nitro**   nitroglycerin
**NK**   natural killer (cells)
**NKA**   no known allergies
**NKDA**   no known drug allergies
**NMDA**   N-methyl-D-aspartate (receptor)
**NNRTI**   non-nucleoside reverse transcriptase inhibitor (drug)
**No.**   number
**NP**   nurse practitioner
    no preservatives (in the trade name of a drug)

**NPH**   neutral protamine Hagedorn

**NPO or n.p.o.**   nothing by mouth (Latin, *nil per os*)

**NR**   no refills (on a prescription blank)

**NRT**   nicotine replacement therapy

**NRTI**   nucleoside reverse transcriptase inhibitor (drug)

**NS**   normal saline (intravenous fluid)
　　　nasal spray

**NSAID**   nonsteroidal anti-inflammatory drug

**NTI**   narrow therapeutic index

**NTP**   nicotine transdermal patch

**NTZ**   nitazoxanide

**NVP**   nevirapine


**OA**   osteoarthritis

**OB**   obstetrics

**OCD**   obsessive-compulsive disorder

**OCP**   oral contraceptive pill

**o.d. or OD■**   once daily

**O.D. or OD■**   right eye (Latin, *oculus dexter*)
　　　　　　Doctor of Optometry
　　　　　　overdose

**ODT**   orally disintegrating tablet

**oint.**   ointment

**OJ■**   orange juice

**OOB**   out of bed

**OPV**   oral poliovirus (vaccine)

**OR**   operating room

**O.S. or OS■**   left eye (Latin, *oculus sinister*)

**OT**   occupational therapy or therapist

**OTC or otc**   over the counter (drug)

**O.U. or OU■**   both eyes (Latin, *oculus unitas*)
　　　　　　each eye (Latin, *oculus uterque*)

**oz.**   ounce


**PA**   physician's assistant

**PAC**   cisplatin (Platinol), Adriamycin, Cytoxan (chemotherapy protocol)
　　　premature atrial contraction

**PACU**   postanethesia care unit

**PAD**   peripheral artery disease

**P&T**   pharmacy and therapeutics (committee)

**p.c. or pc**   after meals (Latin, *post cibum*)

**PCA■**   patient-controlled analgesia

**PCN**   penicillin

**PCP**   primary care physician
　　　phencyclidine/angel dust (street drug)
　　　*Pneumocystis carinii* pneumonia

**PCV**   procarbazine, CeeNu, vincristine (chemotherapy protocol)
　　　pneumococcal vaccine

**PD**   Parkinson's disease
　　　phenylephrine decongestant (in the trade name of a drug)

**PD or P-D**   Parke-Davis (drug company)

**PDR**   *Physicians' Desk Reference*

**PE**   pulmonary embolus
　　　phenylephrine and expectorant (in the trade name of a drug)

**PEG**   polyethylene glycol
　　　percutaneous endoscopic gastrostomy (tube)

**PEJ**   percutaneous endoscopic jejunostomy (tube)

**PF**   preservative free

**PFA**   phosphonoformic acid (foscarnet)

**PFL**   cisplatin (Platinol), fluorouracil, leucovorin (chemotherapy protocol)

**PFS**   preservative-free solution

**PGE**   prostaglandin E

**pharm**   pharmacy

**Pharm.D.**   Doctor of Pharmacy

**PI**   protease inhibitor (drug)

**PICC**   peripherally inserted central line

**PICU**   pediatric intensive care unit

**PID**   pelvic inflammatory disease

**PM, P.M. or P.M.**   afternoon, between noon and midnight (Latin, *post meridiem*)

**PMDD**   premenstrual dysphoric disorder

**PMF**   premenstrual formula (in the trade name of a drug)

**PMMA**   polymethylmethacrylate

**PMS**   premenstrual syndrome

**PO, po, or p.o.**   by mouth (Latin, *per os*)

**PPD**   purified protein derivative

**PPI**   proton pump inhibitor (drug)

**ppm**   parts per million

**PPO**   preferred provider organization

**PPV**   pneumococcal polysaccharide vaccine

**PR**   per rectum
　　　progesterone receptor

**PRN or p.r.n.**   as needed, whenever necessary (Latin, *pro re nata*)

**PSE**   pseudoephedrine

**PT or Pt**   patient
　　　　　prothrombin time
　　　　　physical therapy or therapist

**PTSD**   posttraumatic stress disorder

**PTT**   partial thromboplastin time

**PTU**   propylthiouracil

**PUD**   peptic ulcer disease

**PUVA**   psoralen (drug) and ultraviolet light A

**PVA**   prednisone, vincristine, asparaginase (chemotherapy protocol)

**PVB**   cisplatin (Platinol), vinblastine, bleomycin (chemotherapy protocol)

**PVC**   premature ventricular contraction

**PVD**   peripheral vascular disease

**PVDA**   prednisone, vincristine, daunorublcin, asparaginase (chemotherapy protocol)


**q.**   every (Latin, *quaque*)

**q1d■**   every day

**q.1h. or q1h**   every [one] hour

**q.2h.** or **q2h**   every 2 hours

**q.3h.** or **q3h**   every 3 hours

**q.4h.** or **q4h**   every 4 hours

**q.6h.** or **q6h**   every 6 hours

**q.8h.** or **q8h**   every 8 hours

**q.12h.** or **q12h**   every 12 hours

**Q.A.M.** or **q.a.m.**   every morning, between midnight and noon (Latin, *quaque ante meridiem*)

**Q.D., q.d.** or **qd**\*■   every day (Latin, *quaque die*)

**q.h.** or **qh**   every hour (Latin, *quaque hora*)

**q.h.s.** or **qhs**■   every bedtime, every hours of sleep (Latin *quaque hora somni*)

**Q.I.D.** or **q.i.d.**   four times a day (Latin, *quarter in die*)

**q.n.**■   every night

**Q.O.D.**\* or **q.o.d.**\*■   every other day

**Q.P.M.** or **q.p.m.**   every afternoon, between noon and midnight (Latin, *quaque post meridiem*)

**RA**   rheumatoid arthritis

**R&D**   research and development

**RBC**   red blood cell

**RDA**   recommended dietary allowance

**RDF**   rapid dissolution formula

**rDNA**   recombinant deoxyribonucleic acid (DNA)

**RDS**   respiratory distress syndrome

**RFF**   revised formulation female (in the trade name of a drug)

**RFs**   refills

**RHIA**   registered health information administrator

**RHIT**   registered health information technician

**RIG**   rabies immune globulin

**RL**   Ringer's lactate (intravenous fluid)

**RMS**   rectal morphine sulfate

**RMT**   registered medical transcriptionist

**RN**   registered nurse

**RNA**   ribonucleic acid

**R/O** or **r/o**   rule out

**RPD**   rapid

**RPh**   registered pharmacist

**RR**   recovery room

**RRT**   registered respiratory therapist

**RSV**   respiratory syncytial virus

**RTV**   ritonavir

**Rx**   prescription (Latin, *recipe, take*)

**SA**   sustained action (in the trade name of a drug)

**SAD**   seasonal affective disorder

**SARS**   severe acute respiratory syndrome

**SBE**   subacute bacterial endocarditis

**SC**■   subcutaneous

**SCC**   squamous cell carcinoma

**SCI**   spinal cord injury

**SD**   solvent/detergent (treated)

**SDF**   solvent/detergent free

**SERM**   selective estrogen receptor modulator (drug)

**17-AGG**   17-allylamino-17-demethoxygeldanamycin

**SF**   soy formula (in the trade name of an infant formula)

**SGC**   soft gel capsule

**SI**   International System of Units (French, *Système International d'Unités*)

**SIADH**   syndrome of inappropriate antidiuretic hormone

**Sig.** or **S.**   write or print (these instructions) on the label (Latin, *signetur*)

**6-MP**   6-mercaptopurine (mercaptopurine) (chemotherapy drug)

**SKB**   SmithKline Beecham (drug company)

**SL**   sublingual

**SLE**   systemic lupus erythematosus

**SNF**   skilled nursing facility (pronounced "sniff")

**SNRI**   selective norepinephrine reuptake inhibitor (drug)

**sol.**   solution

**SOM**   serous otitis media

**S/P**   status post

**SPF**   sun protection factor

**SQ**■   subcutaneous

**SQV**   saquinavir

**SR**   slow release or sustained release (in the trade name of a drug)

**ss**■   sliding scale (insulin)

**SSD**   silver sulfadiazine

**SSI**■   sliding scale insulin

**SSKI**   saturated solution (of) potassium iodide

**SSRI**■   selective serotonin reuptake inhibitor (drug)

**stat.**   immediately (Latin, *statim*)

**STD**   sexually transmitted disease

**subcu**   subcutaneous

**subQ** or **sub q**■   subcutaneous

**supp.**   suppository

**susp.**   suspension

**Sx**   symptom

**T**   topical

**tab** or **tabs**   tablet(s)

**TAC**■   triamcinolone

**TACE**   transarterial chemoembolization

**TB**   tuberculin (syringe)
tuberculosis

**Tbsp.**   tablespoon

**TBW**   total body weight

**TCA**   tricyclic antidepressant (drug)

**TCF**   Taxol, cisplatin, fluorouracil (chemotherapy protocol)

**TCH**   Taxotere, carboplatin, Herceptin (chemotherapy protocol)

**Td**   tetanus and diphtheria (vaccine)

**Tdap**   tetanus, diphtheria and acellular pertussis (vaccine)

**TDF**   tenofovir disoproxil fumarate

**TD$_{50}$**   median toxic dose for 50 percent of animals tested

**T.E.N.** or **TEN**   total enteral nutrition

**TESPA**   triethylenethiophosphoramide (thiotepa)

**3TC-TP**   lamivudine triphosphate

**THC**   delta-9-tetrahydrocannabinol (dronabinol)
**TI**   therapeutic index
**TIA**   transient ischemic attack
**T.I.D.** or **t.i.d.**   three times a day (Latin, *ter in die*)
**TIG**   tetanus immune globulin
**tinct.**   tincture (Latin, *tinctura*)
**TIP**   Taxol, ifosfamide, cisplatin (Platinol) (chemotherapy protocol)
**TIV**   trivalent inactivated influenza vaccine
**TIW or t.i.w.**■   three times a week
**TMP/SMX**   trimethoprim and sulfamethoxazole
**TNF**   tumor necrosis factor
**TNM**   tumor, nodes, metastases
**TNT**   tumor necrosis treatment
**TOPV**   trivalent oral polio vaccine
**tPA**   tissue plasminogen activator (drug)
**TPN**   total parenteral nutrition
**TQM**   total quality management
**Tsp.** or **tsp.**   teaspoon
**TST**   tuberculin skin test
**T3**■   triiodothyronine
        Tylenol w/ Codeine No. 3
**TTS**   transdermal therapeutic system (in the trade name of a drug)
**Tx**   treatment

**U*,**■   unit
**U-100**   100 units (of insulin per milliliter)
**U-500**   500 units (of insulin per milliliter)
**UA** or **U/A**   urinalysis
**μ g*,**■   microgram (Greek μ, *micro*)
**ung.**   ointment (Latin, *unguentum*)
**URI**   upper respiratory infection
**USAN**   United States Adopted Names
**USP**   *United States Pharmacopeia*
**UTI**   urinary tract infection

**VAD**   vincristine, Adriamycin, dexamethasone (chemotherapy protocol)
**Vag.**   vaginal

**VBAP**   vincristine, BiCNU, Adriamycin, prednisone (chemotherapy protocol)
**VBCMP**   vincristine, BiCNU, Cytoxan, melphalan, prednisone (chemotherapy protocol)
**VCAP**   vincristine, Cytoxan, Adriamycin, prednisone (chemotherapy protocol)
**VCR**   vincristine (chemotherapy drug)
**VD**   venereal disease
**V fib**   ventricular fibrillation
**VH**   vapor heated (in the trade name of a drug)
**VIP**   VePesid, ifosfamide, cisplatin (Platinol) (chemotherapy protocol)
**VLDL**   very low-density lipoprotein
**VMCP**   vincristine, melphalan, Cytoxan, prednisone (chemotherapy protocol)
**VM-26**   teniposide (chemotherapy drug)
**V.O.** or **VO**   verbal order
**VP-16-213**   etoposide (chemotherapy drug)
**VS**   vital signs
**V tach**   ventricular tachycardia
**VWF**   von Willebrand factor

**w/**   with
**WA** or **W-A**   Wyeth-Ayerst (drug company)
**WBC**   white blood cell
**WHO**   World Health Organization
**WNL**   within normal limits
**w/o**   without

**XDR TB**   extensively drug resistant tuberculosis
**XL**   extended length (extended release)
**XR**   extended release (in the trade name of a drug)
**x3d**■   times 3 doses

**y.o.**   year old

**ZDV**   zidovudine (chemotherapy drug)
**ZMT**   zolmitriptan
**Zn**   zinc
**ZnSO₄**■   zinc sulfate
**ZX**   zinc, extra strength (in the trade name of a drug)

# Symbols

These symbols appear in printed or handwritten prescriptions for drugs or on the physician's order sheet or in other related notes made by healthcare professionals.

| Symbol | Meaning | Symbol | Meaning |
|--------|---------|--------|---------|
| Ⓡ | right | 1° | primary |
| Ⓛ | left | 2° | secondary |
| ♂ | male | 3° | tertiary |
| ♀ | female | + | positive, plus |
| − | negative, minus | ↓ | down, below, decrease |
| ± | plus or minus, slightly more or slightly less | → | to the right, causes or produces |
| = | equal | ← | to the left, in the direction of |
| ≠ | does not equal | / | or, over, out of (diagonal, slant, slash, virgule) |
| ø | none | : | to, is to (ratio sign) |
| < | less than | ° | degree; hour |
| > | greater than | ™ | trademark |
| ≤ | less than or equal to | 3▪ | dram |
| ≥ | greater than or equal to | Σ | sum (Greek, *sum*) |
| × | by, times (times sign) | α | alpha |
| X | magnification | β | beta |
| % | percent | γ | gamma |
| ℅ | complains of | μ | micro |
| # | number, pounds | ℞ | prescription (Latin, *recipe, take*) |
| Δ | change (Greek letter *delta*) | ÷I | one |
| & | and (ampersand) | ÷II | two |
| @ | at | ÷III | three |
| ® | registered | ÷IV | four |
| c̄ | with | ÷V | five |
| s̄ | without | ÷X | ten |
| ↑ | up, above, increase | | |

# *Appendix D*

# Glossary of Generic and Trade Name Drugs, Categories, Indications, Doses, and Drug Pronunciations

*Note:* All drug names listed in this Glossary are prescription drugs, unless specifically designated as over-the-counter drugs.

**A and D Medicated** (Derm) (generic *vitamin A, vitamin D, zinc oxide*).   Combination over-the-counter vitamin and astringent (drying) drug used topically to treat diaper rash and other skin rashes. Ointment. [A and D].

**abacavir** (Ziagen) (Anti-infec).   Nucleoside reverse transcriptase inhibitor antiviral drug used to treat treat HIV and AIDS. Tablet: 300 mg. Oral liquid: 20 mg/mL. [ah-BAK-ah-veer].

**abarelix** (Plenaxis) (Chemo).   Hormonal chemotherapy drug used to treat cancer of the prostate gland. Intramuscular: 113 mg. [AB-ah-RAY-liks].

**abatacept** (Orencia) (Ortho).   Immunomodulator drug used to treat adult and juvenile rheumatoid arthritis. Intravenous (powder to be reconstituted): 250 mg. [ah-BAT-ah-sept].

**abciximab** (ReoPro) (Cardio, Hem).   Platelet aggregation inhibitor drug used to treat patients who are undergoing angioplasty or stent placement. Intravenous: 2 mg/mL. [ab-SIK-sih-mab].

**Abelcet** (Anti-infec).   See *amphotericin B.* [AA-bel-set].

**Abilify, Abilify Discmelt** (Psych).   See *aripiprazole.* [ah-BIL-ih-fy].

**Abraxane** (Chemo).   See *paclitaxel.* [ah-BRAK-sayn].

**Abreva** (Anti-infec, Derm, ENT).   See *docosanol.* [ah-BREE-vah].

**absorbable gelatin** (Gelfilm, Gelfilm Ophthalmic, Gelfoam) (Hem).   Absorbable gelatin used topically to control bleeding during surgical or dental procedures. Film. Dental sponge. Pack. Prostatectomy cone. Sponge. [ab-SOR-bah-bl JEL-ah-tin].

**Absorbine Athlete's Foot, Absorbine Footcare** (Derm).   See *tolnaftate.* [ab-SOR-been].

**Absorbine Power Gel** (Ortho) (generic *alcohol, methol*).   Combination over-the-counter analgesic drug used topically to treat the pain of osteoarthritis and minor muscle injuries. Gel: 4%. [ab-SOR-been].

**Abthrax** (Misc).   Used to treat anthrax from bioterrorism. Orphan drug. [AB-thraks].

**acamprosate** (Campral) (Psych).   Used to deter alcohol consumption in recovering alcoholic patients. Delayed-release tablets: 233 mg. [AH-kam-PROH-sayt].

**acarbose** (Precose) (Endo).   Alpha-glucosidase inhibitor oral antidiabetic drug used to treat type 2 diabetes mellitus. Tablet: 25 mg, 50 mg, 100 mg. [aa-KAR-bohs].

**Accolate** (Pulm).   See *zafirlukast.* [AK-koh-layt].

**Accretropin** (Endo).   See *somatropin.* [AK-reh-TROH-pin].

**AccuNeb** (Pulm).   See *albuterol.* [AK-kyoo-neb].

**Accupril** (Cardio).   See *quinapril.* [AK-kyoo-pril].

**Accuretic** (Cardio) (generic *quinapril, hydrochlorothiazide*).   Combination ACE inhibitor and diuretic drug used to treat hypertension. Tablet: 10 mg/12.5 mg, 20 mg/12.5 mg, 20 mg/25 mg. [AK-kyoo-RET-ik].

**Accutane** (Derm).   See *isotretinoin.* [AK-kyoo-tayn].

**Accuzyme** (Derm).   See *papain.* [AK-kyoo-zime].

**acebutolol** (Sectral) (Cardio).   Cardioselective beta-blocker drug used to treat hypertension and premature ventricular contractions. Capsule: 200 mg, 400 mg. [AA-seh-BYOO-toh-lawl].

**Aceon** (Cardio).   See *perindopril.* [AA-see-awn].

**Acetadote** (Emerg).   See *acetylcysteine.* [ah-SEE-tah-doht].

**acetaminophen** (Anacin Aspirin Free Maximum Strength, Children's Panadol, Children's Tylenol, Children's Tylenol Soft Chews, Comtrex Maximum Strength Sore Throat, Infants' Drops Panadol, Infants' Drops Tylenol, Junior Strength Panadol, Panadol Extra Strength, Tempra 1, Tempra 2, Tempra 3, Tylenol, Tylenol Arthritis, Tylenol Caplets, Tylenol Children's Meltaways, Tylenol 8 Hour, Tylenol Extended Relief, Tylenol Extra Strength, Tylenol Junior Strength, Tylenol Regular Strength, Tylenol Sore Throat) (Analges).   Over-the-counter, non-aspirin analgesic drug used to treat fever and pain from colds, toothaches, headaches, sore throats, backaches, and skin injuries; used to treat the pain of osteoarthritis and menstrual cramps. Caplet: 160 mg, 500 mg, 650 mg. Extended-release caplet: 650 mg. Gelcap: 500 mg. Extended-release geltab: 650 mg. Capsule: 500 mg. Tablet:

325 mg, 500 mg, 650 mg. Chewable tablet: 80 mg, 160 mg. Dispersable tablet: 80 mg. Extended-release tablet: 650 mg. Drops: 100 mg/mL. Liquid: 160 mg/5 mL, 500 mg/15 mL. Elixir: 80 mg/2.5 mL, 80 mg/5 mL, 120 mg/5 mL, 160 mg/5 mL. Suppository: 80 mg, 120 mg, 125 mg, 300 mg, 325 mg, 650 mg. [ah-SEE-tah-MIN-oh-fen].

**Aceta w/ Codeine** (Analges) (generic *acetaminophen, codeine*). Combination Schedule III salicylate and narcotic analgesic drug. Tablet: 300 mg/30 mg. [ah-SEE-tah with KOH-deen].

**acetazolamide** (Diamox Sequels) (Cardio, Neuro, Ophth). Carbonic anhydrase inhibitor drug used to treat glaucoma; used to treat edema from congestive heart failure; used to treat epilepsy; used to treat drug-induced edema; used to treat acute mountain/altitude sickness. Sustained-release capsule: 500 mg. Tablet: 125 mg, 250 mg. Intramuscular or intravenous (powder to be reconstituted): 500 mg. [ah-SEE-tah-ZOH-lah-mide].

**acetic acid** (Uro). Used to irrigate the bladder. Irrigating solution: 0.25%. (ah-SEE-tik AS-id].

**acetohydroxamic acid** (Lithostat) (Uro). Anti-infective drug used to treat urinary tract infections caused by urea-splitting bacteria. Tablet: 250 mg. [ah-SEE-toh-HY-drawks-AM-ik AS-id].

**acetylcholine** (Miochol-E) (Ophth). Miotic drug used to constrict the pupil during eye surgery. Ophthalmic solution: 0.01%. [ah-SEE-til-KOH-leen].

**acetylcysteine** (Acetadote, Mucomyst) (Emerg, Pulm). Antidote drug used to treat acetaminophen overdose (Acetadote); mucolytic drug used to break apart thick mucus in patients with pulmonary disease and cystic fibrosis (Mucomyst). Liquid (oral or by NG tube): 10%, 20%. Intravenous: 200 mg/mL. Nebulizer solution for inhalation: 10%, 20%. [ah-SEE-til-SIS-teen].

**acetylsalicylic acid** (ASA). See *aspirin.* [ah-SEE-til-SAL-ih-SIL-ik AS-id].

**Acid Reducer 200** (GI). See *cimetidine.* [AS-id ree-DOO-ser].

**AcipHex** (GI). See *rabeprazole.* [AS-ih-feks].

**acitretin** (Soriatane) (Derm). Vitamin A-type (retinoid) drug used to treat severe psoriasis. Capsule: 10 mg, 25 mg. [AS-ih-TREH-tin].

**Aclaro** (Derm). See *hydroquinone.* [ah-KLAIR-oh].

**Aclovate** (Derm). See *alclometasone.* [AK-loh-vayt].

**Acne Clear** (Derm). See *benzoyl peroxide.* [AK-nee KLEER].

**ActHIB** (Pulm). Used to prevent *H. influenzae* infection in children. Subcutaneous: Vaccine. [AKT-H-I-B].

**Acthrel** (Endo). Used to help diagnose whether Cushing's syndrome is due to a pituitary gland malfunction or another cause. 100 mcg/5 mL. [AK-threl].

**Acticin** (Derm). See *permethrin.* [AK-tih-sin].

**Acticort 100** (Derm). See *hydrocortisone.* [AK-tih-kort].

**Actidose-Aqua** (Emerg, GI). See *activated charcoal.* [AK-tih-dohs-AW-kwah].

**Actifed Cold & Allergy** (ENT) (generic *pseudoephedrine, triprolidine*). Combination over-the-counter decongestant and antihistamine drug. Tablet: 60 mg/2.5 mg. [AK-tih-fed].

**Actifed Cold & Sinus Maximum Strength** (ENT) (generic *acetaminophen, chlorpheniramine, pseudoephedrine*). Combination over-the-counter analgesic, antihistamine, and decongestant drug. Tablet: 500 mg/2 mg/30 mg. [AK-tih-fed].

**ActiFruit/Cran-Max** (Uro). Dietary supplement of cranberries for urinary tract health. Capsule. Softchew tablet. [AK-tih-froot].

**Actigall** (GI). See *ursodiol.* [AK-tih-gawl].

**Actimmune** (Chem, Derm). See *interferon gamma-1b.* [AK-tih-myoon].

**Actimid** (Chemo). Chemotherapy drug used to treat multiple myeloma. Orphan drug. [AK-tih-mid].

**actinomycin D** (Chemo). See *dactinomycin.* [ak-TIN-oh-MY-sin D].

**Actiq** (Analges). See *fentanyl.* [ak-TEEK].

**Activase** (Cardio, Hem, Neuro). See *alteplase.* [AK-tih-vays].

**activated charcoal** (Actidose-Aqua, CharcoAid, CharcoAid 2000, Liqui-Char) (Emerg, GI). Used to absorb drugs or toxic substances from the GI tract after an accidental drug ingestion or suicide attempt. Oral or nasogastric tube. Granules: 15 g. Liquid: 208 mg/mL. Suspension: 15 g, 30 g. Powder (to be reconstituted). [AK-tih-vay-ted CHAR-kohl].

**Activella** (OB/GYN, Ortho) (generic *norethindrone, estradiol*). Combination hormone drug used to treat the symptoms of menopause; used to prevent postmenopausal osteoporosis. Tablet: 0.5 mg/1 mg. [AK-tih-VEL-ah].

**Actonel** (OB/GYN, Ortho). See *risedronate.* [AK-toh-nel].

**Actonel with Calcium** (Ortho) (generic *risedronate, calcium*). Combination bone resorption inhibitor drug with calcium; used to prevent bone loss and treat osteoporosis in men and postmenopausal women. Tablet: 35 mg/1250 mg. [AK-toh-nel].

**ActoPlus Met** (Endo) (generic *pioglitazone, metformin*). Combination oral antidiabetic drug used to treat type 2 diabetes mellitus. Tablet: 15 mg/500 mg, 15 mg/850 mg. [AK-toh-plus MET].

**Actos** (Endo). See *pioglitazone.* [AK-tohs].

**Acular, Acular LS, Acular PF** (Ophth). See *ketorolac.* [AK-yoo-lar].

**acyclovir** (Zovirax) (Anti-infec, Derm, OB/GYN). Antiviral drug used topically to treat herpes simplex type 1 virus lesions (cold sores) and herpes simplex whitlow infection of the nail; used orally to treat herpes simplex type 2 virus lesions (genital herpes); used to treat herpes varicella-zoster

**Alimentum** (GI).   Lactose-free, sucrose-free infant formula for infants with severe allergies or protein or fat malabsorption. Liquid. [AL-ih-MEN-tum].

**Alimta** (Chemo).   See *pemetrexed.* [ah-LIM-tah].

**Alinia** (GI).   See *nitazoxanide.* [ah-LIN-ee-ah].

**aliskiren** (Tekturna) (Cardio).   Renin inhibitor drug used to treat hypertension. Tablet: 150 mg, 300 mg. [AH-lis-KY-ren].

**alitretinoin** (Panretin) (Chemo, Derm).   Vitamin A-type (retinoid) drug used topically to treat cancerous skin lesions of cutaneous T-cell lymphoma and Kaposi's sarcoma. Gel: 0.1%. [AL-ih-TREH-tih-NOH-in].

**Alka-Mints** (GI).   See *calcium carbonate.* [AL-kah-MINTZ].

**Alka-Seltzer Extra Strength, Alka-Seltzer Original, Alka-Seltzer with Aspirin** (Analges) (generic *aspirin, sodium bicarbonate*).   Combination over-the-counter salicylate and antacid drug used to treat pain. Effervescent tablet: 325 mg/1700 mg, 500 mg/1985 mg. [AL-kah SELT-zer].

**Alkeran** (Chemo).   See *melphalan.* [AL-ker-an].

**allantoin** (Alwextin) (Derm).   Used to treat skin erosions from epidermolysis bullosa. Orphan drug. [AL-lan-TOH-in].

**Allegra** (Derm, ENT).   See *fexofenadine.* [ah-LEG-rah].

**Allegra-D** (ENT) (generic *fexofenadine, pseudoephedrine*).   Combination antihistamine and decongestant drug. Tablet: 60 mg/120 mg, 180 mg/240 mg. [ah-LEG-rah-D].

**AllerMax, AllerMax Maximum Strength** (Derm, ENT, Ophth).   See *diphenhydramine.* [AL-er-maks].

**Allfen Jr** (Pulm).   See *guaifenesin.* [AWL-fen JOO-nyoor].

**Alli** (GI).   See *orlistat.* [AL-lie].

**Alloprim** (Chemo, Ortho, Uro).   See *allopurinol.* [AL-oh-prim].

**allopurinol** (Aloprim, Zyloprim) (Chemo, Ortho, Uro).   Decreases uric acid levels; used to treat gout and gouty arthritis; used to treat patients with recurrent calcium oxalate kidney stones; used as a preservative solution for cadaver kidneys prior to kidney transplantation; used to treat cancer patients whose chemotherapy drugs cause elevated levels of uric acid. Tablet: 100 mg, 300 mg. Intravenous (powder to be reconstituted): 500 mg/30 mL. [AL-oh-PYOOR-ih-nawl].

**Allovectin-7** (Chemo).   Chemotherapy drug used to treat malignant melanoma. Orphan drug. [AL-oh-VEK-tin-7].

**almotriptan** (Axert) (Analges).   Serotonin receptor agonist drug used to treat migraine headaches. Tablet: 6.25 mg, 12.5 mg. [AL-moh-TRIP-tan].

**Alocril** (Ophth).   See *nedocromil.* [AL-oh-kril].

**Alomide** (Ophth).   See *lodoxamide.* [AL-oh-mide].

**Alor** (Analges) (generic *aspirin, hydrocodone*).   Schedule III combination salicylate and narcotic analgesic drug for pain. Tablet: 500 mg/5 mg. [ah-LOR].

**Alora** (OB/GYN, Ortho).   See *estradiol.* [ah-LOR-ah].

**alosetron** (Lotronex) (GI).   Serotonin receptor blocker drug used to treat irritable bowel syndrome. Tablet: 0.5 mg, 1 mg. [ah-LOH-seh-trawn].

**Aloxi** (Chemo, GI).   See *palonosetron.* [ah-LAWK-see].

**alpha-galactosidase A** (Fabrase, Replagal) (Misc).   Used to treat Fabry disease. Orphan drug. [AL-fah-gah-LAK-toh-SY-days A].

**Alphagan P** (Ophth).   See *brimonidine.* [AL-fah-gan P].

**Alphanate** (Hem).   See *factor VIII.* [AL-fah-nayt].

**AlphaNine SD** (Hem).   See *factor IX.* [AL-fah-nine S D].

**alpha₁-proteinase inhibitor** (Aralast, Prolastin, Zemaira) (Pulm).   Enzyme replacement drug for emphysema patients with alpha₁-antitrypsin deficiency. Intravenous: 400 mg/25 mL, 800 mg/50 mL, 500 mg/20 mL, 1000 mg/40 mL. [AL-fah-1-PROH-teen-ace in-HIB-ih-tor].

**alprazolam** (Xanax) (GI, OB/GYN, Psych).   Schedule IV benzodiazepine drug used to treat anxiety and neurosis; used to treat panic disorder; used to treat premenstrual dysphoric disorder; used to treat irritable bowel syndrome. Oral liquid: 1 mg/mL. Tablet: 0.25 mg, 0.5 mg, 1 mg, 2 mg. Extended-release tablet: 0.5 mg, 1 mg, 2 mg, 3 mg. Orally disintegrating tablet: 0.25 mg, 0.5 mg, 1 mg, 2 mg. [al-PRAZ-oh-lam].

**alprostadil** (Caverject, Edex, Muse, Prostin VR Pediatric) (Cardio, Uro).   Prostaglandin drug used to treat impotence due to erectile dysfunction; used to keep the ductus arteriosus open until surgery can be performed on newborns with congenital heart defects. Liquid (for injection into penis): 10 mcg/mL, 20 mg/mL, 40 mcg/mL. Powder (to be reconstituted for injection into penis): 5 mcg/mL, 10 mcg/mL, 20 mcg/mL, 40 mcg/mL. Pellet (inserted into the urethra): 125 mcg, 250 mcg, 500 mcg, 1000 mcg. Intravenous: 500 mcg/mL. [al-PRAWS-tah-dil].

**Alrex** (Ophth).   See *loteprednol.* [AL-reks].

**Altabax** (Derm, ENT).   See *retapamulin.* [AL-tah-baks].

**Altacaine** (Ophth).   See *tetracaine.* [AL-tah-kayn].

**Altace** (Cardio).   See *ramipril.* [AL-tays].

**Altafrin** (Ophth).   See *phenylephrine.* [AL-tah-frin].

**Altastaph** (Anti-infec).   Used to prevent *S. aureus* infections in premature infants. Orphan drug. [AL-tah-staf].

**alteplase** (Activase, Cathflo Activase) (Cardio, Hem, Neuro).   Tissue plasminogen activator drug used to dissolve blood clots that cause a myocardial infarction, pulmonary embolus, or stroke; used to dissolve clots in central venous catheters (Cathflo Activase). Intravenous (powder to be reconstituted): 50 mg (29 million units)/50 mL, 100 mg (58 million units)/100 mL, 2 mg. [AL-teh-plays].

**AlternaGEL** (GI).   See *aluminum hydroxide.* [al-TER-nah-jel].

**Altinac** (Derm).   See *tretinoin.* [AL-tih-nak].

**Altoprev** (Cardio).   See *lovastatin.* [AL-toh-prev].

**Altracin** (Anti-infec).   See *bacitracin.* [al-TRAY-sin].

**altretamine** (Hexalen) (Chemo).   Alkylating chemotherapy drug used to treat ovarian cancer. Capsule: 50 mg. [al-TREE-tah-meen].

**Aludrox** (GI) (generic *aluminum, magnesium, simethicone*).   Combination antacid and anti-gas drug for heartburn. Suspension: 307 mg/103 mg/20 mg. [AL-yoo-drawks].

**aluminum acetate** (Bite Rx, Bluboro, Buro-Sol, Burow's solution, Domeboro, modified Burow's solution, Pedi-Boro Soak) (Derm).   Over-the-counter astringent drug used topically to treat minor skin conditions. Effervescent tablet. Powder. Solution: 0.5%. [ah-LOO-mih-num AS-eh-tayt].

**aluminum chloride** (Drysol, Xerac AC) (Derm).   Astringent and drying drug used topically to treat excessive sweating. Topical liquid: 20%. [ah-LOO-mih-num KLOH-ride].

**aluminum hydroxide** (AlternaGEL, Alu-Tab, Amphojel, Dialume) (GI).   Aluminum-containing antacid drug used to treat heartburn and gastric ulcer. Capsule: 500 mg. Tablet: 500 mg, 600 mg. Oral suspension: 320 mg/5 mL, 450 mg/5mL, 675 mg/5 mL. Oral liquid: 600 mg/5 mL. [ah-LOO-mih-num hy-DRAWK-side].

**Alupent** (Pulm).   See *metaproterenol.* [AL-yoo-pent].

**Alu-Tab** (GI).   See *aluminum hydroxide.* [AL-yoo-tab].

**Alvesco** (Pulm).   See *ciclesonide.* [al-VES-koh].

**alvimopan** (Entereg) (Analges, GI).   Narcotic antagonist drug used to restore intestinal motility after surgery and after treatment with narcotic drugs for pain. Capsule: 12 mg. [AL-vih-MOH-pan].

**Alwextin** (Derm).   See *allantoin.* [al-WEKS-tin].

**amantadine** (Symmetrel) (Anti-infec, Neuro, Pulm).   Antiviral drug used to prevent and treat influenza virus A respiratory tract infection; dopamine receptor stimulant drug used to treat Parkinson's disease; used to treat drug-induced extrapyramidal side effects. Capsule: 100 mg. Syrup: 50 mg/5 mL. Tablet: 100 mg. [ah-MAN-tah-deen].

**Amaryl** (Endo).   See *glimepiride.* [AM-ah-ril].

**Amatine** (Cardio).   See *midodrine.* [AM-ah-teen].

**ambenonium** (Mytelase) (Neuro).   Anticholinesterase drug used to treat myasthenia gravis. Tablet: 10 mg. [AM-beh-NOH-nee-um].

**Ambien, Ambien CR** (Neuro).   See *zolpidem.* [AM-bee-en].

**AmBisome** (Anti-infec).   See *amphotericin B.* [AM-bih-zohm].

**ambrisentan** (Letairis) (Cardio).   Used to treat pulmonary arterial hypertension. Tablet: 5 mg. [AM-brih-SEN-tan].

**amcinonide** (Derm).   Corticosteroid drug used topically to treat inflammation and itching from dermatitis, seborrhea, eczema, psoriasis, and yeast or fungal infections. Cream: 0.1%. Lotion: 0.1%. Ointment: 0.1%. [am-SIN-oh-nide].

**Amerge** (Analges).   See *naratriptan.* [ah-MERJ].

**Americet** (Analges) (generic *acetaminophen, butalbital, caffeine*).   Combination nonsalicylate analgesic, barbiturate sedative, and stimulant drug used to treat pain. Tablet: 325 mg/50 mg/40 mg. [ah-MAIR-ih-set].

**A-Methapred** (Endo, Neuro).   See *methylprednisolone.* [AA-METH-ah-pred].

**Amevive** (Derm).   See *lefacept.* [AM-eh-veev].

**Amicar** (Hem).   See *aminocaproic acid.* [AM-ih-kar].

**Amidate** (Anes).   See *etomidate.* [AM-ih-dayt].

**amifostine** (Ethyol) (Chemo, Uro).   Cytoprotective drug used to prevent toxicity of the kidneys in patients receiving cisplatin or cyclophosphamide chemotherapy; used to protect

against xerostomia after radiation therapy for head and neck cancer. Intravenous (powder to be reconstituted): 500 mg/10mL. [AM-ih-FAWS-teen].

**Amigesic** (Analges).   See *salsalate.* [AM-ih-JEE-sik].

**amikacin** (Amikin) (Anti-infec).   Aminoglycoside antibiotic drug used to treat a variety of serious gram-negative bacterial infections, such as peritonitis, meningitis, and septicemia; used to prevent *Mycobacterium avium-intracellulare* infection in AIDS patients; orphan drug used to treat *P. aeruginosa* lung infections in patients with cystic fibrosis. Intramuscular or intravenous: 50 mg/mL, 250 mg/mL [AM-ih-KAY-sin].

**Amikin** (Anti-infec).   See *amikacin.* [AM-ih-kin].

**amiloride** (Midamor) (Cardio, Pulm, Uro).   Potassium-sparing diuretic drug used to treat hypertension; used to treat edema from congestive heart failure; orphan drug that is inhaled to treat cystic fibrosis. Tablet: 5 mg. Aerosol. [ah-MIL-oh-ride].

**Amin-Aid** (GI, Uro).   Nutritional supplement formulated for patients with acute or chronic renal failure. Powder (to be reconstituted). [AM-in-aid].

**aminobenzoate** (Potaba) (Derm).   Used to treat scleroderma. Tablet: 500 mg. Capsule: 500 mg. Envules (powder): 2 g. [ah-MEE-noh-BEN-zoh-ate].

**aminocaproic acid** (Amicar, Caprogel) (Hem, Ophth).   Hemostatic drug used to treat bleeding in patients with fibrinolysis; used topically to treat traumatic hyphema in the eye. Oral liquid: 250 mg/mL. Tablet: 500 mg, 1000 mg. Intravenous: 250 mg/mL. Orphan drug. [ah-MEE-noh-kap-ROH-ik AS-id].

**aminoglutethimide** (Cytadren) (Chemo, Endo).   Corticosteroid drug used to treat Cushing's syndrome; used to treat breast and prostate cancer. Tablet: 250 mg. [ah-MEE-noh-gloo-TETH-ih-mide].

**aminolevulinic acid** (Levulan Kerastick) (Derm).   Used topically to treat actinic keratoses; used with photodynamic therapy (blue light of a specific wavelength [BLU-U]) to treat skin cancers and Kaposi's sarcoma. Topical solution: 20%. [ah-MEE-noh-LEV-yoo-LIN-ik AS-id].

**aminophylline** (Pulm).   Bronchodilator drug used to treat bronchospasm in asthma and emphysema. Tablet: 100 mg, 200 mg. Intravenous: 25 mg/10 mL, 25 mg/20 mL. [AM-ih-NAW-fih-lin].

**aminosalicylate** (GI).   Used to treat Crohn's disease. Orphan drug. [ah-MEE-noh-sah-LIH-sih-layt].

**aminosalicylic acid** (4-ASA, Pamisyl, Paser, Rezipas) (GI, Pulm).   Antitubercular antibiotic drug used to treat tuberculosis that is resistant to other antitubercular drugs; used to treat Crohn's disease; used to treat ulcerative colitis in patients who cannot tolerate sulfasalazine. Oral granules: 4 g. [ah-MEE-noh-SAL-ih-SIL-ik AS-id].

**aminosidine** (Gabbromicina) (Anti-infec, Pulm).   Used to treat *Mycobacterium avium-intracellulare* infection in AIDS patients; used to treat tuberculosis. Orphan drug. [ah-MEE-noh-SY-deen].

**Aminoxin** (OB/GYN, Pulm).   See *pyridoxine*. [AM-ih-NAWK-sin].

**amiodarone** (Cordarone, Pacerone) (Cardio).   Antiarrhythmic drug used to treat ventricular tachycardia and ventricular fibrillation. Tablet: 100 mg, 200 mg, 400 mg. Intravenous: 50 mg/mL. [AM-ee-OH-dah-rohn].

**Amitiza** (GI).   See *lubiprostone*. [AM-ih-TEE-zah].

**amitriptyline** (Analges, Neuro, Psych).   Tricyclic antidepressant drug used to treat depression; used to treat bulimia; used to treat migraine headaches; used to treat severe laughing and weeping from brain disease; used to treat nerve pain from phantom limb, diabetic neuropathy, peripheral neuropathy, and postherpetic neuralgia; used to treat tic douloureux. Tablet: 10 mg, 25 mg, 50 mg, 75 mg, 100 mg, 150 mg. Intramuscular: 10 mg/mL. [AM-ee-TRIP-tih-leen].

**amlexanox** (Aphthasol) (ENT).   Used topically to treat aphthous ulcers in the mouth. Paste: 5%. [am-LEK-sah-nawks].

**amlodipine** (Amvaz, Norvasc) (Cardio).   Calcium channel blocker drug used to prevent and treat angina pectoris; used to treat hypertension, pulmonary arterial hypertension, and Raynaud's disease. Tablet: 2.5 mg, 5 mg, 10 mg. [am-LOH-dih-peen].

**Ammonul** (Hem) (generic *sodium benzoate, sodium phenylacetate*).   Combination drug used to prevent and treat increased blood levels of ammonia in patients with abnormalities of the enzymes that produce urea; used to treat hepatic encephalopathy. Intravenous: 100 mg/100 mg per mL. [AM-moh-nul].

**Amnesteem** (Derm).   See *isotretinoin*. [AM-nes-steem].

**amobarbital** (Amytal) (Neuro).   Schedule II barbiturate drug used to provide sedation. Intramuscular and intravenous (powder to be reconstituted): 250 mg, 500 mg. [AM-oh-BAR-bih-tawl].

**AMO Vitrax** (Ophth).   See *sodium hyaluronate*. [A-M-O VY-traks].

**amoxapine** (Analges, Neuro, Psych).   Tricyclic antidepressant drug used to treat depression or depression with anxiety; used to treat migraine headaches; used to treat nerve pain from phantom limb, diabetic neuropathy, peripheral neuropathy, and postherpetic neuralgia; used to treat tic douloureux. Tablet: 25 mg, 50 mg, 100 mg, 150 mg. [ah-MAWK-sah-peen].

**amoxicillin** (Amoxil, Amoxil Pediatric, DisperMox, Moxatag, Trimox) (Anti-infec).   Penicillin-type antibiotic drug used to treat bacterial infections of the ears, nose, throat, lungs, genitourinary tract, and skin; used to treat gonorrhea; used to treat *H. pylori* infection of the gastrointestinal tract; used prophylactically to prevent bacterial endocarditis in patients with congenital heart disease, rheumatic heart disease, or prosthetic heart valves who are undergoing dental or surgical procedures. Capsule: 250 mg, 500 mg. Chewable tablet: 125 mg, 200 mg, 250 mg, 400 mg. Extended-release tablet: 775 mg. Tablet: 500 mg, 875 mg. Liquid (powder to be reconstituted): 50 mg/mL, 125 mg/5 mL, 200 mg/5 mL, 250 mg/5 mL, 400 mg/5 mL. Liquid (tablet to be reconstituted): 200 mg, 400 mg. [ah-MAWK-sih-SIL-in].

**Amoxil, Amoxil Pediatric** (Anti-infec).   See *amoxicillin*. [ah-MAWK-sil].

**Amphadase** (Misc).   See *hyaluronidase*. [AM-fah-days].

**Amphocin** (Anti-infec).   See *amphotericin B*. [AM-foh-sin].

**Amphojel** (GI).   See *aluminum hydroxide*. [AM-foh-jel].

**Amphotec** (Anti-infec).   See *amphotericin B*. [AM-foh-tek].

**amphotericin B** (Abelcet, AmBisome, Amphocin, Amphotec, Fungizone Intravenous) (Anti-infec).   Antifungal drug used to treat severe systemic fungal and yeast infections, such as aspergillosis, blastomycosis, coccidioidomycosis, and candidiasis. Intravenous: 100 mg/20 mL. Inhaled powder (orphan drug). [AM-foh-TAIR-ah-sin].

**ampicillin** (Principen) (Anti-infec).   Penicillin-type antibiotic drug used to treat bacterial infections; used to treat infections caused by *E. coli, Salmonella, H. influenzae, S. pneumoniae, and S. aureus;* used to treat gonorrhea, meningitis, endocarditis, and septicemia. Capsule: 250 mg, 500 mg. Liquid: 125 mg/5 mL, 250 mg/5 mL. Intramuscular or intravenous (powder to be reconstituted): 250 mg, 500 mg, 1 g, 2 g. [AM-pih-SIL-in].

**Ampligen** (Anti-infec, Chemo).   Chemotherapy drug used to treat AIDS; used to treat kidney cancer and malignant melanoma; used to treat chronic fatigue syndrome. Orphan drug. [AM-plih-jen].

**Amplimexon** (Chemo).   See *imexon*. [AM-plih-MEK-sawn].

**Amrix** (Ortho).   See *cyclobenzaprine*. [AM-riks].

**amsacrine** (Amsidyl) (Chemo).   Chemotherapy drug used to treat leukemia. Orphan drug. [am-SAK-reen].

**Amsidyl** (Chemo).   See *amsacrine*. [AM-sih-dil].

**Amvaz** (Cardio).   See *amlodipine*. [AM-vaz].

**Amvisc, Amvisc Plus** (Ophth).   See *sodium hyaluronate*. [AM-visk].

**amyl nitrite** (Cardio).   Nitrate drug used to treat angina pectoris. Inhalation (capsule crushed and inhaled): 0.3 mL. [AA-mil NY-trayt].

**Amytal** (Neuro).   See *amobarbital*. [AM-ih-tawl].

**Anacin, Anacin Maximum Strength** (Analges) (generic *aspirin, caffeine*).   Combination over-the-counter salicylate analgesic and stimulant drug used to treat pain and headaches. Caplet, Tablet: 400 mg/32 mg, 500 mg/32 mg. [AN-ah-sin].

**Anacin Aspirin Free Maximum Strength** (Analges).   See *acetaminophen*. [AN-ah-sin].

**Anadrol-50** (Anti-infec, Chemo, Hem).   See *oxymetholone*. [AN-ah-drawl-50].

**Anafranil** (Psych).   See *clomipramine*. [ah-NAF-rah-nil].

**anagrelide** (Agrylin) (Hem).   Antiplatelet drug used to decrease an elevated platelet count in patients with bone marrow disorders. Capsule: 0.5 mg, 1 mg. [an-AH-greh-lide].

**anakinra** (Kineret) (Ortho).   Immunomodulator drug used to treat rheumatoid arthritis. Subcutaneous: 100 mg/0.67 mL. [AN-ah-KIN-rah].

**Analpram-HC** (Derm, GI) (generic *hydrocortisone, pramoxine*) Combination corticosteroid and anesthetic drug used topically to treat pain, itching, and inflammation from hemorrhoids and perianal dermatitis. Cream/lotion: 1%/1%, 2.5%/1%. [AA-nawl-pram-H-C].

**AnaMantle HC** (Derm, GI) (generic *hydrocortisone, lidocaine*). Combination corticosteroid and anesthetic drug used topically to treat pain, itching, and inflammation from hemorrhoids and perianal dermatitis. Gel: 2.5%/3%. [AA-nah-MAN-tl H-C].

**Anaprox, Anaprox DS** (Analges). See *naproxen.* [AN-ah-prawks].

**anaritide** (Auriculin) (Uro). Used to treat renal failure; used to improve kidney function following renal transplantation. Orphan drug. [ah-NAIR-ih-tide].

**Anaspaz** (GI, Uro). See *L-hyoscyamine.* [AN-ah-spaz].

**anastrozole** (Arimidex) (Chemo). Hormonal chemotherapy drug used to treat breast cancer; used to treat male infertility. Tablet: 1 mg. [ah-NAS-troh-zohl].

**anatibant** (Neuro). Used to decrease mortality and increase neurologic function after traumatic brain injury. Orphan drug. [ah-NAT-ih-bant].

**Anbesol, Anbesol Cold Sore Therapy, Anbesol Maximum Strength, Baby Anbesol** (Anes, ENT). See *benzocaine.* [AN-beh-sawl].

**Ancobon** (Anti-infec). See *flucytosine.* [AN-koh-bawn].

**ancrod** (Viprinex) (Hem). Anticoagulant drug used in patients who cannot tolerate heparin during cardiopulmonary bypass. Orphan drug. [AN-krawd].

**Androcur** (Endo). See *cyproterone.* (AN-droh-kyoor].

**Androderm** (Endo). See *testosterone.* [AN-droh-derm].

**AndroGel** (Endo). See *testosterone.* [AN-droh-jel].

**Androgel-DHT** (Endo). See *dihydrotestosterone.* [AN-droh-jel-D-H-T].

**Android** (Chemo, Endo). See *methyltestosterone.* [AN-droyd].

**Androxy** (Chemo, Endo). See *fluoxymesterone.* [an-DRAWK-see].

**Anectine, Anectine Flo-Pack** (Anes, Pulm). See *succinylcholine.* [ah-NEK-teen].

**Anestacon** (Anes, Uro). See *lidocaine.* [ah-NES-tah-kawn].

**Anestafoam** (Anes). See *lidocaine.* [an-NES-tah-fohm].

**Anexsia** (Analges) (generic *acetaminophen, hydrocodone*). Combination Schedule III nonnarcotic and narcotic analgesic drug for pain. Tablet: 325 mg/5 mg, 325 mg/7.5 mg, 500 mg/5 mg, 650 mg/7.5 mg, 650 mg/10 mg. [ah-NEK-see-ah].

**Angeliq** (OB/GYN) (generic *drospirenone, estradiol*). Combination hormone drug used to treat the symptoms of menopause. Tablet: 0.5 mg/1 mg. [AN-jeh-LEEK].

**Angiomax** (Hem). See *bivalirudin.* [AN-jee-oh-maks].

**anidulafungin** (Eraxis) (Anti-infec). Antifungal drug used to treat severe systemic yeast infections and esophageal candidiasis. Intravenous: 50 mg. [ah-NID-yoo-lah-FUN-jin].

**Animi-3** (Cardio). See *omega-3 fatty acids.* [AN-ih-mee-3].

**Ansaid** (Analges). See *flurbiprofen.* [AN-sayd].

**Antabuse** (Psych). See *disulfiram.* [AN-tah-byoos].

**Antara** (Cardio). See *fenofibrate.* [an-TAIR-ah].

**Anthim** (Pulm). Used to treat exposure to anthrax from bioterrorism. Orphan drug. [AN-thim].

**anthralin** (Dritho-Scalp, Psoriatec) (Derm). Used topically to treat psoriasis. Cream: 0.5%, 1%. [AN-trah-lin].

**antiepilepsirine** (Neuro). Anticonvulsant drug used to treat drug-resistant, tonic-clonic seizures. Orphan drug. [AN-tee-EP-ih-LEP-sih-reen].

**antihemophiliac factor** (Hem). See *factor VIII.* [AN-tee-HEE-moh-FIL-ee-ak FAK-tor].

**anti-inhibitor coagulant complex** (Feiba VH) (Hem). Anti-inhibitor drug used to treat hemophiliac patients who produce inhibitors against factor VIII; used during bleeding episodes or surgery. Intravenous: 8 mg/mL. [AN-tee-in-HIB-ih-tor koh-AG-yoo-lant KAWM-pleks].

**Anti-Itch** (Derm) (generic *diphenhydramine, zinc*). Combination over-the-counter antihistamine and astrigent drug used topically to decrease itching and oozing. Cream: 2%. [AN-tee-ITCH].

**Antilirium** (Emerg, Psych). See *physostigmine.* [AN-tee-LEER-ee-um].

**Antiminth** (GI). See *pyrantel.* [AN-tee-minth].

**antithrombin III** (ATnativ, Kybernin P, Thrombate III) (Hem). Used to treat patients with antithrombin III deficiency when they have a blood clot or during surgery or childbirth. Intravenous: 500 IU/10 mL, 1000 IU/20 mL. [AN-tee-THRAWM-bin-3].

**antithymocyte globulin** (Thymoglobulin) (Chemo, Hem). Immunoglobulin drug used to treat rejection of donor organ after organ transplantation; used to treat anemia; used to prevent graft-versus-host disease after bone marrow transplantation. Intravenous (powder to be reconstituted): 25 mg. [AN-tee-THY-moh-site GLAW-byoo-lin].

**Antivert, Antivert/25, Antivert/50** (GI). See *meclizine.* [AN-tee-vert].

**Antivipmyn** (Emerg). See *crotalidae polyvalent immune fab.* [AN-tee-VIP-min].

**Antizol** (Emerg, Psych). See *fomepizole.* [AN-tih-zohl].

**Antril** (Chemo, Ortho). See *interleukin-1 receptor antagonist.* [AN-tril].

**Antrizine** (GI). See *meclizine.* [AN-trih-zeen].

**Antrocol** (GI) (generic *atropine, phenobarbital*). Combination anticholinergic and sedative drug; used to treat irritable bowel syndrome, spastic colon, and peptic ulcer. Elixir: 0.195 mg/16 mg. [AN-troh-kawl].

**Anturane** (Ortho). See *sulfinpyrazone.* [AN-tyoo-rayn].

**Anucort-HC** (Derm, GI). See *hydrocortisone.* [AN-yoo-kort].

**Anusol-HC** (Derm, GI). See *hydrocortisone.* [AN-yoo-sawl].

**Anzemet** (Chemo, GI). See *dolasetron.* [AN-zeh-met].

**Apep** (Chemo). See *mitoguazone.* [AA-pep].

**ApexiCon, ApexiCon E** (Derm). See *diflorasone.* [ah-PEK-sih-con].

**Aphrodyne** (Uro). See *yohimbine*. [AF-roh-dine].

**Aphthaid** (Anti-infec). See *lactic acid*. [AFTH-aid].

**Aphthasol** (ENT). See *amlexanox*. [AF-thah-sawl].

**Apidra** (Endo). See *insulin glulisine*. [ah-PEE-drah].

**Aplenzin** (Psych). See *bupropion*. [ah-PLEN-zin].

**Aplidin** (Chemo). See *plitidepsin*. [AP-lih-din].

**Aplisol** (Pulm). See *tuberculin purified protein derivative*. [AP-lih-sawl].

**Apokyn** (Neuro). See *apomorphine*. [AP-oh-kin].

**apomorphine** (Apokyn) (Neuro). Dopamine receptor stimulant drug used to treat Parkinson's disease. Subcutaneous injection: 10 mg/mL. [AP-oh-MOR-feen].

**apraclonidine** (Iopidine) (Ophth). Alpha receptor stimulator drug used topically to treat glaucoma. Ophthalmic solution: 0.5%, 1%. [AP-rah-KLAWN-ih-deen].

**aprepitant** (Emend) (Chemo, GI). Serotonin blocker drug used to treat nausea and vomiting caused by chemotherapy or radiation therapy; used to prevent postoperative nausea and vomiting. Capsule: 40 mg, 80 mg, 125 mg. Bi-pack and tri-pack. [ah-PREP-ih-tant].

**Apresoline** (Cardio). See *hydralazine*. [aa-PRES-oh-leen].

**Apri** (OB/GYN) (generic *desogestrel, ethinyl estradiol*). Combination monophasic oral contraceptive drug. Pill pack, 28-day: (21 hormone tablets) 0.15 mg/30 mcg; (7 inert tablets). [ah-PREE].

**Aptivus** (Anti-infec). See *tipranavir*. [ap-TEE-vus].

**Aqua-Ban, Maximum Strength** (Uro). See *pamabrom*. [AW-kwah-ban].

**Aquachloral Supprettes** (Neuro). See *chloral hydrate*. [AW-kwah-KLOR-awl soo-PRETZ].

**AquaSite** (Ophth). Over-the-counter artificial tears drug for dry eyes. Ophthalmic solution. [AW-kwah-site].

**Aracmyn** (Emerg). Used to treat black widow spider bite. Orphan drug. [ah-RAK-min].

**Aralast** (Pulm). See *alpha₁-proteinase inhibitor*. [AIR-ah-last].

**Aralen** (Anti-infec). See *chloroquine*. [AIR-ah-len].

**Aranelle** (OB/GYN) (generic *norethindrone, ethinyl estradiol*). Combination triphasic oral contraceptive drug. Pill pack, 28-day: (7 hormone tablets) 0.5 mg/35 mcg; (9 hormone tablets) 1 mg/35 mcg; (5 hormone tablets) 0.5 mg/35 mcg; (7 inert tablets). [AIR-ah-nel].

**Aranesp** (Hem). See *darbepoetin alfa*. [AIR-ah-nesp].

**Arava** (Cardio, GI, Ortho, Uro). See *leflunomide*. [ah-RAV-ah].

**Aramine** (Anes). See *metaraminol*. [AIR-ah-meen].

**Arcalyst** (Misc). See *rilonacept*. [AR-kah-list].

**arcitumomab** (Chemo). Monoclonal antibody drug used to identify the location of thyroid cancer and metastases. Orphan drug. [AR-sih-TOO-moh-mab].

**Aredia** (Chemo, OB/GYN, Ortho). See *pamidronate*. [ah-REE-dee-ah].

**Arestin** (Anti-infec). See *minocycline*. [ah-RES-tin].

**arformoterol** (Brovana) (Pulm). Bronchodilator drug used to treat chronic obstructive pulmonary disease. Inhalation (jet nebulizer): 15 mcg/2 mL. [AR-for-MOH-ter-awl].

**argatroban** (Hem). Thrombin inhibitor drug used to prevent blood clots in patients undergoing coronary artery angioplasty; used to treat heparin-induced thrombocytopenia. Intravenous: 100 mg/mL. [ar-GAH-troh-ban].

**Arginaid Extra** (GI). Nutritional supplement formulated for patients with wounds. Liquid. [AR-jih-naid].

**arginine butyrate** (Hem). Used to treat beta-thalassemia and sickle cell disease. Orphan drug. [AR-jih-neen BYOO-tih-rayt].

**Aricept, Aricept ODT** (Neuro). See *donepezil*. [AIR-ih-sept].

**Arimidex** (Chemo). See *anastrozole*. [ah-RIM-ih-deks].

**arimoclomol** (Neuro). Used to treat amyotrophic lateral sclerosis. Orphan drug. [AR-ih-MOH-kloh-mawl].

**aripiprazole** (Abilify, Abilify Discmelt) (Psych). Quinolone antipsychotic drug used to treat schizophrenia; used to treat mania in children and adults with manic-depressive disorder; orphan drug used to treat Tourette syndrome. Tablet: 2 mg, 5 mg, 10 mg, 15 mg, 20 mg, 30 mg. Orally disintegrating tablet: 10 mg, 15 mg. Liquid: 1 mg/mL. Intramuscular: 7.5 mg/mL. [AIR-ih-PIP-rah-zohl].

**Aristospan Intra-articular, Aristospan Intralesional** (Derm, Ortho). See *triamcinolone*. [ah-RIS-to-span].

**Arixtra** (Hem). See *fondaparinux*. [ah-RIK-strah].

**armodafinil** (Nuvigil) (Neuro). Used to treat narcolepsy. Tablet: 50 mg, 150 mg, 250 mg. [AR-moh-DAF-ih-nil].

**Armour Thyroid** (Endo). See *desiccated thyroid*. [AR-mor THY-royd].

**Aromasin** (Chemo). See *exemestane*. [ah-ROH-mah-sin].

**Arranon** (Chemo). See *nelarabine*. [AIR-rah-nawn].

**arsenic trioxide** (Trisenox) (Chemo). Chemotherapy drug used to treat leukemia; orphan drug used to treat cancer of the brain and liver and multiple myeloma. Intravenous: 1 mg/1 mL. [AR-seh-nik try-AWK-side].

**Arthra-G** (Analges). See *salsalate*. [AR-thrah-G].

**Arthritis Foundation Pain Reliever** (Analges, Ortho). See *aspirin*. [ar-THRY-tis foun-DAY-shun].

**Arthritis Pain Formula** (Analges, Ortho) (generic *aluminum, aspirin, magnesium*). Combination aspirin and antacid drug used to treat the pain of osteoarthritis and rheumatoid arthritis while protecting the mucous membranes of the stomach. Tablet: 27mg/500 mg/100 mg. [ar-THRY-tis PAYN FOR-myoo-lah].

**Arthrotec** (Analges) (generic *diclofenac, misoprostol*). Combination NSAID and prostaglandin drug; used to treat the pain of osteoarthritis and rheumatoid arthritis while protecting the mucous membranes of the stomach. Tablet: 50 mg/200 mcg, 75 mg/200 mcg. [AR-throh-tek].

**articaine** (Septocaine) (Anes, ENT). Anesthetic drug used to produce local anesthesia during dental and oral cavity procedures. Injection: 4% with 1:100,000 epinephrine. [AR-tih-kayn].

**Artiss** (Derm). See *human fibrin sealant*. [AR-tis].

**Asacol** (GI). See *mesalamine*. [AA-sah-kawl].

**Ascomp with Codeine** (Analges) (generic *aspirin, butalbital caffeine, codeine*).    Combination Schedule III salicylate, barbiturate sedative, stimulant, and narcotic analgesic drug for pain. Capsule: 325 mg/ 50 mg/40 mg/30 mg. [AS-kawmp with KOH-deen].

**ascorbic acid** (Uro).    Over-the-counter vitamin C dietary supplement drug used to acidify the urine to treat urinary tract infections. [as-KOR-bik AS-id].

**Ascriptin, Ascriptin A/D, Ascriptin Extra Strength, Ascriptin Maximum Strength** (Analges) (generic *aspirin, aluminum, calcium, magnesium*).    Combination over-the-counter salicylate and antacid drug used to treat the pain and protect the mucous memabranes of the stomach. Tablet: 325 mg/50 mg/ 50 mg/50 mg, 325 mg/75 mg/75 mg/75 mg, 500 mg/ 33mg/237 mg/33 mg, 500 mg/80 mg/80 mg/80 mg. [ah-SKRIP-tin].

**Asmalix** (Pulm).    See *theophylline*. [AZ-mah-liks].

**Asmanex Twisthaler** (Pulm).    See *mometasone*. [AZ-mah-neks twist-HAY-ler].

**asparaginase** (Elspar) (Chemo).    Chemotherapy enzyme drug used to treat leukemia. Intramuscular or intravenous (powder to be reconstituted): 10,000 IU. [ah-SPAIR-ah-jih-nays].

**Aspercreme** (Ortho) (generic *trolamine, alcohol*).    Combination over-the-counter salicylate analgesic and alcohol drug used topically to treat the pain of osteoarthritis and minor muscle injuries. Cream: 10%. [AS-per-kreem].

**Aspergum** (Analges).    See *aspirin*. [AS-per-gum].

**aspirin** (Arthritis Foundation Pain Reliever, Aspergum, Bayer Children's Aspirin, Bayer Low Adult Strength, Ecotrin, Ecotrin Adult Low Strength, Ecotrin Maximum Strength, Empirin, Extended Release Bayer 8-Hour, Extra Strength Bayer Enteric 500, Fasprin, Genuine Bayer Aspirin, Halfprin 81, Heartline, Maximum Bayer Aspirin, Norwich Extra Strength, Norwich Regular Strength, St. Joseph Adult Chewable, ZORprin) (Analges, Cardio, Hem, Ortho). Salicylate drug used to relieve the pain of headaches, toothaches, muscle pain, and menstrual pain; antipyretic drug used to reduce fever; used to treat the pain and inflammation of osteoarthritis, rheumatoid arthritis, and systemic lupus erythematosis; platelet aggregation inhibitor drug used to prevent blood clots, stroke, and myocardial infarction; used to treat chronic angina pectoris. Gum: 227.5 mg. Delayed-release tablet: 81 mg. Enteric-coated tablet: 81 mg, 165 mg, 325 mg, 500 mg, 650 mg. Controlled-release tablet: 800 mg. Orally dissolving tablet: 81 mg. Chewable tablet: 81 mg. Tablet: 325 mg, 500 mg. Suppository: 120 mg, 200 mg, 300 mg, 600 mg. [AS-pih-rin].

**Astelin** (ENT).    See *azelastine*. [AS-teh-lin].

**Astramorph PF** (Analges, Anes).    See *morphine*. [AS-trah-morf].

**Atacand** (Cardio).    See *candesartan*. [AT-ah-kand].

**Atacand HCT** (Cardio) (generic *candesartan, hydrochlorothiazide*).    Combination angiotensin II receptor blocker and diuretic drug used to treat hypertension. Tablet: 16 mg/12.5 mg, 32 mg/12.5 mg. [AT-ah-kand H-C-T].

**atazanavir** (Reyataz) (Anti-infec).    Protease inhibitor antiviral drug used to treat HIV and AIDS. Capsule: 100 mg, 150 mg, 200 mg, 300 mg. [AA-tah-ZAN-oh-veer].

**atenolol** (Tenormin) (Analges, Cardio, GI).    Cardioselective beta-blocker drug used to treat angina pectoris, hypertension, and acute myocardial infarction; used to treat migraine headaches; used to prevent bleeding from esophageal varices in patients with portal hypertension. Tablet: 25 mg, 50 mg, 100 mg. [ah-TEN-oh-lawl].

**Atgam** (Misc).    See *lymphocyte immune globulin*. [AT-gam].

**Atiprimod** (Chemo).    Used to treat multiple myeloma. Orphan drug. [ah-TIP-rih-mawd].

**Ativan** (Anes, GI, Neuro, Psych).    See *lorazepam*. [AT-ih-van].

**ATnativ** (Hem).    See *antithrombin III*. [A-T-NAY-tiv].

**atomoxetine** (Strattera) (Psych).    Selective norepinephrine uptake inhibitor drug used to treat attention-deficit/hyperactivity disorder; orphan drug used to treat Tourette syndrome. Capsule: 10 mg, 18 mg, 25 mg, 40 mg, 60 mg, 80 mg, 100 mg.[AA-toh-MAWK-seh-teen].

**atorvastatin** (Lipitor) (Cardio).    HMG-CoA reductase inhibitor drug used to treat hypercholesterolemia and arteriosclerosis. Tablet: 10 mg, 20 mg, 40 mg, 80 mg. [ah-TOR-vah-STAT-in].

**atovaquone** (Mepron) (Anti-infec).    Antiprotozoal drug used to prevent and treat *Pneumocystis carinii* pneumonia in AIDS patients. Liquid: 750 mg/5 mL. [ah-TOH-vah-kwohn].

**atracurium** (Tracrium) (Anes, Pulm).    Neuromuscular blocker drug used during surgery; used to treat patients who are intubated and on the ventilator. Intravenous: 10 mg/mL. [AH-trah-KYOOR-ee-um].

**Atridox** (Anti-infec).    See *doxycycline*. [AH-trih-dawks].

**Atripla** (Anti-infec) (generic *efavirenz, emtricitabine, tenofovir*).    Combination nonnucleoside reverse transcriptase inhibitor, nucleoside reverse transcriptase inhibitor, and nucleotide analog reverse transcriptase inhibitor antiviral drug used to treat HIV and AIDS. Tablet: 600 mg/ 200 mg/300 mg. [aa-TRIP-lah].

**AtroPen** (Emerg).    See *atropine*. [AH-troh-pen].

**atropine** (AtroPen, Isopto Atropine, Sal-Tropine) (Anes, Cardio, Emerg, GI, Neuro, Ophth, Uro).    Anticholinergic drug used to facilitate endotracheal intubation by decreasing oral and bronchial secretions; used during intra-abdominal surgery to sustain blood pressure; antiarrhythmic drug used to treat bradycardia and atrioventricular heart block; used to treat poisoning from organophosphate pesticides; used to treat spasms of the stomach and intestines; used to treat biliary spasm (colic); used to treat the rigidity and tremors of Parkinson's disease; used to treat crying/laughing episodes in patients with brain damage; mydriatic drug used topically to dilate the pupil to treat eye inflammation; used to treat urinary tract spasms. Tablet: 0.4 mg. Subcutaneous, endotracheal, intramuscular, or intravenous: 0.05 mg/mL, 0.1 mg/mL, 0.3 mg/mL, 0.4 mg/mL, 0.5 mg/mL, 0.8 mg/mL, 1 mg/mL. AtroPen: 0.5 mg, 1 mg, 2 mg. Ophthalmic ointment: 1%. Ophthalmic solution: 0.5%, 1%, 2%. [AH-troh-peen].

**Atrosept** (Uro) (generic *atropine, hyoscyamine, methenamine, methylene blue, phenyl salicylate*).    Combination urinary tract antispasmodic, anti-infective, antiseptic, and analgesic drug used to treat urinary tract infections with pain and spasms. Tablet: 0.03 mg/0.03 mg/40.8 mg/5.4 mg/18.1 mg. [AH-troh-sept].

**Atrovent, Atrovent HFA** (ENT, Pulm).    See *ipratropium*. [AH-troh-vent].

**A/T/S** (Derm).    See *erythromycin*. [A-T-S].

**attapulgite** (Diasorb, Kaopectate Maximum Strength, K-Pek, Parepectolin) (GI).    Over-the-counter absorbent drug used to treat diarrhea. Liquid: 600 mg/15 mL. Suspension: 750 mg/5 mL, 750 mg/15 mL. Capsule: 750 mg. Tablet: 750 mg. [AT-ah-PUL-gite].

**Attenuvax** (Anti-infec).    Used to prevent measles in children. Subcutaneous: Vaccine. [ah-TEN-yoo-vaks].

**Augmentin, Augmentin ES-600** (Anti-infec) (generic *amoxicillin, clavulanic acid*).    Combination penicillin-type antibiotic and penicillinase inhibitor drug used to treat penicillin-resistant bacterial infections. Tablet: 250 mg/125 mg, 500 mg/125 mg, 875 mg/125 mg. Extended-release tablet: 1000 mg/62.5 mg. Chewable tablet: 125 mg/31.25 mg, 200 mg/28.5 mg, 250 mg/62.5 mg, 400 mg/57 mg. Liquid: 125 mg/31.25 mg per 5 mL, 200 mg/28.5 mg per 5 mL, 250 mg/62.5 mg per 5 mL, 400 mg/57 mg per 5 mL. [AWG-men-tin].

**augmerosen** (Genasense) (Chemo).    Chemotherapy drug used to treat leukemia and multiple myeloma. Orphan drug. [awg-MAIR-oh-sen].

**auranofin** (Ridaura) (Ortho).    Gold compound drug used to treat rheumatoid arthritis. Capsule: 3 mg. [aw-RAY-noh-fin].

**Auriculin** (Uro).    See *anaritide*. [aw-RIK-yoo-lin].

**Aurolate** (Ortho).    See *gold sodium thiomalate*. [AW-roh-layt].

**aurothioglucose** (Solganal) (Ortho).    Gold compound drug used to treat rheumatoid arthritis. Intramuscular: 50 mg/mL. [AW-roh-THY-oh-GLOO-kohs].

**Avage** (Derm).    See *tazarotene*. [AA-vaj].

**Avalide** (Cardio) (generic *irbesartan, hydrochlorothiazide*).    Combination angiotensin II receptor blocker and diuretic drug used to treat hypertension. Tablet: 150 mg/12.5 mg, 300 mg/12.5 mg, 300 mg/25 mg. [AV-ah-lide].

**Avandamet** (Endo) (generic *metformin, rosiglitazone*).    Combination oral antidiabetic drug used to treat type 2 diabetes mellitus. Tablet: 500 mg/2 mg, 1000 mg/2 mg, 500 mg/4 mg, 1000 mg/4 mg. [ah VAN-dah-met].

**Avandaryl** (Endo) (generic *glimepiride, rosiglitazone*).    Combination oral antidiabetic drug used to treat type 2 diabetes mellitus. Tablet: 1 mg/4 mg, 2 mg/4 mg, 4 mg/4 mg. [ah-VAN-dah-ril].

**Avandia** (Endo, OB/GYN).    See *rosiglitazone*. [ah-VAN-dee-ah].

**Avapro** (Cardio, Endo, Uro).    See *irbesartan*. [AV-ah-proh].

**Avar, Avar-e, Avar Green** (Derm) (generic *sodium sulfacetamide, sulfur*).    Combination anti-infective and keratolytic drug used topically to treat acne vulgaris. Cream, gel, or cleanser: 10%/5%. [AA-var].

**Avastin** (Chemo, Ophth).    See *bevacizumab*. [ah-VAS-tin].

**AVC** (OB/GYN).    See *sulfanilamide*. [A-V-C].

**Aveeno, Aveeno Moisturizing** (Derm).    See *colloidal oatmeal*. [ah-VEE-noh].

**Avelox, Avelox I.V.** (Anti-infec).    See *moxifloxacin*. [AV-eh-lawks].

**Aventyl** (Analges, Neuro, Psych).    See *nortriptyline*. [ah-VEN-til].

**avian influenza vaccine** (Anti-infec, Pulm).    Inactivated virus vaccine used to protect against strain H5N1 that causes bird flu. Intramuscular: 90 mcg (2-dose regimen with second dose 28 days later). Subcutaneous: Vaccine. [AA-vee-an in-floo-EN-zah vak-SEEN].

**Aviane** (OB/GYN) (generic *levonorgestrel, ethinyl estradiol*).    Combination monophasic oral contraceptive drug. Pill pack, 28-day: (21 hormone tablets) 0.1 mg/20 mcg; (7 inert tablets). [AV-ee-an].

**Avinza** (Analges, Anes).    See *morphine*. [ah-VIN-zah].

**Avita** (Derm).    See *tretinoin*. [ah-VEE-tah].

**Avodart** (Uro).    See *dutasteride*. [AV-oh-dart].

**Avonex** (Neuro).    See *interferon beta-1a*. [AV-oh-neks].

**Axert** (Analges).    See *almotriptan*. [AKS-ert].

**Axid, Axid AR, Axid Pulvules** (GI).    See *nizatidine*. [AK-sid].

**Axocet** (Analges) (generic *acetaminophen, butalbital*).    Combination nonsalicylate analgesic and barbiturate sedative drug for pain. Tablet: 650 mg/50 mg. [AK-soh-set].

**Aygestin** (OB/GYN).    See *norethindrone*. [eye-JES-tin].

**Ayr Saline** (ENT).    See *saline*. [AIR SAY-leen].

**azacitidine** (Vidaza) (Chemo, Hem).    Demethylating chemotherapy drug used to treat leukemia; used to treat anemia, neutropenia, thrombocytopenia, and myelodysplastic syndrome. Intravenous: 100 mg. [AA-zah-SIT-ih-deen].

**Azactam** (Anti-infec).    See *aztreonam*. [aa-ZAK-tam].

**Azasan** (Ortho, Uro).    See *azathioprine*. [AA-zah-san].

**AzaSite** (Anti-infec, Ophth).    See *azithromycin*. [AA-zah-site].

**azathioprine** (Azasan, Imuran) (Ortho, Uro).    Immunosuppressant drug given after kidney transplantation to prevent rejection of the donor kidney; used to treat rheumatoid arthritis; orphan drug used to treat oral lesions from graft-versus-host disease. Tablet: 50 mg, 75 mg, 100 mg. Intravenous: 100 mg/20 mL. [AA-zah-THY-oh-preen].

**AZDU** (Anti-infec).    Antiviral drug used to treat AIDS. Orphan drug. [A-Z-D-U].

**azelaic acid** (Azelex, Finacea) (Derm).   Antibiotic drug used topically to treat acne vulgaris and acne rosacea. Cream: 20%. Gel: 15%. [AA-zeh-LAY-ik AS-id].

**azelastine** (Astelin, Optivar) (ENT, Ophth).   Antihistamine and mast cell stabilizer drug used topically to treat allergic rhinitis (Astelin) and allergy symptoms in the eyes (Optivar). Ophthalmic solution: 0.5 mg/mL. Nasal spray: 137 mcg/spray. [AA-zeh-LAS-teen].

**Azelex** (Derm).   See *azelaic acid.* [AA-zeh-leks].

**azidothymidine** (Anti-infec).   See *zidovudine.* [ah-ZEE-doh-THY-mih-deen].

**Azilect** (Neuro).   See *rasagiline.* [AA-zih-lekt].

**azithromycin** (AzaSite, Zithromax, Zmax) (Anti-infec, Ophth).   Macrolide antibiotic drug used to treat gram-negative and gram-positive bacterial infections; used to treat streptococcal pharyngitis and tonsillitis; used to treat otitis media, sinusitis, bronchitis, and pneumonia due to *S. pneumoniae, H. influenzae,* and *Mycoplasma;* used to treat staphylococcal and streptococcal skin infections; used to treat pelvic inflammatory disease, gonorrhea, syphilis, and *Chlamydia;* used to prevent *Mycobacterium avium-intracellulare* infection in AIDS patients; used topically in the eye to treat bacterial conjunctivitis (AzaSite). Tablet: 250 mg, 500 mg, 600 mg. Liquid (powder to be reconstituted): 100 mg/5 mL, 167 mg/5 mL, 200 mg/5 mL. Intramuscular or intravenous (powder to be reconstituted): 500 mg. Ophthalmic solution: 1% (25 mg/mL). [ah-ZIH-throh-MY-sin].

**Azmacort** (Pulm).   See *triamcinolone.* [AZ-mah-kort].

**Azopt** (Ophth).   See *brinzolamide.* [AA-zawpt].

**Azor** (Cardio) (generic *amlodipine, olmesartan*).Combination calcium channel blocker and angiotensin II receptor blocker drug used to treat hypertension. Tablet: 5 mg/20 mg, 5 mg/40 mg, 10 mg/20 mg, 10 mg/40 mg. [AA-zohr].

**Azo-Standard** (Uro).   See *phenazopyridine.* [AA-zoh-STAN-dard].

**aztreonam** (Azactam) (Anti-infec).   Monobactam antibiotic drug used to treat gram-negative bacterial infections; used to treat urinary tract infections due to *E. coli;* used to treat bronchitis and pneumonia due to *E. coli* and *H. influenzae;* used to treat burns and postoperative wounds; used to treat peritonitis, endometritis, and septicemia; orphan drug inhaled to treat gram-negative bacterial infections of the lung in patients with cystic fibrosis. Intramuscular or intravenous (powder to be reconstituted): 500 mg, 1 g, 2 g. [az-TREE-oh-nam].

**Azulfidine, Azulfidine EN-tabs** (GI, Ortho).   See *sulfasalazine.* [aa-ZUL-fih-deen].

**B&O Supprettes No. 15A, B&O Supprettes No. 16A** (Analges) (generic *opium, belladonna*).   Combination Schedule II narcotic analgesic and antispasmodic drug. Suppository: 30 mg/16.2 mg, 60 mg/16.2 mg. [B and O soo-PRETZ].

**BabyBIG** (GI).   See *botulism immune globulin.* [BAY-bee B-I-G].

**bacitracin** (AK-Tracin, Altracin) (Anti-infec, Derm, Ophth).   Antibiotic drug used to treat staphylococcal pneumonia in infants; included in many combination topical antibiotic drugs to treat skin infections; used topically to treat bacterial infections of the eyes; orphan drug used to treat pseudomembranous enterocolitis associated with antbiotic drugs (Altracin). Intramuscular (powder to be reconstituted): 500,000 units. Ointment: 500 units/g. Ophthalmic ointment: 500 units/g. [BAH-sih-TRAY-sin].

**baclofen** (Kemstro, Lioresal, Lioresal Intrathecal) (Analges, GI, Neuro, Ortho).   Skeletal muscle relaxant drug used to treat trigeminal neuralgia and tic douloureux; used to treat severe muscle spasticity associated with multiple sclerosis, cerebral palsy, stroke, or spinal cord injury; used to treat rigidity associated with Parkinson's disease; used to treat intractable hiccoughs and esophageal reflux; used to prevent migraine headaches. Tablet: 10 mg, 20 mg. Orally dissolving tablet: 10 mg, 20 mg. Intrathecal: 0.05 mg/mL, 10 mg/5 mL, 10 mg/20 mL. [BAK-loh-fen].

**Bactine Maximum Strength** (Derm).   See *hydrocortisone.* [bak-TEEN].

**Bactrim, Bactrim DS, Bactrim IV** (Anti-infec) (generic *sulfamethoxazole, trimethoprim*).   Combination antibiotic and sulfonamide anti-infective drug used to treat bronchitis, otitis media, traveler's diarrhea, urinary tract infection, and prostatitis; used to treat *Pneumocystis carinii* pneumonia in AIDS patients. Oral suspension: 200 mg/40 mg per 5 mL. Tablet: 400 mg/80 mg, 800 mg/160 mg. Intravenous: 80 mg/16 mg per 5 mL, 400 mg/80 mg per 5 mL. [BAK-trim].

**Bactroban, Bactroban Nasal** (Derm, ENT).   See *mupirocin.* [BAK-troh-ban].

**baking soda** (GI).   Antacid home remedy for indigestion and hyperacidity. [BAY-king SOH-dah].

**Balacet** (Analges) (generic *acetaminophen, propoxyphene*).   Combination Schedule IV nonnarcotic and narcotic analgesic drug for pain. Tablet: 325 mg/100 mg. [BAL-ah-set].

**balanced salt solution** (BSS) (Ophth).   Irrigating saline solution used during eye surgery. Ophthalmic solution. [BAL-ansd SALT soh-LOO-shun].

**Balziva** (OB/GYN) (generic *norethindrone, ethinyl estradiol*).   Combination monophasic oral contraceptive drug. Pill pack, 28-day: (21 hormone tablets) 0.4 mg/35 mcg; (7 inert tablets). [bal-ZEE-vah].

**Bancap** (Analges) (generic *acetaminophen, hydrocodone*).   Combination Schedule III nonnarcotic and narcotic analgesic drug for pain. Capsule: 500 mg/5 mg. [BAN-kap].

**Banflex** (Ortho).   See *orphenadrine.* [BAN-fleks].

**BAL In Oil** (Emerg).   See *dimercaprol.* [B-A-L in oil].

**Balnetar** (Derm).   See *coal tar.* [BAL-neh-tar].

**balsalazide** (Colazal) (GI).   Anti-inflammatory drug used to treat ulcerative colitis. Capsule: 750 mg. [bal-SAL-ah-zide].

**Baraclude** (Anti-infec, GI).    See *entecavir.* [BAIR-ah-klewd].

**Baridium** (Uro).    See *phenazopyridine.* [bah-RID-ee-um].

**basiliximab** (Simulect) (GI, Uro).    Immunosuppressant monoclonal antibody drug given after organ transplantation to prevent rejection of a donor liver or kidney. Intravenous: 10 mg/25 mL, 20 mg/50 mL. [BAY-sih-LIK-sih-mab].

**Bayer Buffered Aspirin, Bayer Plus Extra Strength** (Analges) (generic *aspirin, aluminum, calcium, magnesium*). Combination over-the-counter salicylate and antacid drug used to treat pain and protect the mucous membrane of the stomach. Tablet: 325/antacid, 500 mg/antacid. [BAY-er].

**Bayer, Bayer Children's Aspirin, Bayer Extended Release 8-Hour, Bayer Low Adult Strength, Extra Strength Bayer Enteric, Genuine Bayer Aspirin** (Analges).    See *aspirin.* [BAY-er].

**Bayer Extra Strength Back & Body Pain** (Analges) (generic *aspirin, caffeine*).    Combination over-the-counter salicylate analgesic and stimulant drug used to treat pain. [BAY-er].

**Bayer Plus Extra Strength** (Analges) (generic *aspirin, calcium*).    Combination over-the-counter salicylate analgesic and antacid for pain and to protect the mucous membrane of the stomach. [BAY-er].

**Bayer PM Extra Strength Aspirin Plus Sleep Aid** (Analges, Neuro) (generic *aspirin, diphenhydramine*).    Combination salicylate analgesic and antihistamine sedative for pain relief and sleep. Caplet: 500 mg/25 mg. [BAY-er].

**Bayer Select Maximum Strength Night Time Pain Relief** (Analges, Neuro) (generic *acetaminophen, diphenhydramine*).    Over-the-counter combination analgesic and antihistamine drug used for pain and sleep. Tablet: 500 mg/25 mg. [BAY-er].

**BayGam** (Anti-infec, Misc).    See *human immune globulin.* [BAY-gam].

**BayHep B** (GI).    See *hepatitis B immunoglobulin.* [BAY-hep B].

**BayRab** (Misc).    Immunoglobulin drug used to treat patients exposed to rabies. Intramuscular: 150 IU/mL. [BAY-rab].

**BayRho-D Full Dose** (Hem, OB/GYN).    Immunoglobulin drug given to an Rh-negative mother after the birth of an Rh-positive infant; it prevents the mother from making antibodies during the next pregnancy and causing hemolytic disease if the next infant is also Rh positive. Intramuscular: 15% gamma globulin. [BAY-roh-D].

**BayTet** (Misc).    Immunoglobulin drug used to treat patients exposed to tetanus. Intramuscular: 15-18%. [BAY-tet].

**BCG Vaccine** (Pulm).    Used to protect against contracting tuberculosis. Intradermal (liquid with multi-puncture device): Vaccine. [B-C-G].

**BCG** (TheraCys, TICE BCG) (Chemo).    Chemotherapy drug used to treat bladder cancer. Intravesical by catheter (powder to be reconstituted): 50 mg, 81 mg. [B-C-G].

**B-D Glucose** (Endo).    See *glucose.* [B-D GLOO-kohs].

**Beano** (GI).    Anti-gas dietary enzyme supplement to be taken when eating beans, broccoli, brussel sprouts, cabbage, etc. Liquid. Tablet. [BEE-noh].

**Bebulin VH** (Hem).    See *factor IX.* [BEB-yoo-lin V-H].

**becaplermin** (Regranex) (Derm).    Human platelet-derived growth factor drug used topically to stimulate the growth of granulation tissue in skin ulcers, particularly in diabetic patients. Gel: 100 mcg. [bee-KAP-ler-min].

**beclomethasone** (Beconase AQ, QVAR) (ENT, Pulm). Corticosteroid anti-inflammatory drug used to prevent acute asthma attacks; used intranasally to treat allergy symptoms in the nose. Aerosol inhaler: 40 mcg/puff, 80 mcg/puff. Nasal spray: 42 mcg/activation. [BEH-kloh-METH-ah-zohn].

**Beconase AQ** (ENT).    See *beclomethasone.* [BEK-oh-nays-A-Q].

**belladona tincture** (GI, Neuro, OB/GYN, Uro). Anticholinergic antispasmotic drug used to treat GI spasms, dysmenorrhea, noctural enuresis, and Parkinson's disease. Liquid: 27 mg/100 mL. [BEL-ah-DAWN-ah TINK-tyoor].

**Bellamine** (GI) (generic *belladonna, butabarbital*). Combination anticholinergic antispasmodic and barbiturate sedative drug used to treat GI spasm associated with irritable bowel syndrome, spastic colon, diverticulitis, and peptic ulcers. Tablet: 0.2 mg/40 mg. [BEL-ah-meen].

**Benadryl, Benadryl Allergy, Benadryl Children's Allergy** (Derm, ENT, GI, Ophth).    See *diphenhydramine.* [BEN-ah-dril].

**Benadryl Allergy & Cold, Benadryl Allergy & Sinus Headache** (ENT) (generic *acetaminophen, diphenhydramine, phenylephrine*).    Combination over-the-counter analgesic, antihistamine, and decongestant drug. Tablet: 325 mg/12.5 mg/5 mg. [BEN-ah-dril].

**Benadyl Itch Relief, Benadryl Itch Relief Children's, Benadryl Itch Relief Maximum Strength, Benadryl Itch Stopping Extra Strength, Benadryl Itch Stopping Maximum Strength, Benadryl Itch Stopping Original Strength** (Derm) (generic *diphenhydramine, zinc acetate*).    Combination over-the-counter antihistamine and astringent drug used topically to treat allergic skin reactions with itching and oozing. Cream: 1%/0.1%, 2%/0.1%. Gel: 2%/0.1%. Solid stick: 2%/0.1%. Spray: 1%/0.1%, 2%/0.1%. [BEN-ah-dril].

**Benadryl Maximum Strength Severe Allergy & Sinus Headache** (ENT) (generic *acetaminophen, diphenhydramine, pseudoephedrine*).    Combination over-the-counter analgesic, antihistamine, and decongestant drug used to treat allergies and sinus headaches. Tablet: 500 mg/25 mg/30 mg. [BEN-ah-dril].

**benazepril** (Lotensin) (Cardio, Neuro).    ACE inhibitor drug used to treat hypertension; used to treat nondiabetic neuropathy. Tablet: 5 mg, 10 mg, 20 mg, 40 mg. [ben-AA-zeh-pril].

**bendamustine** (Treanda) (Chemo).    Alkylating chemotherapy drug used to treat leukemia. Intravenous (powder to be reconstituted): 100 mg. [BEN-dah-MUS-teen].

**bendroflumethiazide** (Naturetin) (Cardio, Uro). Thiazide diuretic drug used to treat hypertension; used to treat edema from congestive heart failure, liver disease, or kidney disease. Tablet: 10 mg. [BEN-droh-FLOO-meh-THY-ah-zide]

**BeneFix** (Hem). See *factor IX*. [BEN-eh-fiks].

**Ben-Gay Original, Ben-Gay Ultra Strength, Arthritis Formula Ben-Gay** (Ortho) (generic *methyl salicylate, menthol*). Combination over-the-counter salicylate analgesic drug used topically to treat the pain of osteoarthritis and minor muscle injuries. Cream. Gel. Ointment. [ben-GAY].

**Benicar** (Cardio). See *olmesartan*. [BEN-ih-kar].

**Benicar HCT** (Cardio) (generic *olmesartan, hydrochlorothiazide*). Combination angiotensin II receptor blocker and diuretic drug used to treat hypertension. Tablet: 20 mg/12.5 mg, 40 mg/12.5 mg, 40 mg/25 mg. [BEN-ih-kar H-C-T].

**Benoquin** (Derm). See *monobenzone*. [BEN-oh-kwin].

**Bensal HP** (Derm) (generic *benzoic acid, salicylic acid*). Combination antifungal and keratolytic drug used topically to treat tinea (ringworm) fungal infection. Ointment: 6%/3%. [BEN-sawl H-P].

**Bentyl** (GI). See *dicyclomine*. [BEN-til].

**Benylin Expectorant** (ENT) (generic *dextromethorphan, guaifenesin*). Combination nonnarcotic antitussive and expectorant drug. Liquid: 5 mg/100 mg. [BEN-ih-lin].

**Benzac 5, Benzac 10, Benzac AC 2¼, Benzac AC 5, Benzac AC 10, Benzac AC Wash 2½, Benzac AC Wash 5, Benzac AC Wash 10, Benzac W 2½, Benzac W 5, Benzac W 10, Benzac W Wash 5, Benzac W Wash 10** (Derm). See *benzoyl peroxide*. [BEN-zak].

**BenzaClin** (Derm) (generic *benzoyl peroxide, clindamycin*). Combination antibiotic drug used topically to treat acne vulgaris. Gel: 5%/1%. [BEN-zah-klin].

**Benzagel Wash** (Derm). See *benzoyl peroxide*. [BEN-zah-jel].

**benzalkonium** (Pedi-Pro, Zephiran) (Derm). Over-the-counter antiseptic drug used topically on the skin and wounds; used to irrigate the eye, bladder, vagina, and body cavities; preoperative skin prep and wash; powder used to prevent bacterial infections of the skin and feet. Liquid: 1%. Powder: 1%. [BEN-zal-KOH-nee-um].

**Benzamycin, Benzamycin Pak** (Derm) (generic *benzoyl peroxide, erythromycin*). Combination anti-infective and antibiotic drug used topically to treat acne vulgaris. Gel: 5%/3%. [BEN-zah-MY-sin].

**benzphetamine** (Didrex) (GI). Schedule III appetite suppresant drug used to treat obesity. Tablet: 25 mg, 50 mg. [benz-FET-ah-meen].

**benzocaine** (Anbesol, Anebesol Cold Sore Therapy, Anbesol Maximum Strength, Baby Anbesol, Baby Orajel, Benzodent, Cepacol, Chloraseptic Kids Sore Throat, Dermoplast, Hurricaine, Lanacane, Mycinettes, Numzit Teething, Orabase-B, Orajel Mouth-Aid, Solarcaine, Unguentine Maximum Strength, Vagisil, Zilactin-B Medicated) (Anes, Derm, ENT, GI, OB/GYN, Pulm, Uro). Over-the-counter anesthetic drug used topically to treat the pain of abrasions, burns, and sunburn; used to treat the pain of canker sores, cold sores, teething pain, toothache, and pain from braces, dentures, or a sore throat; used to suppress the gag reflex when passing a nasogastric tube; used to treat the pain of hemorrhoids; used to prevent pain during sigmoidoscopy; used to treat vaginal irritation; used to prevent pain during dental and oral anesthesia; placed on the tip of an endotracheal tube or laryngoscope prior to endotracheal intubation; placed on an endoscope prior to endoscopic procedures in the urethra, rectum, or vagina. Aerosol: 5%, 13.6%, 20%. Cream: 5%, 6%. Gel: 6.3%, 20%. Liquid: 6.3%, 20%. Lotion: 8%. Lozenge. Ointment: 5%, 20%. Spray: 5%, 20%. Oral paste: 20%. [BEN-zoh-kayn].

**Benzodent** (Anes, ENT). See *benzocaine*. [BEN-zoh-dent].

**benzoin, benzoin compound** (Derm). Over-the-counter drug used topically on the skin to protect it from irritation. Tincture. [BEN-zoyn].

**benzonatate** (Tessalon) (ENT). Nonnarcotic antitussive drug used to treat nonproductive coughs. Capsule: 100 mg, 200 mg. [ben-ZOH-nah-tayt].

**benzoyl peroxide** (Acne Clear, Benzac 5, Benzac 10, Benzac AC 2½, Benzac AC 5, Benzac AC 10, Benzac AC Wash 2½, Benzac AC Wash 5, Benzac AC Wash 10, Benzac W 2½, Benzac W 5, Benzac W 10, Benzac W Wash 5, Benzac W Wash 10, Benzagel Wash, Brevoxyl Creamy Wash, Brevoxyl-4, Brevoxyl 4 Cleansing. Brevoxyl-8, Brevoxyl 8 Cleansing, Clearasil Maximum Strength Acne Treatment, Clinac BPO, Desquam-E 5, Desquam-E 10, Desquam-X 5, Desquam-X 10, Neutrogena Clear Pore, Oxy Oil-Free Maximum Strength Acne Wash, PanOxyl, PanOxyl 5, PanOxyl 10, PanOxyl AQ 2½, PanOxyl AQ 5, PanOxyl AQ 10, Triaz, Triaz Cleanser, Zoderm) (Derm). Over-the-counter and prescription antibiotic drug used topically to treat acne vulgaris. Bar: 5%, 10%. Cleanser: 4.5%, 6.5%, 8.5%. Cleanser/mask: 3.5%. Cream: 4.5%, 6.5%, 8.5%,10%. Gel: 2.5%, 3%, 4%, 4.5%, 5%, 6%, 6.5%, 7%, 8%, 8.5%, 9%, 10%. Liquid: 2.5%, 3%, 4%, 5%, 6%, 8%, 9%,10%. Lotion: 3%, 4%, 5%, 6%, 8%, 10%. [BEN-zoyl per-AWK-side].

**benztropine** (Cogentin) (Neuro). Anticholinergic drug used to treat Parkinson's disease. Tablet: 0.5 mg, 1 mg, 2 mg. Intramuscular or intravenous: 1 mg/mL. [BENZ-troh-peen].

**benzydamine** (Tantum) (Chemo). Used to prevent oral mucositis in patients receiving radiation therapy for head and neck cancer. Orphan drug. [ben-ZY-dah-meen].

**beractant** (Survanta) (Pulm). Surfactant drug used to prevent and treat respiratory distress syndrome in premature newborns. Liquid (via endotracheal tube): 25 mg/mL. [bair-AK-tant].

**beraprost** (Pulm). Vasodilator drug used to treat pulmonary arterial hypertension. Orphan drug. [BAIR-ah-prawst].

**Berinert P** (Misc). Used to treat hereditary angioedema. Orphan drug. [BAIR-ih-nert P].

**Berocca** (Misc). Prescription multivitamin nutritional supplement. Tablet. (bair-OH-kah].

**Berocca Plus** (Misc). Prescription multivitamin with iron nutritional supplement. Tablet. [bair-OH-kah].

**Berocca Parenteral Nutrition** (I.V.). See *intravenous multivitamins.* [bair-OH-kah pah-REN-ter-al noo-TRIH-shun].

**beta alethine** (Betathine) (Chemo). Chemotherapy drug used to treat multiple myeloma and malignant melanoma. Orphan drug. [BAY-tah AL-eh-theen].

**Betadine** (Derm, Ophth). See *povidone iodine.* [BAY-tah-dine].

**Betadine First Aid Antibiotic** (Derm) (generic *bacitracin, polymyxin B*). Combination over-the-counter antibiotic drug used topically to treat skin infections. Ointment: 500 units/10,000 units per g. [BAY-tah-dine].

**Betadine First Aid Antibiotic and Pain Reliever** (Derm) (generic *bacitracin, polymyxin B, pramoxine*). Combination over-the-counter antibiotic and anesthetic drug used topically to treat skin itching and inflammation. Ointment: 500 units/10,000 units/10 mg per g. [BAY-tah-dine].

**Betagan Liquifilm** (Ophth). See *levobunolol.* [BAY-tah-gan LIH-kwih-film].

**betaine** (Cystadane) (Uro). Used to treat homocystinuria. Powder (to be reconstituted to a liquid): 1 g/1.7 mL. [BEH-tayn].

**betamethasone** (Beta-Val, Celestone, Celestone Soluspan, Diprolene, Diprolene AF, Diprosone, Luxiq, Maxivate, Psorion, Teladar) (Derm, Endo, Ortho). Corticosteroid drug used topically to treat inflammation and itching from dermatitis, seborrhea, eczema, psoriasis, and yeast and fungal infections; used orally to treat severe inflammation in various body systems; injected into a joint to treat osteoarthritis, rheumatoid arthritis, and gouty arthritis; injected near a joint to treat bursitis and tenosynovitis; injected into skin lesions. Aerosol: 0.1%. Cream: 0.05%, 0.1%. Foam: 1.2 mg/g. Gel: 0.05%. Lotion: 0.05%, 0.1%. Ointment: 0.05%, 0.1%. Oral liquid: 0.6 mg/5 mL. Intra-articular: 0.6 mg/5 mL, 3 mg/5 mL. [BAY-tah-METH-ah-sohn].

**Betapace, Betapace AF** (Cardio). See *sotalol.* [BAY-tah-pays].

**BetaRx** (Endo). Encapsulated pig pancreas islet cells used to treat patients with type 1 diabetes mellitus who are on immunosuppressant drugs. Orphan drug. [BAY-tah-R-X].

**Betasept** (Derm). See *chlorhexidine.* [BAY-tah-sept].

**Betaseron** (Anti-infec, Neuro). See *interferon beta-1b.* [BAY-tah-SEER-awn].

**Betathine** (Chemo). See *beta alethine.* [BAY-tah-theen].

**Beta-Val** (Derm). See *betamethasone.* [BAY-tah-VAL].

**betaxolol** (Betoptic, Betoptic S, Kerlone) (Cardio, Ophth). Cardioselective beta-blocker drug used to treat hypertension; used topically in the eye to treat glaucoma. Tablet: 10 mg, 20 mg. Ophthalmic solution: 0.25%, 0.5%. [beh-TAK-soh-lawl].

**Betaxon** (Ophth). See *levobetaxolol.* [beh-TAKS-awn].

**bethanidine** (Cardio). Used to treat ventricular fibrillation. Orphan drug. [beh-THAN-dih-deen].

**bethanechol** (Urecholine) (Uro). Antispasmodic drug used to treat urinary retention. Tablet: 5 mg, 10 mg, 25 mg, 50 mg. [beh-THAN-eh-kawl].

**Betimol** (Ophth). See *timolol.* [BEH-tih-mawl].

**Betoptic, Betoptic S** (Ophth). See *betaxolol.* [beh-TAWP-tik].

**bevacizumab** (Avastin) (Chemo, Ophth). Monoclonal antibody drug used to treat cancer of the brain, lung, pancreas, colon, rectum, kidney, breast, and ovary; used to treat macular degeneration in the eye. Intravenous: 25 mg/mL. [BEV-ah-SIZ-yoo-mab].

**bexarotene** (Targretin) (Chemo, Derm). Chemotherapy vitamin A-type (retinoid) drug used topically and orally to treat cancerous skin lesions of cutaneous T-cell lymphoma. Capsule: 75 mg. Gel: 1%. [bek-SAIR-oh-teen].

**Bexxar** (Chemo) (generic *iodine 131, tositumomab*). Combination radioactive isotope and monoclonal antibody drug used to treat non-Hodgkin's lymphoma. Intravenous: 0.1 mg/14 mg per mL. [BEKS-zar].

**Biavax II** (Anti-infec). Combination drug used to prevent rubella and mumps in children. Subcutaneous: Vaccine. [BY-ah-vaks 2].

**Biaxin, Biaxin XL** (Anti-infec). See *clarithromycin.* [by-AK-sin].

**bicalutamide** (Casodex) (Chemo). Hormonal chemotherapy drug used to treat cancer of the prostate gland in men. Tablet: 50 mg. [BY-kah-LOO-tah-mide].

**Bicillin C-R** (Anti-infec) (generic *penicillin G benzathine, penicillin G procaine*). Combination penicillin antibiotic drug. Intramuscular: 300,000 units/300,000 units per mL. [BY-sil-in C-R].

**Bicillin L-A** (Anti-infec). See *penicillin G benzathine.* [BY-sil-in L-A].

**Bicitra** (Hem) (generic *citric acid, sodium citrate*). Used to increase the alkalinity of body fluids. Oral liquid: 334 mg/500 mg. [by-SIH-trah].

**BiCNU** (Chemo). See *carmustine.* [by-C-N-U].

**Bidhist** (Derm, ENT). See *brompheniramine.* [BID-hist].

**BiDil** (Cardio) (generic *hydralazine, isosorbide dinitrate*). Combination peripheral vasodilator and nitrate drug used to treat angina pectoris. Tablet: 37.5 mg/20 mg. [BY-dil].

**Biltricide** (Misc). See *praziquantel.* [BIL-trih-side].

**bimatoprost** (Lumigan) (Ophth). Prostaglandin F drug used topically in the eye to treat glaucoma. Ophthalmic solution: 0.03%. [bih-MAT-oh-prawst].

**bindarit** (Uro). Used to treat lupus nephritis. Orphan drug. [bin-DAIR-it].

**biocarbonate infusate** (Normocarb HF) (Hem). Used during hemofiltration. Orphan drug. [BY-oh-KAR-boh-nayt in-FYOO-sayt].

**Bioclate** (Hem). See *factor VIII*. [BY oh klayt].

**Bio-Rescue** (Emerg) (generic *deferoxamine, dextran*). Combination drug used to treat iron overdose. Orphan drug [BY-oh-RES-kyoo].

**Biosynject** (Hem). Used to treat blood transfusion or bone marrow transfusion reaction; used to treat hemolytic disease of the newborn. Orphan drug. [BY-oh-SIN-jekt].

**Bio-Throid** (Endo). See *desiccated thyroid*. [BY-oh-throid].

**Biotropin** (Endo). See *somatropin*. [BY-oh-TROH-pin].

**biperiden** (Akineton) (Neuro). Anticholinergic drug used to treat Parkinson's disease. Tablet: 2 mg. [by-PAIR-ih-den].

**bisacodyl** (Correctol, Doxidan, Dulcolax, Dulcolax Bowel Prep Kit, Feen-a-mint, Fleet Bisacodyl Enema, Fleet Laxative, Modane) (GI). Over-the-counter irritant/stimulant laxative drug used to treat constipation. Delayed-release tablet: 10 mg. Enteric-coated tablet: 5 mg. Tablet: 5 mg. Suppository: 10 mg. Enema: 10 mg/30 mL. [BIS-ah-KOH-dil].

**Bismatrol** (GI). See *bismuth*. [BIZ-mah-trawl].

**bismuth** (Bismatrol, Kaopectate, Kaopectate Children's, Kaopectate Extra Strength, Maalox Total Stomach Relief, Pepto-Bismol, Pepto-Bismol Maximum Strength) (GI). Over-the-counter anti-infective drug used to treat diarrhea caused by bacteria and viruses; used to decrease GI inflammation; used to treat *H. pylori* infection associated with peptic ulcers. Liquid: 87 mg/5 mL, 130 mg/15 mL, 262 mg/15 mL, 524 mg/15 mL. Chewable tablet: 262 mg. Tablet: 262 mg. Oral suspension: 262 mg/15 mL, 525 mg/15 mL. [BIZ-mooth].

**Bisolvon** (Ophth). See *bromhexine*. [by-SAWL-von].

**bisoprolol** (Zebeta) (Cardio). Cardioselective beta-blocker drug used to treat hypertension. Tablet: 5 mg, 10 mg. [bih-SOH-proh-lawl].

**Bite Rx** (Derm). See *aluminum acetate*. [BITE R-X].

**bitolterol** (Tornalate) (Pulm). Bronchodilator drug used to prevent and treat asthma and bronchospasm. Liquid for inhalation: 0.2%. [by-TOHL-ter-awl].

**bivalirudin** (Angiomax) (Hem). Thrombin inhibitor drug used to prevent blood clots in patients with unstable angina during coronary artery angioplasty. Intravenous (powder to be reconstituted). [by-VAL-ih-ROO-din].

**Black Draught** (GI). See *sennosides*. [BLAK DRAWT].

**black cohosh** (Remicade) OB/GYN. Over-the-counter herbal drug used to treat the symptoms of menopause. Tablets. [BLAK KOH-hawsh].

**Blenoxane** (Chemo, Pulm). See *bleomycin*. [bleh-NAWK-sayn].

**bleomycin** (Blenoxane) (Chemo, Pulm). Chemotherapy antibiotic drug used to treat cancer of the head and neck, bone, pancreas, cervix, testicle, and penis; used to treat Hodgkin's lymphoma, non-Hodgkin's lymphoma, mycosis fungoides, and Kaposi's sarcoma; sclerosing drug administered via chest tube into the lung to treat malignant pleural effusion. Subcutaneous, intramuscular, or intravenous (powder for reconstitution): 15 units, 30 units. Chest tube (powder to be reconstituted): 15 units, 30 units. [bah-ee-oh-MY-sin]

**Bleph-10** (Anti-Infec, Ophth). See *sulfacetamide*. [BLEF-10].

**Blephamide** (Ophth) (generic *prednisolone, sulfacetamide*). Combination corticosteroid and sulfonamide anti-infective drug used topically in the eyes to treat infection and inflammation. Ophthalmic solution: 0.2%/10%. Ophthalmic ointment: 0.2%/10%. [BLEF-ah-mide].

**Blocadren** (Analges, Cardio). See *timolol*. [BLAW-kah-dren].

**Bluboro** (Derm). See *aluminum acetate*. [bloo-BUR-oh].

**Bonamil Infant Formula with Iron** (GI). Infant formula with iron. Liquid. Powder (to be reconstituted). [BAWN-ah-mil].

**Bonefos** (Chemo). See *disodium clodronate*. [BOH-neh-faws].

**Boniva** (Ortho). See *ibandronate*. [boh-NEE-vah].

**Bontril, Bontril PDM** (GI). See *phendimetrazine*. [BAWN-tril].

**Boost Nutritional** (GI). Nutritional supplement. Pudding. [BOOST].

**Boostrix** (Misc). Combination drug used to prevent diphtheria, pertussis, and tetanus. Subcutaneous: Vaccine. [BOOS-triks].

**Borocell** (Chemo). Chemotherapy drug used to treat brain cancer. Orphan drug. [BOR-oh-sel].

**bortezomib** (Velcade) (Chemo). Chemotherapy drug used to treat multiple myeloma and leukemia. Intravenous (powder to be reconstituted): 3.5 mg. [bor-TEZ-oh-mib].

**bosentan** (Tracleer) (Pulm). Endothelin receptor blocker drug used to dilate pulmonary blood vessels in patients with pulmonary arterial hypertension. Tablet: 62.5 mg, 125 mg. [boh-SEN-tan].

**Botox** (Derm, Ophth, Ortho). See *botulinum toxin type A*. [BOH-tawks].

**botulinum toxin type A** (Botox, Dysport) (Derm, Ophth, Ortho). Toxin drug used to relax muscles and decrease facial wrinkle lines; used to relax eye muscles to treat blepharospasm, nystagmus, and strabismus; used to treat neck pain and abnormal head position of cervical dystonia (torticollis); used to treat excessive sweating in the axillary area; used to relax muscle spasticity in cerebral palsy. Intramuscular (powder to be reconstituted): 100 units. [BAW-tyoo-LY-num TAWK-sin].

**botulinum toxin type B** (Myobloc) (Ortho). Toxin drug used to relax muscles and treat neck pain and abnormal head position of cervical dystonia (torticollis). Intramuscular: 5000 U/ mL. [BAW-tyoo-LY-num TAWK-sin].

**botulinum toxin type F** (Ortho). Toxin drug used to relax eye muscles to treat blepharospasm; used to relax neck muscles to treat cervical dystonia (torticollis). Orphan drug. [BAW-tyoo-LY-num TAWK-sin].

**botulism immune globulin** (BabyBIG) (GI).   Used to treat infant botulism (food poisoning). Orphan drug. [BAW-tyoo-liz-im im-MYOON GLAW-byoo-lin].

**bovine colostrum** (Anti-infec).   Used to treat diarrhea in AIDS patients. Orphan drug. [BOH-vine koh-LAWS-trum].

**bovine immunoglobulin** (Immuno-C, Sporidin-G) (Anti-infec).   Cow immunoglobulin drug used to treat *Cryptosporidium parvum* GI tract infection in immunocompromised patients. Orphan drug. [BOH-vine IM-myoo-noh-GLAW-byoo-lin].

**BRAD 2** (GI).   Nutritional supplement formulated for patients with maple syrup urine disease. Powder (to be reconstituted). [BRAD 2].

**Bravavir** (Anti-infec).   See *sorivudine.* [BRAW-vah-veer].

**Bravelle** (Endo, OB/GYN).   See *urofollitropin.* [braw-VEL].

**Brethine** (Pulm).   See *terbutaline.* [BRETH-een].

**bretylium** (Cardio).   Antiarrhythmic drug used to treat ventricular fibrillation. Intramuscular or intravenous: 2 mg/mL, 4 mg/mL, 50 mg/mL. [breh-TIL-ee-um].

**Brevibloc, Brevibloc Double Strength** (Cardio).   See *esmolol.* [BREV-ih-blawk].

**Brevicon** (OB/GYN) (generic *norethindrone, ethinyl estradiol*).   Combination monophasic oral contraceptive drug. Pill pack (Wallette), 21-day: (21 hormone tablets) 0.5 mg/35 mcg. Pill pack (Wallette), 28-day: (21 hormone tablets) 0.5 mg/35 mcg; (7 inert tablets). [BREV-ih-kawn].

**Brevital** (Anes).   See *methohexital.* [BREV-ih-tawl].

**Brevoxyl Creamy Wash, Brevoxyl-4, Brevoxyl 4 Cleansing, Brevoxyl-8, Brevoxyl 8 Cleansing** (Derm).   See *benzoyl peroxide.* [breh-VAWK-sil].

**brimonidine** (Alphagan P) (Ophth).   Alpha receptor stimulator drug used topically in the eyes to treat glaucoma; orphan drug used to treat optic neuropathy. Ophthalmic solution: 0.1%, 0.15%, 0.2%. [brih-MOH-nih-deen].

**brimvaracetam** (Ortho).   Used to treat myoclonus. Orphan drug. [brim-VAIR-ah-SEE-tam].

**brinzolamide** (Azopt) (Ophth).   Carbonic anhydrase inhibitor drug used topically in the eyes to treat glaucoma. Ophthalmic suspension: 1%. [brin-ZOL-ah-mide].

**Brolene** (Ophth).   Used to treat amoebic infection of the cornea. Ophthalmic solution: 0.1%. Orphan drug. [BROH-leen].

**bromfenac** (Xibrom) (Ophth).   Nonsteroidal anti-inflammatory drug used topically to treat pain and inflammation in the eye after corneal surgery. [BRAWM-feh-nak].

**bromhexine** (Bisolvon) (Ophth).   Used to treat Sjögren's syndrome. Orphan drug. [brom-HEK-seen].

**bromocriptine** (Parlodel, Parlodel Snap Tabs) (Endo, Neuro).   Dopamine receptor stimulant drug used to treat Parkinson's disease; used to decrease elevated levels of prolactin hormone and treat galactorrhea; used to decrease elevated levels of growth hormone in adults to treat acromegaly. Capsule: 5 mg. Tablet: 2.5 mg. [BROH-moh-KRIP-teen].

**Bromo Seltzer** (GI) (generic *acetaminophen, sodium bicarbonate*).   Combination analgesic and antacid drug for pain and heartburn. Effervescent granules: 325 mg/2781 mg. [BROH-moh SELT-zer].

**brompheniramine** (Bidhist, BroveX, BroveX CT, Lodrane 24, Lodrane XR, LoHist 12 Hour, VaZol).   (Derm, ENT). Antihistamine drug used to treat symptoms of seasonal and perennial allergies, allergic rhinitis, and skin allergies and itching. Extended-release capsule: 12 mg. Oral liquid: 2 mg/5 mL, 4 mg/5 mL, 8 mg/5 mL, 10 mg/5 mL, 12 mg/5 mL. Chewable tablet: 12 mg. Extended-release tablet: 6 mg. [BROM-feh-NEER-ah-meen].

**Bronchitol** (Pulm).   See *mannitol.* [BRONG-kih-tawl].

**Bronkaid Dual Action** (ENT, Pulm) (generic *ephedrine, guaifenesin*).   Combination over-the-counter decongestant and expectorant drug. Tablet: 25 mg/400 mg. [BRONG-kayd].

**Bronkodyl** (Pulm).   See *theophylline.* [BRAWN-koh-dil].

**Brovana** (Pulm).   See *arformoterol.* [broh-VAN-ah].

**BroveX, BroveX CT** (Derm, ENT).   See *brompheniramine.* [BROH-veks].

**Broxine** (Chemo).   See *broxuridine.* [BRAWK-seen].

**broxuridine** (Broxine, Neomark) (Chemo).   Radiation sensitizer drug used to treat brain tumors. Orphan drug. [brawks-YOOR-ih-deen].

**BSS** (Ophth).   See *balanced salt solution.* [B-S-S].

**Bucet** (Analges) (generic *acetaminophen, butalbital*).   Combination nonsalicylate analgesic and barbiturate sedative drug for pain. Capsule: 650 mg/50 mg. [BYOO-set].

**budesonide** (Entocort EC, Pulmicort Respules, Pulmicort Turbuhaler, Rhinocort Aqua) (ENT, GI, Pulm). Corticosteroid anti-inflammatory drug used to treat Crohn's disease; used to prevent acute asthma attacks; used intranasally to treat allergy symptoms of the nose. Capsule: 3 mg. Liquid for inhalation (Respule packet): 0.25 mg/2 mL, 0.5 mg/2 mL, 1 mg/2 mL. Turbuhaler device (inhaled powder): 200 mcg/metered dose. Nasal spray: 32 mcg/actuation. [byoo-DES-oh-nide].

**Bufferin, Bufferin Extra Strength** (Analges) (generic *aspirin, calcium, magnesium*).   Combination over-the-counter salicylate and antacid drug used to treat the pain of osteoarthritis and rheumatoid arthritis. Tablet: 325/158 mg, 34 mg, 500 mg/antacid. [BUF-fer-in].

**Bufferin AF Nite Time** (Neuro) (generic *diphenhydramine, magnesium*).   Combination over-the-counter antihistamine and magnesium drug used to induce sleep and relax muscles. Tablet: 25 mg/500 mg. [BUF-fer-in].

**bumetanide** (Bumex) (Cardio, Uro).   Loop diuretic drug used to treat edema from congestive heart failure, liver disease, or kidney disease. Tablet: 1 mg. Intramuscular or intravenous: 0.25 mg/mL. [byoo-MET-ah-nide].

**Bumex** (Cardio, Uro).   See *bumetanide.* [BYOO-meks].

**Bupap** (Analges) (generic *acetaminophen, butalbital*).   Combination nonsalicylate analgesic and barbiturate sedative drug for pain. Tablet: 650 mg/50 mg. [BYOO-pap].

**Buphenyl** (Uro).    See *sodium phenylbutyrate*. [BYOO-feh-nil].

**bupivacaine** (Marcaine, Sensorcaine, Sensorcaine MPF, Sensorcaine MPF Spinal) (Anes, ENT, OB/GYN). Anesthetic drug used to produce local, regional, epidural, and spinal anesthesia; used for local anesthesia during dental and oral surgery; used for epidural anesthesia during labor and vaginal delivery or cesarean section. Injection. 0.25%; 0.25% with 1:200,000 epinephrine; 0.5%; 0.5% with 1:200,000 epinephrine; 0.75%; 0.75% with 1:200,000 epinephrine. [byoo-PIV-ah-kayn].

**Buprenex** (Analges, Psych).    See *buprenorphine*. [BYOO-preh-neks].

**buprenorphine** (Buprenex, Subutex) (Analges, Psych). Schedule III narcotic drug used to treat moderate-to-severe pain (Buprenex); used to treat narcotic addiction (Subutex). Sublingual tablet: 2 mg, 8 mg. Intramuscular or intravenous: 0.3 mg/mL.[BYOO-preh-NOR-feen].

**bupropion** (Aplenzin, Wellbutrin, Wellbutrin SR, Wellbutrin XL, Zyban) (GI, Pulm, Psych).    Antidepressant drug used to treat depression; used to treat obesity; non-nicotine aid used to help stop smoking. Tablet: 75 mg, 100 mg. Extended-release tablet: 150 mg, 300 mg. Sustained-release tablet: 100 mg, 150 mg, 200 mg. [byoo-PROH-pee-awn].

**Buro-Sol** (Derm).    See *aluminum acetate*. [BUR-oh-sawl].

**Burow's solution, modified Burow's solution** (Derm).    See *aluminum acetate*. [BUR-ohs].

**BuSpar** (Psych).    See *buspirone*. [BYOO-spar].

**buspirone** (BuSpar) (Psych).    Benzodiazepine drug used to treat anxiety and neurosis; used to treat premenstrual dysphoric disorder. Tablet: 5 mg, 7.5 mg, 10 mg, 15 mg, 30 mg. [byoo-SPY-rohn].

**busulfan** (Busulfex, Myleran, Partaject, Spartaject) (Chemo).    Alkylating chemotherapy drug used to treat leukemia; used to treat increased platelet count and polycythemia vera; orphan drug (Partaject, Spartaject); used to treat brain cancer and malignancy associated with bone marrow transplantation. Tablet: 2 mg. Intravenous: 6 mg/mL. [boo-SUL-fan].

**Busulfex** (Chemo).    See *busulfan*. [byoo-SUL-feks].

**butabarbital** (Butisol) (Neuro).    Schedule III barbiturate drug used to provide sedation. Tablet: 15 mg, 30 mg, 50 mg, 100 mg. Liquid: 30 mg/5 mL. [BYOO-tah-BAR-bih-tawl].

**butenafine** (Lotrimin Ultra, Mentax) (Derm). Over-the-counter and prescription antifungal drug used topically to treat tinea (ringworm) skin infections. Cream: 1%. [byoo-TEN-ah-feen].

**Butex Forte** (Analges) (generic *acetaminophen, butalbital*). Combination nonsalicylate analgesic and barbiturate sedative drug for pain. Capsule: 650 mg/50 mg. [BYOO-teks].

**Butibel** (GI) (generic *belladonna, butabarbital*).    Combination anticholinergic and barbiturate drug used to reduce spasm and produce sedation; used to treat GI spasm associated with irritable bowel syndrome, spastic colon, diverticulitis, and peptic ulcers. Tablet: 15 mg/15 mg. Elixir. [BYOO-tih-bel].

**Butisol** (Neuro).    See *butabarbital*. [BYOO-tih-sawl].

**butoconazole** (Gynazole-1, Mycelex-3) (Anti-infec, OB/GYN).    Over-the-counter and prescription antiyeast drug used topically to treat vaginal yeast infections caused by *Candida albicans*. Vaginal cream: 2%. [byoo-toh-KAWN-ah-zohl].

**butorphanol** (Stadol) (Analges, Anes).    Schedule IV narcotic analgesic drug used to treat moderate-to-severe pain; used to treat pain during labor and delivery; used as a preoperative drug and to maintain general anesthesia. Nasal spray: 10 mg/mL. Intramuscular or intravenous: 1 mg/mL, 2 mg/mL. [byoo-TOR-fah-nawl].

**Byclomine** (GI).    See *dicyclomine*. [BY-kloh-meen].

**Byetta** (Endo).    See *exenatide*. [by-AA-tah].

**Bystolic** (Cardio).    See *nebivolol*. [by-STAWL-ik].

**cabergoline** (Dostinex) (Endo).    Used to decrease elevated levels of prolactin hormone from the anterior pituitary gland and treat galactorrhea. Tablet: 0.5 mg. [kah-BAIR-goh-leen].

**Cachexon** (Anti-infec).    Used to treat AIDS wasting syndrome. Orphan drug. [kah-KEK-sawn].

**Caduet** (Hem) (generic *amlodipine, atorvastatin*) (Cardio).    Combination antihypertensive and hypercholesterolemia drug. Tablet: 2.5 mg/10 mg, 2.5 mg/20 mg, 2.5 mg/40 mg, 5 mg/10 mg, 5 mg/20 mg, 5 mg/40 mg, 5 mg/80 mg, 10 mg/10 mg, 10 mg/20 mg, 10 mg/40 mg, 10 mg/80 mg. [KAD-oo-et].

**Cafcit** (Neuro, Pulm).    See *caffeine*. [KAF-sit].

**Cafergot** (Analges) (generic *ergotamine, caffeine*). Combination vasoconstrictor amd stimulant drug used to treat migraine headaches. Tablet: 1 mg/100 mg, 2 mg/100 mg. [KAF-er-gawt].

**caffeine** (Cafcit) (Neuro, Pulm).    Stimulant drug used to treat apnea in premature infants; used to prevent mental and physical fatigue. Oral liquid: 20 mg/mL. Intravenous: 20 mg/mL. [kaf-FEEN].

**Caladryl** (Derm) (generic *calamine, diphenhydramine*). Combination over-the-counter astringent and antihistamine drug used topically to decrease oozing and stop itching of the skin. Cream 1%. Lotion 1%. [KAL-ah-dril].

**calamine** (Derm).    Astringent drug used topically to treat oozing skin. Lotion. [KAL-ah-mine].

**Calamycin** (Derm) (generic *benzocaine, calamine, zinc oxide*).    Combination over-the-counter anesthetic and astringent drug used topically to decrease oozing and numb the skin. Lotion. [KAL-ah-MY-sin].

**Calan, Calan SR** (Analges, Cardio).    See *verapamil*. [KAY-lan].

**Calcibind** (Uro).    See *cellulose sodium phosphate*. [KAL-sih-bind].

**Calcijex** (Uro).    See *calcitriol*. [KAL-sih-jeks].

**calcipotriene** (Dovonex) (Derm).    Vitamin D-type drug used topically to treat psoriasis. Cream: 0.005%. Ointment: 0.005%. Topical solution: 0.005%. [kal-SIP-oh-TRY-een].

**calcitonin-human** (Cibacalcin) (Ortho).   Calcium-regulating hormone drug used to treat Paget's disease of the bones. Orphan drug. [KAL-sih-TOH-nin].

**calcitonin-salmon** (Fortical, Miacalcin) (Ortho).   Calcium-regulating hormone drug used to prevent and treat osteoporosis; used to treat Paget's disease of the bones; used to treat hypercalcemia. Nasal spray: 200 units/spray. Injection: 200 units/mL. [KAL-sih-TOH-nin].

**calcitriol** (Calcijex, Rocaltrol) (Uro).   Used to treat hypocalcemia in patients on dialysis. Capsule: 0.25 mcg, 0.5 mcg. Liquid: 1 mcg/mL. Intravenous: 1 mcg/mL, 2 mcg/mL. [KAL-sih-TRY-awl].

**calcium acetate** (Phos-Lo) (Uro).   Used to treat hyperphosphatemia in patients with kidney disease. Orphan drug. [KAL-see-um AS-eh-tayt].

**calcium carbonate** (Alka-Mints, Chooz, Maalox Antacid Barrier Maximum Strength, Mylanta Children's, Os-Cal 500, Rolaids Extra Strength, Tums Ultra (GI, Ortho, Uro).   Antacid drug used to treat heartburn; used as a dietary calcium supplement; orphan drug used to treat hyperphosphatemia in patients with kidney disease. Tablets: 500 mg, 600 mg, 1250 mg, 1500 mg. Chewable tablets: 400 mg, 500 mg, 750 mg, 850 mg, 1000 mg, 1250 mg. Gum: 300 mg, 400 mg, 500 mg. [KAL-see-um KAR-boh-nayt].

**calcium chloride** (Cardiac, Emerg, Ortho).   Used to stimulate a heart contraction during cardiac arrest and resuscitation; used to treat the bone diseases of rickets and osteomalacia. Intracardiac or intravenous: 10%. [KAL-see-um KLOH-ride].

**calcium citrate** (Citracal) (Misc).   Over-the-counter calcium supplement. Tablet: 200 mg. [KAL-see-um SIH-trayt].

**Calcium Disodium Versenate** (Emerg, Neuro).   See *edetate calcium disodium.* [KAL-see-um dy-SOH-dee-um VER-seh-nayt].

**calcium EDTA** (Emerg, Neuro).   See *edetate calcium disodium.* [KAL-see-um E-D-T-A].

**calcium gluconate** (Calgonate, H-F-Gel) (Emerg).   Used topically to treat hydrofluoric acid spilled on the skin. Irrigating wash. Gel: 2%. [KAL-see-um GLOO-koh-nayt].

**Caldecort Maximum Strength** (Derm).   See *hydrocortisone.* [KAL-deh-kort].

**calfactant** (Infasurf) (Pulm).   Surfactant drug used to prevent and treat respiratory distress syndrome in newborn infants. Liquid (via endotracheal tube): 35 mg/mL. [kal-FAK-tant].

**Calgonate** (Emerg).   See *calcium gluconate.* [KAL-goh-nayt].

**Camila** (OB/GYN).   See *norethindrone.* [kah-MIL-ah].

**Campath** (Chemo, Neuro, Ortho).   See *alemtuzumab.* [KAM-path].

**Campho-Phenique Cold Sore and Scab Relief** (Anes, Derm, ENT).   Over-the-counter anesthetic drug used topically to treat the pain of abrasions, burns, insect bites, and cold sores. Gel. Liquid. [KAM-foh-feh-NEEK].

**Campral** (Psych).   See *acamprosate.* [KAM-pral].

**Camptosar** (Chemo).   See *irinotecan.* [KAMP-toh-sar].

**Camvirex** (Chemo).   Chemotherapy drug used to treat pancreatic cancer. Orphan drug. [kam-VY-reks].

**Canasa** (GI).   See *mesalamine.* [kah-NAH-sah].

**Cancidas** (Anti-infec).   See *caspofungin.* [KAN-kih-das].

**candesartan** (Atacand) (Cardio).   Angiotensin II receptor blocker drug used to treat hypertension and congestive heart failure. Tablet: 4 mg, 8 mg, 16 mg, 32 mg [KAN-deh-SAR-tan].

**cannabinoid** (Misc).   See *dronabinol.* [kah-NAB-ih-noyd].

**Cantil** (GI).   See *mepenzolate.* [KAN-til].

**Canvaxin** (Chemo).   Melanoma cell vaccine for cancer. Orphan drug. [kan-VAK-sin].

**Capastat** (Pulm).   See *capreomycin.* [KAP-ah-stat].

**capecitabine** (Xeloda) (Chemo).   Antimetabolite chemotherapy drug used to treat cancer of the colon, rectum, pancreas, and breast. Tablet: 150 mg, 500 mg. [KAP-eh-SY-tah-been].

**Capex** (Derm).   See *fluocinolone.* [KAY-peks].

**Capitrol** (Derm).   See *chloroxine.* [KAP-ih-trawl].

**Capoten** (Cardio).   See *captopril.* [KAP-oh-ten].

**Capozide 25/15, Capozide 25/25, Capozide 50/15, Capozide 50/25** (Cardio) (generic *captopril, hydrochlorothiazide*).   Combination ACE inhibitor and diuretic drug used to treat hypertension. Tablet: 25 mg/15 mg, 25 mg/25 mg, 50 mg/15 mg, 50 mg/25 mg. [KAP-oh-zide].

**capreomycin** (Capastat) (Pulm).   Antitubercular antibiotic drug used to treat tuberculosis that is resistant to other antitubercular drugs. Intramuscular (powder to be reconstituted): 1 g. [KAP-ree-oh-MY-sin].

**Caprogel** (Ophth).   See *aminocaproic acid.* [KAP-roh-jel].

**capsaicin** (Capsin, Zostrix, Zostrix-HP, Zostrix Neuropathy Cream) (Derm, Ortho, Neuro).   Over-the-counter irritant drug used topically to treat the pain of herpes zoster virus lesions (shingles) on the skin; used to treat the pain of arthritis, muscle pain, and neuralgia. Cream: 0.025%, 0.035%, 0.075%, 0.1%, 0.25%. Gel: 0.025%, 0.05%. Lotion: 0.025%, 0.075%. Roll-on applicator. [kap-SAY-ih-sin].

**Capsin** (Derm, Ortho, Neuro).   See *capsaicin.* [KAP-sin].

**Captique** (Derm).   See *hyaluronic acid.* [kap-TEEK].

**captopril** (Capoten) (Cardio, Uro).   ACE inhibitor drug used to treat hypertension; used to treat congestive heart failure and left ventricular failure after a myocardial infarction; used to improve survival after a myocardial infarction; used to treat diabetic nephropathy. Tablet: 12.5 mg, 25 mg, 50 mg, 100 mg. [KAP-toh-pril].

**Carac** (Derm, OB/GYN).   See *fluorouracil.* [KAIR-ak].

**Carafate** (Chemo, GI).   See *sucralfate.* [KAIR-ah-fayt].

**carbachol** (Carbastat, Carboptic, Isopto Carbachol, Miostat) (Ophth).   Miotic drug used topically to constrict the pupil and treat glaucoma; used intraocularly to constrict the pupil during eye surgery. Ophthalmic solution: 0.75%, 1.5%, 2.25%, 3%. [KAR-bah-kawl].

**carbamazepine** (Carbatrol, Epitol, Equetro, Tegretol, Tegretol-XR) (Neuro, Psych).   Anticonvulsant drug used to treat tonic-clonic and complex partial seizures; used to treat trigeminal neuralgia and postherpetic neuralgia; used to treat restless legs syndrome; used to treat bipolar disorder. Extended-release capsule: 100 mg, 200 mg, 300 mg. Chewable tablet: 100 mg. Tablet: 100 mg, 200 mg, 300 mg, 400 mg. Extended-release tablet: 100 mg, 200 mg, 400 mg. Liquid: 100 mg/5 mL, 200 mg/5 mL. [KAR-bah-MAZ-eh-peen].

**carbamide** (Debrox, Murine Ear). Over-the-counter drug used topically to soften hardened earwax. Drops: 6.5%. [KAR-bah-mide].

**Carbastat** (Ophth). See *carbachol*. [KAR-bah-stat].

**Carbatrol** (Neuro, Psych). See *carbamazepine*. [KAR-bah-trawl].

**carbinoxamine** (Histex CT, Histex I/E, Histex Pd, Palgic, Pediatex, Pediatex 12) (Derm, ENT, Ophth). Antihistamine drug used to treat symptoms of seasonal and perennial allergies, allergic rhinitis, allergic conjunctivitis, and skin allergies and itching. Extended-release capsule: 10 mg. Oral liquid: 1.67 mg/5 mL, 4 mg/5 mL. Oral suspension: 3.2 mg/5 mL. Tablet: 4 mg. Timed-release tablet: 8 mg. [KAR-bih-NAWKS-ah-meen].

**Carbocaine** (Anes, ENT, OB/GYN). See *mepivacaine*. [KAR-boh-kayn].

**carboplatin** (Paraplatin) (Chemo). Platinum chemotherapy drug used to treat cancer of the head and neck, lung, ovary, uterus, and testicle; used to treat leukemia. Intravenous (powder to be reconstituted): 10 mg/mL. [KAR-boh-PLAT-in].

**carboprost** (Hemabate) (OB/GYN). Smooth muscle stimulant drug used to produce abortion; used to treat uterine bleeding after delivery. Intramuscular: 250 mcg/ml. [KAR-boh-prawst].

**Carboptic** (Ophth). See *carbachol*. [karb-AWP-tik].

**carbovir** (Anti-infec). Antiviral drug used to treat AIDS. Orphan drug. [KAR-boh-veer].

**Cardene, Cardene I.V., Cardene SR** (Cardio). See *nicardipine*. [KAR-deen].

**Cardio-Green** (Cardio). See *indocyanine green*. [KAR-dee-oh-green].

**cardioplegic solution** (Plegisol) (Cardio). Electrolyte solution used in open heart surgery to induce cardiac arrest. Intra-arterial (into the aortic root): Solution. [KAR-dee-oh-PLEE-jik].

**Cardizem, Cardizem CD, Cardizem LA** (Analges, Cardio). See *diltiazem*. [KAR-dih-zem].

**Cardura, Cardura XL** (Cardio, Uro). See *doxazosin*. [kar-DOOR-ah].

**Carimune F, Carimune NF** (Anti-infec, Misc). See *human immune globulin*. [KAIR-ih-myoon].

**carisoprodol** (Soma) (Ortho). Skeletal muscle relaxant drug used to treat spasm and stiffness associated with minor muscle injuries. Tablet: 350 mg. [kar-EYE-soh-PROH-dawl].

**Carmol 40** (Derm). See *urea*. [KAR-mawl 40].

**Carmol Scalp Treatment** (Anti-infec, Derm). See *sulfacetamide*. [KAR-mawl].

**carmustine** (BiCNU, Gliadel) (Chemo). Alkylating chemotherapy drug used to treat cancer of the brain and colon; used to treat multiple myeloma, Hodgkin's lymphoma, non-Hodgkin's lymphoma, mycosis fungoides, and malignant melanoma. Intracranial wafer: 7.7 mg. Intravenous (powder to be reconstituted): 100 mg. [kar-MUS-teen].

**Carnation Follow-Up, Carnation Good-Start** (GI). Infant formula. Liquid. Powder (to be reconstituted). [kar-NAY-shun].

**Carnitor** (Anti-infec). See *levocarnitine*. [KAR-nih-tor].

**carteolol** (Cartrol, Ocupress) (Cardio, Ophth). Beta-blocker drug used to treat hypertension; used topically in the eye to treat glaucoma. Tablet: 2.5 mg, 5 mg. Ophthalmic solution: 1%. [KAR-tee-oh-lawl].

**Cartia XT** (Analges, Cardio). See *diltiazem*. [KAR-tee-ah X-T].

**Cartrol** (Cardio). See *carteolol*. [KAR-trawl].

**carvedilol** (Coreg, Coreg CR) (Cardio). Alpha-blocker and beta-blocker drug used to treat angina pectoris, congestive heart failure, hypertension, and left ventricular failure after myocardial infarction. Extended-release capsule: 10 mg, 20 mg, 40 mg, 80 mg. Tablet: 3.125 mg, 6.25 mg, 12.5 mg, 25 mg. [kar-VEE-dih-lawl].

**cascara** (GI). Over-the-counter irritant/stimulant laxative drug used to treat constipation. Liquid. Tablet: 325 mg. [kas-KAIR-ah].

**Casodex** (Chemo). See *bicalutamide*. [KAS-oh-deks].

**caspofungin** (Cancidas) (Anti-infec). Antifungal drug used to treat severe systemic fungal and yeast infections, such as candidiasis and aspergillosis in adults and children. Intravenous (powder for reconstitution): 50 mg, 70 mg. [KAS-poh-FUN-jin].

**Castellani Paint Modified** (Derm) (generic *basic fuchsin dye, resorcinol*). Combination antifungal, antipruritic, and antiseptic drug used topically to treat tinea (ringworm) fungal skin infections. Liquid. [KAS-teh-LAW-nee].

**castor oil** (Emulsoil, Neoloid) (GI). Over-the-counter osmotic laxative drug used to treat constipation. Emulsion. Liquid. [KAS-tor OYL].

**Cataflam** (Analges). See *diclofenac*. [KAT-ah-flam].

**Catapres, Catapres-TTS-1, Catapres-TTS-2, Catapres-TTS-3** (Cardio, Derm, Endo, GI, Neuro, OB/GYN, Pulm, Psych). See *clonidine*. [KAT-ah-pres].

**Catatrol** (Neuro). See *viloxazine*. [KAT-ah-trawl].

**Cathflo Activase** (Cardio, Hem). See *alteplase*. [KATH-floh AK-tih-vays].

**catumaxomab** (Removab) (Chemo). Monoclonal antibody drug used to treat ovarian cancer. Orphan drug. [KAH-too-MAK-soo-mab].

**Cavatak** (Chemo).　Chemotherapy drug used to treat malignant melanoma of the skin. Orphan drug. [KAV-ah-tak].

**Caverject** (Uro).　See *alprostadil.* [KAV-er-jekt].

**Cea-Cide** (Chemo).　Monoclonal antibody drug used to treat cancer of the lung, pancreas, and ovary. Orphan drug. [SEE-ah-side].

**Ceclor, Ceclor Pulvules** (Anti-infec).　See *cefaclor.* [SEE-klor].

**Cedax** (Anti-infec).　See *ceftibuten.* [SEE-daks].

**CeeNU** (Chemo).　See *lomustine.* [SEE-N-U].

**cefaclor** (Ceclor, Ceclor Pulvules, Raniclor) (Anti-infec). Cephalosporin antibiotic drug used to treat various bacterial infections, including streptococcal pharyngitis and tonsillitis, oititis media, staphylococcal skin infections, bronchitis and pneumonia due to *S. pneumoniae* and *H. influenzae,* and urinary tract infections caused by *E. coli.* Capsule: 250 mg, 500 mg. Chewable tablet: 125 mg, 187 mg, 250 mg, 375 mg. Extended-release tablet: 375 mg, 500 mg. Liquid: 125 mg/5 mL, 187 mg/5 mL, 250 mg/5 mL, 375 mg/5 mL. [SEF-ah-klor].

**cefadroxil** (Duricef) (Anti-infec).　Cephalosporin antibiotic drug used to treat a variety of bacterial infections, including urinary tract infections caused by *E. coli,* staphylococcal and streptococcal skin infections, and streptococcal pharyngitis and tonsillitis. Capsule: 500 mg. Tablet: 1 g. Liquid: 125 mg/5 mL, 250 mg/5 mL, 500 mg/5 mL. [SEF-ah-DRAWK-sil].

**cefazolin** (Anti-infec).　Cephalosporin antibiotic drug used to treat a variety of bacterial infections; used to treat gallbladder, urinary tract infections, and prostatitis due to *E. coli;* used to treat endocarditis; used to treat pneumonia due to *S. pneumoniae* and *H. influenzae;* used to treat bone infections due to *S. aureus,* staphylococcal and streptococcal skin infections, and septicemia. Intramuscular or intravenous (powder to be reconstituted): 500 mg, 1 g. [SEF-ah-ZOH-lin].

**cefdinir** (Omnicef) (Anti-infec).　Cephalosporin antibiotic drug used to treat a variety of bacterial infections, including bronchitis and pneumonia due to *S. pneumoniae* and *H. influenzae,* sinusitis, streptococcal pharyngitis and tonsillitis, otitis media, and streptococcal and staphylococcal skin infections. Capsule: 300 mg. Liquid: 125 mg/5 mL, 250 mg/5 mL. [SEF-dih-neer].

**cefditoren** (Spectracef) (Anti-infec).　Cephalosporin antibiotic drug used to treat a variety of bacterial infections, including bronchitis and pneumonia due to *S. pneumoniae* and *H. influenzae,* streptococcal pharyngitis and tonsillitis, and staphylococcal or streptococcal skin infections. Tablet: 200 mg. [SEF-dih-TOR-en].

**cefepime** (Maxipime) (Anti-infec).　Cephalosporin antibiotic drug used to treat a variety of bacterial infections, including pneumonia due to *S. pneumoniae,* urinary tract infections due to *E. coli,* staphylococcal and streptococcal skin infec-

tions, and intra-abdominal infections. Intravenous (powder to be reconstituted): 500 mg, 1 g, 2 g. [SEF-eh-peem].

**cefixime** (Suprax) (Anti-infec).　Cephalosporin antibiotic drug used to treat a variety of bacterial infections, including pharyngitis, tonsillitis, bronchitis, otitis media, gonorrhea; used to treat urinary tract infections due to *E. coli.* Oral liquid (powder to be reconstituted): 100 mg/5 mL, 200 mg/5mL. Tablet: 400 mg. [seh-FIK-seem].

**Cefizox** (Anti-infec).　See *ceftizoxime.* [SEF-ih-zawks].

**Cefobid** (Anti-infec).　See *cefoperazone.* [SEF-oh-bid].

**cefoperazone** (Cefobid) (Anti-infec).　Cephalosporin antibiotic drug used to treat a variety of bacterial infections, including respiratory infections due to *S. pneumoniae* and *H. influenzae,* staphylococcal skin infections, pelvic inflammatory disease, urinary tract infections due to *E. coli,* peritonitis, and septicemia. Intravenous (powder to be reconstituted): 1 g, 2 g. [SEF-oh-PAIR-ah-zohn].

**Cefotan** (Anti-infec).　See *cefotetan.* [SEF-oh-tan].

**cefotaxime** (Claforan) (Anti-infec).　Cephalosporin antibiotic drug used to treat a variety of bacterial infections, including pneumonia due to *S. pneumonia* and *H. influenzae,* urinary tract infections due to *E. coli,* endometriosis, pelvic inflammatory disease, staphylococcal and streptococcal skin infections, peritonitis, bone infections, meningitis, and septicemia. Intramuscular or intravenous (powder to be reconstituted): 500 mg, 1 g, 2 g. [SEF-oh-TAK-seem].

**cefotetan** (Cefotan) (Anti-infec).　Cephalosporin antibiotic drug used to treat a variety of bacterial infections, including urinary tract infections due to *E. coli,* respiratory infections, staphylococcal and streptococcal skin infections, gonorrhea, intra-abdominal infections, and bone infections. Intramuscular or intravenous (powder to be reconstituted): 1 g, 2 g. [SEF-oh-TEE-tan].

**cefoxitin** (Mefoxin) (Anti-infec).　Cephalosporin antibiotic drug used to treat a variety of bacterial infections, including pneumonia due to *H. influenzae,* urinary tract infections due to *E. coli,* peritonitis, endometritis, pelvic inflammatory disease, gonorrhea, *Chlamydia,* bone infections, staphylococcal and streptococcal skin infections, and septicemia. Intravenous (powder to be reconstituted): 1 g, 2 g. [seh-FAWK-sih-tin].

**cefpodoxime** (Vantin) (Anti-infec).　Cephalosporin antibiotic drug used to treat a variety of bacterial infections, including urinary tract infections due to *E. coli,* sinusitis and otitis media, streptococcal pharyngitis and tonsillitis, bronchitis and pneumonia due to *S. pneumoniae* or *H. influenzae,* staphylococcal and streptococcal skin infections, and gonorrhea. Tablet: 100 mg, 200 mg. Liquid (granules to be reconstituted): 50 mg/5 mL, 100 mg/5 mL. [SEF-poh-DAWK-seem].

**cefprozil** (Cefzil) (Anti-infec).　Cephalosporin antibiotic drug used to treat a variety of bacterial infections, including streptococcal pharyngitis and tonsillitis, otitis media, sinusitis, bronchitis, and staphylococcal and streptococcal skin infections. Tablet: 250 mg, 500 mg. Liquid: 125 mg/5 mL, 250 mg/5 mL. [sef-PROH-zil].

**ceftazidime** (Ceptaz, Fortaz, Tazicef, Tazidime) (Anti-infec). Cephalosporin antibiotic drug used to treat a variety of bacterial infections, including urinary tract infections, pneumonia due to *S. pneumoniae* and *H. influenzae,* staphylococcal and streptococcal skin infections, bone infections, endometritis, peritonitis, meningitis, and septicemia. Intramuscular or intravenous (powder to be reconstituted): 500 mg, 1 g, 2 g. [sef-TAZ-ih-deem].

**ceftibuten** (Cedax) (Anti-infec). Cephalosporin antibiotic drug used to treat a variety of bacterial infections, including bronchitis due to *S. pneumoniae* and *H. influenzae,* otitis media, and streptococcal pharyngitis and tonsillitis. Capsule: 400 mg. Liquid: 90 mg/5 mL. [SEF-tih-BYOO-tin].

**Ceftin** (Anti-infec). See *cefuroxime.* [SEF-tin].

**ceftizoxime** (Cefizox) (Anti-infec). Cephalosporin antibiotic drug used to treat a variety of bacterial infections, including respiratory infections due to *S. pneumoniae* and *H. influenzae,* urinary tract infections due to *E. coli,* pelvic inflammatory disease, gonorrhea, staphylococcal and strep-tococcal skin infections, bone infections, intra-abdominal infections, meningitis, and septicemia. Intramuscular or intravenous (powder to be reconstituted): 500 mg, 1 g, 2 g. [SEF-tih-ZAWK-seem].

**ceftriaxone** (Rocephin) (Anti-infec). Cephalosporin antibi-otic drug used to treat a variety of bacterial infections, including urinary tract infections due to *E. coli,* respiratory infections due to *S. pneumoniae* and *H. influenzae,* otitis media, staphylococcal and streptococcal skin infections, pelvic inflammatory disease, gonorrhea, bone infections, intra-abdominal infections, meningitis, and septicemia; orphan drug used to treat amyotrophic lateral sclerosis. Intramuscular or intravenous (powder to be reconstituted): 250 mg, 500 mg, 1 g, 2 g. [SEF-try-AK-zohn].

**cefuroxime** (Ceftin, Zinacef) (Anti-infec). Cephalosporin antibiotic drug used to treat a variety of bacterial infections, including streptococcal pharyngitis and tonsillitis, otitis media, sinusitis, bronchitis, staphylococcal and streptococcal skin infections, urinary tract infections due to *E. coli,* gonorrhea, and Lyme's disease. Tablet: 125 mg, 250 mg, 500 mg. Liquid: 125 mg/5 mL, 250 mg/5 mL. Intramuscular or intravenous (powder to be reconstituted): 750 mg, 1.5 g. [SEF-yoor-AWK-seem].

**Cefzil** (Anti-infec). See *cefprozil.* [SEF-zil].

**Celebrex** (Analges, GI). See *celecoxib.* [SEL-eh-breks].

**celecoxib** (Celebrex) (Analges, GI). COX-2 inhibitor NSAID drug used to treat pain and inflammation; used to decrease the number of colonic polyps in patients with familial ade-nomatous polyposis; used to treat the pain of osteoarthritis, rheumatoid arthritis, ankylosing spondylitis, and dysmenor-rhea. Capsule: 50 mg, 100 mg, 200 mg, 400 mg. [SEL-eh-KAWK-sib].

**Celestone, Celestone Soluspan** (Derm, Endo, Ortho). See *betamethasone.* [seh-LES-tohn].

**Celexa** (Psych). See *citalopram.* [seh-LEK-sah].

**CellCept** (Cardio, GI, Neuro, Uro). See *mycophenolate.* [SEL-sept].

**cellulose sodium phosphate** (Calcibind) (Uro). Used to pre-vent the formation of calcium oxalate kidney stones in patients with hypercalciuria. Powder to be taken with each meal. [SEL-yoo-lohs SOH-dee-um FAWS-fayt].

**Celluvisc** (Ophth). Over-the-counter artificial tears drug for dry eyes. Ophthalmic solution. [SELL-yoo-visk].

**Celontin** (Neuro). See *methsuximide.* [seh-LAWN-tin].

**Cena-K** (Uro). See *potassium.* [SEN-ah-K].

**Cenestin** (OB/GYN). See *conjugated estrogens.* [seh-NES-tin].

**Centany** (Derm, ENT). See *mupirocin.* [SEN-tah-nee].

**Centovir** (Anti-infec). Used to treat cytomegalovirus in patients wiith bone marrow transplantation. Orphan drug. [SEN-toh-veer].

**Centoxin** (Anti-infec). See *nebacumab.* [sen-TAWK-sin].

**Centrum, Advanced Formula** (Misc). Over-the-counter multivitamin supplement. Tablet. [SEN-trum].

**centruroides immune fab 2** (Alacramyn) (Emerg). Antivenom drug given after scorpion bites. Orphan drug. [SEN-troo-ROY-deez im-MYOON fab 2].

**Ceo-Two** (GI). Over-the-counter laxative drug that releases carbon dioxide foam to treat constipation. Suppository. [SEE-oh-TOO].

**Cepacol** (ENT). See *benzocaine.* [SEE-pah-kawl].

**cephalexin** (Keflex) (Anti-infec). Cephalosporin antibiotic drug used to treat a variety of bacterial infections, includ-ing pneumonia due to *S. pneumoniae* and *H. influenzae,* otitis media, staphylococcal or streptococcal skin infections, bone infections, and prostatitis. Capsule: 250 mg, 333 mg, 500 mg, 750 mg. Tablet: 250 mg, 500 mg, 1 g. Liquid: 125 mg/5 mL, 250 mg/5 mL. [SEF-ah-LEKS-zin].

**Cephulac** (GI). See *lactulose.* [SEF-yoo-lak].

**Ceprotin** (Hem). See *protein C concentrate.* [seh-PROH-tin].

**Ceptaz** (Anti-infec). See *ceftazidime.* [SEP-taz].

**Cerebyx** (Neuro). See *fosphenytoin.* [SAIR-eh-biks].

**Ceredase** (Misc). See *alglucerase.* [SAIR-eh-days].

**Ceresine** (Neuro). Used to treat severe head injury. Orphan drug. [SAIR-eh-seen].

**Cerezyme** (Misc). See *imiglucerase.* [SAIR-eh-zime].

**Cernevit-12** (I.V.). See *intravenous multivitamins.* [SER-neh-vite-12].

**certolizumab** (Cimzia) (GI). Anti-tumor necrosis factor drug used to treat Crohn's disease. Subcutaneous: 200 mg/mL. [SER-toh-LIZ-yoo-mab].

**Cerubidine** (Chemo). See *daunorubicin.* [seh-ROO-bih-deen].

**Cervidil** (OB/GYN). See *dinoprostone.* [SER-vih-dil].

**Cesamet** (Chemo, GI). See *nabilone.* [SES-ah-met].

**Cesia** (OB/GYN) (generic *desogestrel, ethinyl estradiol*). Combination triphasic oral contraceptive drug. Pill pack, 28-day: (7 hormone tablets) 0.1 mg/25 mcg; (7 hormone tablets) 0.125 mg/25 mcg; (7 hormone tablets) 0.15 mg/25 mcg; (7 inert tablets). [SEE-zee-ah].

**Cetacaine** (Anes, Derm, ENT) (generic *benzocaine, butamben, tetracaine*). Combination anesthetic drug used topically to prevent pain during mouth and throat procedures; used to treat pain from skin irritation or from minor procedures on the skin. Gel, liquid, ointment, spray: 14%/2%/2%. [SEE-tah-kayn].

**Cetacort** (Derm). See *hydrocortisone*. [SEE-tah-kort].

**Cetamide** (Anti-infec, Ophth). See *sulfacetamide*. [SEE-tah-mide].

**Ceta-Plus** (Analges) (generic *acetaminophen, hydrocodone*). Combination Schedule III nonnarcotic and narcotic analgesic drug for pain. Capsule: 500 mg/5 mg. [SEE-tah-PLUS].

**Cethrin** (Neuro). Used to treat spinal cord injury. Orphan drug. [SETH-rin].

**cetiedil citrate** (Hem). Used to treat sickle cell crisis. Orphan drug. [seh-TY-ah dil SIH-trayt].

**cetirizine** (Children's Zyrtec Allergy, Children's Zyrtec Hives Relief, Zyrtec) (Derm, ENT). Over-the-counter and prescription antihistamine drug used to treat seasonal and perennial allergies and allergic rhinitis; used to treat allergic skin reactions with itching. Chewable tablet: 5 mg, 10 mg. Tablet: 5 mg, 10 mg. Syrup: 5 mg/5mL. [seh-TEER-ah-zeen].

**cetrorelix** (Cetrotide) (OB/GYN). Used to inhibit excessive gonadotropin-releasing hormone from the anterior pituitary gland in patients taking ovulation-stimulating drugs for infertility. Subcutaneous: 0.25 mg, 3 mg. [seh-TROH-reh-liks].

**Cetrotide** (OB/GYN). See *cetrorelix*. [SEH-troh-tide].

**cetuximab** (Erbitux) (Chemo). Monoclonal antibody drug used to treat cancer of the head and neck, colon, and rectum. Intravenous: 2 mg/mL. [seh-TUK-sih-mab].

**cevimeline** (Evoxac) (ENT). Used to treat dry mouth due to Sjögren's syndrome. Capsule: 30 mg. [seh-VIM-ih-leen].

**Chantix** (Pulm). See *varenicline*. [CHAN-tiks].

**charcoal** (CharcoCaps) (GI). Adsorbent drug used to treat gas and diarrhea; used as an antidote to neutralize an overdose of an oral drug. Capsule: 250 mg. Tablet: 250 mg. [CHAR-kohl].

**CharcoAid, CharcoAid 2000** (Emerg, GI). See *activated charcoal*. [CHAR-koh-aid].

**CharcoCaps** (GI). See *charcoal*. [CHAR-koh-kaps].

**Chemet** (Emerg, Uro). See *succimer*. [CHEE-met].

**Chenix** (GI). See *chenodiol*. [KEE-niks].

**chenodiol** (Chenix) (GI). Used to dissolve gallstones in patients who cannot undergo gallbladder surgery. Orphan drug. [KEE-noh-DY-awl].

**Cheracol Cough** (ENT) (generic *codeine, guaifenesin*). Combination Schedule V narcotic antitussive and expectorant drug. Syrup: 10 mg/100 mg. [CHAIR-ah-kawl].

**Cheracol D Cough, Cheracol Plus** (ENT) (generic *dextromethorphan, guaifenesin*). Combination over-the-counter antitussive and expectorant drug. [CHAIR-ah-kawl].

**chloral hydrate** (Aquachloral Supprettes) (Neuro). Schedule IV nonbarbiturate drug used to produce sedation in ill and elderly patients; used to treat insomnia. Capsule: 500 mg. Liquid: 250 mg/5 mL, 500 mg/5 mL. Suppository: 325 mg, 500 mg, 650 mg. [KLOR-awl HY-drayt].

**chlorambucil** (Leukeran) (Chemo, Hem). Alkylating chemotherapy drug used to treat leukemia, lymphoma, and cancer of the ovary and breast; used to treat polycythemia vera. Tablet: 2 mg. [klor-AM-byoo-sil].

**chloramphenicol** (Chloromycetin) (Anti-infec, Ophth). Antibiotic drug used to treat a variety of gram-negative bacterial infections, including *H. influenzae, Salmonella,* meningitis, and rickettsiae; used to treat lung infections in patients with cystic fibrosis; antibiotic drug used topically in the eye to treat bacterial infections. Intravenous: 100 mg/mL. Ophthalmic solution: 5 mg/mL. Ophthalmic ointment: 10 mg/g. Powder to be reconstituted. [KLOR-am-FEN-ih-kawl].

**Chloraseptic Kids Sore Throat** (Anes, ENT). See *benzocaine*. [KLOR-ah-SEP-tik].

**chlordiazepoxide** (Librium) (Anes, GI, Psych). Schedule IV benzodiazepine drug used as a preoperative drug to relieve anxiety and provide sedation; used to treat anxiety and neurosis; used to treat alcohol withdrawal; used to treat irritable bowel syndrome. Capsule: 5 mg, 10 mg, 25 mg. Intramuscular or intravenous (powder to be reconstituted): 100 mg. [KLOR-dy-AZ-eh-PAWK-side].

**Chloresium** (Derm). See *chlorophyll derivative*. [klor-EE-see-um].

**chlorhexidine** (Betasept, Exidine, Hibiclens, Hibistat, Peridex, PerioChip, PerioGard) (Derm, ENT). Over-the-counter and prescription drug used topically as an antiseptic hand wash, preoperative surgical skin scrub, wound cleanser; and mouth rinse (Peridex, PerioGard); used as a periodontal implant chip (PerioChip) to treat gingivitis; used to treat oral mucositis caused by chemotherapy drugs (Peridex). Foam: 4%. Liquid: 2%, 4%. Rinse: 0.5%. Sponge/brush: 4%. Mouth rinse: 0.12%. Periodontal chip: 2.5 mg. [klor-HEK-sih-deen].

**Chloromycetin** (Anti-infec, Ophth). See *chloramphenicol*. [KLOR-oh-my-SEE-tin].

**chlorophyll derivative** (Chloresium) (Derm). Over-the-counter drug used topically to promote healing of skin ulcers and wounds and control odors. Ointment: 0.5%. Solution: 0.2%. [KLOR-oh-fil].

**chloroprocaine** (Nesacaine, Nesacaine MPF) (Anes). Used to provide local, regional, lumbar, and epidural anesthesia. Injection: 1%, 2%, 3%. [KLOR-oh-PROH-kayn].

**chloroquine** (Aralen) (Anti-infec). Antiprotozoal drug used to treat malaria and amebiasis. Tablet: 250 mg, 500 mg. [KLOR-oh-kwin].

**chlorothiazide** (Diurigen, Diuril) (Cardio, Uro). Thiazide diuretic drug used to treat hypertension; used to treat edema from congestive heart failure, liver disease, or kidney disease. Oral suspension: 250 mg/5 mL. Tablet: 250 mg, 500 mg. Intravenous: 500 mg/20 mL. [KLOR-oh-THY-ah-zide].

**chloroxine** (Capitrol) (Derm). Anti-infective drug used topically to treat dandruff and seborrheic dermatitis of the scalp. Shampoo: 2%. [klor-AWK-seen].

**chlorpheniramine** (Chlor-Trimeton Allergy, Efidac 24) (ENT). Over-the-counter antihistamine drug used to treat seasonal and perennial allergies and allergic rhinitis. Caplet: 8 mg. Extended-release capsule: 8 mg, 12 mg. Tablet: 4 mg. Chewable tablet: 2 mg. Extended-release tablet: 8 mg, 12 mg, 16 mg. Syrup: 2 mg/5mL. [KLOR-feh-NEER-ah-meen].

**chlorpromazine** (Thorazine) (Analges, Anes, GI, Psych). Phenothiazine antipsychotic drug used to treat the manic phase of manic-depressive disorder and schizophrenia; used to treat hyperactivity; used to treat severe behavior problems and conduct disorders with aggression in children; antiemetic drug used to treat nausea and vomiting and intractable hiccoughs; used preoperatively to decrease anxiety; used to treat migraine headaches; used to treat intermittent porphyria. Tablet: 10 mg, 25 mg, 50 mg, 100 mg, 200 mg. Suppository: 100 mg. Intramuscular: 25 mg/mL. [klor-PROH-mah-zeen].

**chlorpropamide** (Diabinese) (Endo). Sulfonylurea oral antidiabetic drug used to treat type 2 diabetes mellitus; used to treat diabetes insipidus. Tablet: 100 mg, 250 mg. [klor-PROH-pah-mide].

**chlorthalidone** (Hygroton) (Cardio, Uro). Thiazide diuretic drug used to treat hypertension; used to treat edema from congestive heart failure, liver disease, or kidney disease. Tablet: 15 mg, 25 mg, 50 mg, 100 mg. [klor-THAL-ih-dohn].

**Chlor-Trimeton Allergy** (ENT). See *chlorpheniramine*. [klor-TRIM-eh-tawn].

**Chlor-Trimeton Allergy-D** (ENT) (generic *chlorpheniramine, pseudoephedrine*). Combination over-the-counter antihistamine and decongestant drug. Tablet: 4 mg/60 mg, 8 mg/120 mg. [klor-TRIM-eh-tawn].

**chlorzoxazone** (Paraflex, Parafon Forte DSC, Remular-S) (Ortho). Skeletal muscle relaxant drug used to treat spasm and stiffness associated with minor muscle injuries. Tablet: 250 mg, 500 mg. [klor-ZAWK-sah-zohn].

**Choice DM, Choice DM Sugar Free** (Endo, GI). Lactose-free or lactose-free and sugar-free nutritional supplement formulated for patients with diabetes mellitus. Liquid. Shakes. [CHOYS D-M].

**Cholac** (GI). See *lactulose*. [CHOH-lak].

**Cholestrase** (GI). Used to treat deficiency of the enzyme lipase. Orphan drug. [koh-LES-trays].

**cholestyramine** (Prevalite, Questran, Questran Light) (Cardio, Emerg, Endo, GI). Bile acid sequestrant drug used to treat high cholesterol levels; used to treat digitalis toxicity; used to relieve itching in patients with biliary obstruction; used to treat thyroid hormone overdose. Powder (to be reconstituted): 4 g. [kon les TY rah meen].

**Chooz** (GI). See *calcium carbonate*. [CHOOZ].

**choriogonadotropin alfa** (Ovidrel) (Endo, OB/GYN). Luteinizing hormone drug used to mature and release an egg to treat infertility. Subcutaneous: 250 mcg/0.5 mL. [KOR-ee-oh-goh-NAD-oh-TROH-pin AL-fah].

**Choron 10** (Endo, OB/GYN). See *human chorioic gonadotropin*. [KOR-awn 10].

**Chromelin Complexion Blender** (Derm). See *dihydroxyacetone*. [KROH-meh-lin].

**Cialis** (Uro). See *tadalafil*. [see-AL-is].

**Cibacalcin** (Ortho). See *calcitonin-human*. [SEE-bah-KAL-sin].

**ciclesonide** (Alvesco, Omnaris) (ENT, Pulm). Corticosteroid anti-inflammatory drug used to prevent acute asthma attacks (Alvesco); used topically in the nose to treat allergy symptoms (Omnaris). Inhaler: 80 mcg, 160 mcg. Nasal spray: 50 mcg/spray. [sy-KLES-oh-nide].

**ciclopirox** (Loprox, Penlac Nail Lacquer) (Derm). Antifungal drug used topically to treat tinea (ringworm) and other fungal skin infections; used to treat onychomycosis (nail fungus). Cream: 0.77%. Gel: 0.77%. Liquid nail solution: 8%. Lotion: 0.77%. Shampoo: 1%. Liquid: 0.77%. [SY-kloh-PEER-awks].

**cidofovir** (Vistide) (Anti-infec, Ophth). Antiviral drug used to treat cytomegalovirus retinitis. Intravenous: 75 mg/mL. [sih-DOH-foh-veer].

**cilengitide** (Chemo). Chemotherapy drug used to treat brain cancer. Orphan drug. [sih-LEN-gih-tide].

**ciliary neurotrophic factor** (Neuro). Used to treat amyotrophic lateral sclerosis. Orphan drug. [SIL-ee-air-ee NYOOR-oh-TROH-fik FAK-tor].

**cilostazol** (Pletal) (Cardio, Hem). Platelet aggregation inhibitor drug used to prevent blood clots; vasodilator drug used to treat peripheral vascular disease and intermittent claudication. Tablet: 50 mg, 100 mg. [sih-LOH-stah-zawl].

**Ciloxan** (Anti-infec, Ophth). See *ciprofloxacin*. [sy-LAWK-san].

**cimetidine** (Acid Reducer 200, Tagamet, Tagamet HB 200) (GI). Over-the-counter and prescription $H_2$ blocker drug used to treat heartburn, peptic ulcer, GERD, and *H. pylori* infection. Oral liquid: 300 mg/5 mL. Tablet: 200 mg, 300 mg, 400 mg, 800 mg. Intramuscular or intravenous: 150 mg/ 2 mL, 6 mg/mL. [sy-MEH-tih-deen].

**Cimzia** (GI). See *certolizumab*. [SIM-zee-ah].

**cinacalcet** (Sensipar) (Chemo, Endo). Used to decrease elevated levels of parathyroid hormone in patients on dialysis; used to treat hypercalcemia in patients with cancer of the parathyroid glands. Tablet: 30 mg, 60 mg, 90 mg. [SIN-ah-KAL-set].

**cinoxacin** (Anti-infec).   Quinolone antibiotic drug used to treat gram-negative bacterial infections of the urinary tract. Capsule: 250 mg, 500 mg. [sih-NAWK-sah-sin].

**Cipro, Cipro I.V., Cipro XR** (Anti-infec).   See *ciprofloxacin.* [SIP-roh].

**Ciprodex** (ENT) (generic *ciprofloxacin, dexamethasone*)   Combination antibiotic and corticosteroid drug used topically to treat ear infections. Ear drops: 0.3%/0.1%. [SIP-roh-deks].

**ciprofloxacin** (Ciloxan, Cipro, Cipro I.V., Cipro XR, Proquin XR) (Anti-infec, Ophth).   Fluoroquinolone antibiotic drug used to treat gram-negative and gram-positive bacterial infections; used to treat sinusitis, pneumonia due to *S. pneumoniae,* Legionnaire's disease of the lungs, staphylococcal and streptococcal skin infections, bone infections, gonorrhea, traveler's diarrhea, urinary tract infections due to *E. coli,* and prostatitis; used to treat cutaneous or inhaled anthrax from bioterrorism; antibiotic drug used topically in the eye to treat bacterial infections (Ciloxan); used to prevent *Mycobacterium avium-intracellulare* infection in AIDS patients. Powder (to be reconstituted to make oral liquid): 250 mg/5 mL, 500 mg/5 mL. Tablet: 100 mg, 250 mg, 500 mg, 750 mg. Extended-release tablet: 500 mg, 1000 mg. Intravenous: 200 mg/20 mL, 400 mg/40 mL. Ophthalmic solution: 3.5 mg/mL. Ophthalmic ointment: 3.33 mg/g. [sip-roh-FLAWK-sah-sin].

**Cipro HC Otic** (ENT) (generic *ciprofloxacin, dexamethasone*).   Combination antibiotic and corticosteroid drug used topically to treat ear infections. Ear drops: 0.3%/0.1%. [SIP-roh-deks].

**Circadin** (Neuro).   See *melatonin.* [SIR-kah-din].

**cisatracurium** (Nimbex) (Anes, Pulm).   Neuromuscular blocker drug used during surgery; used to treat patients who are intubated and on the ventilator. Intravenous: 2 mg/mL, 10 mg/mL. [sis-ah-trah-KYOOR-ee-um].

**cisplatin** (Chemo).   Platinum chemotherapy drug used to treat cancer of the brain, head and neck, lung, esophagus, liver, bone, adrenal gland, bladder, breast, ovary, uterus, cervix, and testicle. Intravenous: 1 mg/mL. [sis-PLAT-in].

**citalopram** (Celexa) (Psych).   Selective serotonin reuptake inhibitor antidepressant drug used to treat depression; used to treat panic disorder, anxiety, obsessive-compulsive disorder, premenstrual dysphoric disorder, and posttraumatic stress disorder. Tablet: 10 mg, 20 mg, 40 mg. Liquid: 10 mg/5 mL. [sih-TAL-oh-pram].

**Citanest** (Anes, ENT).   See *prilocaine.* [SIT-ah-nest].

**Citracal** (Misc).   See *calcium citrate.* [SIH-trah-kal].

**CitraNatal DHA, CitraNatal Rx** (OB/GYN).   Prenatal vitamins. Tablet. [SIH-trah-NAY-tal].

**Citra pH** (GI).   See *sodium citrate.* [SIH-trah P-H].

**Citrolith** (Uro) (generic *potassium citrate, sodium citrate*).   Combination drug used to prevent the formation of calcium oxalate or uric acid kidney stones. Tablet: 50 mg/950 mg. [SIH-troh-lith].

**Citrotein** (GI).   Cholesterol-free, lactose-free, gluten-free nutritional supplement. Liquid. Powder (to be reconstituted). [SIH-troh-teen].

**citrovorum factor** (Chemo).   See *leucovorin.* [SIH-troh-VOH-rum FAK-tor].

**Citrucel, Citrucel Sugar Free** (GI).   See *methylcellulose.* [SIH-troo-sel].

**civamide** (Zucapsaicin) (ENT).   Used to treat postherpetic neuralgia that affects the trigeminal nerve. Orphan drug. [SIV-ah-mide].

**cladribine** (Leustatin, Mylinax) (Chemo).   Antimetabolite chemotherapy drug used to treat leukemia and non-Hodgkin's lymphoma; orphan drug used to treat multiple sclerosis (Mylinax). Intravenous: 1 mg/mL. [KLAD-rih-been].

**Claforan** (Anti-infec).   See *cefotaxime.* [KLAF-oh-ran].

**Claravis** (Derm).   See *isotretinoin.* [KLAIR-ah-vis].

**Clarinex, Clarinex RediTabs** (Derm, ENT).   See *desloratadine.* [KLAIR-ih-neks].

**Clarinex-D** (ENT) (generic *desloratadine, pseudoephedrine*).   Combination antihistamine and decongestant drug used to treat allergies. [KLAIR-ih-neks].

**Claripel** (Derm).   See *hydroquinone.* [KLAIR-ih-pel].

**clarithromycin** (Biaxin, Biaxin XL) (Anti-infec).   Macrolide antibiotic drug used to treat gram-negative and gram-positive bacterial infections; used to treat streptococcal pharyngitis and tonsillitis, otitis media, sinusitis, bronchitis, and pneumonia due to *S. pneumonia, H. influenzae,* and *Mycoplasma;* used to treat staphylococcal and streptococcal skin infections; used to treat gonorrhea and *Chlamydia;* used to prevent *Mycobacterium avium-intracellulare* in AIDS patients; used to treat gastric ulcers due to *H. pylori* infection. Tablet: 250 mg, 500 mg. Extended-release tablet: 500 mg, 1000 mg. Liquid (granules to be reconstituted): 125 mg/5 mL, 250 mg/5 mL. [KLAIR-ih-throh-MY-sin].

**Claritin, Claritin Chilren's Allergy, Claritin Hives Relief, Claritin Reditabs, Claritin 24-Hour Allergy** (Derm, ENT).   See *loratadine.* [KLAIR-ih-tin].

**Claritin-D** (ENT) (generic *loratadine, pseudoephedrine*).   Combination over-the-counter antihistamine and decongestant drug. Tablet: 5 mg/120 mg, 10 mg/240 mg. [KLAIR-ih-tin].

**clazosentan** (Erajet) (Neuro).   Used to treat vasospasm after subarachnoid hemorrhage in the brain. Orphan drug. [klah-ZOH-sen-tan].

**Clearasil Acne-Fighting Pads, Clearasil Clearstick, Clearasil Double Clear, Clearasil Medicated Deep Cleanser** (Derm).   See *salicylic acid.* [KLEER-ah-sil].

**Clearasil Antibacterial Soap, Clearasil Daily Face Wash** (Derm).   See *triclosan.* [KLEER-ah-sil].

**Clearasil Maximum Strength Acne Treatment** (Derm).   See *benzoyl peroxide.* [KLEER-ah-sil].

**Clearly Cala-gel** (Derm) (generic *benzocaine, zinc acetate*). Combination over-the-counter anesthetic and astringent drug used topically to numb the skin and decrease oozing. [KLEER-lee KAL-ah-jel].

**clemastine** (DayHist-1, Tavist Allergy) (Derm, ENT). Over-the-counter and prescription antihistamine drug used to treat the symptoms of seasonal and perennial allergies, allergic rhinitis, and skin allergies with itching. Syrup: 0.67 mg/5 mL. Tablet: 1.34 mg, 2.68 mg. [KLEM-as-teen].

**Clenia** (Derm) (generic *sodium sulfacetamide, sulfur*). Combination anti-infective and keratolytic drug used topically to treat acne vulgaris. Cream: 10%/5%. Cream and foam: 10%/5%. [KLEN-ee-ah].

**Cleocin, Cleocin Pediatric, Cleocin T** (Derm). See *clindamycin*. [KLEE-oh-sin].

**clevidipine** (Cleviprex) (Cardio). Calcium channel blocker drug used to treat hypertension. Intravenous: 0.5 mg/mL. [kleh-VID-ih-peen].

**Cleviprex** (Cardio). See *clevidipine*. [KLEV-ih-preks].

**Climara** (OB/GYN, Ortho). See *estradiol*. [kly-MAIR-ah].

**ClimaraPro** (OB/GYN, Ortho) (generic *levonorgestrel, estradiol*). Combination hormone drug used to treat the symptoms of menopause; used to prevent osteoporosis. Transdermal patch: 0.015 mg/0.04 mg (22 cm$^2$). [kly-MAIR-ah-PROH].

**Clinac BPO** (Derm). See *benzoyl peroxide*. [KLIN-ak B-P-O].

**Clindagel** (Derm). See *clindamycin*. [KLIN-dah-jel].

**ClindaMax** (Derm). See *clindamycin*. [KLIN-dah-maks].

**clindamycin** (Cleocin, Cleocin Pediatric, Cleocin T, Clindagel, ClindaMax, Clindesse, Clindets, Evoclin) (Anti-infec, Derm, OB/GYN). Antibiotic drug used to treat gram-positive bacterial infections; used to treat staphylococcal and streptococcal infections of the skin, bones, and lungs; used to treat endometriosis and intra-abdominal infections; used to treat septicemia; used to treat serious infections caused by anaerobic bacteria; used to treat CNS toxoplasmosis and *Pneumocystis carinii* pneumonia in AIDS patients; antibiotic drug used topically to treat acne vulgaris; used vaginally to treat bacterial vaginosis. Capsule: 75 mg, 150 mg, 300 mg. Liquid (granules to be dissolved): 75 mg/5 mL. Intramuscular or intravenous: 150 mg/mL. Foam: 1%. Gel: 1%. Lotion: 1%. Liquid: 1%. Cream: 2%. Vaginal suppository: 100 mg. [KLIN-dah-MY-sin].

**Clindesse** (OB/GYN). See *clindamycin*. [klin-DES].

**Clindets** (Derm). See *clindamycin*. [KLIN-dets].

**Clinoril** (Analges). See *sulindac*. [KLIN-oh-ril].

**Clivarine** (Hem). See *reviparin*. [klih-VAIR-een].

**clobetasol** (Clobex, Cormax, Olux, Olux-E, Temovate) (Derm). Corticosteroid drug used topically to treat inflammation and itching from dermatitis, seborrhea, eczema, psoriasis, and yeast or fungal infections. Cream: 0.05%. Foam: 0.05%. Gel: 0.05%. Liquid: 0.05%. Lotion: 0.05%. Ointment: 0.05%. Scalp solution: 0.05%. Shampoo: 0.05%. Spray: 0.05%. [kloh-BAY-tah-sawl].

**Clobex** (Derm). See *clobetasol*. [KLOH-beks].

**clocortolone** (Cloderm) (Derm). Corticosteroid drug used topically to treat inflammation and itching from dermatitis, seborrhea, eczema, psoriasis, and yeast or fungal infections. Cream (metered-dose pump): 0.1%. [kloh-KOR-toh-lohn].

**Cloderm** (Derm). See *clocortolone*. [KLOH-derm].

**clofarabine** (Clofarex, Clolar) (Chemo). Antimetabolite chemotherapy drug used to treat leukemia. Intravenous: 1 mg/mL. [kloh-FAIR-ah-been].

**Clofarex** (Chemo). See *clofarabine*. [kloh-FAIR-eks].

**clofazimine** (Lamprene) (Derm). Used to treat leprosy. Orphan drug. [kloh-FAZ-ih-meen].

**Clolar** (Chemo). See *clofarabine*. [KLOH-lar].

**Clomid** (OB/GYN). See *clomiphene*. [KLOH-mid].

**clomiphene** (Clomid, Milophene, Serophene) (OB/GYN). Ovulation-stimulating hormone drug used to treat infertility. Tablet: 50 mg. [KLOH-mih-feen].

**clomipramine** (Anafranil) (Psych). Antidepressant drug used to treat obsessive-compulsive disorder; used to treat panic attacks; used to treat premenstrual dysphoric disorder. Capsule: 25 mg, 50 mg, 75 mg. [kloh-MIP-rah-meen].

**clonazepam** (Klonopin) (Neuro, Psych). Schedule IV benzodiazepine antianxiety and anticonvulsant drug used to treat absence and myoclonic seizures; used to treat Parkinson's disease; used to treat neuralgia; used to treat the manic phase of manic-depressive disorder; used to treat panic disorder; orphan drug used to treat startle disease. Tablet: 0.5 mg, 1 mg, 2 mg. Orally disintegrating tablets: 0.125 mg, 0.25 mg, 0.5 mg, 1 mg, 2 mg. [kloh-NAZ-eh-pam].

**clonidine** (Catapres, Catapres-TTS-1, Catapres-TTS-2, Catapres-TTS-3, Duraclon) (Analges, Cardio, Chemo, Derm, Endo, GI, Neuro, OB/GYN, Pulm, Psych, Uro). Alpha$_2$ receptor stimulator drug used to treat hypertension, atrial fibrillation, and hypertensive emergency; nonnarcotic drug used to treat severe pain in cancer patients; used to treat excessive sweating; used to decrease postoperative shivering; used to diagnose pheochromocytoma of the adrenal medulla; used to treat growth delay in children; used to treat ulcerative colitis; used to treat restless legs syndrome and postherpetic neuralgia/shingles; used to treat hot flashes of menopause; used to treat attention deficit-hyperactivity disorder; used to treat withdrawal from alcohol and methadone; used to treat Tourette's syndrome; used to treat schizophrenia; used to help stop smoking; used to treat cyclosporine-induced nephrotoxicity. Tablet: 0.1 mg, 0.2 mg, 0.3 mg. Transdermal patch: 0.1 mg/24 hr, 0.2 mg/24 hr, 0.3 mg/24 hr. Epidural injection: 100 mcg/mL, 500 mcg/mL. [KLAWN-ih-deen].

**clopidogrel** (Plavix) (Cardio, Hem, Neuro). Platelet aggregation inhibitor drug used to prevent a second heart attack or stroke; used to treat peripheral arterial disease and acute coronary syndrome. Tablet: 75 mg, 300 mg. [kloh-PID-oh-grel].

**clorazepate** (Tranxene, Tranxene-SD, Tranxene-SD Half Strength, Tranxene T-tab) (GI, Psych). Schedule IV benzodiazepine drug used to treat anxiety; used to treat alcohol withdrawal; used to treat irritable bowel syndrome. Tablet: 3.75 mg, 7.5 mg, 15 mg. Extended-release tablet: 11.25 mg, 22.5 mg. [klor-AA-zeh-payt].

**cloretazine** (Chemo). Used to treat leukemia. Orphan drug. [klor-ET-ah-zeen].

**Clorpactin WSC-90** (Derm). See *oxychlorosene*. [klor-PAK-tin W-S-C-90].

**Clorpres** (Cardio) (generic *clonidine, chlorthalidone*). Combination alpha-receptor blocker and diuretic drug used to treat hypertension. Tablet: 0.1 mg/15 mg, 0.2 mg/15 mg, 0.3 mg/15 mg. [KLOR-pres].

**clotrimazole** (Cruex Cream, Desenex Cream, Gyne-Lotrimin 3 Gyne-Lotrimin 7, Lotrimin AF 1%, Mycelex, Mycelex-7) (Derm, ENT, OB/GYN). Over-the-counter and prescription antifungal and antiyeast drug used topically to treat tinea (ringworm) and other fungal skin infections; used to treat skin, mouth, and vaginal yeast infections caused by *Candida albicans;* orphan drug used to treat sickle cell disease and Huntington disease. Cream: 1%. Liquid: 1%. Lotion: 1%. Oral troche: 10 mg. Vaginal cream: 1%, 2%. Vaginal suppository: 100 mg, 200 mg. [kloh-TRIM-ah-zohl].

**clozapine** (Clozaril, FazaClo) (Psych). Dibenzapine antipsychotic drug used to treat psychosis and schizophrenia; used to treat the mania of manic-depressive disorder; used to treat suicidal behavior; used to treat psychosis and agitation in patients with Alzheimer's disease. Tablet: 12.5 mg, 25 mg, 50 mg, 100 mg, 200 mg. Orally disintegrating tablet: 25 mg, 100 mg. [KLAW-zah-peen].

**Clozaril** (Psych). See *clozapine*. [KLAW-zah-ril].

**Coagulin-B** (Hem). Gene drug for clotting factor IX that is carried on a virus vector; used to treat severe hemophilia. Intrahepatic. Intramuscular. Orphan drug. [koh-AG-yoo-lin B].

**coal tar** (Balnetar, Creamy Tar, Cutar Emulsion, DHS Tar, Doak Tar, Doak Tar Oil, Fototar, Ionil T Plus, Medotar, MG 217 Medicated Tar, Neutrogena T/Gel Original, Oxipor VHC, Packer's Pine Tar, PC-Tar, Pentrax, Polytar, Psorent, Taraphilic, Tera-Gel, Zetar) (Derm). Over-the-counter coal tar drug used topically to treat psoriasis, seborrheic dermatitis, and eczema. Bath liquid: 1.5%, 2.5%. Bath oil: 2%. Cream: 2%. Lotion: 5%, 25%. Topical liquid: 15%. Ointment: 1%, 2%. Shampoo: 0.5%, 1%, 1.2%, 2%, 4.5%, 5%, 6.6%. Soap: 2.5%. [KOHL tar].

**COBARTin** (GI). Used to treat steatorrhea in patients with short bowel syndrome. [koh-BAR-tin].

**cocaine** (Cocaine Viscous) (ENT). Schedule II anesthetic and vasoconstrictor drug used topically to decrease pain and bleeding of the mucous membranes during nose and throat procedures. Topical solution: 4%, 10%. Powder. [koh-KAYN].

**Cocaine Viscous** (ENT). See *cocaine*. [koh-KAYN VIS-kuhs].

**codeine** (Analges, ENT). Schedule II narcotic analgesic drug used to treat pain; antitussive drug used to treat chronic, dry cough. Tablet: 15 mg, 30 mg, 60 mg. Oral liquid: 15 mg/5 mL. Subcutaneous or intramuscular: 15 mg/mL, 30 mg/mL. [KOH-deen].

**Coease** (Ophth). See *sodium hyaluronate*. [KOH-eez].

**CoFactor** (Chemo). Chemotherapy drug used to treat pancreatic cancer. Orphan drug. [koh-FAK-tor].

**Cogentin** (Neuro). See *benztropine*. [koh-JEN-tin].

**Co-Gesic** (Analges) (generic *acetaminophen, hydrocodone*). Schedule III combination nonnarcotic and narcotic analgesic drug for pain. Tablet: 500 mg/5 mg. [koh-JEE-sik].

**Cognex** (Neuro). See *tacrine*. [KAWG-neks].

**Colace** (GI). See *docusate*. [KOH-lays].

**Colace Infant/Child, Colace Suppository** (GI). See *glycerin*. [KOH-lays].

**Colazal** (GI). See *balsalazide*. [KOL-ah-zal].

**colchicine** (Derm, GI, Ortho). Used to decrease uric acid levels to treat gout and gouty arthritis; used to treat hepatic and biliary cirrhosis; used to treat scleroderma; orphan drug used to treat multiple sclerosis. Tablet: 0.6 mg. Injection: 0.5 mg/mL. [KOHL-chih-seen].

**colesevelam** (WelChol) (Cardio, Endo). Bile acid sequestrant drug used to treat hypercholesterolemia; used to improve blood glucose control in patients with type 2 diabetes mellitus. Tablet: 625 mg. [KOH-leh-SEV-eh-lam].

**Colestid** (Cardio, GI). See *colestipol*. [koh-LES-tid].

**colestipol** (Colestid) (Cardio, GI). Bile acid sequestrant drug used to treat high cholesterol levels; used to treat digitalis toxicity; used to relieve itching in patients with biliary obstruction. Granules: 5 g. Tablet: 1 g. [koh-LES-tih-pohl].

**colfosceril** (Exosurf, Exosurf Neonate) (Pulm). Surfactant drug used to treat adult respiratory distress syndrome; used to prevent and treat respiratory distress syndrome in premature newborns. Liquid (via endotracheal tube). Orphan drug. [kohl-FAWS-keh-ril].

**colistimethate** (Coly-Mycin M) (Anti-infec). Antibiotic drug used to treat gram-negative bacterial infections. Intramuscular or intravenous (powder to be reconstituted): 150 mg. [koh-LIS-tih-METH-ate].

**collagen** (Colloral) (Ortho). Used to treat juvenile rheumatoid arthritis. Orphan drug. [KAWL-ah-jen].

**collagenase** (Plaquase, Santyl) (Derm, Uro). Enzyme drug used topically to debride burns and wounds (Santyl); orphan drug used to treat Peyronie disease (chordee of the penis (Plaquase). Ointment: 250 units. [koh-LAJ-eh-nays].

**colloidal oatmeal** (Aveeno, Aveeno Moisturizing) (Derm). Over-the-counter antipruritic drug used topically to treat itching and soothe the skin. Cream: 1%. Lotion: 1%. [koh-LOY-dal OHT-meel].

**Colloral** (Ortho). See *collagen*. [kawl-OR-al].

**Colomed** (Chemo, GI). Used to treat proctitis caused by radiation therapy; used to treat ulcerative colitis. Enema. Solution. Orphan drug. [KOH-loh-med].

**Coly-Mycin M** (Anti-infec). See *colistimethate*. [KOH-lee-MY-sin M].

**Coly-Mycin S Otic** (ENT) (generic *hydrocortisone, neomycin*). Combination antibiotic and corticosteroid drug used topically to treat inflammation and bacterial infection of the ear. Ear drops: 1%/3 mg/4.71 mg. [KOH-lee-MY-sin S OH-tik].

**CoLyte** (GI) (generic *polyethylene glycol, electrolyte solution*). Combination bowel evacuant and bowel prep. Oral liquid (powder to be reconstituted). [KOH-lite]

**Combigan** (Ophth) (generic *brimonidine, timolol*). Combination alpha receptor stimulant and beta-blocker drug used to treat glaucoma. Ophthalmic solution: 0.2%/0.5%. [KAWM-bih-gan].

**CombiPatch** (OB/GYN) (generic *norethindrone, estradiol*). Combination hormone drug used to treat the symptoms of menopause; used to treat primary ovarian failure. Transdermal patch: 0.14 mg/0.05 mg (9 cm$^2$), 0.25 mg/0.05 mg (16 cm$^2$). [KAWM-bih-patch].

**Combivent** (Pulm) (generic *albuterol, ipratropium*). Combination bronchodilator drug used to treat bronchospasm with chronic obstructive pulmonary disease. Aerosol inhaler: 103 mcg/18 mcg per puff. [KAWM-bih-vent].

**Combivir** (Anti-infec) (generic *lamivudine, zidovudine*). Combination nucleoside reverse transcriptase inhibitor antiviral drug used to treat HIV and AIDS. Tablet: 150 mg/300 mg. [KAWM-bih-veer].

**Combunox** (Analges) (generic *acetaminophen, oxycodone*). Combiantion Schedule II nonnarcotic and narcotic drug used to treat pain. Capsule: 325 mg/5 mg. [KAWM-byoo-nawks].

**Commit** (Pulm, Psych). See *nicotine*. [koh-MIT].

**Compazine** (Analges, GI, Psych). See *prochlorperazine*. [KAWM-pah-zeen].

**Compleat Modified Formula** (GI). Lactose-free nutritional supplement. Liquid. [kawm-PLEET].

**Compound 347** (Anes). See *eflorane*. [KAWM-pound 347].

**Compound W, Compound W for Kids** (Derm). See *salicylic acid*. [KAWM-pound W].

**Compoz Nighttime Sleep Aid** (Neuro). See *diphenydramine*. [com-POHZ].

**Compro** (Analges, GI, Psych). See *prochlorperazine*. [KAWM-proh].

**Comtan** (Neuro). See *entacapone*. [KAWM-tan].

**Comtrex Acute Head Cold Maximum Strength, Comtrex Nighttime Acute Head Cold Maximum Strength, Comtrex Nighttime Flu Therapy Maximum Strength** (ENT) (generic *acetaminophen, brompheniramine, pseudoephedrine*). Combination over-the-counter analgesic, antihistamine, and decongestant drug used to treat allergies and sinus pain. Liquid: 166.7 mg/0.67 mg/10 mg. Tablet: 500 mg/2 mg/30 mg. [KAWM-treks].

**Comtrex Cold and Cough Relief Multisymptom, Comtrex Maximum Strength Nighttime Cold & Cough** (ENT) (generic *acetaminophen, chlorpheniramine, dextromethorphan, pseudoephedrine*). Combination over-the-counter analgesic, antihistamine, nonnarcotic antitussive, and decongestant drug used to treat allergies and colds. Liquid: 166.7 mg/0.67 mg/5 mg/10 mg. Tablet: 500 mg/2 mg/15 mg/30 mg. [KAWM-treks].

**Comtrex Multi-Symptom Deep Chest Cold** (ENT) (generic *acetaminophen, dextromethorphan, guaifenesin, pseudoephedrine*). Combination analgesic, antitussive, expectorant, and decongestant drug used to treat colds with productive coughs. Softgel: 250 mg/10 mg/100 mg/30 mg. [KAWM-treks].

**Comtrex Multi-Symptom Maximum Strength Non-Drowsy Cold & Cough Relief** (ENT) (generic *acetaminophen, dextromethorphan, pseudoephedrine*). Combination over-the-counter analgesic, nonnarcotic antitussive, and decongestant drug used to treat coughs and colds. Tablet: 500 mg/15 mg/30 mg. [KAWM-treks].

**Comtrex Maximum Strength Sore Throat** (Analges, ENT). See *acetaminophen*. [KAWM-treks].

**Comtrex Sinus & Nasal Decongestant Maximum Strength** (ENT) (generic *acetaminophen, chlorpheniramine, pseudoephedrine*). Combination analgesic, antihistamine, and decongestant drug used to treat nasal and sinus allergies and colds. Tablet: 500 mg/2 mg/30 mg. [KAWM-treks].

**Comvax** (Misc). Combination drug used to prevent *H. influenzae* and hepatitis B infection in children. Subcutaneous: Vaccine. [KAWM-vaks].

**Concerta** (Neuro, Psych). See *methylphenidate*. [kawn-SER-tah].

**Condylox** (Derm. OB/GYN). See *podofilox*. [KAWN-dih-lawks].

**conivaptan** (Vaprisol) (Endo). Antagonist drug used to block the hormone vasopressin and treat syndrome of inappropriate ADH (SIADH). Intravenous: 5 mg/mL. [koh-NY-vap-tan].

**conjugated estrogens** (Cenestin, Enjuvia, Premarin, Premarin Intravenous, Premarin Vaginal) (Chemo, OB/GYN, Ortho). Hormone drug used to treat hot flashes and vaginal dryness of menopause; used to treat abnormal uterine bleeding; used to prevent osteoporosis in postmenopausal women; palliative chemotherapy for advanced breast and prostate cancer. Tablet: 0.3 mg, 0.45 mg, 0.625 mg, 0.9 mg, 1.25 mg. Cream: 0.625 mg. Intramuscular or intravenous: 25 mg/5 mL. [KAWN-joo-gay-ted ES-troh-jens].

**Constulose** (GI). See *lactulose*. [KAWNS-tyoo-lohs].

**Contact Severe Cold & Flu** (ENT) (generic *acetaminophen, chlorpheniramine, dextromethorphan, pseudoephedrine*). Combination over-the-counter analgesic, antihistamine, nonnarcotic antitussive, and decongestant drug for colds and flu. Tablet: 500 mg/2 mg/15 mg/30 mg. [KAWN-takt].

**Contraceptrol** (OB/GYN). See *nonoxynol-9*. [KAWN-trah-SEP-trawl].

**Copaxone** (Neuro). See *glatiramer*. [koh-PAK-zohn].

**Copegus** (Anti-infec, GI, Pulm). See *ribavirin*. [KOH-peh-gus].

**Coramsine** (Chemo) (generic *solasonine, solamargine*). Combination chemotherapy drug used to treat malignant melanoma and kidney cancer. Orphan drug. [koh-RAM-ih-seen].

**Coraz** (Derm). See *hydrocortisone*. [KOR-az].

**Cordarone** (Cardio). See *amiodarone*. [KOR-dah-rohn].

**Cordox** (Hem). Used to treat sickle cell disease. Orphan drug. [KOR-dawks].

**Cordran, Cordran SP** (Derm). See *flurandrenolide*. [KOR-dran].

**Coreg, Coreg CR** (Cardio). See *carvedilol*. [KOH-reg].

**Corgard** (Analges, Cardio, GI, Neuro). See *nadolol*. [KOR-gard].

**Coricidin D Cold, Flu, and Sinus** (ENT) (generic *acetaminophen, chlorpheniramine, pseudoephedrine*). Combination over-the-counter analgesic, antihistamine, and decongestant drug for colds and sinus. Tablet: 325 mg/2mg/30 mg. [KOR-ih-SEE-din].

**Coricidin HBP Maximum Strength Flu** (ENT) (generic *acetaminophen, chlorpheniramine, dextromethorphan*). Combination over-the-counter analgesic, antihistamine, and nonnarcotic antitussive drug for colds, flu, and coughs. Tablet: 500 mg/2 mg/4 mg. [KOR-ih-SEE-din].

**Corlopam** (Cardio). See *fenoldopam*. [KOR-loh-pam].

**Cormax** (Derm). See *clobetasol*. [KOR-maks].

**Correctol** (GI). See *bisacodyl*. [koh-REK-tawl].

**CortaGel Extra Strength** (Derm). See *hydrocortisone*. [KOR-tah-jel].

**Cortaid Faststick Maximum Strength, Cortaid Intensive Therapy, Cortaid Maximum Strength, Cortaid with Aloe** (Derm). See *hydrocortisone*. [KORT-aid].

**Cort-Dome, Cort-Dome High Potency** (Derm, GI). See *hydrocortisone*. [KORT-dohm].

**Cortef** (Endo, Ortho). See *hydrocortisone*. [KOR-tef].

**Cortef Feminine Itch** (Derm). See *hydrocortisone*. [KOR-tef].

**Corticaine** (Derm). See *hydrocortisone*. [KOR-tih-kayn].

**corticotrophin** (Endo). See *respository corticotropin*. [KOR-tih-koh-TROH-pin].

**corticotropin-releasing factor** (Xerecept) (Neuro). Used to treat edema from a brain tumor. Orphan drug. [KOR-tih-koh-TROH-pin].

**Cortifoam** (GI). See *hydrocortisone*. [KOR-tih fohm].

**cortisone** (Derm, Endo, GI, Hem, Ortho). Corticosteroid anti-inflammatory drug used as replacement therapy for Addison's disease; used to treat severe inflammation in various body systems; used to treat collagen diseases, skin diseases, regional enteritis, and ulcerative colitis; used to

treat thrombocytopenia and some types of anemia; used to treat the pain and inflammation of osteoarthritis and rheumatoid arthritis. Tablet: 25 mg. [KOR-tih-sohn].

**Cortisporin** (Derm) (generic *neomycin, hydrocortisone*). Combination antibiotic and corticosteroid drug used topically to treat inflammation and infection of the skin. Cream: 0.5%/0.5%. Ointment: 0.5%/1%. [KOR-tih-SPOR-in].

**Cortisporin Otic** (ENT) (generic *hydrocortisone, neomycin, polymyxin B*). Combination corticosteroid and antibiotic drug used topically to treat ear infections. Ear drops: 1%/5 mg/10,000 units. [KOR-tih-SPOR-in OH-tik].

**Cortizone-5, Cortizone for Kids, Cortizone-10, Cortizone-10 External Anal Itch, Cortizone-10 Plus, Cortizone-10 Quickshot** (Derm). See *hydrocortisone*. [KOR-tih-zohn].

**Cortrosyn** (Endo). See *cosyntropin*. [KOR-troh-sin].

**Corvert** (Cardio). See *ibutilide*. [KOR-vert].

**Corzide 40/5, Corzide 80/5** (Cardio) (generic *nadolol, bendroflumethiazide*). Combination beta-blocker and diuretic drug used to treat hypertension. Tablet: 40 mg/5 mg, 80 mg/5 mg. [KOR-zide].

**Cosmegen** (Chemo). See *dactinomycin*. [KAWS-meh-jen].

**CosmoDerm** (Derm). See *human collagen*. [KAWS-moh-derm].

**CosmoPlast** (Derm). See *human collagen*. [KAWS-moh-plast].

**Cosopt** (Ophth) (generic *dorzolamide, timolol*). Combination carbonic anhydrase inhibitor and beta-blocker drug used topically in the eye to treat glaucoma. Ophthalmic solution: 2%0.5%. [KOH-sawpt].

**cosyntropin** (Cortrosyn) (Endo). Corticotropin (ACTH) drug used in diagnostic testing to assess adrenal cortex function. Intramuscular or intravenous (powder to be reconstituted): 0.25 mg. [KOH-sin-TROH-pin].

**Cotrim Pediatric** (Anti-infec) (generic *sulfamethoxazole, trimethoprim*). Combination antibiotic and sulfonamide anti-infective drug used to treat bronchitis, otitis media, traveler's diarrhea, and urinary tract infections. Oral suspension: 200 mg/40 mg per 5 mL. [KOH-trim PEE-dee-AH-trik].

**Coumadin** (Cardio, Hem, Neuro). See *warfarin*. [KOO-mah-din].

**coumarin** (Onkolox) (Chemo). Chemotherapy drug used to treat cancer of the kidney. Orphan drug. [KOO-mah-rin].

**Covera-HS** (Analges, Cardio). See *verapamil*. [koh-VAIR-ah-H-S].

**Cozaar** (Cardio). See *losartan*. [KOH-zar].

**Creamy Tar** (Derm). See *coal tar*. [KREE-mee tar].

**Creapure** (Neuro). See *creatine*. [KREE-ah-pyoor].

**creatine** (Creapure) (Neuro). Used to treat amyotrophic lateral sclerosis and Huntingdon disease. Orphan drug. [KREE-ah-teen].

**Creon 5, Creon 10, Creon 20** (GI) (generic *amylase, lipase, protease*). Combination digestive enzyme drug used as replacement therapy. Delayed-release capsule: 16,000 units/5000 units/18,750 units; 33,200 units/10,000 units/37,500 units; 66,400 units/20,000 units/75,000 units. [KREE-awn].

**Crestor** (Cardio). See *rosuvastatin*. [KRES-tor].

**Crinone** (OB/GYN). See *progesterone*. [KRY-nohn].

**Criticare HN** (GI). Lactose-free nutritional supplement. Liquid. [KRIT-ih-kair H-N].

**Crixivan** (Anti-infec). See *indinavir*. [KRIK-sih-van].

**CroFab** (Emerg). See *crotalidae polyvalent immune fab*. [KROH-fab]

**Crolom** (Ophth). See *cromolyn*. [KROH-lawm].

**cromolyn** (Crolom, Gastrocrom, Intal, Nasalcrom, Opticrom) (ENT, GI, Ophth, Pulm). Prescription and over-the-counter mast cell stabilizer drug used topically to treat allergic symptoms in the nose; inhaled to prevent asthma and bronchospasm; given orally to prevent the release of histamine in patients with food allergies; used topically to treat allergy symptoms in the eyes. Aerosol: 800 mcg/puff. Inhalation solution: 20 mg/2 mL. Oral liquid: 100 mg/5 mL. Nasal solution: 40 mg/mL, 5.2 mg/spray. Ophthalmic solution: 4%. [KROH-moh-lin].

**Cronassial** (Ophth). See *gangliosides*. [kroh-NAZ-ee-al].

**crotalidae polyvalent immune fab** (Antivipmyn, CroFab) (Emerg). Antivenom drug given after a rattlesnake bite. Intravenous (powder to be reconstituted): 1 g. [kroh-TAL-ih-dee PAWL-ee-VAY-lent im-MYOON FAB].

**crotamiton** (Eurax) (Derm). Scabicide drug used topically to treat parasitic infection from scabies (mites). Cream: 10%. Lotion: 10%. [kroh-TAM-ih-ton].

**Cruex** (Derm). See *clotrimazole*. [KROO-eks].

**Cruex Aerosol, Cruex Powder** (Derm). See *undecylenic acid*. [KROO-eks].

**cryoprecipitate** (I.V.). Plasma product that contains no blood cells; used to replace plasma proteins and clotting factors in hemophiliacs and patients with von Willebrand's disease. Intravenous. [KRY-oh-pree-SIP-ih-tayt].

**Cryptaz** (GI). See *nitazoxanide*. [KRIP-taz].

**Cryselle** (OB/GYN) (generic *norgestrel, ethinyl estradiol*). Combination monophasic oral contraceptive drug. Pill pack (Pilpak), 21-day: (21 hormone tablets) 0.3 mg/30 mcg. Pill pack (Pilpak), 28-days: (21 hormone tablets) 0.3 mg/30 mcg; (7 inert tablets). [krih-SEL].

**crystalloid** (I.V.). Normal saline and lactated Ringer's intravenous fluids. Intravenous. [KRIS-tay-loyd].

**Crystamine** (Hem). See *cyanocobalamin*. [KRIS-tah-meen].

**Crysti 1000** (Hem). See *cyanocobalamin*. [KRIS-tee 1000].

**Cubicin** (Anti-infec). See *daptomycin*. [KYOO-bih-sin].

**Cuprimine** (Ortho, Uro). See *penicillamine*. [KOO-prih-meen].

**Curosurf** (Pulm). See *poractant alfa*. [KYOOR-oh-surf].

**Cutar Emulsion** (Derm). See *coal tar*. [KYOO-tar ee-MUL-shun].

**Cutivate** (Derm). See *fluticasone*. [KYOO-tih-vayt].

**cyanocobalamin** (Crystamine, Crysti 1000, Cyanoject, Cyomin, Nascobal, Rubesol-1000) (Hem). Vitamin $B_{12}$ drug used to treat pernicious anemia. Intranasal spray: 500 mcg/0.1 mL. Tablet: 500 mcg, 1000 mcg. Intramuscular or subcutaneous: 100 mcg/mL, 1000 mcg/mL. [sy-AN-oh-koh-BAWL-ah-min].

**Cyanoject** (Hem). See *cyanocobalamin*. [sy-AN-oh-jekt].

**Cyanokit** (Emerg). See *hydroxocobalamin*. [sy-AN-oh-kit].

**Cyclessa** (OB/GYN) (generic *desogestrel, ethinyl estradiol*). Combination triphasic oral contraceptive drug. Pill pack, 28-day: (7 hormone tablets) 0.1 mg/25 mcg; (7 hormone tablets) 0.125 mg/25 mcg; (7 hormone tablets) 0.15 mg/25 mcg; (7 inert tablets). [sy-KLES-sah].

**cyclizine** (Marezine) (GI). Antiemetic drug used to treat nausea and vomiting; used to treat motion sickness. Tablet: 50 mg. [SY-klih-zeen].

**cyclobenzaprine** (Amrix, Flexeril) (Ortho). Skeletal muscle relaxant drug used to treat spasm and stiffness associated with minor muscle injuries; used to treat fibromyalgia. Extended-release capsule: 15 mg, 30 mg. Tablet: 5 mg, 10 mg. [SY-kloh-BEN-zah-preen].

**Cyclogyl** (Ophth). See *cyclopentolate*. [SY-kloh-jel].

**Cyclomydril** (Ophth) (generic *cyclopentolate, phenylephrine*). Combination mydriatic drug used topically to dilate the pupil before eye examinations or surgery. Ophthalmic solution: 0.2%/1%. [SY-kloh-MY-dril].

**cyclopentolate** (AK-Pentolate, Cyclogyl, Pentolair) (Ophth). Mydriatic drug used topically to dilate the pupil prior to eye examination or surgery. Ophthalmic solution: 0.5%, 1%, 2%. [SY-kloh-PEN-toh-layt].

**cyclophosphamide** (Cytoxan, Cytoxan Lyophilized, Neosar) (Chemo, Uro). Alkylating chemotherapy drug used to treat Hodgkin's lymphoma, non-Hodgkin's lymphoma, multiple myeloma, leukemia, mycosis fungoides, and cancer of the eye, breast, and ovary; used to treat nephrotic syndrome in children. Tablet: 25 mg, 50 mg. Intravenous: 100 mg. [SY-kloh-FAWS-fah-mide].

**Cycloprostin** (Hem). See *epoprostenol*. [SY-kloh-PRAWS-tin].

**cycloserine** (Seromycin Pulvules) (Pulm). Antitubercular antibiotic drug used to treat tuberculosis that has become resistant to other antitubercular drugs. Capsule: 250 mg. [SY-kloh-SEER-een].

**Cyclospire** (Hem). See *liposomal cyclosporin A*. [SY-kloh-spyr].

**cyclosporine A** (Neuro). Used to treat amyotrophic lateral sclerosis. Orphan drug. [SY-kloh-SPOR-een A].

**cyclosporine** (Gengraf, Neoral, Optimmune, Restasis, Sandimmune) (Cardio, Derm, GI, Hem, Ophth, Ortho, Uro). Immunosuppressant drug used to treat severe psoriasis; used to treat rheumatoid arthritis; used after transplantation to prevent rejection of the donor heart, liver, or kidney; used after bone marrow transplantation to prevent graft-versus-host disease; used topically to treat dry eyes (Restasis); orphan drug used to treat the dry eyes of Sjögren's syndrome (Optimmune). Capsule: 25 mg, 100 mg. Gel capsule: 25 mg, 50 mg, 100 mg. Oral liquid: 100 mg/mL. Injection: 50 mg/mL. Ophthalmic emulsion: 0.05%. [SY-kloh-SPOR-een].

**Cyklokapron** (Hem). See *tranexamic acid*. [SY-kloh-KAP-rawn].

**Cymbalta** (Neuro, Psych). See *duloxetine*. [sim-BAL-tah].

**Cylexin** (Pulm).  To promote pulmonary reperfusion after cardiopulmonary bypass surgery. Orphan drug. [sy-LEK-sin].

**Cyomin** (Hem).  See *cyanocobalamin.* [SY-oh-min].

**cyproheptadine** (Derm, ENT, Ophth).  Antihistamine drug used to treat allergic skin reactions and itching; used to treat the symptoms of seasonal and perennial allergies, allergic rhinitis, and allergic conjunctivitis. Syrup: 2 mg/5 mL. Tablet: 4 mg. [SIH-proh-HEP-tah-deen].

**cyproterone** (Androcur) (Endo).  Used to treat severe hirsutism. Orphan drug. [sy-PROH-teh-rohn].

**Cystadane** (Uro).  See *betaine.* [SIS-tah-dayn].

**Cystagon** (Uro).  See *cysteamine.* [SIS-tah-gawn].

**cysteamine** (Cystagon) (Uro).  Used to treat nephropathic cystinosis. Capsule: 50 mg, 150 mg. [sis-TEE-ah-meen].

**Cystex** (Uro) (generic *methenamine, sodium salicylate*).  Combination antibiotic and analgesic drug used to treat urinary tract infections. Tablet. [SIS-teks].

**Cystospaz** (GI, Uro).  See *L-hyoscyamine.* [SIS-toh-spaz].

**Cytadren** (Chemo, Endo).  See *aminoglutethimide.* [SY-tah-dren].

**cytarabine** (DepoCyt, Tarabine PFS) (Chemo).  Antimetabolite chemotherapy drug used to treat leukemia, Hodgkin's lymphoma, and cancerous meningitis. Subcutaneous, intravenous, or intrathecal: 10 mg/mL, 20 mg/mL. [sy-TAIR-ah-been].

**CytoGam** (Anti-infec).  See *cytomegalovirus immunoglobulin.* [SY-toh-gam].

**Cytoimplant** (Chemo).  Chemotherapy drug used to treat pancreatic cancer. Orphan drug. [SY-toh-IM-plant].

**cytomegalovirus immunoglobulin** (CytoGam) (Anti-infec).  Antiviral drug used to prevent cytomegalovirus infection in AIDS patients and organ transplant patients. Intravenous: 10 mg/mL. [SY-toh-MEG-ah-loh-VY-rus IM-myoo-noh-GLAW-byoo-lin).

**Cytomel** (Endo).  See *liothyronine.* [SY-toh-mel].

**Cytotec** (GI, OB/GYN).  See *misoprostol.* [SY-toh-tek].

**Cytovene** (Anti-infec).  See *ganciclovir.* [SY-toh-veen].

**Cytoxan, Cytoxan Lyophilized** (Chemo, Uro).  See *cyclophosphamide.* [sy-TAWK-san].

**dacarbazine** (DTIC-Dome) (Chemo).  Alkylating chemotherapy drug used to treat cancer of the thyroid gland, pancreas, and bone; used to treat malignant melanoma, Hodgkin's lymphoma, Kaposi's sarcoma, and pheochromocytoma of the adrenal gland. Intravenous (powder to be reconstituted): 100 mg, 200 mg. [dah-KAR-bah-zeen].

**daclizumab** (Zenapax) (Chemo, Uro).  Monoclonal antibody drug used to prevent rejection of the kidney after organ transplantation; orphan drug used to prevent graft-versus-host disease after bone marrow transplanation. Intravenous: 25 mg/5 mL. [dah-KLIZ-yoo-mab].

**Dacogen** (Chemo).  See *decitabine.* [DAY-koh-jen].

**dactinomycin** (Cosmegen) (Chemo).  Chemotherapy antibiotic drug used to treat bone and testicular cancer; used to treat rhabdomyosarcoma, malignant melanoma, and Wilm's tumor. Intravenous (powder to be reconstituted): 500 mcg. [dak-TIN-oh-MY-sin].

**Dairy Ease** (Misc).  See *lactase.* [DAIR-ee-EEZ].

**Dakin's solution** (Derm).  Over-the-counter antiseptic solution used topically on the skin. [DAY-kinz].

**Dalmane** (Neuro).  See *flurazepam* [dal-MAYN].

**dalteparin** (Fragmin) (Cardio, Hem, Uro).  Low molecular weight heparin anticoagulant drug used to prevent deep venous thrombosis in patients undergoing abdominal or joint replacement surgery or those wth poor mobility; used to prevent a blood clot in patients with acute coronary syndrome, unstable angina, and myocardial infarction; used to provide anticoagulation during hemodialysis for patients in chronic renal failure. Subcutaneous: 2500 units/0.2 mL; 5000 units/0.2 mL; 7500 units/0.3 mL; 10,000 units/0.4 mL; 10,000 units/1 mL; 12,500 units/0.5 mL; 15,000 units/0.6 mL; 18,000 units/0.72 mL; 95,000 units/3.8 mL; 95,000 units/9.5 mL. [DAL-teh-PAIR-in].

**danazol** (Endo, OB/GYN).  Male sex hormone used to treat precocious puberty; used to treat gynecomastia in males; used to treat endometriosis and fibrocystic breast disease in females; used to treat hereditary angioedema. Capsule: 50 mg, 100 mg, 200 mg. [DAN-ah-zohl].

**Dantrium** (Anes, Ortho, Psych).  See *dantrolene.* [DAN-tree-um].

**dantrolene** (Dantrium) (Anes, Ortho, Psych).  Skeletal muscle relaxant drug used to treat severe muscle spasticity associated with multiple sclerosis, cerebral palsy, stroke, or spinal cord injury; used to treat intraoperative malignant hyperthermia; used to treat neuroleptic malignant syndrome caused by antipsychotic drugs. Capsule: 25 mg, 50 mg, 100 mg. Intravenous (powder to be reconstituted): 20 mg/70 mL. [DAN-troh-leen].

**dapiprazole** (Rev-Eyes) (Ophth).  Used topically in the eyes to reverse the effects of a mydriatic drug. Ophthalmic solution: 0.5%. [dah-PY-prah-zohl].

**dapsone** (Anti-infec, Ortho).  Antibiotic drug used to treat *Pneumocystis carinii* pneumonia and toxoplasmosis in AIDS patients; used to treat leishmaniasis and leprosy; used to treat rheumatoid arthritis. Tablet: 25 mg, 100 mg. [DAP-sohn].

**Daptacel** (Misc).  Combination drug used to prevent diphtheria, pertussis, and tetanus. Subcutaneous: Vaccine. [DAP-tah-sel].

**daptomycin** (Cubicin) (Anti-infec).  Used to treat staphylococcal and streptococcal skin and blood infections. Intravenous: 500 mg/10 mL. [DAP-toh-MY-sin].

**Daraprim** (Anti-infec).  See *pyrimethamine.* [DAIR-ah-prim].

**darbepoetin alfa** (Aranesp) (Hem).  Recombinant DNA technology erythropoietin-type drug that stimulates red blood cell production to treat anemia associated with chronic renal failure and chemotherapy. Subcutaneous or intravenous: 25 mcg/0.42 mL, 25 mcg/1 mL, 40 mcg/0.4 mL, 40 mcg/1 mL, 60 mcg/0.3 mL, 60 mcg/1 mL, 100 mcg/0.5 mL, 100 mcg/1 mL, 150 mcg/0.3 mL,

150 mcg/0.75 mL, 200 mcg/0.4 mL, 200 mcg/1 mL, 300 mcg/0.6 mL, 300 mcg/1 mL, 500 mcg/1 mL. [DAR-bee-POH-eh-tin AL-fah].

**darifenacin** (Enablex) (Uro). Anticholinergic drug used to treat the urgency and frequency of overactive bladder. Extended-release tablet: 7.5 mg, 15 mg. [DAR-ih-FEN-oh-sin]

**darunavir** (Prezista) (Anti-infec). Protease inhibitor antiviral drug used to treat HIV and AIDS. Tablet: 300 mg, 600 mg. [dah-ROO-nah-veer].

**Darvocet-N 50, Darvocet-N 100, Darvocet A500** (Analges) (generic *acetaminophen, propoxyphene*). Combination Schedule IV nonsalicylate and narcotic analgesic drug for pain. Tablet: 325 mg/50 mg, 500 mg/100 mg, 650 mg/100 mg. [DAR-voh-set].

**Darvon-N, Darvon Pulvules** (Analges). See *propoxyphene*. [DAR-vawn].

**dasatinib** (Sprycel) (Chemo). Chemotherapy drug used to treat leukemia. Tablet: 20 mg, 50 mg, 70 mg. [dah-SAT-ih-nib].

**daunorubicin** (Cerubidine, DaunoXome) (Chemo). Chemotherapy antibiotic drug used to treat leukemia and Kaposi's sarcoma. Intravenous: 5 mg/mL. [DAW-noh-ROO-bih-sin].

**DaunoXome** (Chemo). See *daunorubicin*. [DAW-noh-zohm].

**DayHist-1** (Derm, ENT). See *clemastine*. [DAY-hist-1].

**Daypro, Daypro ALTA** (Analges). See *oxaprozin*. [DAY-proh].

**Daytrana** (Neuro, Psych). See *methylphenidate*. [day-TRAN-ah].

**DCVax-Brain** (Chemo). Vaccine used to treat brain cancer. Orphan drug. [D-C-vaks-BRAYN].

**DDAVP** (Endo, Hem). See *desmopressin*. [D-D-A-V-P].

**Debacterol** (ENT) (generic *sulfuric acid, sulfonated phenolics*). Combination chemical cautery and antiseptic drug used topically to treat canker sores and ulcerating mouth lesions. Topical liquid: 30%/50%. [deh-BAK-teh-rawl].

**debrase** (Debridase) (Derm). Used to debride deep burns. Orphan drug. [dee-BRAYS].

**Debridase** (Derm). See *debrase*. [deh-BREE-days].

**Debrisan** (Derm). See *dextranomer*. [deh-BREE-san].

**Debrox** (ENT). See *carbamide*. [dee-BRAWKS].

**Decadron** (Chemo, Derm, Endo, Ophth, Ortho). See *dexamethasone*. [DEK-ah-drawn].

**Decapeptyl** (Chemo). See *triptorelin*. [DEK-ah-PEP-til].

**Decaspray** (Derm). See *dexamethasone*. [DEK-ah-spray].

**decitabine** (Dacogen) (Chemo). Demethylating chemotherapy drug used to treat leukemia; used to treat myelodysplastic syndrome and anemia. Intravenous: 50 mg. [deh-SIT-ah-been].

**Declomycin** (Anti-infec, Endo). See *demeclocycline*. [DEK-loh-MY-sin].

**Deconamine, Deconamine SR** (ENT) (generic *chlorpheniramine, pseudoephedrine*). Combination antihistamine and decongestant drug used to treat allegies and colds. Capsule: 8 mg/120 mg. Syrup: 2 mg/30 mg. Tablet: 4 mg/60 mg. [deh-KAWN-ah-meen].

**deferasirox** (Exjade) (Hem). Chelating drug used to treat high levels of iron in patients receiving repeated blood transfusions. Tablet: 125 mg, 250 mg, 500 mg. [deh-FAIR-ah-SY-rawks].

**deferiprone** (Ferriprox) (Hem). Chelating drug used to treat high levels of iron in patients receiving repeated blood transfusions. Orphan drug. [dě-FAIR-ih-prohn].

**deferoxamine** (Desferal) (Emerg). Chelating drug used to treat iron or aluminum toxicity. Intravenous, intramuscular: 500 mg. [DEH-fair-AWK-sah-meen].

**defibrotide** (Hem). Used to treat thrombocytopenia purpura. Orphan drug. [dee-FIB-roh-tide].

**Defy** (Anti-infec, Ophth). See *tobramycin*. [dee-FY].

**Degas** (GI). See *simethicone*. [dee-GAS].

**Dehydrex** (Ophth). See *dextran 70*. [dee-HY-dreks].

**dehydroepiandrosterone** (DHEA, Fidelin) (Endo). Used to treat lupus erythematosus, adrenal insufficiency, and severe burns. Orphan drug. [dee-HY-droh-EP-ee-an-DRAWS-teh-rohn].

**Delatestryl** (Chemo, Endo). See *testosterone*. [DEL-ah-TES-tril].

**delavirdine** (Rescriptor) (Anti-infec). Nonnucleoside reverse transcriptase inhibitor antiviral drug used to treat HIV and AIDS. Tablet: 100 mg, 200 mg. [DEL-ah-VEER-deen].

**Delcort** (Derm). See *hydrocortisone*. [DEL-kort].

**Delestrogen** (Chemo, OB/GYN). See *estradiol*. [del-ES-troh-jen].

**Delfen** (OB/GYN). See *nonoxynol-9*. [DEL-fen].

**Deltasone** (Chemo, Endo, Ortho, Pulm, Neuro). See *prednisone*. [DEL-tah-zohn].

**Delta-Tritex** (Derm). See *triamcinolone*. [DEL-tah-TRY-teks].

**Demadex** (Cardio, Uro). See *torsemide*. [DEM-ah-deks].

**demeclocycline** (Declomycin) (Anti-infec, Endo). Tetracycline antibiotic drug used to treat infection due to gram-negative and gram-positive bacteria; used to treat pelvic inflammatory disease; used to treat intestinal infection caused by amoebas; used to treat pneumonia due to *S. pneumoniae, H. influenzae,* or *Mycoplasma;* used to treat Rocky Mountain spotted fever and *Chlamydia;* used to treat gonorrhea and syphilis; used to treat ulcerative gingivitis (trench mouth); used to treat the endocrine disorder of syndrome of inappropriate ADH. Tablet: 150 mg, 300 mg. [deh-MEK-loh-SY-kleen].

**Demerol** (Analges, Anes). See *meperidine*. [DEM-eh-rawl].

**Demser** (Endo). See *metyrosine*. [DEM-ser].

**Demulen 1/35** (OB/GYN) (generic *ethynodiol, ethinyl estradiol*). Combination monophasic oral contraceptive drug. Pill pack (Compack), 21-day: (21 hormone tablets) 1 mg/35 mcg. Pill pack (Compack), 28-day: (21 hormone tablets) 1 mg/35 mcg; (7 inert tablets). [DEM-yoo-len].

**Demulen 1/50** (OB/GYN) (generic *ethynodiol, ethinyl estradiol*). Combination monophasic oral contraceptive drug. Pill pack (Compack), 21-day: (21 hormone tablets) 1 mg/50 mcg.

Pill pack (Compack), 28-day: (21 hormone tablets) 1 mg/50 mcg; (7 inert tablets). [DEM-yoo-len].

**Denavir** (Anti-infec, Derm).    See *penciclovir.* [DEN-ah-veer].

**denileukin** (Ontak) (Chemo).    Chemotherapy recombinant DNA drug that combines interleukin-2 and diphtheria toxin protein to treat cutaneous T-cell lymphoma. Intravenous: 150 mcg/mL. [DEN-ih-LOO-kin].

**Denorex Everyday Dandruff** (Derm).    See *pyrithione zinc.* [DEN-oh-reks].

**Dentipatch** (Anes, Dent).    See *lidocaine.* [DEN-tih patch].

**Depacon** (Neuro).    See *valproic acid.* [DEP-ah-kawn].

**Depakene** (Neuro).    See *valproic acid.* [DEP-ah-keen].

**Depakote, Depakote ER** (Neuro).    See *valproic acid.* [DEP-ah-koht].

**Depen** (Ortho, Uro).    See *penicillamine.* [DEE-pen].

**Deplin** (Hem, OB/GYN).    See *folic acid.* [DEP-lin].

**DepoCyt** (Chemo).    See *cytarabine.* [DEP-oh-sit].

**DepoDur** (Analges, Anes).    See *morphine.* [DEP-oh-DYOOR].

**Depo-Estradiol** (OB/GYN).    See *estradiol.* [DEP-oh-ES-trah-DY-awl].

**Depo-Medrol** (Derm, Endo, Ortho, Pulm).    See *methylprednisolone.* [DEP-oh-MED-rawl].

**Depo-Provera** (Chemo, OB/GYN).    See *medroxyprogesterone.* [DEP-oh-proh-VAIR-ah].

**Depo-Sub Q Provera 104** (OB/GYN).    See *medroxyprogesterone.* [DEP-oh-sub Q proh-VAIR-ah 104].

**Depo-Testosterone** (Endo).    See *testosterone.* [DEP-oh-tehs-TAWS teh-rohn].

**depsipeptide** (Chemo).    Chemotherapy drug used to treat mycosis fungoides. Orphan drug. [DEP-sih-PEP-tide].

**Dermaflex** (Anes, Derm, GI).    See *lidocaine.* [DER-mah-fleks].

**Dermamycin** (Derm).    See *diphenhydramine.* [DER-mah-MY-sin].

**Dermarest, Dermarest Plus** (Derm).    See *diphenhydramine.* [DER-mah-rest].

**Derma-Smoothe/FS** (Derm).    See *fluocinolone.* [DER-mah-smooth-F-S].

**Dermatop E** (Derm).    See *prednicarbate.* [DER-mah-top E].

**Dermazinc** (Derm).    See *pyrithione zinc.* [DER-mah-zink].

**Dermol HC** (GI).    See *hydrocortisone.* [DER-mawl H-C].

**Dermolate** (Derm).    See *hydrocortisone.* [DER-moh-layt].

**Dermoplast** (Anes, Derm).    See *benzocaine.* [DER-moh-plast].

**Desenex Cream** (Derm).    See *clotrimazole.* [DES-eh-neks].

**Desenex Powder, Desenex Soap** (Derm).    See *undecylenic acid.* [DES-eh-neks].

**Desenex Prescription Strength** (Derm).    See *miconazole.* [DES-eh-neks].

**DesenexMyax** (Derm).    See *terbinafine.* [DES-eh-neks-MY-aks].

**Desferal** (Emerg).    See *deferoxamine.* [des-FAIR-al].

**desflurane** (Suprane) (Anes).    Anesthetic drug used to induce and maintain general anesthesia. Inhaled gas. [DES-floor-ayn].

**desiccated thyroid** (Armour Thyroid, Bio-Throid, Nature-Throid, Westhroid) (Endo).    Thyroid hormone replacement drug used to treat hypothyroidism. Capsule: 7.5 mg (1/8 grain), 15 mg (¼; grain), 30 mg (½; grain), 60 mg (1 grain), 90 mg (1½ grains), 120 mg (2 grains), 150 mg (2½ grains), 180 mg (3 grains), 240 mg (4 grains). Tablet: 15 mg (¼ grain), 30 mg or 32.5 mg (½ grain), 60 mg or 65 mg (1 grain), 90 mg (1½ grains), 120 mg or 130 mg (2 grains), 180 mg or 195 mg (3 grains), 240 mg (4 grains), 300 mg (5 grains). [DES-ih-kay-ted THY-royd]

**desipramine** (Norpramin) (Analges, Neuro, Psych, Uro).    Tricyclic antidepressant drug used to treat depression, anxiety, panic attacks, bulimia, and premenstrual dysphoric disorder; used to treat withdrawal from cocaine addiction; used to treat attention-deficit hyperactivity disorder; used to treat Tourette syndrome; used to treat nerve pain from phantom limb, diabetic neuropathy, peripheral neuropathy, and postherpetic neuralgia; used to treat enuresis; used to treat migraine headaches; used to treat tic douloureux. Tablet: 10 mg, 25 mg, 50 mg, 75 mg, 100 mg, 150 mg. [des-IP-rah-meen].

**desirudin** (Iprivask) (Hem).    Thrombin inhibitor drug used to prevent deep venous thrombosis during joint replacement surgery. Subcutaneous (powder to be reconstituted): 15 mg/0.6 mL. [deh-SIH-roo-din].

**Desitin** (Derm) (generic *vitamin A, vitamin E, zinc oxide*).    Combination over-the-counter vitamin and astringent drug used topically to treat skin irritation, diaper rash, and dry, oozing skin. [DES-ih-tin].

**desloratadine** (Clarinex, Clarinex RediTabs) (Derm, ENT).    Antihistamine drug used to treat seasonal and perennial allergies and allergic rhinitis; used to treat allergic skin reactions with itching. Syrup: 2.5 mg/5 mL. Tablet: 5 mg. Rapidly disintegrating tablet: 2.5 mg, 5 mg. [DES-lor-AT-ah-deen].

**desmopressin** (DDAVP, Minirin, Stimate) (Endo, Hem).    Vasopressin antidiuretic hormone (ADH) drug used as replacement therapy to treat diabetes insipidus; orphan drug used to treat hemophilia A and von Willibrand disease. Tablet: 0.1 mg, 0.2 mg. Nasal solution or spray (via spray pump or nasal tube delivery system): 0.1 mg/mL (10 mcg/spray), 1.5 mg/mL (150 mcg/spray). Subcutaneous or intravenous: 4 mcg/mL. [DEZ-moh-PRES-sin].

**Desogen** (OB/GYN) (generic *desogestrel, ethinyl estradiol*).    Combination monophasic oral contraceptive drug. Pill pack, 28-day: (21 hormone tablets) 0.15 mg/30 mcg; (7 inert tablets). [DES-oh-jen].

**desonide** (Desonate, DesOwen, LoKara, Verdeso) (Derm).    Corticosteroid drug used topically to treat inflammation and itching from dermatitis, seborrhea, eczema, psoriasis, and yeast or fungal infections. Cream: 0.05%. Foam: 0.05%. Gel: 0.05%. Lotion: 0.05%. Ointment: 0.05%. [DES-oh-nide]

**Desonate** (Derm).    See *desonide.* [DES-oh-nayt].

**DesOwen** (Derm).    See *desonide.* [des-OH-wen].

**desoximetasone** (Topicort, Topicort LP) (Derm).    Corticosteroid drug used topically to treat inflammation and itching from dermatitis, seborrhea, eczema, psoriasis, and yeast or fungal infections. Cream: 0.05%, 0.25%. Gel: 0.05%. Ointment: 0.25%. [deh-SAWK-sih-MET-ah-zohn].

**Desoxyn** (GI, Psych). See *methamphetamine*. [des-AWK-sin].

**Desquam-E 5, Desquam-E 10, Desquam-X 5, Desquam-X 10** (Derm). *benzoyl peroxide*. [DES-kwam].

**dessicated thyroid** (Armour Thyroid, Bio-Throid, Nature Throid, Westhroid) (Endo). Thyroid hormones $T_3$ and $T_4$ replacement drug used to treat hypothyroidism; used to suppress pituitary gland secretion of TSH to treat Hashimoto's thyroiditis and thyroid cancer. Tablet: 15 mg (¼ gr), 30 mg (½ gr), 32.4 mg, 32.5 mg, 60 mg (1 gr), 64.8 mg, 65 mg, 90 mg (1½ gr), 120 mg (2 gr), 129.6 mg, 130 mg, 180 mg (3 gr), 194.4 mg, 195 mg, 240 mg (4 gr), 300 mg (5 gr). Capsule: 7.5 mg (1/8 gr), 15 mg (¼ gr), 30 mg (½ gr), 60 mg (1 gr), 90 mg (1½ gr), 120 mg (2 gr), 150 mg (2½ gr), 180 mg (3 gr), 240 mg (4 gr). [DES-ih-kay-ted THY-royd].

**desvenlafaxine** (Pristiq) (Psych). Serotonin and norepinephrine reuptake inhibitor (SNRI) drug used to treat depression. Tablet: 50 mg, 100 mg. [des-VEN-lah-FAK-seen].

**Detrol, Detrol LA** (Uro). See *tolterodine*. [DEH-trawl].

**dexamethasone** (Decadron, Decaspray, Dexamethasone Intensol, Dexasol, Hexadrol, Maxidex, Posurdex) (Chemo, Derm, Endo, ENT, GI, Hem, Neuro, Ophth, Ortho, Pulm, Uro). Corticosteroid anti-inflammatory drug used to treat severe inflammation and edema in various body systems; used to decrease inflammation in allergic states and drug hypersensitivity reactions; used to treat collagen diseases; used to decrease cerebral edema; used to treat flareups of ulcerative colitis and regional enteritis; used to treat thrombocytopenia and some types of anemia; used to decrease the white blood cell count in leukemia and lymphoma; used to treat hypercalcemia associated with cancer; used as part of a chemotherapy protocol to decrease inflammation or to prevent nausea and vomiting; used to treat osteoarthritis and rheumatoid arthritis; injected near joints to treat bursitis and tenosynovitis; used topically in the eye to treat inflammation, choroiditis, and corneal injuries (Dexasol, Maxidex); orphan drug used to treat idiopathic uveitis (Posurdex); used to treat inflammation in the external ear canal; used topically to treat severe inflammation and itching from dermatitis, seborrhea, eczema, psoriasis, and yeast or fungal infections (Decaspray); used to treat inflammation associated with respiratory distress syndrome and aspiration pneumonitis; used to relieve edema from nephrotic syndrome and lupus erythematosus; used diagnostically to test the functioning of the adrenal gland cortex. Topical ophthalmic solution or suspension: 0.1%. Topical aerosol skin spray: 0.04%. Topical skin cream: 0.1%. Otic solution: 0.1%. Elixir: 0.5 mg/5 mL. Oral liquid: 0.5 mg/5 mL, 1 mg/mL. Tablet: 0.25 mg, 0.5 mg, 0.75 mg, 1 mg, 1.5 mg, 2 mg, 4 mg, 6 mg. Intramuscular, intravenous, intra-articular, soft tissue injection, or skin lesion injection: 4 mg/mL, 10 mg/mL, 20 mg/mL. [DEK-sah-METH-ah-zohn].

**Dexamethasone Intensol** (Chemo, Endo). See *dexamethasone*. [DEK-sah-METH-ah-sohn in-TEN-sawl].

**dexamabinol** (Neuro). Used to improve neurologic function after traumatic brain injury. Orphan drug. [DEKS-am-AB-ih-nawl].

**Dexasol** (Ophth). See *dexamethasone*. [DEK-sah-sawl].

**dexchlorpheniramine** (Derm, ENT, Ophth). Antihistamine drug used to treat symptoms of seasonal and perennial allergies, allergic rhinitis, allergic conjunctivitis, and skin allergies and itching. Syrup: 2 mg/5 mL. Extended-release tablet: 4 mg, 6 mg. [DEKS-klor-feh-NEER-ah-meen].

**Dexedrine, Dexedrine Spansules** (Neuro, Psych). See *dextroamphetamine*. [DEK-seh-dreen].

**DexFerrum** (Hem). See *iron dextran*. [deks-FAIR-um].

**Dex4 Glucose** (Endo). See *glucose*. [DEKS-4 GLOO-kohs].

**dexmedetomidine** (Precedex) (Anes, Pulm). Sedative drug used to sedate patients who are intubated and on the ventilator; used to prevent shivering during surgery; used with regional or general anesthesia. Intravenous: 100 mcg/mL. [DEKS-med-eh-TOH-mih-deen].

**dexmethylphenidate** (Focalin, Focalin XR) (Psych). Schedue II central nervous system stimulant drug used to treat attention-deficit/hyperactivity disorder. Tablet: 2.5 mg, 5 mg, 10 mg. Extended-release capsule: 5 mg, 10 mg, 15 mg, 20 mg. [deks-METH-il-FEN-ih-dayt].

**dexpanthenol** (Ilopan, Panthoderm) (Derm, GI). Over-the-counter and prescription drug used topically to treat itching skin (Panthoderm); gastric stimulant drug given after abdominal surgery to decrease the risk of postoperative ileus (Ilopan). Cream: 2%. Intramuscular or intravenous: 250 mg/mL. [deks-PAN-theh-nawl].

**dexrazoxane** (Zinecard) (Cardio, Chemo). Cytoprotective drug used to prevent cardiac toxicity in patients receiving doxorubicin or epirubicin chemotherapy; orphan drug used to treat skin sloughing from intravenous anthracyline. Intravenous (powder to be reconstituted): 10 mg/mL. [DEKS-rah-ZAWK-sayn].

**dextran 1** (Promit) (I.V.). Given intravenously before a dextran infusion to prevent an anaphylactic reaction; orphan drug used to treat cystic fibrosis. Intravenous: 150 mg/mL. [DEKS-tran 1].

**dextran 40** (Gentran 40, Rheomacrodex) (I.V.). Low molecular weight dextran, a nonblood plasma volume expander. Intravenous. [DEKS-tran 40].

**dextran 70** (Dehydrex, Gentran 70, Macrodex) (Emerg, Ophth). High molecular weight dextran used as a nonblood plasma volume expander; used topically in the eye to treat corneal erosion (Dehydrex). Orphan drug. [DEKS-trans 70].

**dextran 75** (I.V.) High molecular weight dextran; a nonblood plasma volume expander. [DEKS-tran 75].

**dextranomer** (Debrisan) (Derm). Over-the-counter debriding drug used topically to remove necrotic tissue from burns, skin ulcers, and wounds. Beads. Paste. [deks-TRAN-oh-mer].

**dextran sulfate** (Uendex) (Anti-infec, Pulm). Used to treat HIV and AIDS; inhaled to treat cystic fibrosis. Aerosol inhaler. Orphan drug. [DEKS-tran SUL-fayt].

**dextroamphetamine** (Dexedrine, Dexedrine Spansules, DextroStat, Liquadd). (Neuro, Psych). Schedule II amphetamine stimulant drug used to treat attention-deficit/hyperactivity disorder; used to treat narcolepsy. Extended-release capsule: 5 mg, 10 mg, 15 mg. Tablet: 5 mg, 10 mg. Oral liquid: 5 mg/5mL. [DEKS-troh-am-FET-ah-meen].

**dextromethorphan** (Robitussin CoughGels, Robitussin Pediatric Cough, PediaCare Infants' Cough, Vicks 44 Cough Relief) (ENT). Over-the-counter nonnarcotic anti-tussive drug used to treat nonproductive coughs. Gelcap: 15 mg, 30 mg. Orally disintegrating strip: 7.5 mg, 15 mg. Liquid/syrup: 5 mg/5 mL, 7.5 mg/5 mL, 10 mg/5 mL, 10 mg/15 mL, 15 mg/5 mL. Lozenge: 5 mg, 7.5 mg. [DEKS-troh-meh-THOR-fan].

**dextrose 2.5% in water** (D-2.5-W) (I.V.). Intravenous fluid of dextrose and water. [DEKS-trohs].

**dextrose 5% in water** (D-5-W) (I.V.). Intravenous fluid of dextrose and water. [DEKS-trohs].

**dextrose 10% in water** (D-10-W) (I.V.). Intravenous fluid of dextrose and water. [DEKS-trohs].

**dextrose 20% in water, dextrose 25% in water, dextrose 30% in water, dextrose 40% in water, dextrose 50% in water, dextrose 60% in water, dextrose 70% in water** (I.V.). Concentrated intravenous fluid of dextrose and water. [DEKS-trohs].

**dextrose 5% with lactated Ringer's** (D5/LR) (I.V.). Combination intravenous fluid of dextrose and water with sodium, potassium, calcium, chloride and lactate. [DEKS-trohs with LAK-tay-ted RING-erz].

**dextrose 5% with half normal saline** (D5/0.45% NaCl) (I.V.). Combination intravenous fluid of dextrose and water with normal saline. [DEKS-trohs with HAF NOR-mal SAY-leen].

**dextrose 5% with normal saline** (D5/0.9% NaCl, D5%/NS) (I.V.). Combination intravenous fluid of dextrose and water with normal saline. [DEKS-trohs with NOR-mal SAY-leen].

**dextrose 10% with half normal saline** (D10/0.45% NaCl) (I.V.) Combination intravenous fluid of dextrose and water with normal saline. [DEKS-trohs with HAF NOR-mal SAY-leen].

**dextrose 10% with normal saline** (D10/NS) (I.V.) Combination intravenous fluid of dextrose and water with normal saline. [DEKS-trohs with NOR-mal SAY-leen].

**Dextrostat** (Neuro, Psych). See *dextroamphetamine*. [DEKS-troh-stat].

**D.H.E. 45** (Analges). See *dihydroergotamine*. [D-H-E 45].

**DHS Tar** (Derm). See *coal tar*. [D-H-S TAR].

**DHS Zinc** (Derm). See *pyrithione zinc*. [D-H-S ZINK].

**DiaBeta** (Endo). See *glyburide*. [DY-ah-BAY-tah].

**Diabetic Tussin** (Pulm). See *guaifenesin*. [DY-ah-BEH-tik TUS-sin].

**Diabinese** (Endo). See *chlorpropamide*. [dy-AB-ih-nees].

**Dialume** (GI). See *aluminum hydroxide*. [DY-ah-loom].

**Diamox Sequels** (Cardio, Neuro, Ophth). See *acetazolamide*. [DY-ah-mawks].

**Diasorb** (GI). See *attapulgite*. [DY-ah-sorb].

**Diastat** (Neuro, Ortho, Psych). See *diazepam*. [DY-ah-stat].

**diazepam** (Diastat, Diazepam Intensol, Valium) (Anes, GI, Neuro, Ortho, Psych). Schedule IV benzodiazepine drug used to treat anxiety disorders; used to treat alcohol with-drawal; used as a skeletal muscle relaxant drug to treat spasm and stiffness from muscle injuries; used to treat severe muscle spasticity associated with multiple sclerosis, cerebral palsy, stroke, or spinal cord injury; used to treat status epilepticus; used to treat irritable bowel syndrome; used preoperatively to decrease anxiety and provide seda-tion. Oral liquid: 5 mg/mL, 5 mg/5 mL. Tablet: 2 mg, 5 mg, 10 mg. Rectal gel: 2.5 mg, 10 mg, 20 mg. Intramuscular or intravenous: 5 mg/mL. [dy-AZ-eh-pam].

**Diazepam Intensol** (Neuro, Ortho, Psych). See *diazepam*. [dy-AZ-eh-pam in-TEN-sawl].

**diaziquone** (Chemo). Chemotherapy drug used to treat brain cancer. Orphan drug. [dy-AZ-ih-kwon].

**diazoxide** (Hyperstat IV, Proglycem) (Cardio, Endo). Peripheral vasodilator drug used to treat hypertensive crisis; insulin-inhibiting drug used to treat severe hypoglycemia. Capsule: 50 mg. Oral liquid: 50 mg. Intravenous: 15 mg/mL. [DY-ah-ZAWK-side].

**Dibent** (GI). See *dicyclomine*. [DY-bent].

**dibucaine** (Nupercainal) (Derm, GI). Over-the-counter anes-thetic drug used topically to treat the pain and itching of sunburn, bites, cuts, and hemorrhoids. Ointment: 1%. [DY-byoo-kayn].

**diclofenac** (Cataflam, Flector, Solaraze, Voltaren, Voltaren Emugel, Voltaren-XR) (Analges). Nonsteroidal anti-inflammatory drug used systemically and topically to treat pain and inflammation; used to treat osteoarthritis, rheuma-toid arthritis, and ankylosing spondylitis; used to treat dysmenorrhea; keratolytic drug used topically to treat actinic keratoses on the skin (Solaraze); used topically in the eye to treat pain, inflammation, and photophobia after corneal surgery (Voltaren). Tablet: 50 mg. Delayed-release tablet: 25 mg, 50 mg, 75 mg. Extended-release tablet: 100 mg. Emulgel tube: 20 g, 50 g, 100 g. Gel: 1%, 3%. Ophthalmic solution: 0.1%. Topical patch (Flector): 180 mg. [dy-KLOH-feh-nak].

**dicloxacillin** (Anti-infec). Penicillin-type antibiotic drug used to treat staphylococcal bacterial infections. Capsule: 250 mg, 500 mg. [dy-KLAWK-sah-SIL-in).

**dicyclomine** (Bentyl, Byclomine, Dibent, Dilomine, Di-Spaz, Or-Tyl) (GI). Anticholinergic antispasmodic drug used to decrease acid production and stop spasm; used to treat irritable bowel syndrome and spastic colon. Capsule: 10 mg, 20 mg. Tablet: 20 mg. Syrup: 10 mg/5 mL. Intramuscular: 10 mg/mL. [dy-SY-kloh-meen].

**didanosine** (Videx, Videx EC) (Anti-infec).   Nucleoside reverse transcriptase inhibitor antiviral drug used to treat HIV and AIDS. Delayed-release capsule: 125 mg, 200 mg, 250 mg, 400 mg. Tablet: 25 mg, 50 mg, 100 mg, 200 mg. Oral liquid (powder to be reconstituted): 100 mg, 250 mg. [dy-DAN-oh-seen].

**dideoxyinosine** (ddI) (Anti-infec).   See *didanosine.* [DY-dee-AWK-see-IN-oh-seen].

**Didrex** (GI).   See *benzphetamine.* [DY-dreks].

**Didronel** (Chemo, Ortho).   See *etidronate.* [DIH-droh-nel].

**diethyldithiocarbamate** (Imuthiol) (Anti-infec).   Used to treat HIV and AIDS. Orphan drug. [dy-ETH-il-dy-THY-oh-KAR-bah-mayt].

**diethylpropion** (GI).   Schedule IV appetite suppressant drug used to treat obesity. Tablet: 25 mg. Controlled-release tablet: 75 mg. [dy-ETH-il-PROH-pee-awn].

**Differin** (Derm).   See *adapalene.* [DIF-er-in].

**diflorasone** (ApexiCon, ApexiCon E, Florone, Florone E, Maxiflor, Psorcon E).   Corticosteroid drug used topically to treat inflammation and itching from dermatitis, seborrhea, eczema, psoriasis, and yeast or fungal infections. Cream: 0.05%. Ointment: 0.05%. [dy-FLOR-ah-zohn].

**Diflucan** (Anti-infec).   See *fluconazole.* [dy-FLOO-kan].

**diflunisal** (Dolobid) (Analges).   Salicylate analgesic drug used to treat pain and inflammation; used to treat osteoarthritis and rheumatoid arthritis. Tablet: 250 mg, 500 mg. [dy-FLOO-nih-sawl].

**difluprednate** (Durezol) (Ophth).   Corticosteroid drug used to treat inflammation and pain after eye surgery. Ophthalmic emulsion: 0.05%. [DY-floo-PRED-nayt].

**"dig"** (Cardio).   Slang. See *digoxin.* [DIJ].

**Di-Gel** (GI) (generic *aluminum, magnesium, simethicone*).   Combination antacid and anti-gas drug used to treat heartburn and gas. Liquid: 200 mg/20 mg. [DY-jel].

**Di-Gel Advanced Formula** (GI) (generic *calcium, magnesium, simethicone*).   Combination antacid and anti-gas drug used to treat heartburn and gas. Tablet: 280 mg/128 mg/20 mg. [DY-jel].

**Digibind** (Cardio, Emerg).   See *digoxin immune Fab.* [DIJ-ih-bind].

**Digidote** (Cardio, Emerg).   See *digoxin immune Fab.* [DIJ-ih-doht].

**DigiFab** (Cardio, Emerg).   See *digoxin immune Fab.* [DIJ-ih-FAB].

**Digitek** (Cardio).   See *digoxin.* [DIJ-ih-tek].

**digitoxin** (Chemo, Pulm).   Used to treat cancer of the ovary and sarcoma; used to treat cystic fibrosis. Orphan drug. [DIH-jih-TAWK-sin].

**digoxin** (Digitek, Lanoxicaps, Lanoxin) (Cardio).   Digitalis drug used to treat atrial fibrillation and congestive heart failure. Capsule: 0.05 mg, 0.1 mg, 0.2 mg. Elixir: 0.05 mg/mL. Tablet: 0.125 mg, 0.25 mg, 0.5 mg. Intravenous: 0.1 mg/mL, 0.25 mg/mL. [dij-AWK-sin].

**digoxin immune Fab** (Digibind, Digidote, DigiFab) (Cardio, Emerg)   Antidote drug used to reverse the effects of digitalis overdose or toxicity. Intravenous (powder to be reconstituted): 38 mg/vial, 40 mg/vial. [dij-AWK-sin ih-MYOON FAB].

**dihydroergotamine** (D.H.E. 45, Migranal) (Analges).   Ergotamine drug used to treat migraine headaches. Nasal spray: 0.5 mg/spray. Subcutaneous, intramuscular, or intravenous: 1 mg/mL. [dy-HY-droh-er-GAW-tah-meen].

**dihydrotestosterone** (Androgel-DHT) (Endo).   Male hormone drug used to treat AIDS wasting syndrome. Orphan drug. [dy-HY-droh-tes-TAWS-teh-rohn].

**dihydroxyacetone** (Chromelin Complexion Blender) (Derm).   Over-the-counter drug used topically to darken depigmented areas of skin in patients with vitiligo. Suspension: 5%. [DY-hy-DRAWK-see-AS-eh-tohn].

**Dilacor XR** (Analges, Cardio).   See *diltiazem.* [DIL-ah-kor X-R].

**Dilantin Infatabs, Dilantin Kapseals, Dilantin-125** (Neuro).   See *phenytoin.* [dy-LAN-tin].

**Dilatrate-SR** (Cardio).   See *isosorbide dinitrate.* [DIL-ah-trayt-S-R].

**Dilaudid, Dilaudid HP** (Analges).   See *hydromorphone.* [dy-LAW-did].

**Dilaudid Cough** (ENT) (generic *guaifenesin, hydromorphone*).   Combination Schedule II expectorant and narcotic antitussive drug used to treat a severe productive cough. Syrup: 100 mg/1 mg. [dy-LAW-did].

**Dilomine** (GI).   See *dicyclomine.* [DY-loh-meen].

**Dilor-G** (Pulm) (generic *dyphylline, guaifenesin*).   Combination bronchodilator and expectorant drug used to treat asthma and bronchitis with a productive cough. Liquid: 300 mg/300 mg. [DY-lor-G].

**Dilt-CD, Dilt-XR** (Analges, Cardio).   See *diltiazem.* [DILT].

**Diltia XT** (Analges, Cardio).   See *diltiazem.* [dil-TY-ah X-T].

**diltiazem** (Cardizem, Cardizem CD, Cardizem LA, Cartia XT, Dilacor XR, Dilt-CD, Dilt-XR, Diltia XT, Taztia XT, Tiazac) (Analges, Cardio).   Calcium channel blocker drug used to prevent and treat angina pectoris; used to treat hypertension, pulmonary arterial hypertension, and Raynaud's disease; used to treat atrial flutter, atrial fibrillation, and ventricular tachycardia; used to prevent migraine headaches. Extended-release capsule: 60 mg, 90 mg, 120 mg, 180 mg, 240 mg, 300 mg, 360 mg, 420 mg. Tablet: 30 mg, 60 mg, 90 mg, 120 mg. Extended-release tablet: 120 mg, 180 mg, 240 mg, 300 mg, 360 mg, 420 mg. Intravenous: 5 mg/mL. [dil-TY-ah-zem].

**dimenhydrinate** (Children's Dramamine, Dimetabs, Dinate, Dramamine, Dramanate, Dymenate) (ENT, GI).   Over-the-counter and prescription antihistamine drug used to treat nausea and vomiting, vertigo, and motion sickness.

Liquid: 12.5 mg/4 mL, 15.6 mg/5 mL. Chewable tablet: 50 mg. Tablet: 50 mg. Intramuscular or intravenous: 50 mg/mL. [DY-men-HY-drih-nayt].

**dimercaprol** (BAL In Oil) (Emerg).    Chelating drug used to treat mercury, arsenic, or gold poisoning. Intramuscular: 100 mg/mL. [DY-mer-KAH-prawl].

**Dimetabs** (GI).    See *dimenhydrinate.* [DIME-tabz].

**Dimetapp Children's Decongestant Plus Cough** (ENT) (generic *dextromethorphan, pseudoephedrine*). Combination over-the-counter nonnarcotic antitussive and decongestant drug used to treat colds and coughs. Oral drops: 2.5 mg/7.5 mg. [DY-meh-tap].

**Dimetapp Children's ND Non-Drowsy Allergy** (Derm, ENT). See *loratadine.* [DY-meh-tap].

**Dimetapp Children's Non-Drowsy Flu** (ENT) (generic *acetaminophen, dextromethorphan, pseudoephedrine*). Combination over-the-counter analgesic, nonnarcotic antitussive, and decongestant drug used to treat colds and coughs. Liquid: 5 mg/15 mg. [DY-meh-tap].

**Dimetapp Decongestant Pediatric, Dimetapp Maximum Strength Non-Drowsy** (ENT).    See *pseudoephedrine.* [DY-meh-tap].

**Dimetapp Long Acting Cough & Cold** (ENT) (generic *dextromethorphan, pseudoephedrine*).    Combination over-the-counter antitussive and decongestant drug used to treat colds and coughs. Syrup: 7.5 mg/15 mg. [DY-meh-tap].

**dimethyl sulfoxide** (DMSO, Rimso-50) (Uro).    Urinary tract analgesic drug used topically to treat pain. Solution (instilled via catheter into the bladder): 50%. [dy-METH-il sul-FAWK-side].

**Dinate** (GI).    See *dimenhydrinate.* [DY-nayt].

**dinoprostone** (Cervidil, Prepidil, Prostin E2) (OB/GYN).    Smooth muscle stimulant drug used to ripen the cervix for delivery; used to induce abortion (Prostin E2). Vaginal gel: 0.5 mg. Vaginal insert: 10 mg. Vaginal suppository: 20 mg. [DY-noh-PRAWS-tohn].

**Diovan** (Cardio).    See *valsartan.* [DY-oh-van].

**Diovan HCT** (Cardio) (generic *valsartan, hydrochlorothiazide*).    Combination angiotensin II receptor blocker and diuretic drug used to treat hypertension. Tablet: 80 mg/12.5 mg, 160 mg/12.5 mg, 160 mg/25 mg, 320 mg/12.5 mg, 320 mg/25 mg. [DY-oh-van H-C-T].

**Dipentum** (GI).    See *olsalazine.* [dy-PEN-tum].

**diphenhydramine** (AllerMax, AllerMax Maximum Strength, Benadryl, Benadryl Allergy, Benadryl Children's Allergy, Compoz Nighttime Sleep Aid, Dermamycin, Dermarest, Dermarest Plus, Genahist, Hydramine Cough, Midol PM, Miles Nervine, Nytol, Nytol Maximum Strength, PediaCare Children's Nighttime Cough, Scot-Tussin Allergy Relief Formula Clear, Siladryl, Silphen Cough, Sominex, Triaminic Cough & Runny Nose, Triaminic Multisymptom, Tusstat, Unisom Maximum Strength SleepGels (Derm, Emerg, ENT, GI, Neuro, Ophth).    Over-the-counter antihistamine drug used to treat the symptoms of seasonal and perennial allergies, allergic rhinitis and coughing, allergic conjunctivitis; used topically to treat skin allergies and itching; used to treat allergic skin reactions from foods and other allergens; used to control the severity of an allergic reaction to blood products; used to prevent or treat nausea and vomiting associated with motion sickness; side effect of drowsiness used to induce sleep. Capsule: 25 mg, 50 mg. Chewable tablet: 12.5 mg, 25 mg. Cream: 1%, 2%. Elixir: 12.5 mg/5 mL. Gel: 1%, 2%. Gel capsule: 25 mg. Intramuscular or intravenous: 50 mg/mL. Liquid: 12.5 mg/5 mL. Liqui Gels: 25 mg. Orally disintegrating strip: 12.5 mg, 25 mg. Orally disintegrating tablet: 12.5 mg. Spray: 1%, 2%. Oral suspension: 25 mg/5 mL. Syrup: 12.5 mg/5 mL. Tablet: 25 mg, 50 mg. [DY-fen-HY-drah-meen].

**dipivefrin** (Propine) (Ophth).    Sympathomimetic drug used topically to treat glaucoma. Ophthalmic solution: 0.1%. [dy-PIH-veh-frin].

**Diprivan** (Anes, Pulm).    See *propofol.* [DIP-rih-van].

**Diprolene, Diprolene AF** (Derm).    See *betamethasone.* [DIP-roh-leen].

**Diprosone** (Derm).    See *betamethasone.* [DIP-roh-sohn].

**dipyridamole** (Persantine) (Cardio, Hem).    Coronary artery vasodilator drug used as a diagnostic aid to provoke angina in patients with coronary artery disease who cannot tolerate exercise stress testing; platelet aggregation inhibitor drug used to prevent a blood clot after cardiac valve replacement surgery. Tablet: 25 mg, 50 mg, 75 mg. Intravenous: 5 mg/mL. [DY-pih-RID-ah-mohl].

**Diskets** (Analges).    See *methadone.* [dis-KETZ].

**disodium clodronate** (Bonefos) (Chemo).    Used to treat hypercalcemia and osteoporosis caused by cancer. Orphan drug. [di-SOH-dee-um KLOH-droh-nayt].

**disopyramide** (Norpace, Norpace CR) (Cardio).    Antiarrhythmic drug used to treat ventricular tachycardia. Capsule: 100 mg, 150 mg. Extended-release capsule: 100 mg, 150 mg. [DY-soh-PEER-ah-mide].

**DisperMox** (Anti-infec).    See *amoxicillin.* [DIS-per-mawks].

**Di-Spaz** (GI).    See *dicyclomine.* [DY-spaz].

**disulfiram** (Antabuse) (Psych).    Used to deter alcohol consumption in recovering alcoholic patients. Tablet: 250 mg, 500 mg. [dy-SUL-fih-ram].

**Ditropan, Ditropan XL** (Uro).    See *oxybutynin.* [DIH-troh-pan].

**Diurigen** (Cardio, Uro).    See *chlorothiazide.* [dy-YOOR-ih-jen].

**Diuril** (Cardio, Uro).    See *chlorothiazide.* [DY-yoor-il].

**Divigel** (OB/GYN).    See *estradiol.* [DIV-ih-jel].

**DMSO** (Uro).    See *dimethyl sulfoxide.* [D-M-S-O].

**Doak Tar, Doak Tar Oil** (Derm).    See *coal tar.* [DOH-ak TAR].

**Doan's, Doan's Extra Strength** (Analges).    See *magnesium salicylate.* [DOHNZ].

**Doan's P.M., Extra Strength** (Neuro) (generic *diphenhydramine, magnesium*).    Combination over-the-counter antihistamine and magnesium drug to induce sleep and relax muscles. Tablet: 25 mg/500 mg. [DOHNZ].

**dobutamine** (Cardio).    Vasopressor drug used to treat severe congestive heart failure. Intravenous: 12.5 mg/mL. [doh-BYOO-tah-meen].

**docetaxel** (Taxotere) (Chemo).    Mitosis inhibitor chemotherapy drug used to treat cancer of the head and neck, breast, lung, esophagus, stomach, ovary, prostate gland, and urinary tract. Intravenous. 20 mg/0.5 mL, 80 mg/2 mL. [DOH-see-TAK-sel].

**docosanol** (Abreva) (Anti-infec, Derm, ENT).    Over-the-counter antiviral drug used topically on the skin to treat herpes simplex type 1 viral infections (cold sores). Cream:10%. [doh-KOH-sah-nawl].

**Dr Scholl's Cracked Heel Relief** (Anes, Derm).    See *lidocaine.* [DOK-tor SHOLZ].

**Dr Scholl's Clear Away OneStep, Dr Scholl's Corn/Callus Remover, Dr Scholl's Wart Remover Kit** (Derm).    See *salicylic acid.* [DOK-tor SHOLZ].

**Docu** (GI).    See *docusate.* [DAW-kyoo].

**docusate** (Colace, Docu, Dulcolax Stool Softener, ex-lax Stool Softener, Genasoft, Phillips' Liqui-Gels, Silace, Surfak Liquigels) (GI).    Over-the-counter stool-softener laxative drug used to treat constipation. Capsule: 50 mg, 100 mg, 240 mg, 250 mg. Gel capsule: 50 mg, 100 mg, 240 mg, 250 mg. Liquid: 10 mg/mL, 150 mg/15 mL. Syrup: 20 mg/5 mL, 50 mg/15 mL, 60 mg/15 mL, 100 mg/30 mL. Tablet: 100 mg. [DAW-kyoo-sayt].

**dofetilide** (Tikosyn) (Cardio).    Antiarrhythmic drug used to treat atrial flutter and atrial fibrillation. Capsule: 0.125 mg, 0.25 mg, 0.5 mg. [doh-FET-ih-lide].

**dolasetron** (Anzemet) (Chemo, GI).    Serotonin blocker drug used to treat nausea and vomiting caused by chemotherapy. Tablet: 50 mg, 100 mg. Intravenous: 20 mg/mL. [doh-LAS-eh-trawn].

**Dolgic** (Analges) (generic *acetaminophen, butalbital*). Combination nonsalicylate analgesic and barbiturate sedative drug for pain. Tablet: 650 mg/50 mg. [DOL-jik].

**Dolobid** (Analges).    See *diflunisal.* [DOH-loh-bid].

**Dolophine** (Analges).    See *methadone.* [DOH-loh-feen].

**Dolsed** (Uro) (generic *atropine, hyoscyamine, methenamine, methylene blue, phenyl salicylate*).    Combination urinary tract antispasmodic, anti-infective, antiseptic, and analgesic drug; used to treat urinary tract infections with pain and spasms. Tablet: 0.03 mg/0.03 mg/40.8 mg/5.4 mg18.1mg. [DOL-sed].

**Domeboro** (Derm).    See *aluminum acetate.* [DOHM-bur-oh].

**donepezil** (Aricept, Aricept ODT) (Neuro).    Cholinesterase inhibitor drug used to treat mild-to-severe Alzheimer's disease. Tablet: 5 mg, 10 mg. Orally disintegrating tablet: 5 mg, 10 mg. Liquid: 1 mg/mL. [doh-NEP-eh-zil].

**Donnatal, Donnatal Extentabs** (GI) (generic *atropine, hyoscyamine, scopolamine, phenobarbital*).    Combination anticholinergic and barbiturate sedative drug; used to treat GI spasm associated with irritable bowel syndrome, spastic colon, diverticulitis, and peptic ulcers. Tablet:

0.0194mg/0.1037 mg/0.0065 mg/16.2 mg. Extended-release tablet: 0.0582 mg/0.0195 mg/0.3111 mg/48.6 mg. Elixir: 0.0194 mg/0.1037 mg/0.0065 mg/16.2 mg. [DAWN-ah-tawl].

**dopamine** (Cardio, Emerg).    Vasopressor drug used to treat severe congestive heart failure; used to treat hypotension during cardiac resuscitation and shock. Intravenous: 40 mg/mL, 80 mg/mL, 160 mg/mL. [DOH-pah-meen]

**Dopram** (Anes, Pulm).    See *doxapram.* [DOH-pram].

**Doral** (Neuro).    See *quazepam.* [doh-RAL].

**Doribax** (Anti-Infec).    See *doripenem.* [DOOR-ih-baks].

**doripenem** (Doribax) (Anti-Infec).    Carbapenem antibiotic drug used to treat severe bacterial infections of the intra-abdominal cavity or urinary tract; orphan drug used to treat *Pseudomonas aeruginosa* infection of the lung in patients with cystic fibrosis. Intravenous: 500 mg/10 mL. Orphan drug. [DOOR-ih-PEN-em].

**dornase alfa** (Pulmozyme) (Pulm).    Enzyme that thins the thick mucus in patients with cystic fibrosis. Liquid for nebulizer: 1 mg/mL. [DOR-nays AL-fah].

**Doryx** (Anti-infec).    See *doxycycline.* [DOOR-iks].

**dorzolamide** (Trusopt) (Ophth).    Carbonic anhydrase inhibitor drug used topically in the eye to treat glaucoma. Ophthalmic solution: 2%. [door-ZOL-ah-mide].

**Dostinex** (Endo).    See *cabergoline.* [DOS-tih-neks].

**Dovonex** (Derm).    See *calcipotriene.* [DOH-voh-neks].

**doxapram** (Dopram) (Anes, Pulm).    Central nervous system stimulant drug used to treat respiratory depression following general anesthesia; used to treat apnea in premature infants. Intravenous: 20 mg/mL. [DAWK-sah-pram].

**doxazosin** (Cardura, Cardura XL) (Cardio, Uro).    Alpha-blocker drug used to treat hypertension; used to treat benign prostatic hypertrophy. Tablet: 1 mg, 2 mg, 4 mg, 8 mg. Extended-release tablet: 4 mg, 8 mg. [dawk-SAY-zoh-sin].

**doxepin** (Sinequan, Zonalon) (Analges, Derm, Neuro, Psych). Tricyclic antidepressant drug used to treat depression; used to treat anxiety associated with alcoholism or brain disease; used to treat migraine headaches; used to treat nerve pain from phantom limb, diabetic neuropathy, peripheral neuropathy, and postherpetic neuralgia; used to treat tic douloureux; antihistamine drug used topically to treat skin itching (Zonalon). Capsule: 10 mg, 25 mg, 50 mg, 75 mg, 100 mg, 150 mg. Oral liquid: 10 mg/mL. Cream: 5%. [DAWK-seh-pin].

**doxercalciferol** (Hectorol) (Endo).    Used to treat hyperparathyroidism in patients with kidney disease. Capsule: 0.5 mcg, 2.5 mcg. Injection (during hemodialysis): 2 mcg/mL. [DAWK-ser-kal-SIF-eh-rawl].

**Doxidan** (GI).    See *bisacodyl.* [DAWK-sih-dan].

**Doxil** (Chemo).    See *doxorubicin.* [DAWK-sil].

**doxorubicin** (Adriamycin PFS, Adriamycin RDF, Doxil) (Chemo).    Chemotherapy antibiotic drug used to treat cancer of the thyroid gland, lung, esophagus, stomach, liver, pancreas, breast, ovary, uterus, bone, and bladder; used to treat leukemia, Hodgkin's lymphoma, non-Hodgkin's lymphoma, Wilm's tumor, multiple myeloma, and Kaposi's sarcoma. Intravenous: 2 mg/mL, 20 mg/10 mL, 50 mg/30 mL. [DAWK-soh-ROO-bih-sin].

**doxycycline** (Adoxa, Atridox, Doryx, Doxy 100, Doxy 200, Monodox, Oracea, Periostat, Vibramycin, Vibra-Tabs) (Anti-infec).   Tetracycline antibiotic drug used to treat infections due to gram-negative and gram-positive bacteria; used orally to treat severe acne vulgaris; used to treat gonorrhea, syphilis, *Chlamydia,* and nongonococcal urethritis; used to treat pneumonia due to *S. pneumoniae, H. influenzae,* and *Mycoplasma;* used to treat Lyme disease and Rocky Mountain spotted fever; used to treat intestinal amebiasis; used to treat ulcerative gingivitis (trench mouth); used to prevent and treat malaria; used to treat inhaled and cutaneous anthrax from bioterrorism. Capsule: 40 mg, 50 mg, 100 mg. Capsule (coated pellets): 75 mg, 100 mg. Delayed-release tablet: 75 mg, 100 mg. Tablet: 20 mg, 50 mg, 75 mg, 100 mg. Liquid (powder to be reconstituted): 25 ml/5 mL. Syrup: 50 mg/5 mL. Intravenous (powder to be reconstituted): 100 mg, 200 mg. [DAWK-see-SY-kleen].

**Doxy 100, Doxy 200** (Anti-infec).   See *doxycycline.* [DAWK-see].

**doxylamine** (Unisom Nighttime Sleep-Aid) (Neuro).   Over-the-counter antihistamine drug used to induce sleep. Tablet: 25 mg. [dawk-SIL-ah-meen].

**Dramamine, Children's Dramamine** (GI).   See *dimenhydrinate.* [DRAM-ah-meen].

**Dramamine Less Drowsy Formula** (GI).   See *meclizine.* [DRAM-ah-meen].

**Dramanate** (GI).   See *dimenhydrinate.* [DRAM-ah-nayt].

**Drepanol** (Hem).   Used to treat sickle cell disease. Orphan drug. [DREH-pah-nawl].

**Dristan Cold Multi-Symptom Formula** (ENT) (generic *acetaminophen, chlorpheniramine, phenylephrine*).   Combination over-the-counter analgesic, antihistamine, and decongestant drug used to treat colds and allergies. Tablet: 325 mg/2 mg/5 mg. [DRIS-tan].

**Dristan Fast Acting Formula** (ENT) (generic *pheniramine, phenylephrine*).   Combination over-the-counter antihistamine and decongestant drug used topically in the nose to treat colds and allergies. Nasal spray: 0.2%/0.5%. [DRIS-tan].

**Dristan Sinus** (Analges, ENT) (generic *ibuprofen, pseudoephedrine*).   Combination over-the-counter analgesic and decongestant drug used to treat colds and sinus congestion. Tablet: 200 mg/30 mg. [DRIS-tan].

**Dristan 12-Hr Nasal** (ENT).   See *oxymetazoline.* [DRIS-tan].

**Dritho-Scalp** (Derm).   See *anthralin.* [DRITH-oh-skalp].

**Drixoral Allergy Sinus** (ENT) (generic *acetaminophen, dexbrompheniramine, pseudoephedrine*).   Combination over-the-counter analgesic, antihistamine, and decongestant drug used to treat colds and allergies. Tablet: 500 mg/30 mg/60 mg. [driks-OR-al].

**Drixoral Cold & Allergy** (ENT) (generic *dexbrompheniramine, pseudoephedrine*).   Combination over-the-counter

antihistamine and decongestant drug used to treat colds and allergies. Tablet: 6 mg/120 mg. [driks-OR-al].

**Drixoral 12 Hour Non-Drowsy Formula** (ENT).   See *pseudoephedrine.* [driks-OR-al].

**dronabinol** (Marinol) (Anti-infec, Chemo, GI).   Schedule III cannabinoid drug used to stimulate the appetite in AIDS patients; antiemetic drug used to treat nausea and vomiting caused by chemotherapy. Capsule. 2.5 mg, 5 mg, 10 mg. [droh-NAB-ih-nawl].

**droperidol** (Inapsine) (Anes, GI, Chemo).   Sedative drug used to prevent nausea and vomiting during surgery or after chemotherapy. Intravenous: 2.5 mg/mL. [droh-PAIR-ih-dawl].

**drotrecogin alfa** (Xigris) (Hem).   Recombinant DNA activated protein C-type thrombolytic drug used to treat patients with severe sepsis. Intravenous (powder to be reconstituted): 5 mg, 20 mg. [DROH-treh-KOH-jin AL-fah].

**Droxia** (Chemo, Derm, Hem).   See *hydroxyurea.* [DRAWK-see-ah].

**Dr. Scholl's Clear Away OneStep, Dr. Scholl's Corn/Callus Remover, Dr. Scholl's Wart Remover Kit** (Derm).   See *salicylic acid.* [DAWK-tor SHOWLZ].

**Dr. Scholl's Cracked Heel Relief** (Derm).   See *lidocaine.* [DAWK-tor SHOWLZ].

**Dr. Smith's Adult Care, Dr. Smith's Diaper Ointment** (Derm).   See *zinc oxide.* [DAWK-tor SMITH].

**Drysol** (Derm).   See *aluminum chloride.* [DRY-sawl].

**Drytex** (Derm).   Keratolytic drug used topically on the skin to treat acne vulgaris. Lotion. [DRY-teks].

**DTIC-Dome** (Chemo).   See *dacarbazine.* [D-T-I-C-dohm].

**Duac** (Derm) (generic *benzoyl peroxide, clindamycin*).   Combination antibiotic drug used topically on the skin to treat acne vulgaris. Gel: 5%/1%. [DOO-ak].

**Duetact** (Endo) (generic *pioglitazone, glimepiride*).   Combination oral antidiabetic drug used to treat type 2 diabetes mellitus. Tablet: 30 mg/20 mg, 30 mg/4 mg. [DOO-et-akt].

**DuetDHA**[ec] (OB/GYN).   Prenatal vitamin and mineral supplement with DHA and omega-3 fatty acids. Daily packet: Enteric-coated tablet and softgel. [DOO-et-D-H-A-e-c].

**Dulcolax, Dulcolax Bowel Prep Kit** (GI).   See *bisacodyl.* [DUL-koh-laks].

**Dulcolax Stool Softener** (GI).   See *docusate.* [DUL-koh-laks].

**duloxetine** (Cymbalta) (Neuro, Psych).   Serotonin and norepinephrine reuptake inhibitor (SNRI) drug used to treat depression and anxiety; used to treat diabetic neuropathy; used to treat fibromyalgia. Delayed-release capsule: 20 mg, 30 mg, 60 mg. [doo-LAWK-seh-teen].

**Duocaine** (Anes) (generic *bupivacaine, lidocaine*).   Combination anesthetic drug used to provide local or regional anesthesia. Injection: 3.75 mg/10 mg per mL. [DOO-oh-kayn].

**DuoDerm** (Derm).   Over-the-counter drug used topically to absorb drainage from burns, skin ulcers, and wounds. Gauze dressing containing gel. Granules. Paste. [DOO-oh-derm].

**Duodopa** (Neuro) (generic *carbidopa, levodopa*).
Combination drug used to treat Parkinson's disease. Orphan
drug. [DOO-oh-DOH-pah].

**DuoFilm** (Derm). See *salicylic acid*. [DOO-oh-film].

**DuoNeb** (Pulm) (generic *albuterol, ipratropium*).
Combination bronchodilator drug used to treat bronchospasm with chronic obstructive pulmonary disease.
Liquid for inhalation: 3 mg/0.5 mg per 3 mL. [DOO-oh-neb].

**DuoPlant** (Derm). See *salicylic acid*. [DOO-oh-plant].

**Duraclon** (Analges, Chemo). See *clonidine*. [DUR-ah-klawn].

**Duradrin** (Analges) (generic *acetaminophen, dichloralphenazone, isometheptene*). Combination analgesic,
sedative, and vasoconstrictor drug used to treat migraine
headaches. Capsule: 325 mg/100 mg/65 mg.[DUR-ah-drin].

**Duragesic-12, Duragesic-25, Duragesic-50, Duragesic-75,
Duragesic-100** (Analges). See *fentanyl*. [DUR-ah-JEE-sik].

**Duramorph** (Analges, Anes). See *morphine*. [DUR-ah-morf].

**duramycin** (Pulm). Used to treat cystic fibrosis. Orphan
drug. [DUR-ah-MY-sin].

**Duratears Naturale** (Ophth). Used to lubricate dry eyes.
Ophthalmic ointment. [DUR-ah-teerz].

**Duration** (ENT). See *oxymetazoline*. [dur-AY-shun].

**Durezol** (Ophth). See *difluprednate*. [DUR-eh-zohl].

**Duricef** (Anti-infec). See *cefadroxil*. [DUR-ah-sef].

**dutasteride** (Avodart) (Uro). Male hormone inhibitor drug
used to treat benign prostatic hypertrophy. Capsule: 0.5 mg.
[doo-TAS-teh-ride].

**Dyazide** (Cardio, Uro) (generic *hydrochlorothiazide,
triamterene*). Combination thiazide diuretic and potassium-sparing diuretic drug used to treat hypertension; used
to treat edema from congestive heart failure, liver disease,
or kidney disease. Capsule: 25 mg/ 37.5 mg. [DY-ah-zide].

**dyclonine** (Sucrets Children's Sore Throat) (ENT).
Anesthetic drug used topically to treat sore throats.
Lozenge: 1.2 mg. [DY-kloh-neen].

**Dyfil-G Forte** (Pulm) (generic *dyphylline, guaifenesin*).
Combination bronchodilator and expectorant drug used to
treat a productive cough. Liquid: 300 mg/300 mg. [DY-fil-G
FOR-tay].

**Dy-G** (Pulm) (generic *dyphylline, guaifenesin*). Combination
bronchodilator and expectorant drug used to treat a productive cough. Liquid: 300 mg/300 mg. [dy-G].

**Dylex-G** (Pulm) (generic *dyphylline, guaifenesin*).
Combination bronchodilator and expectorant drug used to treat
a productive cough. Syrup: 300 mg/300 mg. [DY-leks-G].

**Dyline G. G.** (Pulm) (generic *dyphylline, guaifenesin*).
Combination bronchodilator and expectorant drug used to treat
a productive cough. Tablet: 200 mg/200 mg. [DY-leen G-G].

**Dylix** (Pulm). See *dyphylline*. [DY-liks].

**Dylor-G** (Pulm) (generic *dyphylline, guaifenesin*).
Combination bronchodilator and expectorant drug used to
treat a productive cough. Liquid: 300 mg/300 mg. [DY-lor-G].

**Dymenate** (GI). See *dimenhydrinate*. [DY-meh-nayt].

**Dynacin** (Anti-infec). See *minocycline*. [DY-nah-sin].

**DynaCirc, DynaCirc CR** (Cardio). See *isradipine*.
[DY-nah-sirk].

**dynamine** (Ortho). Used to treat Eaton-Lambert syndrome.
Orphan drug. [DY-nah-meen].

**dyphylline** (Tryllin, Lufyllin) (Pulm). Bronchodilator drug
used to treat bronchospasm associated with asthma, chronic
bronchitis, and emphysema. Tablet: 200 mg, 400 mg.
Elixir: 100 mg/15 mL. [DY-fih-lin].

**Dyrenium** (Cardio, GI, Uro). See *triamterene*.
[dy-REE-nee-um].

**Dysport** (Ophth, Ortho). See *botulinum toxin type A*.
[DIS-port].

**echothiophate iodide** (Phospholine Iodide) (Ophth).
Cholinesterase inhibitor drug used topically in the eye to
treat glaucoma. Ophthalmic solution: 0.125%.
[EK-oh-THY-oh-fayt EYE-oh-dide].

**econazole** (Spectazole) (Derm). Antifungal drug used topically to treat tinea (ringworm) and other fungal infections
of the skin. Cream: 1%. [ee-KAWN-ah-zohl].

**Econopred Plus** (Ophth). See *prednisolone*.
[ee-KAWN-oh-pred].

**Ecotrin, Ecotrin Adult Low Strength, Ecotrin Maximum
Strength** (Analges, Ortho). See *aspirin*. [EK-oh-trin].

**Ecovia** (Neuro). See *remacemide*. [eh-KOH-vee-ah].

**eculizumab** (Soliris) (Heme, Uro). Monoclonal antibody
drug used to treat paroxysmal nocturnal hemoglobinuria
from the destruction of red blood cells. Intravenous:
300 mg/30 mL. [EE-kyoo-LIZ-yoo-mab].

**Edecrin** (Cardio, Uro). See *ethacrynic acid*. [ED-eh-krin].

**edetate** (Endrate) (Cardio). Used to treat ventricular
arrhythmias caused by digitalis toxicity; used to treat
hypercalcemia. Intravenous: 150 mg/mL. [ED-eh-tayt].

**edetate calcium disodium** (calcium EDTA) (Calcium
Disodium Versenate) (Emerg, Neuro). Chelating drug
used to treat lead poisoning and lead encephalopathy.
Intramuscular, intravenous: 200 mg/mL.
[ED-eh-tayt KAL-see-um di-SOH-dee-um].

**Edex** (Uro). See *alprostadil*. [EE-deks].

**edotreotide** (OctreoTher) (Chemo). Chemotherapy drug
used to treat gastrointestinal cancer. Orphan drug.
[EE-doh-TREE-oh-tide].

**edrophonium** (Enlon, Reversol, Tensilon) (Anes, Neuro).
Anticholinesterase drug used to diagnose myasthenia
gravis; used to reverse the effect of neuromuscular blocker
drugs given during general anesthesia. Intramuscular or
intravenous: 10 mg/mL. [ED-roh-FOH-nee-um].

**ED-SPAZ** (GI, Uro). See *L-hyoscyamine*. [E-D-SPAZ].

**E.E.S. 200, E.E.S. 400** (Anti-infec). See *erythromycin*. [E-E-S].

**efalizumab** (Raptiva) (Derm). Immunosupressant monoclonal antibody drug used to treat severe psoriasis.
Subcutaneous: 125 mg/1.25 mL. [EH-fah-LIZ-yoo-mab].

**efaproxiral** (Chemo). Chemotherapy drug used to treat brain metastases from breast cancer. Orphan drug. [EF-ah-PRAWK-ih-ral].

**efavirenz** (Sustiva) (Anti-infec). Nonnucleoside reverse transcriptase inhibitor antiviral drug used to treat HIV and AIDS. Capsule: 50 mg, 100 mg, 200 mg. Tablet: 600 mg. [oh-FAV-ih-renz].

**Effer K** (Uro). See *potassium* [EF-fer K].

**Effexor, Effexor XR** (OB/GYN, Psych). See *venlafaxine*. [ee-FEK-sor].

**Efidac 24** (ENT). See *chlorpheniramine*. [EF-ih-dak 24].

**eflornithine** (Ornidyl, Vaniqa) (Anti-infec, Derm). Used topically to slow the growth of unwanted facial hair in women (Vaniqa); orphan drug used to treat *Pneumocystis carinii* pneumonia in AIDS patients (Ornidyl). Cream: 13.9%. Intravenous: 200 mg/mL [ee-FLOOR-nih-theen].

**Efudex** (Derm, OB/GYN). See *fluorouracil*. [EF-yoo-deks].

**8-MOP** (Derm). See *methoxsalen*. [8-MAWP].

**Elaprase** (Misc). See *idursulfase*. [EL-ah-prays].

**elcatonin** (Analges). Used to treat severe pain. Orphan drug. Intrathecal injection. [EL-kah-TOH-nin].

**Eldecort** (Derm). See *hydrocortisone*. [EL-deh-kort].

**Eldepryl** (Neuro). See *selegiline*. [EL-deh-pril].

**Eldopaque, Eldopaque Forte** (Derm). See *hydroquinone*. [EL-doh-payk].

**Eldoquin-Forte** (Derm). See *hydroquinone*. [EL-doh-kwin].

**Elestat** (Ophth). See *epinastine*. [EL-eh-stat].

**Elestrin** (OB/GYN, Ortho). See *estradiol*. [eh-LES-trin].

**eletriptan** (Relpax) (Analges). Serotonin receptor agonist drug used to treat migraine headaches. Tablet: 24.2 mg, 48.5 mg. [EL-eh-TRIP-tan].

**Elidel** (Derm). See *pimecrolimus*. [EL-ih-del].

**Eligard** (Chemo, Endo). See *leuprolide*. [EL-ih-gard].

**Elimite** (Derm). See *permethrin*. [EE-lih-mite].

**Elitek** (Chemo). See *rasburicase*. [EL-ih-tek].

**Elixophyllin** (Pulm). See *theophylline*. [ee-LIK-soh-FIL-in, EE-lik-SAW-fih-lin].

**Elixophyllin GG** (Pulm) (generic *theophylline, guaifenesin*). Combination bronchodilator and expectorant drug used to treat asthma and bronchitis with a productive cough. Liquid: 100 mg/100 mg. [ee-LIK-soh-FIL-in, EE-lik-SAW-fih-lin].

**Elixophyllin-KI** (Pulm) (generic *theophylline, potassium iodide [KI]*). Combination bronchodilator and expectorant drug used to treat asthma and bronchitis with a productive cough. Elixir: 80 mg/130 mg. [ee-LIK-soh-FIL-in, EE-lik-SAW-fih-lin].

**Ellence** (Chemo). See *epirubicin*. [el-LENS].

**Elliotts B Solution** (Chemo). Dextrose solution used to dilute the chemotherapy drugs methotrexate or cytarabine for intrathecal administration. Orphan drug. [EL-ee-awts B].

**Elmiron** (Uro). See *pentosan*. [EL-mih-rawn].

**Elocon** (Derm). See *mometasone*. [EL-oh-kawn].

**Eloxatin** (Chemo). See *oxaliplatin*. [eh-LAWK-sah-tin].

**Elspar** (Chemo). See *asparaginase*. [EL-spar].

**Emadine** (Ophth). See *emedastine*. [EM-ah-deen].

**Emcyt** (Chemo). See *estramustine*. [EM-sit].

**emedastine** (Emadine) (Ophth). Antihistamine drug used topically in the eyes to treat allergy symptoms. Ophthalmic solution: 0.05%. [eh-MED-ah-steen].

**Emend** (Chemo, GI). See *aprepitant*. [eh-MEND].

**Emend Injection** (Chemo, GI). See *fosaprepitant*. [eh-MEND].

**Emetrol** (GI). See *phosphorated carbohydrate solution*. [EM-eh-trawl].

**Emgel** (Derm). See *erythromycin*. [EM-jel].

**EMLA** (Derm) (generic *lidocaine, prilocaine*). Combination anesthetic drug used topically to prevent pain during skin procedures, such as a biopsy or insertion of an intravenous line. Cream: 2.5%/2.5%. Disc: 2.5%/2.5%, 10 cm². [EM-lah].

**Empirin** (Analges, Ortho). See *aspirin*. [EM-pih-rin].

**Empirin w/ Codeine No. 3** (Analges) (generic *aspirin, codeine*). Combination Schedule III salicylate and narcotic analgesic drug for pain. Tablet: 325 mg/30 mg. [EM-pih-rin with KOH-deen].

**Empirin w/ Codeine No. 4** (Analges) (generic *aspirin, codeine*). Schedule III combination salicylate and narcotic analgesic drug for pain. Tablet: 325 mg/60 mg. [EM-pih-rin with KOH-deen].

**Emsam** (Neuro). See *selegiline*. [EM-sam].

**emtricitabine** (Emtriva) (Anti-infec). Nucleoside reverse transcriptase inhibitor antiviral drug used to treat treat HIV and AIDS. Capsule: 200 mg. Oral liquid: 10 mg/mL. [EM-trih-SY-tah-been].

**Emtriva** (Anti-infec). See *emtricitabine*. [em-TREE-vah].

**Emulsoil** (GI). See *castor oil*. [ee-MULS-oyl].

**Enablex** (Uro). See *darifenacin*. [en-AA-bleks].

**enadoline** (Neuro). Used to treat severe head injury. Orphan drug. [eh-NAD-oh-leen].

**enalapril** (Enalaprilat, Vasotec) (Cardio). ACE inhibitor drug used to treat hypertension and congestive heart failure. Tablet: 2.5 mg, 5 mg, 10 mg, 20 mg. Intravenous: 1.25 mg/mL. [eh-NAL-ah-pril].

**Enalaprilat** (Cardio). See *enalapril*. [eh-NAL-ah-PRIL-at].

**Enbrel** (Derm, GI, Ortho). See *etanercept*. [EN-brel].

**Endocet** (Analges) (generic *acetaminophen, oxycodone*). Combination Schedule II nonnarcotic and narcotic analgesic drug for pain. Tablet: 325 mg/5 mg, 325 mg/7.5 mg, 325 mg/10 mg, 500 mg/7.5 mg, 650 mg/10 mg. [EN-doh-set].

**Endometrin** (OB/GYN). See *progesterone*. [EN-doh-MEE-trin].

**Endrate** (Cardio). See *edetate*. [EN-drayt].

**Enduron** (Cardio, GI, Uro). See *methyclothiazide*. [EN-dyoor-awn].

**EnfaCare** (GI). Infant formula with iron. Liquid. Powder (to be reconstituted). [EN-fah-kair].

**Enfamil, Enfamil Human Milk Fortifier, Enfamil LactoFree, Enfamil LIPIL with Iron, Enfamil Next Step, Enfamil with Iron, Enfamil Premature Formula** (GI). Milk-based or lactose-free infant formula. Liquid. Liquid concentrate. Powder (to be reconstituted). [EN-fah-mil].

**enflurane** (Compound 347, Ethrane) (Anes). Anesthetic drug used to induce and maintain general anesthesia. Inhaled gas. [EN-floo-rayn].

**enfuvirtide** (Fuzeon) (Anti-infec). Fusion inhibitor antiviral drug used to treat HIV and AIDS. Subcutaneous: 108 mg/mL. [en-FYOO-vir-tide].

**Engerix-B** (GI). See *hepatitis B vaccine*. [EN-jeh-riks-B].

**eniluracil** (Chemo). Chemotherapy drug used to treat liver cancer. Orphan drug. [EH-nil-YOOR-ah-sil].

**enisoprost** (Uro). Used to treat kidney transplant patients who have nephrotoxicity caused by cyclosporine. Orphan drug. [eh-NEE-soh-prawst].

**Enjuvia** (OB/GYN). See *conjugated estrogens*. [en-JOO-vee-ah].

**Enlive** (GI). Lactose-free, gluten-free nutritional supplement. Liquid. [en-LIVE].

**Enlon** (Anes). See *edrophonium*. [EN-lawn].

**Enlon-Plus** (Anes) (generic *edrophonium, atropine*). Combination drug used to reverse the effect of neuromuscular blocker drugs given during general anesthesia. Intravenous: 10 mg/0.14 mg per 5 mL. [EN-lawn-PLUS].

**enoxaparin** (Lovenox) (Cardio, Hem). Low molecular weight heparin anticoagulant drug used to prevent deep venous thrombosis in patients who are undergoing abdominal or joint replacement surgery or who have poor mobility; used to prevent a blood clot in patients with acute coronary syndrome, unstable angina, and myocardial infarction. Subcutaneous: 30 mg/0.3 mL, 40 mg/0.4 mL, 60 mg/0.6 mL, 80 mg/0.8 mL, 100 mg/mL, 120 mg/0.8 mL, 150 mg/1 mL, 300 mg/3 mL. [eh-NAWK-sah-PAIR-in].

**Enpresse** (OB/GYN) (generic *levonorgestrel, ethinyl estradiol*). Combination triphasic oral contraceptive drug. Pill pack, 28-day: (6 hormone tablets) 0.05 mg/30 mcg; (5 hormone tablets) 0.075 mg/40 mcg; (10 hormone tablets) 0.125 mg/30 mcg; (7 inert tablets). [en-PRES].

**Ensure, Ensure HN, Ensure High Protein, Ensure with Fiber, Ensure Plus, Ensure Plus HN** (GI). Milk-based or lactose-free nutritional supplement. Liquid. Powder. Pudding. [en-SHOOR].

**entacapone** (Comtan) (Neuro). COMT inhibitor drug used to treat Parkinson's disease. Tablet: 200 mg. [en-TAK-ah-pohn].

**entecavir** (Baraclude) (Anti-infec, GI). Antiviral drug used to treat hepatitis B viral infection. Tablet: 0.5 mg, 1 mg. Oral liquid: 0.05 mg/mL. [en-TEK-ah-veer].

**Entereg** (Analges, GI). See *alvimopan*. [EN-ter-eg].

**Entex ER, Entex LA, PSE** (ENT) (generic *guaifenesin, pseudoephedrine*). Combination expectorant and decongestant drug used to treat colds with productive coughs. Capsule: 300 mg/10 mg, 400 mg/30 mg, 400 mg/120 mg. Tablet: 600 mg/30 mg, 600 mg/120 mg. [EN-teks].

**Entex HC** (ENT) (generic *guaifenesin, hydrocodone, phenylephrine*). Schedule III combination expectorant, narcotic antitussive, and decongestant drug used to treat colds with severe, productive coughing. Liquid: 100 mg/5 mg/7.5 mg. [EN-teks H-C].

**Entocort EC** (GI). See *budesonide*. [EN-toh-kort E-C].

**Entrition 0.5** (GI). Lactose-free nutritional supplement. Liquid. [en-TRII-shun].

**Enuclene** (Ophth). See *tyloxapol*. [ee-NOO-kleen].

**Enulose** (GI). See *lactulose*. [EN-yoo-lohs].

**enzastaurin** (Chemo). Chemotherapy drug used to treat brain cancer. Orphan drug. [en-ZAS-tar-in].

**ephedrine** (Cardio, Neuro, Pulm). Bronchodilator drug used to treat bronchial asthma; vasopressor drug used to treat complete heart block; stimulant drug used to treat narcolepsy and myasthenia gravis. Capsule: 25 mg. Subcutaneous, intramuscular, intravenous: 50 mg/mL. [eh-FED-drin].

**"epi"** (Emerg). Slang. See *epinephrine*. [EP-ee].

**epidermal growth factor** (Derm, Ophth). Used to treat corneal ulcers and burns. Orphan drug. [EP-ih-DER-mal GROWTH FAK-tor].

**epinastine** (Elestat) (Ophth). Antihistamine and mast cell stabilizer drug used topically to treat allergy symptoms in the eyes. Ophthalmic solution: 0.05%. [EP-ih-NAS-teen].

**epinephrine** (Adrenalin, EpiPen, EpiPen Jr, microNefrin, Primatene Mist, S2) (Cardio, Emerg, Pulm). Used to increase the blood pressure and initiate or increase the heart rate during emergency resuscitation; self-administered epinephrine used to prevent anaphylactic shock after an insect bite or food allergy; used to dilate the bronchi in patients with bronchial asthma. Liquid (for nebulizer for inhalation): 1:100 (10 mg/mL), 2.25%. Aerosol inhaler: 0.22 mg/spray. Endotracheal, subcutaneous, intramuscular, intracardiac, or intravenous: 1:1000 (1 mg/mL), 1:2000 (0.5 mg/mL), 1:10,000 (0.1 mg/mL). [EP-ih-NEF-rin].

**EpiPen, EpiPen Jr** (Emerg). See *epinephrine*. [EP-ee-pen].

**EpiQuin Micro** (Derm). See *hydroquinone*. [EP-ih-kwin MY-kroh].

**epirubicin** (Ellence) (Chemo). Chemotherapy antibiotic drug used to treat cancer of the breast, esophagus, and lung; used to treat Hodgkin's lymphoma and non-Hodgkin's lymphoma. Intravenous: 2 mg/mL. [EP-ee-ROO-bih-sin].

**Epitol** (Neuro). See *carbamazepine*. [EP-ih-tawl].

**Epivir, Epivir-HBV** (Anti-infec, GI). See *lamivudine*. [EP-ih-veer].

**eplerenone** (Inspra) (Cardio). Aldosterone receptor inhibitor drug used to treat hypertension; used to treat congestive heart failure; used to prevent death after myocardial infarction. Tablet: 25 mg, 50 mg. [eh-PLAIR-eh-nohn].

**epoetin alfa** (Epogen, Procrit) (Hem). Recombinant DNA technology erythropoietin-type drug that stimulates red blood cell production; used to treat anemia associated with AIDS, chronic renal failure, or chemotherapy; used to treat anemia in premature babies; used to treat myelodysplastic syndrome. Subcutaneous or intravenous: 2000 units/mL;

3000 units/mL; 4000 units/mL; 10,000 units/mL; 20,000 units/mL; 40,000 units/mL. [eh-POY-eh-tin AL-fah].

**epoetin beta** (Marogen) (Hem). Recombinant DNA technology erythropoietin-type drug that stimulates red blood cell production; used to treat anemia in patients with chronic renal failure. Orphan drug. [eh-POY-eh-tin BAY-tah].

**epoetin beta-methoxy polyethylene glycol** (Mircera) (Hem, Uro). Recombinant DNA technology erythropoietin-type drug that stimulates red blood cell production to treat anemia in patients with chronic renal failure. Intravenous: 50 mg/mL, 100 mg/mL, 200 mg/mL, 300 mg/mL, 400 mg/mL, 600 mg/mL, 1000 mg/mL. Subcutaneous with prefilled syringe: 50 mg/0.3 mL, 75 mg/0.3 mL, 100 mg/0.3 mL, 150 mg/0.3 mL, 200 mg/0.3 mL, 250 mg/0.3 mL. [eh-POY-eh-tin BAY-tah-meh-THAWK-see PAWL-ee-ETH-ih-leen GLY-kawl].

**Epogen** (Hem). See *epoetin alfa*. [EP-oh-jen].

**epoprostenol** (Cycloprostin, Flolan) (Hem, Pulm). Vasodilator drug used to treat pulmonary arterial hypertension; orphan drug used instead of heparin for hemodialysis. Intravenous (via a central venous catheter) (powder to be reconstituted): 0.5 mg, 1.5 mg. [EE-poh-PRAWS-teh-nawl].

**epratuzumab** (LymphoCIDE) (Chemo). Monoclonal antibody drug used to treat non-Hodgkin's lymphoma. Orphan drug. [EP-rah-TOOZ-yoo-mab].

**eprodisate** (Fibrillex) (Misc). Used to treat amyloidosis. Orphan drug. [eh-PROH-dih-sayt].

**eprosartan** (Teveten) (Cardio). Angiotensin II receptor blocker drug used to treat hypertension. Tablet: 600 mg. [EP-roh-SAR-tan].

**Epsom salt** (GI). Over-the-counter magnesium-containing laxative drug used to treat constipation. Granules. [EP-som].

**eptifibatide** (Integrilin) (Cardio, Hem). Platelet aggregation inhibitor drug used to treat acute coronary syndrome in patients undergoing angioplasty or stent placement. Intravenous: 0.75 mg/mL, 2 mg/mL. [ep-TIF-ih-bah-tide].

**Epzicom** (Anti-infec) (generic *abacavir, lamivudine*). Combination nucleoside reverse transcriptase inhibitor antiviral drug used to treat HIV and AIDS. Tablet: 600 mg/300 mg. [EP-zih-kawm].

**Equalactin** (GI). See *polycarbophil*. [EE-kwah-LAK-tin].

**Equetro** (Psych). See *carbamazepine*. [EE-kweh-troh].

**Erajet** (Neuro). See *clazosentan*. [AIR-ah-jet].

**Eraxis** (Anti-infec). See *anidulafungin*. [eh-RAK-sis].

**Erbitux** (Chemo). See *cetuximab*. [ER-bih-tuks].

**ergoloid mesylates** (Neuro). Used to treat the dementia of Alzheimer's disease. Tablet: 1 mg. Sublingual tablet: 1 mg. [AIR-goh-loyd MEH-sih-laytz].

**Ergomar** (Analges). See *ergotamine*. [ER-goh-mar].

**ergonovine** (Ergotrate) (OB/GYN). Used to treat postpartum or postabortion uterine bleeding. Tablet: 0.2 mg. [AIR-goh-NOH-veen].

**ergotamine** (Ergomar) (Analges). Used to treat migraine headaches. Sublingual tablet: 2 mg. [er-GAW-tah-meen].

**Ergotrate** (OB/GYN). See *ergonovine*. [AIR-goh-trayt].

**erlotinib** (Tarceva) (Chemo). Chemotherapy drug used to treat cancer of the brain, head and neck, lung, and pancreas. Tablet: 25 mg, 100 mg, 150 mg. [er-LOH-tih-nib].

**Errin** (OB/GYN). See *norethindrone*. [AIR-rin].

**Ertaczo** (Derm). See *sertaconazole*. [er-TAK-zoh].

**ertapenem** (Invanz) (Anti-infec). Carbapenem antibiotic drug used to treat gram-positive and gram-negative bacterial infections; used to treat staphylococcal and streptococcal skin infections; used to treat intra-abdominal infections, postpartum infections, and septic abortion; used to treat pyelonephritis from *E. coli;* used to treat pneumonia from *S. pneumoniae* and *H. influenzae*. Intramuscular or intravenous: 1 g. [ER-tah-PEN-em].

**Erwinase** (Chemo). See *erwinia L-asparaginase*. [ER-wih-nays].

**erwinia L-asparaginase** (Erwinase) (Chemo). Chemotherapy enzyme drug used to treat leukemia. Orphan drug. [er-WIN-ee-ah L-ah-SPAIR-ah-jih-nays].

**Eryc** (Anti-infec). See *erythromycin*. [AIR-ik].

**Eryderm 2%** (Anti-infec, Derm). See *erythromycin*. [AIR-ee-derm].

**Ery Pads** (Anti-infec, Derm). See *erythromycin*. [AIR-ee PADS].

**EryPed, EryPed 200, EryPed 400** (Anti-infec). See *erythromycin*. [AIR-ee-PEED].

**Ery-Tab** (Anti-infec). See *erythromycin*. [AIR-ee-TAB].

**Erythrocin** (Anti-infec). See *erythromycin*. [eh-REE-throh-sin].

**erythromycin** (A/T/S, E.E.S. 200, E.E.S. 400, Emgel, Eryc, Eryderm 2%, Ery Pads, EryPed, EryPed 200, EryPed 400, Ery-Tab, Erythrocin, Ilotycin, PCE Dispertab) (Anti-infec, Derm, Ophth). Macrolide antibiotic drug used to treat gram-negative and gram-positive bacterial infections; used to treat bronchitis and pneumonia due to *S. pneumoniae* , *H. influenzae,* and *Mycoplasma;* used to treat Legionnaire's disease of the lungs; used to treat pelvic inflammatory disease; used to treat gonorrhea, syphilis, *Chlamydia,* and nongonococcal urethritis; used to treat Lyme disease; used to treat intestinal amebiasis; used to prevent subacute bacterial endocarditis; used to treat staphylococcal and streptococcal skin infections; used topically on the skin to treat acne vulgaris (Emgel, Eryderm 2%, Ery Pads); used to treat bacterial infections in the eyes; used to prevent gonorrhea-caused blindness and *Chlamydia* eye infections in newborns (Ilotycin). Topical gel: 2%. Topical liquid: 2%. Topical ointment: 2%. Pledgets: 2%. Ophthalmic ointment: 0.5%. Tablet: 250 mg, 400 mg, 500 mg. Delayed-release tablet: 250 mg, 333 mg, 500 mg. Delayed-release capsule: 250 mg. Oral liquid: 100 mg/mL, 125 mg/5 mL, 200 mg/5 mL, 250 mg/5 mL, 400 mg/5 mL. Intravenous (powder to be reconstituted): 500 mg, 1 g. [eh-RITH-roh-MY-sin].

**erythropoietin** (Hem). See *epoetin alfa.* [eh-RITH-roh-POY-eh-tin].

**Eryzole** (Anti-infec) (generic *erythromycin, sulfisoxazole*). Combination antibiotic and sulfonamide drug used to treat otitis media. Liquid (granules to be reconstituted), 200 mg/600 mg per 5 mL. [AIR-uh-zohl]

**escitalopram** (Lexapro) (Psych). Selective serotonin reuptake inhibitor (SSRI) drug used to treat depression, anxiety, and panic attacks. Tablet: 5 mg, 10 mg, 20 mg. Liquid: 5 mg/5 mL. [ES-sih-TAL-oh-pram].

**Esclim** (OB/GYN, Ortho). See *estradiol.* [ES-klim].

**Esgic** (Analges) (generic *acetaminophen, butalbital, caffeine*). Combination nonsalicylate, barbiturate, and stimulant analgesic and sedative drug for pain. Capsule: 325 mg/50 mg/40 mg. Tablet: 325 mg/50 mg/40 mg. [ES-jik].

**Esgic Plus** (Analges) (generic *acetaminophen, butalbital, caffeine*). Combination nonsalicylate analgesic, barbiturate sedative, and stimulant drug for pain. Capsule: 500 mg/50 mg/40 mg. Tablet: 500 mg/50 mg/40 mg. [ES-jik PLUS].

**esmolol** (Brevibloc, Brevibloc Double Strength) (Cardio). Cardioselective beta-blocker drug used to treat ventricular tachycardia. Intravenous: 10 mg/mL, 20 mg/mL. [EZ-moh-lawl].

**esomeprazole** (Nexium, Nexium I.V.) (GI). Proton pump inhibitor drug used to treat heartburn, peptic ulcer, GERD (in children and adults), esophagitis, and *H. pylori* infection. Delayed-release capsule: 20 mg, 40 mg. Delayed-release oral powder: 20 mg, 40 mg. Intravenous (powder to be reconstituted): 20 mg, 40 mg. [EH-soh-MEH-prah-zohl].

**Esoterica Facial, Esoterica Regular** (Derm). See *hydroquinone.* [ES-oh-TAIR-ih-kah].

**estazolam** (ProSom) (Neuro). Schedule IV benzodiazepine drug used to treat insomnia. Tablet: 1 mg, 2 mg. [es-TAZ-oh-lam].

**esterified estrogens** (Menest) (Chemo, OB/GYN). Hormone drug used to treat hot flashes and vaginal dryness of menopause; palliative therapy used to treat advanced cancer of the breast and prostate gland. Tablet: 0.3 mg, 0.625 mg, 1.25 mg, 2.5 mg. [es-TAIR-ih-fied ES-troh-jens].

**Estrace, Estrace Vaginal** (Chemo, OB/GYN, Ortho). See *estradiol.* [ES-trays].

**Estraderm** (OB/GYN, Ortho). See *estradiol.* [ES-trah-derm].

**estradiol** (Alora, Climara, Delestrogen, Depo-Estradiol, Divigel, Elestrin, Esclim, Estrace, Estrace Vaginal, Estraderm, Estrasorb, Estring, Estrogel, Evamist, Femring, Femtrace, Gynodiol, Menostar, Vagifem, Vivelle, Vivelle-Dot) (Chemo, OB/GYN, Ortho). Hormone replacement therapy used to treat hot flashes and vaginal dryness of menopause; palliative therapy for advanced cancer of the breast and prostate gland; used to prevent osteoporosis in postmenopausal women. Tablet: 0.45 mg, 0.5 mg, 0.9 mg, 1 mg, 1.5 mg, 1.8 mg, 2 mg. Intramuscular: 5 mg/mL, 10 mg/mL, 20 mg/mL, 40 mg/mL. Vaginal gel (metered-dose pump): 0.87 g/pump. Topical skin gel: 0.06%; 0.25 mg, 0.5 mg, 1 mg. Topical skin emulsion: 2.5 mg pouch. Transdermal patch: 0.014 mg/day, 0.025 mg/day, 0.0375 mg/day, 0.05 mg/day, 0.06 mg/day, 0.075 mg/day, 0.1 mg/day. Transdermal spray: 1.53 mg/spray. Vaginal cream: 0.1 mg. Vaginal ring: 0.05 mg/day, 0.1 mg/day, 2 mg/day. Vaginal tablet: 25 mcg. [ES-trah-DY-awl].

**estramustine** (Emcyt) (Chemo). Alkylating chemotherapy drug used to treat cancer of the prostate gland and kidney. Capsule: 140 mg. [ES-trah-MUS-teen].

**Estrasorb** (OB/GYN). See *estradiol.* [ES-trah-sorb].

**Estratest, Estratest H.S.** (OB/GYN) (generic *methyltestosterone, esterified estrogens*). Combination hormone drug used to treat the symptoms of menopause. Tablet: 1.25 mg/0.625 mg, 2.5 mg/1.25 mg. [ES-trah-test].

**Estring** (OB/GYN). See *estradiol.* [ES-tring].

**Estrogel** (OB/GYN). See *estradiol.* [ES-troh-jel].

**estrogen** (OB/GYN). See *esterified estrogens* or *conjugated estrogens.*

**estropipate** (Ogen, Ortho-Est) (OB/GYN, Ortho). Hormone replacement therapy drug used to treat hot flashes and vaginal dryness of menopause; used to prevent osteoporosis in postmenopausal women; used to treat primary ovarian failure. Tablet: 0.625 mg, 1.25 mg, 2.5 mg, 5 mg. [ES-troh-PIH-payt].

**Estrostep 21** (Derm, OB/GYN) (generic *norethindrone, ethinyl estradiol*). Combination triphasic oral contraceptive drug; used to treat acne vulgaris. Pill pack, 21-day: (5 hormone tablets) 1 mg/20 mcg; (7 hormone tablets) 1 mg/30 mcg; (9 hormone tablets) 1 mg/35 mcg. [ES-troh-step].

**Estrostep Fe** (Derm, OB/GYN) (generic *norethindrone, ethinyl estradiol, ferrous fumarate*). Combination triphasic oral contraceptive drug with iron supplement; used to treat acne vulgaris. Pill pack, 28-day: (5 hormone tablets) 1 mg/20 mcg; (7 hormone tablets) 1 mg/30 mcg; (9 hormone tablets) 1 mg/35 mcg; (7 iron [Fe] tablets) 75 mg. [ES-troh-step F-E].

**eszopiclone** (Lunesta) (Neuro). Schedule IV drug used to treat insomnia. Tablet: 1 mg, 2 mg, 3 mg. [es-ZOP-ih-klohn].

**etanercept** (Enbrel) (Derm, GI, Ortho). Immunomodulator drug that blocks tumor necrosis factor; used to treat severe psoriasis and psoriatic arthritis; used to treat ankylosing spondylitis and rheumatoid arthritis; used to treat Crohn's disease. Subcutaneous: 50 mg/mL. [eh-TAN-er-sept].

**ethacrynic acid** (Edecrin) (Cardio, Uro). Loop diuretic drug used to treat edema from congestive heart failure, liver disease, or kidney disease. Tablet: 25 mg, 50 mg. Intravenous: 50 mg/50 mL. [ETH-ah-KRIN-ik AS-id].

**ethambutol** (Myambutol) (Anti-infec, Pulm). Antitubercular antibiotic drug used to treat tuberculosis; used to prevent

*Mycobacterium avium-intracellulare* infection in AIDS patients. Tablet: 100 mg, 400 mg. [eth-AM-byoo-tawl].

**Ethamolin** (GI). See *ethanolamine.* [eh-THAM-oh-lin].

**ethanolamine** (Ethamolin) (GI). Sclerosing drug used to prevent rebleeding from esophageal varices. Injection (into esophageal varix): 5%. [ETH-ah-NOH-lah-meen].

**Ethezyme, Ethezyme 830** (Derm). See *papain.* [ETH-eh-zime].

**ethinyl estradiol** (Misc, OB/GYN). Hormone drug that is a component of oral contraceptive drugs; orphan drug used to treat Turner syndrome. (ETH-ih-nil ES-trah-DY-awl].

**ethiofos** (Chemo). Cytoprotective drug used to prevent toxicity in patients receiving cisplatin or cyclophosphamide chemotherapy. Orphan drug. [ETH-ee-oh-faws].

**ethionamide** (Trecator-SC) (Pulm). Antitubercular antibiotic drug used to treat tuberculosis that is resistant to other antitubercular drugs. Tablet: 250 mg. [eh-thy-AWN-ah-mide].

**Ethmozine** (Cardio). See *moricizine.* [ETH-moh-zeen].

**ethosuximide** (Zarontin) (Neuro). Anticonvulsant drug used to treat absence seizures. Capsule: 250 mg. Liquid: 250 mg/5mL. [ETH-oh-SUK-sih-mide].

**Ethrane** (Anes). See *enflurane.* [EE-thrayn].

**Ethyol** (Chemo, Uro). See *amifostine.* [ETH-ee-awl].

**etidronate** (Didronel) (Chemo, Ortho). Bone resorption inhibitor drug used to treat Paget's disease of the bone; used to prevent abnormal bone formation following hip replacement surgery; used to treat osteoporosis caused by corticosteroid drugs; used to treat hypercalcemia of malignancy. Tablet: 200 mg, 400 mg. [eh-TIH-droh-nayt].

**etodolac** (Analges). Nonsteroidal anti-inflammatory drug used to treat pain and inflammation; used to treat osteoarthritis, rheumatoid arthritis, bursitis, tendinitis, and gout. Capsule: 200 mg, 300 mg. Tablet: 400 mg, 500 mg. Extended-release tablet: 400 mg, 500 mg, 600 mg. [ee-TOH-doh-lak].

**etomidate** (Amidate) (Anes). Sedative drug used to induce and maintain general anesthesia. Intravenous: 2 mg/mL. [eh-TAWM-ih-dayt].

**etonogestrel** (OB/GYN). Progestin hormone contraceptive drug used to prevent pregnancy. Subdermal implant (placed on the inner side of the upper arm, effective for 3 years): 68 mg. [eh-TON-oh-JES-trel].

**Etopophos** (Chemo). See *etoposide.* [eh-TOH-poh-faws].

**etoposide** (Etopophos, Toposar, VePesid) (Chemo). Mitosis inhibitor chemotherapy drug used to treat cancer of the brain, lung, bone, muscle, ovary, testicle, and bladder; used to treat Hodgkin's lymphoma, leukemia, Kaposi's sarcoma, and Wilm's tumor. Capsule: 50 mg. Intravenous: 20 mg/mL. [eh-TOH-poh-side].

**Etrafon, Etrafon-A, Etrafon-Forte, Etrafon 2-10** (Psych) (generic *amitriptyline, perphenazine*). Combination antidepressant and antipsychotic drug. Tablet: 10 mg/2 mg, 25 mg/2 mg, 10 mg/4 mg, 25 mg/4 mg, 50 mg/4 mg. [EH-trah-fawn].

**etravirine** (Intelence) (Anti-infec). Nonnucleoside reverse transcriptase inhibitor antiviral drug used to treat HIV and AIDS. Tablet: 100 mg. [EH-trah-VY-reen].

**Eucalyptamint, Eucalyptamint Maximum Strength** (Ortho) (generic *menthol, eucalyptus oil*). Combination analgesic drug used topically to treat the pain of osteoarthritis and minor muscle injuries. Gel. Ointment. [yoo-kah-LIP-tah-mint].

**Eucerin Plus** (Derm) (generic *lanolin, urea*). Combination over-the-counter debridement and emollient drug used topically to treat minor skin irritation. Lotion. [YOO-seh-rin PLUS].

**Euflexxa** (Ortho). See *hyaluronic acid.* [yoo-FLEKS-zah].

**Eurax** (Derm). See *crotamiton.* [YOOR-aks].

**Evac-u-gen** (GI). See *sennosides.* [ee-VAK-yoo-jen].

**Evamist** (OB/GYN). See *estradiol.* [EE-vah-mist].

**Evicel** (Hem). See *fibrin.* [EV-ih-sel].

**Evista** (Chemo, OB/GYN, Ortho). See *raloxifene.* [ee-VIS-tah].

**Evithrom** (Hem). See *thrombin.* [EV-ih-thrawm].

**Evoclin** (Derm). See *clindamycin.* [EV-oh-klin].

**Evolence** (Derm). See *human collagen.* [EV-oh-lens].

**Evoxac** (ENT). See *cevimeline.* [ee-VAWK-sak].

**Exact** (Derm). Keratolytic drug used topically on the skin to treat acne vulgaris. Liquid. [eks-ZACT].

**Excedrin Aspirin Free, Excedrine Tension Headache, Excedrin QuickTabs** (Analges) (generic *acetaminophen, caffeine*). Combination over-the-counter nonsalicylate analgesic and stimulant drug used to treat pain and headaches. Caplet, geltab: 500 mg/65 mg. [ek-SED-rin].

**Excedrin Extra Strength, Excedrin Migraine** (Analges) (generic *acetaminophen, aspirin, caffeine*). Combination over-the-counter nonsalicylate and salicylate analgesic and stimulant drug used to treat pain and migraine headaches. Caplet, gelcap, tablet: 250 mg/250 mg/65 mg. [ek-SED-rin].

**Excedrin P.M., Excedrin P.M. Liquigels** (Analges, Neuro) (generic *acetaminophen, diphenhydramine*). Combination over-the-counter nonsalicylate analgesic and antihistamine drug used to relieve pain and induce sleep. Capsule: 500 mg/25 mg. Tablet: 500 mg/25 mg. Liquid: 167 mg/8.3 mg per 5 mL, 1000 mg/50 mg per 30 mL. [ek-SED-rin].

**Excedrin Sinus Headache** (Analges, ENT) (generic *acetaminophen, phenylephrine*). Combination over-the-counter nonsalicylate analgesic and decongestant drug used to treat sinus headaches. Tablet: 325 mg/5 mg. [ek-SED-rin].

**Exelderm** (Derm). See *sulconazole.* [EK-sel-derm].

**Exelon, Exelon Oral Solution, Exelon Patch** (Neuro). See *rivastigmine.* [EK-seh-lawn].

**exemestane** (Aromasin) (Chemo). Hormonal chemotherapy drug used to treat breast cancer; used to treat prostate gland cancer in men. Tablet: 25 mg. [EK-seh-MES-tayn].

**exenatide** (Byetta) (Endo). Incretin mimetic antidiabetic drug used to treat type 2 diabetes mellitus. Subcutaneous: 5 mcg/1.2 mL, 10 mcg/2.4 mL. [ek-SEN-ah-tide].

**Exforge** (Cardio) (generic *amlodipine, valsartan*). Combination calcium channel blocker and angiotensin II receptor blocker drug used to treat hypertension. Tablet: 160 mg/5 mg, 160 mg/10 mg, 320 mg/5 mg, 320 mg/10 mg. [EKS-forj].

**Exidine** (Derm).    See *chlorhexidine*. [EK-sih-dine].

**exisulind** (GI).    Used to treat colonic polyps in patients with adenomatous polyps of the colon. Orphan drug. [ek-SIS-oo-lind].

**Exjade** (Hem).    See *deferasirox*. [EKS-jayd].

**ex•lax, ex•lax chocolated, Maximum Relief ex•lax** (GI).    See *sennosides*. [EKS-laks].

**ex•lax Gentle Strength** (GI) (generic *docusate, senna*). Combination over-the-counter stool softener and irritant/stimulant laxative drug used to treat constipation. Caplet: 65 mg/10 mg. [EKS-laks].

**ex•lax Stool Softener** (GI).    See *docusate*. [EKS-laks].

**Exosurf Neonate** (Pulm).    See *colfosceril*. [EK-soh-surf NEE-oh-nayt].

**Extina** (Derm).    See *ketoconazole*. [eks-TEE-nah].

**ezetimibe** (Zetia) (Cardio).    Used to treat hypercholesterolemia and hypertriglyceridemia. Tablet: 10 mg. [ek-SET-ih-mibe].

**Ezide** (Cardio, Uro).    See *hydrochlorothiazide*. [EE-zide].

**4-aminopyridine** (Neuro).    Used to treat motor and sensory deficits in Guillain-Barré syndrome. Orphan drug. [4-ah-MEE-noh-PY-rih-deen].

**4-aminosalicylic acid**. See *aminosalicylic acid*. [4-ah-MEE-noh-SAL-ih-SIL-ik AS-id].

**4-Way Fast Acting** (ENT).    See *phenylephrine*. [4-WAY].

**5-aminosalicylic acid** (5-ASA) (GI).    See *mesalamine*. [5-ah-MEE-noh-SAL-ih-SIL-ik AS-id].

**Fabrase** (Misc).    See *alpha-galactosidase A*. [FAB-rays].

**Fabrazyme** (Misc).    See *agalsidase beta*. [FAB-rah-zime].

**Factive** (Anti-infec).    See *gemifloxacin*. [FAK-tiv].

**factor VIIa** (NovoSeven, NovoSeven RT) (Hem).    Clotting factor VIIa used to treat bleeding episodes in hemophiliac patients who produce inhibitors to factor VIII or factor IX. Intravenous (powder to be reconstituted): 1.2 mg/2.2 mL, 2.4 mg/4.3 mL, 4.8 mg/8.5 mL. [FAK-tor 7-a].

**factor VIII** (Advate, Alphanate, Bioclate, Helixate FS, Hemofil M, Hyate:C, Koate-DVI, Kogenate FS, Monarc-M, Monoclate-P, Recombinate, ReFacto, Xyntha) (Hem).    Clotting factor VIII used to treat bleeding episodes in hemophiliac patients with factor VIII deficiency; orphan drug used to treat von Willebrand disease. Intravenous (powder to be reconstituted). [FAK-tor 8].

**factor IX** (AlphaNine SD, Bebulin VH, BeneFix, Mononine, Profilnine SD, Proplex T) (Hem).    Clotting factor IX used to treat hemophilia B patients with factor IX deficiency (Christmas disease); used to treat factor VII deficiency (Proplex T). Intravenous (powder to be reconstituted). [FAK-tor 9].

**factor XII** (Fibrogammin P) (Hem).    Clotting factor XII used to treat patients with factor XII deficiency. Orphan drug. [FAK-tor 12].

**Factrel** (Misc).    See *gonadorelin*. [fak-TREL].

**Falkochol** (GI).    Used to treat incorrect synthesis and metabolism of cholesterol and bile acids due to genetic mutation. Orphan drug. [FAL-koh-kawl].

**famciclovir** (Famvir) (Anti-infec, Derm, ENT, OB/GYN). Antiviral drug used to treat herpes zoster (shingles) on the skin; used to treat herpes simplex type 1 virus (cold sores) on the mouth in immunocompromised patients; used to treat herpes simplex type 2 virus (genital herpes). Tablet: 125 mg, 250 mg, 500 mg. [fam-SY-kloh-veer].

**famotidine** (Pepcid, Pepcid AC, Pepcid AC Maximum Strength, Pepcid RPD) (GI).    Over-the-counter and prescription $H_2$ blocker drug to treat heartburn, peptic ulcer, GERD, and *H. pylori* infection. Chewable tablet: 10 mg. Orally disintegrating tablet: 20 mg, 40 mg. Gelcap: 10 mg. Oral liquid (powder to be reconstituted): 40 mg/5 mL. Tablet: 10 mg, 20 mg, 40 mg. Intravenous: 10 mg/mL, 20 mg/50 mL. [fah-MOH-tih-deen].

**fampridine** (Neurelan) (Neuro).    Used to treat symptoms of multiple sclerosis and spinal cord injury. Orphan drug. [FAM-prih-deen].

**Famvir** (Anti-infec, Derm, ENT, OB/GYN).    See *famciclovir*. [FAM-veer].

**Fansidar** (Anti-infec).    See *sulfadoxine*. [FAN-sih-dar].

**Fareston** (Chemo).    See *toremifene*. [FAIR-es-ton].

**Faslodex** (Chemo).    See *fulvestrant*. [FAS-loh-deks].

**Fasprin** (Analges).    See *aspirin*. [FAS-prin].

**FazaClo** (Psych).    See *clozapine*. [FAY-zah-kloh].

**Feen-a-mint** (GI).    See *bisacodyl*. [FEEN-ah-mint].

**Feiba VH** (Hem).    See *anti-inhibitor coagulant complex*. [FEE-bah V-H].

**felbamate** (Felbatol) (Neuro).    Anticonvulsant drug used to treat severe seizures not controlled by other anticonvulsant drugs; orphan drug used to treat Lennox-Gastaut syndrome. Tablet: 400 mg, 600 mg. Liquid: 600 mg/5 mL. [FEL-bah-mayt].

**Felbatol** (Neuro).    See *felbamate*. [FEL-bah-tawl].

**Feldene** (Analges).    See *piroxicam*. [FEL-deen].

**felodipine** (Plendil) (Cardio).    Calcium channel blocker drug used to treat hypertension, pulmonary arterial hypertension, and Raynaud's disease. Tablet: 2.5 mg, 5 mg, 10 mg. [feh-LOH-dih-peen].

**Femara** (Chemo).    See *letrozole*. [feh-MAIR-ah].

**Femcon Fe** (OB/GYN) (generic *norethindrone, ethinyl estradiol; ferrous fumarate*).    Combination monophasic oral contraceptive drug with iron supplement. Pill pack, 28-day: (21 hormone tablets) 0.4 mg/35 mcg; (7 iron [Fe] tablets) 75 mg. [FEM-kawn F-E].

**Femhrt** (OB/GYN, Ortho) (generic *norethindrone, estradiol*).    Combination hormone drug used to treat the symptoms of menopause; used to prevent osteoporosis in postmenopausal women. Tablet: 0.5 mg/2/5 mcg, 1 mg/5 mcg. [FEM-H-R-T].

**Femring** (OB/GYN).    See *estradiol*. [FEM-ring].

**Femtrace** (OB/GYN).    See *estradiol*. [FEM-trays].

**fenofibrate** (Antara, Fenoglide, Lipofen, Lofibra, Tricor,Triglide) (Cardio).    Used to treat hypercholesterolemia by decreasing serum cholesterol and LDL; used to treat hypertriglyceridemia by decreasing serum triglyercides; increases HDL. Capsule: 43 mg, 50 mg, 67 mg, 130 mg, 134 mg, 150 mg, 200 mg Tablet: 48 mg, 50 mg, 54 mg, 107 mg, 145 mg, 160 mg. MeltDose tablet: 40 mg, 120 mg. [FEN-oh-FY-brayt].

**Fenoglide** (Cardio).    See *fenofibrate*. [FEN-oh-glide].

**fenoldopam** (Corlopam) (Cardio).    Peripheral vasodilator drug used to treat hypertensive crisis. Intravenous: 10 mg/mL. [feh-NOL-doh-pam].

**fenoprofen** (Nalfon) (Analges).    Nonsteroidal anti-inflammatory drug used to treat pain and inflammation; used to treat osteoarthritis and rheumatoid arthritis; used to prevent migraine headaches. Capsule: 200 mg, 300 mg. Tablet: 600 mg. [FEN-oh-PROH-fen].

**fenretinide** (Chemo).    Chemotherapy drug used to treat brain cancer. Orphan drug. [fen-RET-ih-nide].

**fentanyl** (Actiq, Duragesic-12, Duragesic-25, Duragesic-50, Duragesic-75, Duragesic-100, Ionsys, Sublimaze) (Analges, Anes).    Schedule II narcotic drug used to treat severe pain; used to induce and help maintain general anesthesia (Sublimaze). Transdermal patch: 12.5 mcg/hour, 25 mcg/hour, 50 mcg/hour, 75 mcg/hour, 100 mcg/hour. Transdermal patch with self-administered button: 40 mcg/dose. Intramuscular and intravenous: 0.05 mg/mL. [FEN-tah-nil].

**Feosol** (Hem).    See *ferrous sulfate*. [FEE-oh-sawl].

**Feratab** (Hem).    See *ferrous sulfate*. [FAIR-ah-tab].

**Fergon** (Hem).    See *ferrous gluconate*. [FAIR-gawn].

**Fer-Gen-Sol** (Hem).    See *ferrous sulfate*. [FAIR-jen-sawl].

**Fer-In-Sol** (Hem).    See *ferrous sulfate*. [FAIR-in-sawl].

**Ferralet 90** (Hem) (generic *iron, minerals, vitamins, docusate*).    Combination iron, multivitamin, mineral, and stool softener drug used to treat anemia. Tablet: 90 mg (of iron). [FAIR-ah-let 90].

**Ferrets** (Hem).    See *ferrous fumarate*. [FAIR-ets].

**Ferriprox** (Hem).    See *deferiprone*. [FAIR-ih-prawks].

**Ferrlecit** (Hem, Uro).    See *sodium ferric gluconate*. [FAIR-leh-sit].

**Ferro-Sequels** (Hem).    See *ferrous fumarate*. [FAIR-oh-SEE-kwels].

**ferrous fumarate** (Ferrets, Ferro-Sequels, Hemocyte, Nephro-Fer) (Hem).    Over-the-counter, iron-containing drug used to treat iron deficiency and iron deficiency anemia. Tablet: 90 mg, 325 mg, 350 mg. Timed-release tablet: 150 mg. [FAIR-uhs FYOO-mah-rayt].

**ferrous gluconate** (Fergon) (Hem).    Over-the-counter, iron-containing drug used to treat iron deficiency and iron deficiency anemia. Tablet: 225 mg, 300 mg, 325 mg. [FAIR-uhs GLOO-koh-nayt].

**ferrous sulfate** (Feratab, Feosol, Fer-Gen-Sol, Fer-In-Sol, Slow FE) (Hem).    Over-the-counter iron-containing drug used to treat iron deficiency and iron deficiency anemia. Tablet: 200 mg, 300 mg, 325 mg. Slow-release tablet: 160 mg. Elixir: 220 mg/5 mL. Drops: 75 mg/0.6 mL. Oral liquid: 300 mg/5 mL. [FAIR-uhs SUL-fayt].

**Fertinex** (Endo, OB/GYN).    See *urofollitropin*. [FER-tih-neks].

**fexofenadine** (Allegra, Allegra ODT) (Derm, ENT).    Antihistamine drug used to treat seasonal and perennial allergies and allergic rhinitis; used to treat allergic skin reactions with itching. Tablet: 30 mg, 60 mg, 180 mg. Oral suspension: 6 mg/mL. Orally disintegrating tablet: 30 mg. [FEKS-oh-FEN-ah-deen].

**Fiberall** (GI).    See *psyllium*. [FY-ber-awl].

**FiberCon** (GI).    See *polycarbophil*. [FY-ber-kawn].

**Fiber-Lax** (GI).    See *polycarbophil*. [FY-ber-laks].

**Fibrillex** (Misc).    See *eprodisate*. [FIB-rih-leks].

**fibrin** (Evicel) (Hem).    Hemostatic drug used topically to control bleeding during surgery. Liquid sealant. [FY-brin].

**Fibrogammin P** (Hem).    See *factor XII*. [FY-broh-GAM-min P].

**Fidelin** (Endo).    See *dehydroepiandrosterone*. [FY-deh-lin].

**filgrastim** (Neupogen) (Anti-infec, Chemo, Hem).    Granulocyte colony-stimulating factor drug used to increase the neutrophil count in patients undergoing chemotherapy or bone marrow transplantation and in patient with AIDS; used to treat aplastic anemia. Subcutaneous or intravenous: 300 mcg/mL. [fil-GRAH-stim].

**Finacea** (Derm).    See *azelaic acid*. [fih-NAS-ee-ah].

**finasteride** (Propecia, Proscar) (Derm, Uro).    Male hormone inhibitor drug used to treat male pattern baldness (Propecia); used to treat benign prostatic hypertrophy (Proscar). Tablet: 1 mg, 5 mg. [fin-AS-ter-ide].

**Fioricet** (Analges) (generic *acetaminophen, butalbital, caffeine*).    Combination nonsalicylate analgesic, barbiturate sedative, and stimulant drug for pain. Tablet: 325 mg/50 mg/40 mg. [fee-OR-ih-set].

**Fioricet w/ Codeine** (Analges) (generic *acetaminophen, butalbital, caffeine, codeine*).    Combination Schedule III nonsalicyliate analgesic, barbiturate sedative, stimulant, and narcotic analgesic drug for pain. Capsule: 325 mg/50 mg/40 mg/30 mg. [fee-OR-ih-set with KOH-deen].

**Fiorinal** (Analges) (generic *aspirin, butalbital, caffeine*).    Combination salicylate analgesic, barbiturate sedative, and stimulant drug. Capsule: 325 mg/50 mg/40 mg. [fee-OR-ih-nawl].

**Fiorinal w/ Codeine** (Analges) (generic *aspirin, butalbital, caffeine, codeine*).    Combination Schedule III salicylate analgesic, barbiturate sedative, stimulant, and narcotic analgesic drug for pain. Capsule: 325 mg/ 50 mg/40 mg/30 mg. [fee-OR-ih-nawl with KOH-deen].

**Flagyl, Flagyl ER, Flagyl 375, Flagyl IV** (Anti-infec, GI, OB/GYN).    See *metronidazole*. [FLAJ-il].

**Flammacerium** (Derm).    Used to prevent death in burn patients. Orphan drug. [FLAM-mah-SEH-ree-um].

**Flarex** (Ophth). See *fluorometholone*. [FLAIR-eks].

**Flatulex** (GI) (generic *charcoal, simethicone*). Combination antiflatulent drug for intestinal gas. [FLAH-tyoo-leks].

**flavoxate** (Urispas) (Uro). Antispasmodic drug used to treat urinary frequency, urgency, and spasms from dysuria or urinary tract infections. Tablet: 100 mg. [fluh-VAWK-sayt].

**Flebogamma 5%** (Anti-infec, Misc). See *human immune globulin*. [FLEE-boh-GAM-mah 5%].

**flecainide** (Tambocor) (Cardio). Antiarrhythmic drug used to treat atrial fibrillation and ventricular tachycardia. Tablet: 50 mg, 100 mg, 150 mg. [FLEK-ah-nide].

**Flector** (Analges). See *diclofenac*. [FLEK-tor].

**Fleet Enema** (GI). See *sodium phosphate*. [FLEET EN-eh-mah].

**Fleet Babylax** (GI). See *glycerin*. [FLEET BAY-bee-laks].

**Fleet Bisacodyl Enema, Fleet Laxative** (GI). See *bisacodyl*. [FLEET BIS-ah-KOH-dil].

**Fleet Mineral Oil Enema** (GI). See *mineral oil*. [FLEET].

**Fleet Phospho-soda** (GI). See *sodium phosphate*. [FLEET FAWS-foh-SOH-dah].

**Fleet Prep Kit 1, Fleet Prep Kit 2, Fleet Prep Kit 3** (GI) (generic *phosphosoda, bisacodyl*). Combination over-the-counter bowel evacuant and bowel prep kit. Oral liquid, oral tablets, suppository or enema. [FLEET].

**Fletcher's Castoria** (GI). See *sennosides*. [FLET-churz kas-TOR-ee-ah].

**Flexall Ultra Plus, Maximum Strength Flexall 454** (Ortho) (generic *menthol, methyl salicylate*). Combination analgesic drug used topically to treat the pain of osteoarthritis and minor muscle injuries. Gel. [FLEKS-all].

**Flexaphen** (Ortho) (generic *chlorzoxazone, acetaminophen*). Combination skeletal muscle relaxant and analgesic drug used to treat the pain, spasm, and stiffness of minor muscle injuries. Capsule: 250 mg/300 mg. [FLEK-sah-fen].

**Flexeril** (Ortho). See *cyclobenzaprine*. [FLEK-zeh-ril].

**FlexiGel Strands** (Derm). Over-the-counter drug used topically to absorb drainage from burns, skin ulcers, and wounds. Absorbent gauze dressing. [FLEKS-ee-jel].

**Flexon** (Ortho). See *orphenadrine*. [FLEKS-awn].

**Flocor** (Derm, Hem, Neuro). See *poloxamer 188*. [FLOH-kor].

**Flolan** (Pulm). See *epoprostenol*. [FLOH-lan].

**Flomax** (Uro). See *tamsulosin*. [FLOH-maks].

**Flonase** (ENT). See *fluticasone*. [FLOH-nays].

**Flo-Pred** (Endo, Pulm). See *prednisolone*. [FLOH-pred].

**Florinef** (Endo). See *fludrocortisone*. [FLOOR-ih-nef].

**Florone, Florone E** (Derm). See *diflorasone*. [FLOOR-ohn].

**Flovent, Flovent Diskus, Flovent Rotadisk** (Pulm). See *fluticasone*. [FLOH-vent].

**Floxin, Floxin Otic** (Anti-infec, ENT). See *ofloxacin*. [FLAWK-sin].

**floxuridine** (FUDR) (Chemo). Antimetabolite chemotherapy drug used to treat cancer of the stomach, liver, kidney, or ovary. Intra-arterial (powder to be reconstituted): 500 mg. [flawks-YOOR-ih-deen].

**Fluarix** (Anti-infec, Pulm). See *influenza virus vaccine*. [floo-AIR-iks].

**fluconazole** (Diflucan) (Anti-infec). Antifungal and antiyeast drug used to treat severe systemic fungal and yeast infections; used to treat cryptococcal meningitis in AIDS patients. Tablet: 50 mg, 100 mg, 150 mg, 200 mg. Oral liquid (powder to be reconstituted): 10 mg/mL, 40 mg/mL. Intravenous: 2 mg/mL. [floo-KAWN-ah-zohl].

**flucytosine** (Ancobon) (Anti-infec). Antifungal drug used to treat severe systemic fungal and yeast infections. Capsule: 250 mg, 500 mg. [floo-SY-toh-seen].

**Fludara** (Chemo). See *fludarabine*. [floo-DAIR-ah].

**fludarabine** (Fludara) (Chemo). Antimetabolite chemotherapy drug used to treat leukemia and non-Hodgkin's lymphoma. Intravenous: 25 mg/mL. [floo-DAIR-ah-been].

**fludrocortisone** (Florinef) (Endo). Corticosteroid drug used as hormone replacement to treat Addison's disease. Tablet: 0.1 mg. [FLOO-droh-KOHR-tih-zohn].

**FluLaval** (Anti-infec, Pulm). See *influenza virus vaccine*. [floo-LAY-val].

**Flumadine** (Anti-infec, Pulm). See *rimantadine*. [FLOO-mah-deen].

**flumazenil** (Romazicon) (Emerg, Psych). Benzodiazepine antagonist drug used as an antidote to reverse an overdose of a benzodiazepine antianxiety drug or postoperatively to revise a benzodiazepine drug given preoperatively. Intravenous: 0.1 mg/mL. [floo-MAY-zeh-nil].

**flumecinol** (Zixoryn) (Hem). Used to treat hyperbilirubine-mia in newborns when phototherapy is not effective. Orphan drug. [floo-MEK-ih-nawl].

**FluMist** (Anti-infec, Pulm). See *influenza virus vaccine*. [FLOO-mist].

**flunarizine** (Sibelium) (Neuro). Used to treat alternating hemiplegia. Orphan drug. [floo-NAIR-ih-zeen].

**flunisolide** (AeroBid, AeroBid-M, AeroSpan, Nasalide) (ENT, Pulm). Corticosteroid anti-inflammatory drug used to prevent acute asthma attacks; used topically in the nose to treat allergy symptoms (Nasalide). Aerosol inhaler: 80 mcg/puff, 250 mcg/puff. Nasal spray: 25 mcg/spray. [floo-NIS-oh-lide].

**flunitrazepam** (Rohypnol) (Psych). Illegal drug not approved for use in the United States. One of the so-called "date-rape drugs." [FLOO-nih-TRAZ-eh-pam].

**fluocinolone** (Capex, Derma-Smoothe/FS, Retisert, Synalar) (Derm, Ophth). Corticosteroid drug used topically to treat inflammation and itching from dermatitis, seborrhea, eczema, psoriasis, and yeast or fungal infections; implant inserted in the vitreous humor of the eye to treat uveitis (Retisert). Cream: 0.01%, 0.025%. Liquid: 0.01%. Oil: 0.01%. Ointment: 0.025%. Shampoo: 0.01%. Eye implant: 0.59 mg. [FLOO-oh-SIN-oh-lohn].

**fluocinonide** (Fluonex, Lidex, Lidex-E, Vanos) (Derm). Corticosteroid drug used topically to treat inflammation and itching from dermatitis, seborrhea, eczema, psoriasis, and yeast or fungal infections. Cream: 0.05%, 0.1%. Gel: 0.05%. Liquid: 0.05%. Ointment: 0.05%. [floo-oh-SIN-oh-nide].

**Fluonex** (Derm). See *fluocinonide*. [FLOO-oh-neks].

**Fluoracaine** (Ophth) (generic *fluorescein, proparacaine*). Combination ophthalmic dye and anesthetic drug used topically in the eye. Ophthalmic solution: 0.25%/0.5%. [FLOOR-ah-kayn].

**fluorescein** (Fluorescite, Fluorets, Ful-Glo) (Ophth). Dye used topically to detect corneal abrasions, corneal ulcers, and ill-fitting contact lens; given intravenously during angiography to show yellow-green color of blood vessels during examination of the retina. Ophthalmic solution: 2%. Ophthalmic strips: 0.6 mg, 1 mg. Intravenous: 10%, 25%. [FLOOR-eh-seen].

**Fluorescite** (Ophth). See *fluorescein*. [FLOOR-eh-site].

**Fluoresoft** (Ophth). See *fluorexon*. [FLOOR-eh-sawft].

**Fluorets** (Ophth). See *fluorescein*. [FLOOR-etz].

**fluorexon** (Fluoresoft) (Ophth). Dye used topically to assist in fitting contact lenses. Ophthalmic solution: 0.35%. [floor-EK-sawn].

**fluorometholone** (Flarex, FML, FML Forte, FML S.O.P.) (Ophth). Corticosteroid drug used topically to treat inflammation of the eyes. Ophthalmic suspension: 0.1%, 0.25%. Ophthalmic ointment: 0.1%. [FLOOR-oh-METH-oh-lohn].

**Fluoroplex** (Derm, OB/GYN). See *fluorouracil*. [FLOOR-oh-pleks].

**fluorouracil** (5-FU, Adrucil, Carac, Efudex, Fluoroplex) (Chemo, Derm. OB/GYN). Antimetabolite chemotherapy drug used to treat cancer of the brain, head and neck, breast, ovary, uterus, cervix, esophagus, stomach, pancreas, liver, colon, prostate gland, and bladder; used topically to treat actinic keratoses on the skin; used topically to treat condylomata acuminata (genital warts). Cream: 0.5%, 1%, 5%. Topical solution: 2%, 5%. Intravenous: 50 mg/mL. [FLOOR-oh-YOOR-ah-sil].

**fluoxetine** (Prozac, Prozac Weekly, Sarafem, Selfemra) (Analges, Cardio, OB/GYN, Psych). Selective serotonin reuptake inhibitor (SSRI) drug used to treat depression, anxiety disorder, obsessive-compulsive disorder, panic attacks, posttraumatic stress disorder, and bulimia; used to treat premenstrual dysphoric disorder (Sarafem, Selfemra; orphan drug used to treat autism and body dysmorphic syndrome; used to treat the hot flashes of menopause; used to treat migraine headaches; used to treat Raynaud's disease. Tablet: 10 mg, 20 mg. Capsule/Pulvule: 10 mg, 20 mg, 40 mg. Delayed-release capsule: 90 mg. Liquid: 20 mg/5 mL. [floo-AWK-seh-teen].

**fluoxymesterone** (Androxy) (Chemo, Endo). Schedule III male hormone used as testosterone hormone replacement for patients with cryptorchidism or orchiectomy; used to treat delayed puberty in boys; hormonal chemotherapy drug used to treat breast cancer in women. Tablet: 10 mg. [floo-AWK-see-MES-teh-rohn].

**fluphenazine** (GI, Psych). Phenothiazine antipsychotic drug used to treat psychosis and schizophrenia; used to treat nausea and vomiting. Tablet: 1 mg, 2.5 mg, 5 mg, 10 mg. Liquid: 2.5 mg/mL, 5 mg/mL. Subcutaneous or intramuscular: 2.5 mg/mL, 25 mg/mL. [floo-FEN-ah-zeen].

**flurandrenolide** (Cordran, Cordran SP) (Derm). Corticosteroid drug used topically to treat inflammation and itching from dermatitis, seborrhea, eczema, psoriasis, and yeast or fungal infections. Cream: 0.05%. Lotion: 0.05%. Ointment: 0.05%. Tape: 4 mcg/cm$^2$. [FLOOR-an-DREN-oh-lide].

**Flurate** (Ophth) (generic *benoxinate, fluorescein*). Combination ophthalmic anesthetic and dye drug used topically in the eye. Ophthalmic solution: 0.4%/0.25%. [FLOOR-ate].

**flurazepam** (Dalmane) (Neuro). Schedule IV benzodiazepine drug used to treat insomnia. Capsule: 15 mg, 30 mg. [floor-AA-zeh-pam].

**flurbiprofen** (Ansaid, Ocufen) (Analges, Ophth). Nonsteroidal anti-inflammatory drug used to treat pain and inflammation; used to treat osteoarthritis, rheumatoid arthritis, dysmenorrhea, and gout; used topically to prevent constriction of the pupil during eye surgery (Ocufen). Tablet: 50 mg, 100 mg. Ophthalmic solution: 0.03%. [FLOOR-bih-PROH-fen].

**Fluress** (Ophth) (generic *benoxinate, fluorescein*). Combination anesthetic and dye drug used topically in the eye. Ophthalmic solution: 0.4%/0.25%. [floor-ES].

**Flurox** (Ophth) (generic *benoxinate, fluorescein*). Combination anesthetic and dye drug used topically in the eye. Ophthalmic solution: 0.4%/0.25%. [FLOOR-awks].

**flu shot** (Anti-infec, Pulm). See *influenza virus vaccine*. [FLOO SHAWT].

**flutamide** (Chemo, Endo). Hormonal chemotherapy drug used to treat cancer of the prostate gland in men; used to treat hirsutism in women. Capsule: 125 mg. [FLOO-tah-mide].

**Flutex** (Derm). See *triamcinolone*. [FLOO-teks].

**fluticasone** (Cutivate, Flonase, Flovent, Flovent Diskus, Flovent Rotadisk, Veramyst) (Derm, ENT, Pulm). Corticosteroid anti-inflammatory drug used topically in the nose to treat treat allergic rhinitis (seasonal and perennial allergies) (Flonase, Veramyst); used topically on the skin to treat inflammation and itching from dermatitis, seborrhea, eczema, psoriasis, and yeast or fungal infections (Cutivate); inhaled to prevent acute asthma attacks (Flovent). Cream: 0.05%. Lotion: 0.05%. Nasal spray: 27.5 mcg/spray, 50 mcg/spray. Ointment: 0.005%. Aerosol inhaler: 44 mcg/dose, 110 mcg/dose, 220 mcg/dose. Diskus (inhaled powder) or Rotadisk (inhaled powder): 50 mcg/dose, 100 mcg/dose, 250 mcg/dose. [floo-TIK-ah-zohn].

**fluvastatin** (Lescol, Lescol XL) (Cardio). HMG-CoA reductase inhibitor drug used to treat hypercholesterolemia and arteriosclerosis. Capsule: 20 mg, 40 mg. Extended-release tablet: 80 mg. [FLOO-vah-STAT-in].

**Fluvirin** (Anti-infec, Pulm). See *influenza virus vaccine*. [floo-VY-rin].

**fluvoxamine** (Luvox, Luxor CR) (Psych). Selective serotonin reuptake inhibitor (SSRI) drug used to treat depression, bulimia, obsessive-compulsive disorder, social anxiety disorder, and panic disorder. Controlled-release capsule: 100 mg, 150 mg. Tablet: 25 mg, 50 mg, 100 mg. [floo-VAWK-sah-meen].

**Fluzone** (Anti-infec, Pulm). See *influenza virus vaccine*. [FLOO-zohn].

**FML, FML Forte, FML S.O.P.** (Ophth). See *fluorometholone*. [F-M-L].

**Foamicon** (GI) (generic *aluminum, magnesium, sodium bicarbonate*). Combination antacid drug for heartburn. Tablet: 80 mg/20 mg/1000 mg. [FOH-mih-kawn].

**Focalin, Focalin XR** (Psych). See *dexmethylphenidate*. [FOH-kah-lin].

**folic acid** (Deplin, Folvite) (Hem, OB/GYN). Vitamin B drug that stimulates red blood cell production to treat folic acid (megaloblastic) anemia; prenatal vitamin supplement. Tablet: 0.4 mg, 0.8 mg, 1 mg, 7.5 mg. Subcutaneous, intramuscular, or intravenous: 5 mg/mL. [FOH-lik AS-id].

**folinic acid** (Chemo). See *leucovorin*. [foh-LIN-ik AS-id].

**Follistim AQ** (Endo, OB/GYN). See *follitropin beta*. [FOH-lih-stim A-Q].

**follitropin alfa** (Gonal-f, Gonal-f RFF Pen) (Endo, OB/GYN). Follicle-stimulating hormone drug created by recombinant DNA technology; used to treat infertility in women by stimulating ovulation; used during assisted reproduction to develop multiple follicles; used to treat male infertility caused by a lack of follicle-stimulating hormone. Subcutaneous: 300 units/0.5 mL, 450 units/0.75 mL, 900 units/1.5 mL, 82 units, 600 units, 1200 units. [FOH-lih-TROH-pin AL-fah].

**follitropin beta** (Follistim AQ) (Endo, OB/GYN). Follicle-stimulating hormone drug used to stimulate ovulation to treat infertility. Subcutaneous or intramuscular: 0.75 units/0.21 mL, 350 units/0.42 mL, 650 units/0.78 mL, 975 units/1.17 mL, 0.75 units/0.5 mL, 150 units/0.5 mL. [FOH-lih-TROH-pin BAY-tah].

**Folvite** (Hem, OB/GYN). See *folic acid*. [FOL-vite].

**fomepizole** (Antizol) (Emerg, Psych). Used to reverse the effects of poisoning with ethylene glycol (antifreeze) or methanol (wood alcohol). Intravenous: 1 g/mL. [foh-MEP-eh-zohl].

**fondaparinux** (Arixtra) (Hem). Anticoagulant drug that inhibits blood clotting factor X; used to prevent or treat deep venous thrombosis or pulmonary embolism in patients undergoing joint replacement surgery or abdominal surgery. Subcutaneous: 2.5 mg/0.5 mL, 5 mg/0.4 mL, 7.5 mg/0.6 mL, 10 mg/0.8 mL. [FAWN-dah-PAIR-ih-nuks].

**Foradil Aerolizer** (Pulm). See *formoterol*. [FOR-ah-dil AIR-oh-ly-zer].

**Forane** (Anes). Anesthetic drug used to induce and maintain general anesthesia. Inhaled gas. [FOR-ayn].

**formoterol** (Foradil Aerolizer) (Pulm). Bronchodilator drug used to prevent and treat asthma and bronchospasm; used to treat chronic obstructive pulmonary disease. Capsule with powder for inhalation: 12 mcg. [for-MOH-ter-awl].

**Formulation R** (GI). See *phenylephrine*. [FOR-myoo-LAY-shun R].

**Forta Drink, Forta Shake** (GI). Lactose-free nutritional supplement. Power (to be reconstituted). [FOR-tah].

**Fortamet** (Endo, OB/GYN). See *metformin*. [FOR-tah-met].

**Fortaz** (Anti-infec). See *ceftazidime*. [FOR-taz].

**Forteo** (Endo, Ortho). See *teriparatide*. [for-TAY-oh].

**Fortical** (Ortho). See *calcitonin-salmon*. [FOR-tih-kal].

**Fortovase** (Anti-infec). See *saquinavir*. [FOR-toh-vays].

**Fosamax** (OB/GYN, Ortho). See *alendronate*. [FAWS-ah-maks].

**Fosamax Plus D** (Ortho) (generic *alendronate, vitamin D*). Combination bone resorption inhibitor and vitamin D drug; used to prevent bone loss and treat osteoporosis in men and postmenopausal women. Tablet: 70 mg/70 mcg. [FAWS-ah-maks PLUS D].

**fosamprenavir** (Lexiva) (Anti-infec). Protease inhibitor antiviral drug used to treat HIV and AIDS. Tablet: 700 mg. [FAWS-am-PREN-ah-veer].

**fosaprepitant** (Emend Injection) (Chemo, GI). Serotonin blocker drug used to treat nausea and vomiting caused by chemotherapy. Intravenous: 115 mg. [FAW-sah-PREP-ih-tant].

**Foscan** (Chemo). See *temoporfin*. [FAWS-kan].

**foscarnet** (Foscavir) (Anti-infec). Antiviral drug used to treat cytomegalovirus infection of the retina in AIDS patients; used to treat acyclovir-resistant herpes simplex virus infection. Intravenous: 24 mg/mL. [faws-KAR-net].

**Foscavir** (Anti-infec). See *foscarnet*. [FAWS-kah-veer].

**fosfomycin** (Monurol) (Uro). Anti-infective drug used to treat urinary tract infections. Granules (taken with water or food): 3 g packet. [FAWS-foh-MY-sin]

**fosinopril** (Monopril) (Cardio). ACE inhibitor drug used to treat hypertension and congestive heart failure. Tablet: 10 mg, 20 mg, 40 mg. [foh-SIN-oh-pril].

**fosphenytoin** (Cerebyx) (Neuro). Anticonvulsant drug used to treat status epilepticus; used to prevent or treat seizures during brain surgery. Intramuscular or intravenous: 150 mg/2 mL, 750 mg/10 mL. [FAWS-fen-ih-TOH-in].

**Fosrenol** (Uro). See *lanthanum*. [FAWS-reh-nawl].

**Fostex Acne Cleansing Cream, Fostex Medicated Cleanser Pads** (Derm). See *salicylic acid*. [FAWS-teks].

**Fototar** (Derm). See *coal tar*. [FOH-toh-tar].

**Fragmin** (Cardio, Hem, Uro). See *dalteparin*. [FRAG-min].

**Freezone** (Derm). See *salicylic acid*. [FREE-zohn].

**fresh frozen plasma (FFP)** (I.V.). Blood product that contains no cellular components and is used to replace plasma proteins and clotting factors. Intravenous. [FRESH FROH-zen PLAZ-mah].

**Frova** (Analges). See *frovatriptan*. [FROH-vah].

**frovatriptan** (Frova) (Analges). Serotonin receptor agonist drug used to treat migraine headaches. Tablet: 2.5 mg [FROH-vah-TRIP-tan].

**FUDR** (Chemo). See *floxuridine*. [F-U-D-R].

**Ful-Glo** (Ophth). See *fluorescein*. [FUL-gloh].

**fulvestrant** (Faslodex) (Chemo). Hormonal chemotherapy drug used to treat breast cancer. Intravenous: 50 mg/mL. [ful-VES-trant].

**Fungi-Nail** (Derm) (generic *resorcinol, salicylic acid*). Combination over-the-counter antiseptic and keratolytic drug used topically to treat fungal infections of the skin and nails (onychomycosis). Liquid: 1%/2%. [FUN-jih-nayl].

**Fungizone Intravenous** (Anti-infec). See *amphotericin B*. [FUN-jih-zohn].

**Fungoid, Fungoid Crème, Fungoid Tincture** (Derm). See *triacetin*. [FUN-goyd].

**Fungoid AF** (Derm). See *undecylenic acid*. [FUN-goyd A-F].

**Furacin** (Derm). See *nitrofurazone*. [FYOOR-ah-sin].

**Furadantin** (Anti-infec, Uro). See *nitrofurantoin*. [FYOOR-ah-DAN-tin].

**furosemide** (Lasix) (Cardio, GI, Uro). Loop diuretic drug used to treat hypertension; used to treat edema from congestive heart failure, liver disease, or kidney disease. Oral liquid: 10 mg/mL, 40 mg/5 mL. Tablet: 20 mg, 40 mg, 80 mg. Intramuscular or intravenous: 10 mg/mL. [fyoor-OH-seh-mide].

**Fusilev** (Chemo). See *levoleucovorin*. [FYOO-sih-lev].

**Fuzeon** (Anti-infec). See *enfuvirtide*. [FYOO-zee-awn].

**gabapentin** (Gabarone, Neurontin) (Analges, Neuro, Psych). Used to treat simple partial seizures; used to treat postherpetic neuralgia, trigeminal neuralgia, and diabetic neuropathy; used to treat multiple sclerosis; orphan drug used to treat amyotrophic lateral sclerosis; used to treat migraine headaches; used to treat bipolar disorder. Capsule: 100 mg, 300 mg, 400 mg. Tablet: 600 mg, 800 mg. Liquid: 250 mg/5 mL. [GAB-ah-PEN-tin].

**Gabarone** (Analges, Neuro, Psych). See *gabapentin*. [GAB-ah-rohn].

**Gabitril Filmtabs** (Neuro). See *tiagabine*. [GAB-ah-tril].

**Gabbromicina** (Anti-infec, Pulm). See *aminosidine*. [GAB-roh-my-SIN-ah].

**galantamine** (Razadyne, Razadyne ER, Razadyne Oral Solution) (Neuro). Cholinesterase inhibitor drug used to treat mild-to-moderate Alzheimer's disease. Capsule: 8 mg, 16 mg, 24 mg. Extended-release capsule: 8 mg, 16 mg, 24 mg. Tablet: 4 mg, 8 mg, 12 mg. Liquid: 4 mg/mL. [gah-LAN-tah-meen].

**Galardin** (Ophth). Used to treat corneal ulcers. Orphan drug. [gah-LAR-din].

**gallium nitrate** (Ganite) (Chemo). Used to treat hypercalcemia caused by cancer. Intravenous: 25 mg/mL. [GAL-ee-um NY-trayt].

**galsulfase** (Naglazyme) (Misc). Used to treat mucopolysaccharidosis. Intravenous: 1 mg/mL. [gal-SUL fays].

**Galzin** (Misc). See *zinc acetate*. [GAL-zin].

**Gamimune N** (Anti-infec, Misc). See *human immune globulin*. [GAM-ih-myoon N].

**Gammagard** (Anti-infec, Misc). See *human immune globulin*. [GAM-mah-gard].

**gamma hydroxybutyrate** (GHB) (Neuro). Schedule I drug with no medical uses but now an orphan drug used to treat narcolepsy; also one of the so-called "date-rape drugs." Orphan drug. [GAM-mah hy-DRAWK-see-BYOO-tih-rayt].

**gammalinolenic acid** (Ortho). Used to treat juvenile rheumatoid arthritis. Orphan drug. [GAM-mah-LIN-oh-LEN-ik AS-id].

**Gamunex** (Anti-infec, Misc). See *human immune globulin*. [GAM-yoo-neks].

**ganciclovir** (Cytovene, Vitrasert) (Anti-infec, Ophth). Antiviral drug used to treat cytomegalovirus infection of the retina; used to treat cytomegalovirus infection in organ transplantation and AIDS patients. Capsule: 250 mg, 500 mg. Intravenous (powder to be reconstituted): 500 mg/10 mL. Ocular implant: 4.5 mg. [gan-SY-kloh-veer].

**gangliosides** (Cronassial) (Ophth). Used to treat retinitis pigmentosa. Orphan drug. [GANG-lee-oh-sides].

**ganirelix** (Endo, OB/GYN). Used to inhibit excessive gonadotropin-releasing hormone from the anterior pituitary gland of patients taking ovulation-stimulating drugs for infertility. Subcutaneous: 250 mcg/0.5 mL. [gah-NEER-eh-liks].

**Ganite** (Chemo). See *gallium nitrate*. [GAN-ite].

**Gantrisin Pediatric** (Anti-infec). See *sulfisoxazole*. [GAN-trih-sin PEE-dee-AT-rik].

**Garamycin** (Ophth). See *gentamicin*. [GAIR-ah-MY-sin].

**Gardisil** (Anti-infec, OB/GYN). Vaccine used to prevent genital warts in females ages 9 to 26; used to prevent cervical cancer caused by the human papillomavirus. Intramuscular: 0.5 mL. [GAR-dih-sil].

**Gas Relief** (GI). See *simethicone*. [GAS ree-LEEF].

**Gastrocrom** (GI). See *cromolyn*. [GAS-troh-krawm].

**Gas-X, Gas-X Extra Strength** (GI). See *simethicone*. [GAS-X].

**gatafloxacin** (Zymar) (Ophth). Fluoroquinolone antibiotic drug used topically in the eyes to treat bacterial infections. Ophthalmic solution: 0.3% (3 mg/mL). [GAT-ah-FLAWK-sah-sin].

**gavilimomab** (Hem). Used to treat graft-versus-host disease. Orphan drug. [GAV-ih-LIH-moh-mab].

**Gaviscon Liquid** (GI) (generic *aluminum, magnesium*). Combination over-the-counter antacid drug used to treat heartburn. Liquid: 31 mg/119 mg. [GAV-is-kawn].

**Gaviscon Tablet, Gaviscon Extra Strength Antacid, Gaviscon-2 Double Strength** (GI) (generic *aluminum, magnesium, sodium bicarbonate*). Combination over-the-counter antacid drug used to treat heartburn. Tablet: 80 mg/40 mg/1000 mg, 180 mg/40 mg/1000 mg, 180 mg/105 mg/1000 mg. [GAV-is-kawn]

**Gaviscon Extra Strength Relief Formula** (GI) (generic *aluminum, magnesium, simethicone*). Combination antacid and anti-gas drug used to treat heartburn and gas. Liquid: 254 mg/237 mg/20 mg. [GAV-is-kawn].

**gefitinib** (Iressa) (Chemo). Chemotherapy drug used to treat cancer of the head and neck and lung. Tablet: 250 mg. [geh-FIH-tih-nib].

**Gelfilm, Gelfilm Ophthalmic** (Hem). See *absorbable gelatin*. [JEL-film].

**Gelfoam** (Hem). See *absorbable gelatin*. [JEL-fohm].

**Gelusil** (GI) (generic *aluminum, magnesium, simethicone*). Combination antacid and anti-gas drug for heartburn and indigestion. Tablet: 200 mg/200 mg/25 mg. [JEL-yoo-sil].

**gemcitabine** (Gemzar) (Chemo). Antimetabolite chemotherapy drug used to treat cancer of the head and neck, breast, ovary, lung, bile ducts, pancreas, bladder, and testicles. Intravenous (powder to be reconstituted): 200 mg/10 mL. [jem-SY-tah-been].

**gemfibrozil** (Lopid) (Cardio). Used to treat hypertriglyceridemia by decreasing serum triglyercide and VLDL levels. Tablet: 600 mg. [jem-FY-broh-zil].

**gemifloxacin** (Factive) (Anti-infec). Fluoroquinolone antibiotic drug used to treat gram-negative and gram-positive bacterial infections; used to treat bronchitis and pneumonia due to *S. pneumonia* and *H. influenzae*. Tablet: 320 mg. [JEM-ih-FLAWK-sah-sin].

**gemtuzumab** (Mylotarg) (Chemo). Monoclonal antibody drug used to treat leukemia. Intravenous (powder to be reconstituted): 5 mg. [jem-TOOZ-yoo-mab].

**Gemzar** (Chemo). See *gemcitabine*. [JEM-zar].

**Genahist** (Derm, ENT). See *diphenhydramine*. [JEN-ah-hist].

**Genasense** (Chemo). See *augmerosen*. [JEN-ah-sens].

**Genasoft** (GI). See *docusate*. [JEN-ah-sawft].

**Genasyme** (GI). See *simethicone*. [JEN-ah-sime].

**geneticin** (Anti-infec). Used to treat amoebiasis. Orphan drug. [jeh-NET-ih-sin].

**Genfiber** (GI). See *psyllium*. [jen-FY-ber].

**Gengraf** (Cardio, Derm, GI, Hem, Ortho, Uro). See *cyclosporine*. [JEN-graf].

**Gen-K** (Uro). See *potassium*. [JEN-K].

**Genoptic, Genoptic S.O.P.** (Ophth). See *gentamicin*. [jen-AWP-tik].

**Genotropin, Genotropin Miniquick** (Endo). See *somatropin*. [JEE-noh-TROH-pin].

**Gentacidin** (Ophth). See *gentamicin*. [JEN-tah-SY-din].

**Gentak** (Ophth). See *gentamicin*. [JEN-tak].

**gentamicin** (Garamycin, Genoptic, Genoptic S.O.P., Gentacidin, Gentak, Septopal) (Anti-infec). Aminoglycoside antibiotic drug used to treat a variety of serious gram-negative infections, such as peritonitis, meningitis, septicemia, and burns; used topically to treat bacterial skin infections; used topically in the eye to treat bacterial infections (Garamycin, Genoptic, Gentacidin, Gentak); antibiotic beads on a wire implanted surgically to treat posttraumatic or postoperative osteomyelitis (Septopal). Cream: 0.1%. Ointment: 0.1%. Ophthalmic solution: 3 mg/mL. Ophthalmic ointment: 3 mg/g. Intravenous: 10 mg/mL, 40 mg/mL. Beads on a wire. [JEN-tah-MY-sin].

**gentamicin liposomal** (Maitec) (Anti-infec). Antibiotic drug used to treat *Mycobacterium avium-intracellulare* in AIDS patients. Orphan drug. [JEN-tah-MY-sin LY-poh-SOH-mal].

**gentian violet** (Derm). Over-the-counter purple dye antibacterial and antifungal drug used topically on the skin for cuts and fungal infections; applied to the umbilical cords of newborns. Liquid: 1%, 2%. [JEN-shee-an VY-oh-let].

**Gentran 40** (I.V.). See *dextran 40*. [JEN-tran 40].

**Gentran 70** (I.V.). See *dextran 70*. [JEN-tran 70].

**Geodon** (Neuro, Psych). See *ziprasidone*. [GEE-oh-dohn].

**Gerbauer's Spray and Stretch** (Anes, Ortho). Anesthetic drug used topically on the skin to produce a temporary anesthesia to treat the pain and swelling of muscle spasm or athletic injuries. Spray. [GER-bow-erz].

**Gerber Soy Formula** (GI). Infant formula with soy protein. Liquid. [GER-ber].

**Geref** (Endo). (Anti-infec, Endo, OB/GYN). See *sermorelin*. [JAIR-if].

**Geridium** (Uro). See *phenazopyridine*. [jeh-RID-ee-um].

**Geritol Complete, Geritol Extend, Geritol Tonic** (Misc). Over-the-counter multivitamin with iron nutritional supplement. Caplet. Liquid. Tablet. [JAIR-ih-tawl].

**Gets-It** (Derm). Over-the-counter keratolytic drug used topically on the skin to treat acne vulgaris. Liquid. [GETZ-it].

**Gimatecan** (Chemo). Chemotherapy drug used to treat brain cancer. Orphan drug. [gih-MAT-eh-kan].

**Gladase, Gladase-C** (Derm). See *papain*. [GLAD-ace].

**glatiramer** (Copaxone) (Neuro). Immunosuppressant drug used to treat multiple sclerosis. Subcutaneous: 20 mg/mL. [glah-TEER-ah-mer].

**Gleevec** (Chemo). See *imatinib*. [GLEE-vek].

**Gliadel** (Chemo). See *carmustine*. [GLEE-ah-del].

**glimepiride** (Amaryl) (Endo). Sulfonylurea oral antidiabetic drug used to treat type 2 diabetes mellitus. Tablet: 1 mg, 2 mg, 4 mg. [gly-MEP-ih-ride].

**glipizide** (Glucotrol, Glucotrol XL) (Endo). Sulfonylurea oral antidiabetic drug used to treat type 2 diabetes mellitus. Tablet: 5 mg, 10 mg. Extended-release tablet: 2.5 mg, 5 mg, 10 mg. [GLIP-ih-zide].

**GlucaGen** (Endo). See *glucagon*. [GLOO-kah-jen].

**glucagon** (GlucaGen) (Endo). Hormone drug used to treat severe hypoglycemia. Subcutaneous, intramuscular, intravenous: 1 mg/1mL. [GLOO-kah-gawn].

**glucarpidase** (Voraxaze) (Chemo). Cytoprotective drug used to treat methotrexate toxicity. Orphan drug. [gloo-KAR-pih-days].

**Glucerna, Glucerna Select, Glucerna Weight Loss** (Endo, GI). Lactose-free or lactose-free and gluten-free nutritional supplement formulated for patients with diabetes mellitus. Liquid. Shake. [gloo-SIR-nah].

**Glucophage, Glucophage XR** (Endo). See *metformin.* [GLOO-koh-fawj].

**glucose** (B-D Glucose, Dex4 Glucose, Insta-Glucose, Insulin Reaction) (Endo). Oral glucose drug used to treat hypoglycemia. Gel. Tablet. Chewable tablet: 5 g. [GLOO-kohs].

**Glucotrol, Glucotrol XL** (Endo). See *glipizide.* [GLOO-koh-trawl].

**Glucovance** (Endo) (generic *glyburide, metformin*). Combination oral antidiabetic drug used to treat type 2 diabetes mellitus. Tablet: 1.25 mg/250 mg, 2.5 mg/500 mg, 5 mg/500 mg. [GLOO-koh-vans].

**Glumetza** (Endo). See *metformin.* [gloo-MET-zah].

**glutamine** (NutreStore) (GI). Used to treat short bowel syndrome. Orphan drug. [GLOO-tah-meen].

**glyburide** (DiaBeta, Glynase PresTab, Micronase) (Endo). Sulfonylurea oral antidiabetic drug used to treat type 2 diabetes mellitus. Tablet: 1.25 mg, 2.5 mg, 5 mg. Micronized tablet: 1.5 mg, 3 mg, 4.5 mg, 6 mg. [GLY-byoo-ride].

**glycerin** (Colace Infant/Child, Colace Suppository, Fleet Babylax, Osmoglyn) (GI, Ophth). Over-the-counter osmotic laxative drug used to treat constipation; osmotic diuretic drug used to decrease intraocular pressure and treat glaucoma (Osmoglyn). Rectal liquid: 4 mL/ applicator. Suppository. Ophthalmic solution: 50%. [GLIS-er-in]

**glycine** (Uro). Used to irrigate during urologic surgery. Irrigating solution: 1.5%. [GLY-seen].

**GlycoLax** (GI). See *polyethylene glycol.* [GLY-koh-laks].

**glycopyrrolate** (Robinul, Robinul Forte) (GI). Anticholinergic antispasmodic drug used to decrease acid production and relieve spasms in patients with peptic ulcers; used preoperatively to decrease secretions from the mouth and throat. Tablet: 1 mg, 2 mg. Intramuscular or intravenous: 0.2 mg/mL. [GLY-koh-PY-roh-layt].

**Glynase PresTab** (Endo). See *glyburide.* [GLY-nays PRES-tab].

**Glypressin** (GI). See *terlipressin.* [gly-PRES-sin].

**Glyquin, Glyquin-XM** (Derm). See *hydroquinone.* [GLY-kwin].

**Glyset** (Endo). See *miglitol.* [GLY-set].

**gold sodium thiomalate** (Aurolate, Myochrysine) (Ortho). Gold compound used to treat rheumatoid arthritis. Intramuscular: 50 mg/mL. [GOLD SOH-dee-um THY-oh-MAL-ate].

**GoLYTELY** (GI) (generic *polyethylene glycol, electrolyte solution*). Combination bowel evacuant and bowel prep. Oral liquid (powder to be reconstituted). [go-LITE-lee].

**golimumab** (Ortho). Used to treat sarcoidosis. Orphan drug. [goh-LIM-yoo-mab].

**gonadorelin** (Lutrepulse) (Misc, OB/GYN). Hormone drug used to correct the absence of gonadotropin-releasing hormone from the hypothalamus (Lutrepulse); used to treat primary hypothalamic amenorrhea; used to diagnose the function of the anterior pituitary gland (Factrel). Intravenous test: 100 mcg, 500 mcg. Intravenous (via Lutrepulse pump). [goh-NAD-oh-REL-in].

**Gonak** (Ophth). See *hydroxypropyl methylcellulose.* [GOH-nak].

**Gonal-f, Gonal-f RFF Pen** (Endo, OB/GYN). See *follitropin alfa.* [GOH-nawl- F].

**Gonic** (Endo, OB/GYN). See *human chorioic gonadotropin.* [GOH-nik].

**Gonioscopic** (Ophth). See *hydroxyethylcellulose.* [GOH-nee-oh-SKAW-pik].

**Goniosol** (Ophth). See *hydroxypropyl methylcellulose.* [GOH-nee-oh-sawl].

**goserelin** (Zoladex) (Chemo, OB/GYN). Hormonal chemotherapy drug used to treat cancer of the breast and prostate gland; used to treat endometriosis. Subcutaneous implant: 3.6 mg, 10.8 mg. [GOH-seh-REL-in].

**gossypol 9** (Chemo). Used to treat cancer of the adrenal cortex. Orphan drug. [GAWS-ih-pohl].

**granisetron** (Granisol, Kytril) (Chemo, GI). Serotonin blocker drug used to treat nausea and vomiting caused by chemotherapy or radiation therapy. Tablet: 1 mg. Intravenous: 1 mg/mL. [grah-NIH-seh-trawn].

**Granisol** (Chemo, GI). See *granisetron.* [GRAN-ih-sawl].

**Granulderm** (Derm). See *trypsin.* [GRAN-yool-derm].

**Granulex** (Derm). See *trypsin.* [GRAN-yoo-leks].

**Grifulvin V** (Anti-infec, Derm). See *griseofulvin.* [grih-FUL-vin V].

**griseofulvin** (Grifulvin V, Gris-PEG) (Anti-infec, Derm). Antifungal drug used to treat severe fungal infections of the nails and skin. Tablet: 125 mg, 250 mg, 500 mg. Oral liquid: 125 mg/5 mL. [GRIZ-ee-oh-FUL-vin].

**Gris-PEG** (Anti-infec, Derm). See *griseofulvin.* [GRIZ-peg].

**guaifenesin** (Allfen Jr, Diabetic Tussin, Humibid Maximum Strength, Liquibid, Mucinex Children's, Mucinex Junior Strength, Naldecon Senior EX, Organidin NR, Robitussin) (Pulm). Over-the-counter and prescription expectorant drug used to thin mucus; used to treat a productive cough so that sputum can be expelled. Liquid/syrup: 100 mg/5 mL, 200 mg/5 mL. Tablet: 200 mg, 400 mg. Extended-release tablet: 600 mg, 1200 mg. Granules: 50 mg/packet, 100 mg/packet. [GWY-ih-FEN-eh-sin].

**Guaifenex PSE** (ENT) (generic *guaifenesin, pseudoephedrine*). Combination expectorant and decongestant drug. Tablet: 600 mg/60 mg.[GWY-ih-FEN-eks P-S-E].

**guanabenz** (Wytensin) (Cardio). Alpha$_2$ receptor stimulator drug used to dilate the blood vessels and treat hypertension. Tablet: 4 mg, 8 mg. [GWAN-ah-benz].

**guanethidine** (Ismelin) (Neuro). Blocks the release of hormones from the adrenal medulla and is used to treat sympathetic reflex dystrophy and causalgia. Orphan drug. [gwan-ETH-ih-deen].

**guanfacine** (Tenex) (Cardio, Psych). Alpha$_2$ receptor stimulator drug that is used to treat hypertension, used to treat withdrawal from heroin, orphan drug used to treat fragile X syndrome. Tablet: 1 mg, 2 mg. [GWAN-fah-seen].

**guanidine** (Neuro). Anticholinesterase drug used to treat Eaton-Lambert syndrome. Tablet: 125 mg. [GWAN-ih-deen].

**gusperimus** (Spanidin) (Hem). Used to treat graft-versus-host disease. Orphan drug. [guhs-PAIR-ih-mus].

**Gynazole-1** (Anti-infec, OB/GYN). See *butoconazole*. [GY-nah-zohl-1].

**Gynecort Feminine Crème** (Derm). See *hydrocortisone*. [GY-neh-kort].

**Gyne-Lotrimin 3, Gyne-Lotrimin 7** (OB/GYN). See *clotrimazole*. [GY-nee-LOH-trih-min].

**Gynodiol** (Chemo, OB/GYN, Ortho). See *estradiol*. [GY-noh-DY-awl].

**Gynol II** (OB/GYN). See *nonoxynol-9*. [GY-nawl].

**H5N1 Influenza Vaccine** (Anti-infec). Used to prevent bird flu in adults. Intramuscular: Vaccine. [H-5-N-1 IN-floo-EN-zah].

**halcinonide** (Halog, Halog-E) (Derm). Corticosteroid drug used topically on the skin to treat inflammation and itching from dermatitis, seborrhea, eczema, psoriasis, and yeast or fungal infections. Cream: 0.1%. Liquid: 0.1%. Ointment: 0.1%. [hal-SIN-oh-nide].

**Halcion** (Neuro). See *triazolam*. [HAL-see-awn].

**Haldol Decanoate 50, Haldol Decanoate 100** (GI, Psych). See *haloperidol*. [HAL-dawl].

**Haley's M-O** (GI) (generic *magnesium, mineral oil*). Combination over-the-counter osmotic and oil laxative drug used to treat constipation. Liquid: 900 mg/15 mL. [HAY-leez M-O].

**Halfan** (Misc). See *halofantrine*. [HAL-fan].

**HalfLytely and Bisacodyl Bowel Prep Kit** (GI) (generic *bisacodyl, potassium, sodium bicarbonate*). Combination irritant/stimulant and electrolyte bowel evacuant. Powder (to be reconstituted to oral solution) and tablet (bisacodyl) 5 mg. [haf-LITE-lee and BIS-ah-KOH-dil].

**half normal saline (0.45% NaCl)** (I.V.). Intravenous fluid of sodium and water at half the concentration of tissue fluids. Intravenous. [HAF NOR-mal SAY-leen].

**Halfprin 81** (Analges, Cardio, Hem, Neuro). See *aspirin*. [HAF-prin].

**halobetasol** (Ultravate) (Derm). Corticosteroid drug used topically on the skin to treat inflammation and itching from dermatitis, seborrhea, eczema, psoriasis, and yeast or fungal infections. Cream: 0.05%. Ointment: 0.05%. [HAL-oh-BAY-tah-sawl].

**halofantrine** (Halfan) (Misc). Used to treat malaria. Orphan drug. [HAL-oh-FAN-treen].

**halofuginone** (Stenorol) (Derm). Used to treat systemic sclerosis. Orphan drug. [HAL-oh-FYOO-jih-nohn].

**Halog, Halog-E** (Derm). See *halcinonide*. [HAL-awg]

**haloperidol** (Haldol Decanoate 50, Haldol Decanoate 100) (GI, Psych). Drug used to treat psychosis and schizophrenia, used to treat psychosis with agitation in patients with Alzheimer's disease; used to treat severe, combative or aggressive behavior problems in children; used to treat Tourette's syndrome; used to treat chemotherapy-induced nausea and vomiting and intractable hiccoughs. Tablet: 0.5 mg, 1 mg, 2 mg, 5 mg, 10 mg, 20 mg. Liquid: 2 mg/mL. Intramuscular or intravenous: 5 mg/mL, 50 mg/mL, 100 mg/mL. [HAL-oh-PAIR-ih-dawl].

**halothane** (Anes). Anesthetic drug used to induce and maintain general anesthesia. Inhaled gas. [HAL-oh-thayn].

**Havrix** (GI). See *hepatitis A vaccine*. [HAV-riks].

**Head & Shoulders, Head & Shoulders Dry Scalp** (Derm). See *pyrithione zinc*. [HED and SHOL-derz].

**Head & Shoulders Intensive Treatment** (Derm). See *selenium sulfide*. [HED and SHOL-derz].

**Healon, Healon GV** (Ophth). See *sodium hyaluronate*. [HEE-lawn].

**Healon Yellow** (Ophth) (generic *fluorescein dye, sodium hyaluronate*). Combination aqueous humor replacement and yellow dye drug injected to help visualize the anterior chamber during eye surgery. Ophthalmic solution: 0.005 mg/10 mg per mL. [HEE-lawn YEL-oh].

**Heartline** (Analges, Cardio, Hem, Neuro). See *aspirin*. [HART-line].

**Hectorol** (Endo). See *doxercalciferol*. [HEK-toh-rawl].

**Helidac** (GI) (generic *bismuth, metronidazole, tetracycline*). Combination antibacterial and antiprotozoal drug used to treat peptic ulcers caused by *H. pylori*. Bismuth tablet: 262.4 mg. Metronidazole tablet: 250 mg. Tetracycline capsule: 500 mg capsule. [HEE-lih-dak].

**Helixate FS** (Hem). See *factor VIII*. [HEE-lik-sayt].

**Hemabate** (OB/GYN). See *carboprost*. [HEE-mah-bayt].

**Hematrol** (Hem). See *medroxyprogesterone*. [HEE-mah-trawl].

**Hemex** (Uro). See *hemin*. [HEE-meks].

**hemin** (Hemex, Panhematin) (Uro). Used to treat acute intermittent porphyria. Intravenous (powder to be reconstituted): 7 mg/mL. [HEE-min].

**Hemocitrate** (Hem). Used during leukapheresis. Orphan drug. [HEE-moh-SIH-trayt].

**Hemocyte** (Hem). See *ferrous fumarate*. [HEE-moh-site].

**Hemofil M** (Hem). See *factor VIII*. [HEE-moh-fil M].

**Hemopad** (Hem). See *microfibrillar collagen hemostat*. [HEE-moh-pad].

**Hemotene** (Hem). See *microfibrillar collagen hemostat*. [HEE-moh-teen].

**Hemoxin** (Hem). See *niprisan*. [hee-MAWK-sin].

**Hem-Prep** (GI). See *phenylephrine*. [HEM-prep].

**Hemril-HC Uniserts** (GI). See *hydrocortisone*. [HEM-ril-H-C].

**Hepacid** (Chemo). Chemotherapy drug used to treat liver cancer. Orphan drug. [HEP-ah-sid].

**Hepandrin** (GI). See *oxandrolone*. [hep-AN-drin].

**heparin** (Hem). Anticoagulant drug used to prevent deep venous thrombosis; used to provide anticoagulation during open heart surgery and hemodialysis; orphan drug used to treat cystic fibrosis and sickle cell disease. Subcutaneous or intravenous: 1000 units/mL, 2000 units/mL, 2500 units/mL, 5000 units/mL, 7500 units/mL, 10,000 units/mL, 20,000 units/mL, 40,000 units/mL. [HEP-ah-rin].

**Hepatic-Aid II** (GI). Nutritional supplement formulated for patients with chronic liver disease. Powder (to be reconstituted). [heh-PAT-ik AID].

**hepatitis A vaccine** (Havrix, Vaqta). Vaccine to protect against hepatitis A virus. Intramuscular: 25 U/0.5 mL, 50 U/1 mL, 720 EL.U./0.5 mL, 1440 EL.U./1 mL. [HEP-ah-TY-tis A vak-SEEN].

**hepatitis B immunoglobulin** (BayHep B, Nabi-HB) (GI). Immunoglobulin drug given to prevent hepatitis B after exposure to hepatitis B; orphan drug used to prevent hepatitis B in liver transplant patients. Intramuscular: 50 mg/mL. [HEP-ah-TY-tis B IM-myoo-noh-GLAW-byoo-lin].

**hepatitis B vaccine** (Engerix-B, Recombivax HB). Vaccine to protect against hepatitis B. Intramuscular: 5 mcg/0.5 mL, 10 mcg/0.5 mL, 10 mcg/3 mL, 20 mcg/mL, 40 mcg/mL. [HEP-ah-TY-tis B vak-SEEN].

**Hepsera** (Anti-infec, GI). See *adefovir*. [hep-SEER-ah].

**Herceptin** (Chemo). See *trastuzumab*. [her-SEP-tin].

**herpes simplex virus gene** (Chemo). Chemotherapy drug used to treat brain cancer. Orphan drug. [HER-peez SIM-pleks VY-rus JEEN].

**Herrick Lacrimal Plug** (Ophth). Plug inserted in the lacrimal duct to eliminate tear loss in patients with dry eyes. Silicon plug. [HAIR-ik LAK-rih-mal PLUG.

**Hespan** (I.V.). See *hetastarch*. [HES-pan].

**hetastarch** (Hespan) (I.V.). Nonblood plasma volume expander. Intravenous: 6 g/100 mL. [HET-ah-starch].

**hexachlorophene** (pHisoHex) (Derm). Antibacterial skin cleanser and surgical scrub used topically. Liquid: 3%. [HEK-sah-KLOR-ah-feen].

**Hexadrol** (Derm, Endo, Ortho). See *dexamethasone*. [HEK-sah-drawl].

**Hexalen** (Chemo). See *altretamine*. [HEK-sah-len].

**H-F Gel** (Emerg). See *calcium gluconate*. [H-F-jel].

**Hibiclens** (Derm). See *chlorhexidine*. [HIB-ih-klenz].

**Hibistat** (Derm). See *chlorhexidine*. [HIB-ih-stat].

**HibTITER** (Misc). Used to prevent *H. influenzae* infection in children. Subcutaneous: Vaccine. [hib-TY-ter].

**Hiprex** (Anti-infec, Uro). See *methenamine*. [HIP-reks].

**histamine** (Maxamine) (Chemo). Used to treat leukemia and malignant melanoma. Orphan drug. [HIS-tah-meen].

**Histex CT, Histex I/E, Histex Pd** (Derm, ENT, Ophth). See *carbinoxamine*. [HIS-teks].

**histrelin** (Supprelin, Supprelin LA, Vantas) (Chemo, Endo). Hormonal chemotherapy drug used to treat cancer of the prostate gland in men (Vantas); orphan drug used to treat precocious puberty. Subcutaneous implant: 50 mg. [his-TREL-in].

**HIV immune globulin** (Hivig) (Anti-infec). Used to treat HIV and AIDS. Orphan drug. [H-I-V ih-MYOON GLAW-byoo-lin].

**Hivid** (Anti-infec). See *zalcitabine*. [HIV-id].

**Hivig** (Anti-infec). See *HIV immunoglobulin*. [HIV-ig].

**HIV neutralizing antibodies** (Immupath) (Anti-infec). Antibody drug used to treat HIV and AIDS. Orphan drug. [H-I-V NOO-trah-ly-zing AN-tih baw-deez].

**homatropine** (Isopto Homatropine) (Ophth). Mydriatic drug used topically to dilate the pupil to treat eye inflammation. Ophthalmic solution: 2%, 5%. [HOH-mah-TROH-peen].

**homoharringtonine** (Chemo). Chemotherapy drug used to treat leukemia. Orphan drug. [HOH-moh-HAIR-ring-TOH-neen].

**H.P. Acthar Gel** (Endo). See *respository corticotropin*. [H-P-AK-thar JEL].

**Humalog** (Endo). See *insulin lispro*. [HYOO-mah-lawg].

**Humalog Mix 75/25** (Endo) (generic *NPH insulin, regular insulin lispro*). Combination insulin drug used to treat type 1 diabetes mellitus. Subcutaneous: 100 units/mL. KwikPen: 60 units. [HYOO-mah-lawg].

**human chorionic gonadotropin** (HCG) (Choron 10, Gonic, Novarel, Pregnyl, Profasi) (Endo, OB/GYN). Luteinizing hormone drug used to treat infertility in women and men; used to cause testicular descent in children. Intramuscular: 500 units/mL, 1000 units/mL, 2000 units/mL. [HYOO-man KOR-ee-AW-nik goh-NAH-doh-TROH-pin].

**human collagen** (CosmoDerm, CosmoPlast, Evolence) (Derm). Human collagen dermal filler drug used to fill in skin wrinkles. Intra-dermal injection. [HYOO-man KAWL-oh-jen].

**human fibrin sealant** (Artiss) (Derm). Human fibrinogen and thrombin drug used topically to help skin grafts adhere to and seal burned skin. Liquid spray. [HYOO-man FY-brin SEE-lant].

**human immune globulin** (BayGam, Carimune F, Carimune NF, Flebogamma 5%, Gamimune N, Gammagard, Gamunex, Immuno, Iveegam, Iveegam EN, Octagam, Polygam S/D, Vivaglobin, Vivaglobin P) (Anti-infec, Misc). Immunoglobulin drug used to treat primary humoral immunodeficiency; used to prevent infection after exposure to hepatitis A virus; used to prevent measles in unvaccinated patients; given subcutaneously to treat immune deficiency in patients who cannot tolerate this drug intravenously (Vivaglobin); orphan drug used to treat Guillain-Barré syndrome (Carimune NF) and demyelinating polyneuropathy (Gamunex); orphan drug used to prevent infection in children with HIV (Gamimne N); orphan drug used to treat multifocal motor neuropathy (Gammagard); orphan drug used to treat severe inflammation from myocarditis, polymyositis, dermatomyositis, and rheumatoid arthritis (Immuno, Iveegam). Intramuscular: 15%/2 mL. Intravenous: 5%. Subcutaneous. [HYOO-man im-MYOON GLAW-byoo-lin].

**Human Surf** (Pulm).   Surfactant drug used to treat respiratory distress syndrome in newborns. Orphan drug. [HYOO-man SURF].

**Humate-P** (Hem) (generic *antihemophiliac factor* [*clotting factor VIII*], *von Willebrand factor*).   Combination clotting factor drug used to treat bleeding episodes in hemophiliac patients with factor VIII deficiency or von Willebrand disease. Intravenous: (powder to be reconstituted): 250 units AHF/500 units VWF, 500 units AHF/1000 units VWF, 1000 units AHF/2000 VWF. [HYOO-mayt-P].

**Humatrope** (Endo).   See *somatropin*. [HYOO-mah-trohp].

**HuMax-CD4** (Chemo).   Monoclonal antibody drug used to treat mycosis fungoides cancer of the skin. Orphan drug. [HYOO-maks C-D-4].

**Humibid DM** (ENT) (generic *dextromethorphan, guaifenesin*). Combination nonnarcotic antitussive and expectorant drug used to treat productive coughs. Capsule: 15 mg/300 mg. Tablet: 30 mg/600 mg. [HYOO-mih-bid D-M].

**Humibid Maximum Strength** (Pulm).   See *guaifenesin*. [HYOO-mah-bid].

**Humira** (Derm, GI, Ortho).   See *adalimumab*. [hyoo-MAIR-ah].

**Humulin 50/50** (Endo) (generic *NPH insulin, regular insulin*). Combination insulin drug used to treat type 1 diabetes mellitus. Subcutaneous: 100 units/mL. [HYOO-myoo-lin].

**Humulin 70/30** (Endo) (generic *NPH insulin, regular insulin*).   Combination insulin drug used to treat type 1 diabetes mellitus. Subcutaneous: 100 units/mL [HYOO-myoo-lin].

**Humulin N** (Endo).   See *NPH insulin*. [HYOO-myoo-lin N].

**Humulin R, Humulin R Regular U-500** (Endo).   See *regular insulin*. [HYOO-myoo-lin R].

**Hurricane** (Anes, Derm, ENT).   See *benzocaine*. [HER-ih-kayn].

**Hyalgan** (Ortho).   See *hyaluronic acid*. [hy-AL-gan].

**hyaluronidase** (Amphadase, Hydase, Hylenex, Vitrase) (Misc).   Additive to help an injected drug disperse through the tissues; used during subcutaneous procedures to improve absorption of radiopaque drug. Solution: 150 units/mL, 200 units/mL. [HY-al-yoo-RAWN-ih-days].

**hyaluronic acid** (Captique, Euflexxa, Hyalgan, Hylaform, Juvéderm 24HV, Juvéderm 30, Juvéderm 30HV, Orthovisc, Restylane, Supartz, Synvisc) (Derm, Ortho, Pulm).   Gel-like filler drug used to provide fullness and minimize wrinkle lines (Captique, Hylaform, Juvederm, Restylane); used to improve the viscosity and lubricating quality of synovial fluid in patients with osteoarthritis (Euflexxa, Hyalgan, Orthovisc, Supartz, Synvisc); orphan drug used to treat lung problems caused by

alpha-1-antitrypsin deficiency. Gel (for injection): 5.5 mg/mL, 20 mg/mL, 24 mg/mL. Intra-articular injection: 8 mg/mL, 10 mg/mL, 15 mg/mL. [HY-al-yoo-RAWN-1k AS-1d].

**Hyate:C** (Hem).   See *factor VIII*. [HY-ate C].

**Hycamtin** (Chemo).   See *topotecan*. [hy-KAM-tin].

**Hycet** (Analges) (generic *acetaminophen, hydrocodone*).   Combination Schedule III nonnarcotic and narcotic analgesic drug for pain. Liquid: 108 mg/2.5 mg. [HY-set].

**Hycodan** (ENT).   See *hydrocodone*. [HY-koh-dan].

**Hycort** (Derm).   See *hydrocortisone*. [HY-kort].

**Hycotuss** (ENT) (generic *guaifenesin, hydrocodone*).   Combination Schedule III expectorant and narcotic antitussive drug used to treat severe, productive coughs. Syrup: 100 mg/5 mg. [HY-koh-tus].

**Hydase** (Misc).   See *hyaluronidase*. [HY-days].

**hydralazine** (Apresoline) (Cardio).   Peripheral vasodilator drug used to treat hypertension. Tablet: 10 mg, 25 mg, 50 mg, 100 mg. Intramuscular or intravenous: 20 mg/mL. [hy-DRAL-ah-zeen].

**Hydramine Cough** (ENT).   See *diphenhydramine*. [HY-drah-meen CAWF].

**Hydrea** (Chemo, Derm, Hem).   See *hydroxyurea*. [hy-DREE-ah].

**Hydrocet** (Analges) (generic *acetaminophen, hydrocodone*).   Combination Schedule III nonnarcotic and narcotic analgesic drug for pain. Capsule: 500 mg/5 mg. [HY-droh-set].

**hydrochlorothiazide** (Ezide, HCTZ, HydroDIURIL, Hydro-Par, Microzide) (Cardio, Uro).   Thiazide diuretic drug used to treat hypertension; used to treat edema from congestive heart failure, liver disease, or kidney failure. Capsule: 12.5 mg. Tablet: 25 mg, 50 mg, 100 mg. [HY-droh-KLOR-oh-THY-ah-zide].

**Hydrocil Instant** (GI).   See *psyllium*. [HY-droh-sil].

**hydrocodone** (Hycodan) (ENT).   Schedule III narcotic antitussive drug used to treat severe, nonproductive coughs. Tablet: 5 mg. Syrup: 5 mg/5 mL. [HY-droh-KOH-dohn].

**Hydrocort** (Derm).   See *hydrocortisone*. [HY-droh-kort].

**hydrocortisone** (Acticort 100, A-Hydrocort, Ala-Cort, Ala-Scalp, Anucort-HC, Anusol-HC, Bactine Maximum Strength, Caldecort Maximum Strength, Cetacort, Coraz, CortaGel Extra Strength, Cortaid Faststick Maximum Strength, Cortaid Intensive Therapy, Cortaid Maximum Strength, Cortaid with Aloe, Cort-Dome, Cort-Dome High Potency, Cortef, Cortef Feminine Itch, Corticaine, Cortifoam, Cortizone-5, Cortizone for Kids, Cortizone-10, Cortizone-10 External Anal Itch, Cortizone-10 Plus, Cortizone-10 Quickshot, Delcort, Dermol HC, Dermolate, Eldecort, Gynecort Female Crème, Hemril-HC Uniserts, Hycort, Hydrocort, HydroSkin, HydroTex, Hytone, KeriCort-10 Maximum Strength, LactiCare-HC,

Lanacort-5, Lanacort-10, Locoid, Locoid Lipocream, Orabase HCA, Pandel, Penecort, Procort, Proctocort, Scalpicin, Solu-Cortef, Synacort, Tegrin-HC, Texacort, T/Scalp, Tucks, U-cort, Westcort) (Derm, Endo, GI, Ortho). Over-the-counter and prescription corticosteroid drug; used orally as replacement therapy for Addison's disease; used to treat severe inflammation in various body systems; used to treat acute multiple sclerosis; used topically to treat inflammation and itching from dermatitis, atopic dermatitis, seborrhea, eczema, psoriasis, hemorrhoids, and yeast or fungal infections; retention enema used to treat ulcerative colitis; used topically to treat inflammation and sores in the mouth. Cream: 0.1%, 0.2%, 0.5%, 1%, 2.5%. Gel: 1%. Lotion: 0.1%, 0.25%, 0.5%, 1%, 2%, 2.5%. Foam: 10%. Topical liquid: 0.1%, 1%, 2.5%. Ointment: 0.1%, 0.2%, 0.5%, 1%, 2.5%. Spray: 1%. Stick roll-on: 1%. Tablet: 5 mg, 10 mg, 20 mg. Rectal aerosol foam: 10%, 90 mg/applicator. Suppository: 25 mg, 30 mg. Oral paste: 0.5%. Intramuscular or intravenous: 100 mg/2 mL, 250 mg/2 mL, 500 mg/4 mL, 1000 mg/8 mL. [HY-droh-KOR-tih-zohn].

**Hydro-Crysti-12** (Hem). See *hydroxocobalamin*. [HY-droh-KRIS-tee 12].

**HydroDIURIL** (Cardio, Uro). See *hydrochlorothiazide*. [HY-droh-DY-yoo-ril].

**hydroethyl starch** (Voluven) (I.V.). Nonblood plasma volume expander. Intravenous: 6%. [HY-droh-ETH-il STARCH].

**hydrogen peroxide** (Peroxyl) (ENT). Over-the-counter antiseptic mouth wash. Oral liquid: 1.5%. [HY-droh-jen per-AWK-side].

**Hydrogesic** (Analges) (generic *acetaminophen, hydrocodone*). Combination Schedule III nonnarcotic and narcotic analgesic drug for pain. Capsule: 500 mg/5 mg. [HY-droh-JEE-sik].

**hydromorphone** (Dilaudid, Dilaudid HP) (Analges). Schedule II narcotic analgesic drug used to treat moderate-to-severe pain. Tablet: 2 mg, 4 mg, 8 mg. Oral liquid: 1 mg/mL. Suppository: 3 mg. Subcutaneous, intramuscular, or intravenous: 1 mg/mL, 2 mg/mL, 4 mg/mL, 10 mg/mL. [HY-droh-MOR-fohn].

**Hydro-Par** (Cardio, Uro). See *hydrochlorothiazide*. [HY-droh-par].

**Hydrophed** (Pulm) (generic *theophylline, ephedrine, hydroxyzine*). Combination bronchodilator and antihistamine drug used to treat asthma and bronchitis. Tablet: 130 mg/25 mg/10 mg. [HY-droh-fed].

**hydroquinone** (Aclaro, Claripel, Eldopaque, Eldopaque Forte, Eldoquin-Forte, EpiQuin Micro, Esoterica Facial, Esoterica Regular, Glyquin, Glyquin-XM, Lustra, Lustra-AF, Melpaque HP, Melquin HP, NeoStrata, Nuquin HP, Solaquin, Solaquin Forte) (Derm). Over-the-counter and prescription drug used topically to lighten areas of hyperpigmented skin, freckles, and chloasma. Cream: 2%, 4%. Emulsion: 4%. Gel: 2%, 3%, 4%. Solution: 3%. [HY-droh-KWIH-nohn].

**HydroSkin** (Derm). See *hydrocortisone*. [HY-droh-skin].

**HydroTex** (Derm). See *hydrocortisone*. [HY-droh-teks].

**hydroxocobalamin** (Cyanokit, Hydro-Crysti-12) (Emerg, Hem). Vitamin $B_{12}$ drug used to treat pernicious anemia; emergency kit used to treat cyanide poisoning. Intramuscular: 1000 mcg/mL. Intravenous: 2.5 g/250 mL. [hy-DRAWK-soh-koh-BAWL ah min].

**hydroxychloroquine** (Plaquenil) (Anti-Infec, Derm, Ortho). Used to treat malaria; used to treat rheumatoid arthritis and systemic lupus erythematosis. Tablet: 200 mg. [hy-DRAWK-see-KLOR-oh-kwin].

**hydroxyethylcellulose** (Gonioscopic) (Ophth). Used during eye surgery. Ophthalmic solution: 0.004%. [hy-DRAWK-see-ETH-il-SEL-yoo-lohs].

**hydroxypropyl methylcellulose** (Gonak, Goniosol, OcuCoat, OcuCoat PF) (Ophth). Solution used during gonioscopy in the eye. Ophthalmic solution: 2%, 2.5%. [hy-DRAWK-see-PROH-pil METH-il-SEL-yoo-lohs].

**hydroxyurea** (Droxia, Hydrea) (Chemo, Derm, Hem). Chemotherapy drug used to treat sickle cell anemia and crisis; used to treat an elevated platelet count; used to treat psoriasis; used to treat malignant melanoma, leukemia, and cancer of the brain, head and neck, ovary, and cervix. Capsule: 200 mg, 300 mg, 400 mg, 500 mg. [hy-DRAWK-see-yoo-REE-ah].

**hydroxyzine** (Vistaril) (Anes, Derm, Psych). Antihistamine drug used to treat severe itching; used preoperatively to produce sedation and relieve anxiety; used to treat neurosis and anxiety. Capsule: 25 mg, 50 mg, 100 mg. Liquid: 25 mg/5 mL. Tablet: 10 mg, 25 mg, 50 mg. Syrup: 10 mg/5 mL. Intramuscular: 25 mg/mL, 50 mg/mL. [hy-DRAWK-sih-zeen].

**Hygroton** (Cardio, Uro). See *chlorthalidone*. [HY-groh-ton].

**Hylaform** (Derm). See *hyaluronic acid*. [HY-lah-form].

**Hylenex** (Misc). See *hyaluronidase*. [HY-leh-neks].

**hyoscyamine** (Uro). See *L-hyoscyamine*. [HY-oh-SY-ah-meen].

**hyperalimentation solution** (I.V.). Total parenteral nutrition. [HY-per-AL-ih-men-TAY-shun].

**hypericin** (Chemo). Chemotherapy drug used to treat brain cancer and cutaneous T-cell lymphoma. Orphan drug. [hy-PAIR-ih-sin].

**Hypermune RSV** (Anti-infec, Pulm). See *respiratory syncytial virus immunoglobulin*. [HY-per-myoon R-S-V].

**HyperRHO S/D Mini-Dose** (Hem, OB/GYN). Immunoglobulin drug given to an Rh-negative mother after the birth of an Rh-positive infant; it prevents the mother from making antibodies during the next pregnancy to cause hemolytic disease if the next infant is Rh positive. Intramuscular: 15% gamma globulin. [HY-per-roh S-D].

**Hyperstat IV** (Cardio). See *diazoxide*. [HY-per-stat I-V].

**HypoTears, HypoTears PF** (Ophth). Over-the-counter artificial tears for dry eyes. Ophthalmic solution. Ophthalmic ointment. [HY-poh-teerz].

**Hyskon** (OB/GYN) (generic *dextran, dextrose*).    Used intraoperatively to distend the uterus and facilitate visualization of its interior. Solution. [HIS-kawn].

**Hytone** (Derm).    See *hydrocortisone*. [HY-tohn].

**Hytrin** (Cardio, Uro).    See *terazosin*. [HY-trin].

**Hyzaar** (Cardio) (generic *losartan, hydrochlorothiazide*).    Combination angiotensin II receptor blocker and diuretic drug used to treat hypertension. Tablet: 50 mg/12.5 mg, 100 mg/12.5 mg, 100 mg/25 mg. [HY-zar].

**ibandronate** (Boniva) (Ortho).    Bone resorption inhibitor drug used to prevent bone loss and treat osteoporosis in postmenopausal women. Tablet (once daily): 2.5 mg. Tablet (once monthly): 150 mg. Intravenous: 1 mg/mL. [eye-BAN-droh-nayt].

**iboctadekin** (Chemo).    Chemotherapy drug used to treat kidney cancer. Orphan drug. [ih-BAWK-tah-DEK-in].

**ibritumomab** (Zevalin) (Chemo).    Chemotherapy drug used to treat non-Hodgkin's lymphoma. Orphan drug. [IB-rih-TOO-moh-mab].

**IB-Stat** (GI, Uro).    See *L-hyoscyamine*. [I-B-stat].

**Ibudone** (Analges) (generic *hydrocodone, ibuprofen*).    Combination Schedule III narcotic and NSAID analgesic drug for pain. Tablet: 5 mg/200 mg. [EYE-byoo-dohn].

**ibuprofen** (Advil, Advil Migraine, Children's Advil, Children's Motrin, Infants' Motrin, Junior Strength Advil, Junior Strength Motrin, Midol Maximum Strength Cramp Formula, Motrin, Motrin IB, Motrin Migraine Pain, Pediatric Advil Drops, PediaCare Fever, Salprofen) (Analges).    Prescription and over-the-counter nonsteroidal anti-inflammatory drug used to treat fever, pain, and inflammation; used to treat osteoarthritis, rheumatoid arthritis, dysmenorrhea, and migraine headaches; orphan drug given intravenously to treat patent ductus arteriosus (Salprofen). Capsule/Liqui-Gel: 200 mg. Chewable tablet: 50 mg, 100 mg. Drops: 40 mg/mL. Liquid: 100 mg/2.5 mL, 100 mg/5 mL. Tablet: 100 mg, 200 mg, 400 mg, 600 mg, 800 mg. Intravenous (orphan drug). [EYE-byoo-PROH-fen].

**ibuprofen lysine** (Neoprofen) (Cardio).    Used to treat newborn infants with congenital heart defects to keep the ductus arteriosus open until surgical correction can be done. Intravenous: 10 mg/mL. [EYE-byoo-PROH-fen LY-seen].

**ibutilide** (Corvert) (Cardio).    Antiarrhythmic drug used to treat atrial flutter or atrial fibrillation. Intravenous: 0.1 mg/mL. [eye-BYOO-tih-lide].

**icatibant** (Derm).    Used to treat angioedema and burns. Orphan drug. [eye-CAT-ih-bant].

**IC-Green** (Ophth).    See *indocyanine green*. [I-C-green].

**Icy Hot, Icy Hot Arthritis Therapy** (Ortho) (generic *methyl salicylate, menthol*).    Combination analgesic drug used topically on the skin to treat the pain of osteoarthritis and minor muscle injuries. Cream. Gel. Chill stick. [EYE-see HOT].

**Idamycin PFS** (Chemo).    See *idarubicin*. [EYE-dah-MY-sin P-F-S].

**idarubicin** (Idamycin PFS) (Chemo).    Chemotherapy antibiotic drug used to treat leukemia. Intravenous: 1 mg/mL. [EYE-dah-ROO-bih-sin].

**idoxuridine** (Chemo).    Chemotherapy drug used to treat sarcoma. Orphan drug. [EYE-dawks-YOOR-ih-deen].

**idursulfase** (Elaprase) (Misc).    Used to treat mucopolysaccharidosis, type 2 (Hunter syndrome). Intravenous: 2 mg/mL. [EYE-dur-SUL-fays].

**Ifex** (Chemo).    See *ifosfamide*. [EYE-feks].

**ifosfamide** (Ifex) (Chemo).    Alkylating chemotherapy drug used to treat cancer of the lung, stomach, breast, ovary, cervix, testicle, bone, and bladder; used to treat leukemia and non-Hodgkin's lymphoma. Intravenous (powder to be reconstituted): 1 g, 3 g. [ih-FAWS-fah-mide].

**Ilopan** (GI).    See *dexpanthenol*. [EYE-loh-pan].

**iloprost** (Ventavis) (Cardio).    Used to treat pulmonary arterial hypertension; orphan drug used to treat heparin-induced thrombocytopenia and Raynaud's disease. Inhaled solution: 10 mcg/mL. [EYE-loh-prawst].

**Ilotycin** (Anti-infec, Ophth).    See *erythromycin*. [EYE-loh-TY-sin].

**imatinib** (Gleevec) (Chemo).    Chemotherapy drug used to treat leukemia. Tablet: 100 mg. [ih-MAT-ih-nib].

**Imdur** (Cardio).    See *isosorbide mononitrate*. [IM-dur].

**imexon** (Amplimexon) (Chemo).    Chemotherapy drug used to treat cancer of the pancreas and ovary; used to treat multiple myeloma and malignant melanoma. Orphan drug. [eye-MEK-sawn].

**imiglucerase** (Cerezyme) (Misc).    Enzyme drug used to treat Gaucher disease. Intravenous (powder to be reconstituted): 200 units, 400 units. [IM-ee-GLOO-sair-ace].

**imipramine** (Tofranil, Tofranil-PM) (Analges, Neuro, Psych, Uro).    Tricyclic antidepressant drug used to treat depression, panic attacks, withdrawal from cocaine addiction, and bulimia; used to treat enuresus (childhood bed-wetting); used to treat migraine headaches; used to treat nerve pain from phantom limb, diabetic neuropathy, peripheral neuropathy, and postherpetic neuralgia; used to treat tic douloureux. Capsule: 75 mg, 100 mg, 125 mg, 150 mg. Tablet: 10 mg, 25 mg, 50 mg. [ih-MIP-rah-meen].

**imiquimod** (Aldara) (Derm, OB/GYN, Onco).    Immunomodulator drug used topically to treat condylomata acuminata (genital warts), actinic keratoses, and superficial basal cell carcinoma of the skin. Cream: 5%. [ih-MIH-kwih-mawd].

**Imitrex** (Analges).    See *sumatriptan*. [IM-ih-treks].

**ImmTher** (Chemo).    Chemotherapy drug used to treat metastases in patients with colon or rectal cancer; used to treat bone cancer. Orphan drug. [IM-thair].

**ImmuDyn** (Hem).    Used to treat thrombocytopenia purpura. Orphan drug. [IM-myoo-dine].

**Immun-Aid** (GI). Nutritional supplement formulated for immunocompromised patients. Powder (to be reconstituted). [IM-myoon-aid].

**Immuno** (Anti-infec, Misc). See *human immune globulin.* [im-MYOO-noh].

**Immuno-C** (Anti-infec). See *bovine immunoglobulin.* [IM-myoo-noh-C].

**Immupath** (Anti-infec). See *HIV neutralizing antibodies.* [IM-myoo-path].

**Imodium A-D** (GI). See *loperamide.* [ih-MOH-dee-um A-D].

**Imogam Rabies-HT** (Anti-infec). Immunoglobulin drug used to treat patients exposed to rabies. Intramuscular: 150 IU/mL. [IM-oh-gam RAY-beez-H-T].

**Impact** (GI). Lactose-free nutritional supplement. Liquid. [IM-pakt].

**Implanon** (OB/GYN). See *etonogestrel.* [im-PLAN-awn].

**implitapide** (Cardio). Used to treat hypercholesterolemia. Orphan drug. [im-PLIH-tah-pide].

**Imuran** (Ortho, Uro). See *azathioprine.* [IM-yoor-an].

**Imuthiol** (Anti-infec). See *diethyldithiocarbamate.* [IM-yoo-THY-awl].

**Imuvert** (Chemo). Chemotherapy drug used to treat brain cancer. Orphan drug. [IM-yoo-vert].

**inamrinone** (Cardio). Used to treat congestive heart failure that has not responded to treatment with digoxin. Intravenous: 5 mg/mL. [in-AM-rih-nohn].

**Inapsine** (Anes, GI, Chemo). See *droperidol.* [in-AP-seen].

**Increlex** (Endo). See *mecasermin.* [IN-kreh-leks].

**indapamide** (Lozol) (Cardio, Uro). Thiazide diuretic drug used to treat hypertension; used to treat edema from congestive heart failure. Tablet: 1.25 mg, 2.5 mg. [in-DAP-ah-mide].

**Inderal, Inderal LA** (Analges, Cardio, Endo, GI, Neuro, Psych). See *propranolol.* [IN-der-awl].

**Inderide 40/25** (Cardio) (generic *propranolol, hydrochloro-thiazide*). Combination beta-blocker and diuretic drug used to treat hypertension. Tablet: 40 mg/25 mg. [IN-deh-ride].

**indinavir** (Crixivan) (Anti-infec). Protease inhibitor antiviral drug used to treat HIV and AIDS. Capsule: 100 mg, 200 mg, 333 mg, 400 mg. [in-DIN-ah-veer].

**indium 111** (NeuroendoMedix, SomatoTher) (Endo). Radioactive drug used to treat neuroendocrine tumors. Orphan drug. [IN-dee-um 111].

**Indocin, Indocin I.V., Indocin SR** (Analges, Cardio). See *indomethacin.* [IN-doh-sin].

**indocyanine green** (Cardio-Green, IC-Green) (Cardio, Ophth). Dye used during angiography to determine cardiac output; used during angiography of the eye. Intravenous (powder to be reconstituted). [IN-doh-SY-ah-neen GREEN].

**indomethacin** (Indocin, Indocin I.V., Indocin SR) (Analges, Cardio). Nonsteroidal anti-inflammatory drug used to treat the pain and inflammation of osteoarthritis, rheumatoid arthritis, bursitis, tendinitis, gout, and ankylosing spondylitis; used to close a persistent patent ductus arteriosus in newborns. Capsule: 25 mg, 50 mg. Sustained-release capsule: 75 mg. Oral liquid: 25 mg/5 mL. Suppository: 50 mg. Intravenous: 1 mg. [IN-doh-METH-ah-sin].

**Infalyte** (GI). Electrolyte solution given to children to replace water and electrolytes lost from vomiting and diarrhea. Liquid. [IN-fah-lite].

**Infanrix** (Misc). Combination drug used to prevent diphtheria, pertussis, and tetanus. Subcutaneous. Vaccine. [in-FAN-riks].

**Infasurf** (Pulm). See *calfactant.* [IN-fah-surf].

**InFeD** (Hem). See *iron dextran.* [IN-feh-D].

**Infergen** (GI). See *interferon alfacon-1.* [IN-fer-jen].

**infliximab** (Remicade) (Derm, GI, Ortho). Immunosuppressant monoclonal antibody drug used to treat psoriasis; used to treat Crohn's disease and ulcerative colitis; used to treat rheumatoid arthritis, psoriatic arthritis, and ankylosing spondylitis. Intravenous: 100 mg/20 mL. [in-FLIK-sih-mab].

**influenza virus vaccine** (Afluria, Fluarix, FluLaval, FluMist, Fluvirin, Fluzone) (Anti-infec, Pulm). Vaccine to prevent influenza A and B infections. Intramuscular (split virus): 15 mcg/mL. Nasal spray. [IN-floo-EN-zah VY-rus vak-SEEN].

**Infumorph 200, Infumorph 500** (Analges, Anes). See *morphine.* [IN-fyoo-morf].

**Infuvite Adult, Infuvite Pediatric** (I.V.). Combination 9 water-soluble and 3 fat-soluble vitamins drug. Intravenous. [IN-fyoo-vite].

**Innohep** (Hem). See *tinzaparin.* [EYE-noh-hep].

**InnoPran XL** (Analges, Cardio, Endo, GI, Neuro, Psych). See *propranolol.* [EYE-noh-pran X-L].

**inolimomab** (Leukotac) (Hem). Used to prevent graft-versus-host disease. Orphan drug. [EYE-noh-LIH-moh-mab].

**INOmax** (Pulm). See *nitric oxide.* [EYE-noh-maks].

**Inspra** (Cardio). See *eplerenone.* [IN-sprah].

**Insta-Glucose** (Endo). See *glucose.* [IN-stah-GLOO-kohs].

**insulin aspart** (NovoLog) (Endo). Rapid-acting insulin analog drug created by recombinant DNA technology used to treat type 1 diabetes mellitus. Subcutaneous: 100 units/mL. [IN-soo-lin AS-part].

**insulin detemir** (Levemir) (Endo). Long-acting insulin analog drug created by recombinant DNA technology used to treat type 1 diabetes mellitus. Subcutaneous: 100 units/mL. Penfill cartridge: 3 mL. FlexPen and Innolet prefilled syringes. [IN-soo-lin DET-eh-meer].

**insulin glargine** (Lantus) (Endo). Long-acting insulin analog drug created by recombinant DNA technology used to treat type 1 diabetes mellitus. Subcutaneous: 100 units/mL. SoloSTAR prefilled pen: 80 units. [IN-soo-lin GLAR-jeen].

**insulin glulisine** (Apidra) (Endo). Rapid-acting insulin analog drug created by recombinant DNA technology that is used to treat type 1 diabetes mellitus. Subcutaneous: 100 units/mL. [IN-soo-lin gloo-LIS-een].

**insulin lispro** (Humalog) (Endo).    Rapid-acting insulin analog drug created by recombinant DNA technology that is used to treat type 1 diabetes mellitus. Subcutaneous: 100 units/mL. [IN-soo-lin LIS-proh].

**Insulin Reaction** (Endo).    See *glucose*. [IN-soo-lin ree-AK-shun].

**Intal** (Pulm).    See *cromolyn*. [IN-tawl].

**Integrilin** (Cardio, Hem).    See *eptifibatide*. [in-TEG-reh-lin].

**Intelence** (Anti-infec).    See *etravirine*. [in-TEL-ens].

**interferon alfa-1b** (Chemo).    Chemotherapy drug used to treat multiple myeloma. Orphan drug. [IN-ter-FEER-awn AL-fah-1-b].

**interferon alfa-2b** (Intron A) (Chemo, Derm, GI).    Immunomodulator drug used to treat hepatitis B and hepatic C virus; used topically on the skin to treat condylomata acuminata (genital warts); used to treat cancer of the ovary, cervix, kidney, and bladder; used to treat malignant melanoma, leukemia, Hodgkin's lymphoma, non-Hodgkin's lymphoma, Kaposi's sarcoma, mycosis fungoides, and multiple myeloma. Subcutaneous or intramuscular: 22.5 million IU/mL, 37.5 million IU/mL, 75 million IU/mL. [IN-ter-FEER-awn AL-fah-2-b].

**interferon alfa-n1** (Wellferon) (Anti-infec).    Used to treat Kaposi's sarcoma; used to treat human papillomavirus. Orphan drug. [IN-ter-FEER-awn AL-fah-n-1].

**interferon alfa-n3** (Alferon N) (Derm, OB/GYN).    Immunomodulator and antiviral drug used to treat condylomata acuminata (genital warts). Intralesional injection: 5 million IU/mL. [IN-ter-FEER-awn AL-fah-n-3].

**interferon alfacon-1** (Infergen) (GI).    Immunomodulator drug used to treat hepatitis C virus. Subcutaneous: 9 mcg/0.3 mL, 15 mcg/0.5 mL. [IN-ter-FEER-awn AL-fah-kawn-1].

**interferon beta-1a** (Avonex, Rebif) (Anti-infec, Chemo, GI, Neuro).    Immunomodulator drug used to treat HIV and AIDS; used to treat malignant melanoma, mycosis fungoides, and Kaposi's sarcoma; used to treat non-A non-B hepatitis; used to treat multiple sclerosis. Intramuscular (powder to be reconstituted): 8.8 mcg/0.2 mL, 22 mcg/0.5 mL, 30 mcg/0.5 mL. [IN-ter-FEER-awn BAY-tah-1-a].

**interferon beta-1b** (Betaseron) (Anti-infec, Neuro).    Immunomodulator drug used to treat multiple sclerosis; used to treat AIDS. Subcutaneous (powder to be reconstituted): 0.3 mg/3 mL. [IN-ter-FEER-awn BAY-tah-1-b].

**interferon gamma-1b** (Actimmune) (Chemo, Derm).    Used to treat the skin infections of chronic granulomatous disease; used to treat malignant osteopetrosis; used to treat kidney cancer. Subcutaneous: 100 mcg/0.5 mL. [IN-ter-FEER-awn GAM-mah-1-b].

**interleukin-1 receptor antagonist** (Antril) (Chemo, Ortho).    Used to prevent or treat graft-versus-host disease; used to treat juvenile rheumatoid arthritis. Orphan drug. [IN-ter-LOO-kin-1].

**interleukin-2** (Chemo).    See *aldesleukin*. [IN-ter-LOO-kin-2].

**IntraChol** (Misc).    Used to treat choline deficiency. [IN-trah-KOHL].

**IntraDose** (Chemo) (generic *cisplatin, epinephrine*).    Combination chemotherapy and epinephrine drug used to treat head and neck cancer and malignant melanoma. Orphan drug. [IN-trah-DOHS].

**Intralipid 10%, Intralipid 20%** (I.V.).    See *intravenous lipids*. [IN-trah-LIP-id].

**IntraSite** (Derm).    Over-the-counter drug used topically to absorb drainage from burns, skin ulcers, and wounds. Gauze dressing containing gel. [IN-trah-site].

**intravenous lipids** (Intralipid 10%, Intralipid 20%, Liposyn II 10%, Liposyn II 20%, Liposyn III 10%, Liposyn III 20%) (I.V.).    Lipid (fat) solution. Intravenous. [IN-trah-VEE-nuhs LIP-ids].

**intravenous multivitamins** (Berocca Parenteral Nutrition, Cernevit-12, M.V.I.-12) (I.V.).    Combination 9 water-soluble and 3 fat-soluble multivitamin drug. Intravenous. [IN-trah-VEE-nuhs MUL-tee-VY-tah-mins].

**Introlite** (GI).    Lactose-free nutritional supplement. Liquid. [IN-troh-lite].

**Intron A** (Chemo, Derm, GI).    See *interferon alfa-2b*. [IN-trawn A].

**Invanz** (Anti-infec).    See *ertapenem*. [IN-vanz].

**Invega** (Psych).    See *paliperidone*. [in-VEG-ah].

**Inversine** (Cardio, Psych).    See *mecamylamine*. [IN-ver-seen].

**Invirase** (Anti-infec).    See *saquinavir*. [in-VY-rays].

**iobenguane** (Ultratrace) (Chemo).    Radioactive chemotherapy drug used to treat brain cancer. Orphan drug. [EYE-oh-BEN-gwayn].

**iodine** (Lugol's solution, ThyroShield) (Endo, Derm).    Over-the-counter antibacterial, antiviral, antifungal, and antiyeast drug used topically as a surgical skin prep; used to treat hyperthyroidism and thyrotoxicosis prior to thyroidectomy (Thyroshield). Oral liquid: 65 mg/mL. Topical solution: 2%, 5%, 7%. [EYE-oh-dine].

**iodoquinol** (Yodoxin) (Anti-Infec).    Amebicide drug used to treat intestinal amebiasis. Tablet: 210 mg, 650 mg. Powder. [eye-OH-doh-KWIH-nohl].

**Iodotope** (Chemo, Endo).    See *sodium iodide-131*. [eye-OH-doh-tohp].

**Ionamin** (GI).    See *phentermine*. [eye-AWN-ah-min].

**Ionax Astringent Cleanser** (Derm).    Keratolytic drug used topically on the skin to treat acne vulgaris. Liquid. [EYE-oh-naks].

**Ionil T Plus** (Derm).    See *coal tar*. [EYE-oh-nil T PLUS].

**Ionsys** (Analges).    See *fentanyl*. [eye-AWN-sis].

**Iopidine** (Ophth).    See *apraclonidine*. [eye-OH-peh-deen].

**Iosopan** (GI) (generic *aluminum, magnesium*).    Combination antacid drug used to treat heartburn. Liquid: 540 mg/5 mL. [eye-OH-soh-pan].

**Iosopan Plus** (GI) (generic *aluminum, magnesium, simethicone*).    Combination antacid and anti-gas drug used to treat heartburn and gas. Liquid: 540 mg/20 mg. [eye-OH-soh-pan PLUS].

**ipecac syrup** (Emerg, GI). Emetic drug used to induce vomiting to treat poisoning and drug overdose. Syrup: 15 mL, 30 mL. [IP-eh-kak-SIR-ip].

**Iplex** (Endo). See *mecasermin*. [EYE-pleks].

**IPOL** (Anti-infec). Used to prevent polio in children. Subcutaneous: Vaccine. [I-P-O-L].

**ipratropium** (Atrovent, Atrovent HFA) (ENT, Pulm). Bronchodilator drug used to treat bronchospasm with chronic obstructive pulmonary disease and chronic bronchitis; used to treat allergic rhinitis. Aerosol inhaler: 17 mg/puff, 18 mcg/puff. Liquid for inhalation: 0.02% (500 mcg/2.5 mL). Nasal spray: 0.03%, 0.06%. [IH-prah-TROH-pee-um].

**Iprivask** (Hem). See *desirudin*. [IP-rih-vask].

**Ipstyl** (Endo). See *lanreotide*. [IP-stil]

**irbesartan** (Avapro) (Cardio, Endo, Uro). Angiotensin II receptor blocker drug used to treat hypertension; used to treat diabetic nephropathy. Tablet: 75 mg, 150 mg, 300 mg. [IR-beh-SAR-tan].

**Iressa** (Chemo). See *gefitinib*. [ih-RES-sah].

**irinotecan** (Camptosar) (Chemo). Mitosis inhibitor chemotherapy drug used to treat cancer of the brain, lung, stomach, colon, rectum, or cervix. Intravenous: 20 mg/mL. [eye-RIN-oh-TEE-kan].

**irofulvin** (Chemo). Used to treat cancer of the ovary and kidney. Orphan drug. [EYE-roh-FUL-vin].

**iron dextran** (DexFerrum, InFeD) (Hem). Iron compound drug used to treat iron deficiency anemia. Intramuscular or intravenous: 50 mg/mL. [EYE-ern DEKS-tran].

**iron sucrose** (Venofer) (Hem, Uro). Iron compound drug used to treat iron deficiency anemia in patients with chronic renal failure and those on hemodialysis or peritoneal dialysis. Intravenous: 20 mg/mL. [EYE-ern SOO-krohs].

**Isentress** (Anti-infec). See *raltegravir*. [eye-SEN-tress].

**Ismelin** (Neuro). See *guanethidine*. [IS-meh-lin].

**ISMO** (Cardio). See *isosorbide mononitrate*. [IS-moh].

**Ismotic** (Ophth). See *isosorbide*. [is-MAW-tik].

**isobutyramide** (Hem). Used to treat sickle cell disease and beta-thalassemia. Orphan drug. [EYE-soh-byoo-TY-rah-mide].

**Isocal HCN, Isocal HN** (GI). Lactose-free nutritional supplement. Liquid. [EYE-soh-kal].

**isocarboxazid** (Marplan) (Psych). MAO inhibitor drug used to treat depression. Tablet: 10 mg. [EYE-soh-kar-BAWK-sah-zid].

**Isochron** (Cardio). See *isosorbide dinitrate*. [EYE-soh-krawn].

**isoetharine** (Pulm). Bronchodilator drug used to prevent and treat asthma and bronchospasm. Liquid for inhalation: 1%. [EYE-soh-ETH-ah-reen].

**isofagomine** (Misc). Used to treat Gaucher disease. Orphan drug. [EYE-soh-FAG-oh-meen].

**isoflurane** (Forane, Terrell) (Anes). Anesthetic drug used to induce and maintain general anesthesia. Inhaled gas. [EYE-soh-FLOO-rayn].

**Isomil, Isomil DF, Isomil SF** (GI). Lactose-free, sucrose-free infant formula with soy protein for infants with allergies or diarrhea. Liquid. Powder (to be reconstituted). [EYE-soh-mil]

**IsonaRif** (Pulm) (generic *isoniazid, rifampin*). Combination antitubercular antibiotic drug used to treat tuberculosis. Capsule: 150 mg/300 mg [EYE-soh-NAIR-if].

**isoniazid** (INH) (Nydrazid) (Pulm). Antitubercular antibiotic drug used to treat tuberculosis. Syrup: 50 mg/5 mL. Tablet: 100 mg, 300 mg. Intramuscular: 100 mg/mL. [EYE-soh-NY-ah-zid].

**isoproterenol** (Isuprel) (Cardio, Emerg, Pulm). Vasopressor drug used to treat heart block; used to treat hypotension during cardiac resuscitation and shock; used to treat brochospasm during anesthesia/surgery. Intravenous: 1:5000 (0.2 mg/mL), 1:50,000 (0.02 mg/mL). [EYE-soh-proh-TAIR-eh-nawl].

**Isoptin SR** (Analges, Cardio). See *verapamil*. [eye-SAWP-tin S-R]

**Isopto Atropine** (Ophth). See *atropine*. [eye-SAWP-toh AH-troh-peen].

**Isopto Carbachol** (Ophth). See *carbachol*. [eye-SAWP-toh KAR-bah-kawl].

**Isopto Carpine** (Ophth). See *pilocarpine*. [eye-SAWP-toh KAR-peen].

**Isopto Homatropine** (Ophth). See *homatropine*. [eye-SAWP-toh HOH-mah-TROH-peen].

**Isopto Hyoscine** (Ophth). See *scopolamine*. [eye-SAWP-toh HY-oh-seen].

**Isopto Plain, Isopto Tears** (Ophth). Over-the-counter artificial tears for dry eyes. Ophthalmic solution. [eye-SOP-toh].

**Isordil Titradose** (Cardio). See *isosorbide dinitrate*. [EYE-sohr-dil TY-trah-dohs].

**isosorbide** (Ismotic) (Ophth). Osmotic diuretic drug used to temporarily decrease intraocular pressure prior to eye surgery. Oral liquid: 45% solution. [EYE-soh-SOR-bide].

**isosorbide dinitrate** (Dilatrate-SR, Isochron, Isordil Titradose) (Cardio). Nitrate drug used to prevent and treat angina pectoris. Sustained-release capsule: 40 mg. Sublingual tablet: 2.5 mg, 5 mg. Tablet: 5 mg, 10 mg, 20 mg, 30 mg, 40 mg. Extended-release tablet: 40 mg. [EYE-soh-SOR-bide dy-NY-trayt].

**isosorbide mononitrate** (Imdur, ISMO, Monoket) (Cardio). Nitrate drug used to prevent and treat angina pectoris. Tablet: 10 mg, 20 mg. Extended-release tablet: 30 mg, 60 mg, 120 mg. [EYE-soh-SOR-bide MAWN-noh-NY-trayt].

**Isosource, Isosource HN** (GI). Lactose-free or lactose-free and gluten-free nutritional supplement. Liquid. [EYE-soh-sors].

**Isotein HN** (GI). Lactose-free, gluten-free nutritional supplement. Powder (to be reconstituted). [EYE-soh-teen H-N].

**isotretinoin** (Accutane, Amnesteem, Claravis, Sotret) (Derm). Oral vitamin A-type (retinoid) drug used to treat severe cystic acne vulgaris. Capsule: 10 mg, 20 mg, 30 mg, 40 mg.

Gel capsule: 10 mg, 20 mg, 30 mg, 40 mg.
[EYE-soh-TREE-tih-NOH-in].

**Isovorin** (Chemo). See *L-leucovorin*. [EYE-soh-VOR-in].

**isoxsuprine** (Vasodilan) (Cardio). Peripheral vasodilator drug used to treat peripheral vascular disease, Raynaud's disease, arteriosclerosis obliterans, and Buerger's disease; used to treat preterm labor in women. Tablet: 10 mg, 20 mg. [eye-SAWK-soo-preen].

**isradipine** (DynaCirc, DynaCirc CR) (Cardio). Calcium channel blocker drug used to treat hypertension and Raynaud's disease. Capsule: 2.5 mg, 5 mg. Controlled-release tablet: 5 mg, 10 mg. [is-RAD-ih-peen].

**Istalol** (Ophth). See *timolol*. [IS-tah-lawl].

**Isuprel** (Cardio, Emerg, Pulm). See *isoproterenol*. [EYE-soo-prel].

**itraconazole** (Sporanox) (Anti-infec). Antifungal drug used to treat severe systemic fungal and yeast infections, such as aspergillosis, blastomycosis, histoplasmosis, onychomycosis, and esophageal candidiasis. Capsule: 100 mg. Oral liquid: 10 mg/mL. [IH-trah-KAWN-ah-zohl].

**Iveegam, Iveegam EN** (Anti-infec, Misc). See *human immune globulin*. [EYE-vee-gam].

**ivermectin** (Stromectol) (Misc). Used to treat worm infestations. Tablet: 3 mg, 6 mg. [EYE-ver-MEK-tin].

**ixabepilone** (Ixempra) (Chemo). Chemotherapy drug used to treat breast cancer. Intravenous: 15 mg, 45 mg. [IK-sab-EP-ih-lohn].

**Ixempra** (Chemo). See *ixabepilone*. [ik-SEM-prah].

**Jantoven** (Cardio, Hem, Neuro). See *warfarin*. [JAN-toh-ven].

**Janumet** (Endo) (generic *sitagliptin, metformin*). Combination antidiabetic drug used to treat type 2 diabetes mellitus. Tablet: 50 mg/500 mg, 50 mg/1000 mg. [JAN-yoo-met].

**Januvia** (Endo). See *sitagliptin*. [jah-NOO-vee-ah].

**Jevity, Jevity 1.5 Cal** (GI). Milk-based or lactose-free nutritional supplement. Liquid. [JEH-vih-tee].

**Jolessa** (OB/GYN) (generic *levonorgestrel, ethinyl estradiol*). Combination monophasic oral contraceptive drug. Pill pack, 28-day: (21 hormone tablets) 0.15 mg/30 mcg; (7 inert tablets). [joh-LES-sah].

**Jolivette** (OB/GYN). See *norethindrone*. [JOH-lih-VET].

**Junel 21 Day 1/20, Junel 21 Day 1.5/30** (OB/GYN) (generic *norethindrone, ethinyl estradiol*). Combination monophasic oral contraceptive drug. Pill pack, 21-day: (21 hormone tablets) 1 mg/20 mcg. Pill pack, 21-day: (21 hormone tablets) 1.5 mg/30 mcg. [joo-NEL].

**Junel Fe 1/20, Junel Fe 1.5/30** (OB/GYN) (generic *norethindrone, ethinyl estradiol; ferrous fumarate*). Combination monophasic oral contraceptive drug with iron supplement. Pill pack, 28-day: (21 hormone tablets) 1 mg/20 mcg; (7 iron [Fe] tablets) 75 mg. Pill pack, 28-day: (21 hormone tablets) 1.5 mg/30 mcg; (7 iron [Fe] tablets) 75 mg. [joo-NEL].

**Juvederm 24HV, Juvederm 30, Juvederm 30HV** (Derm). See *hyaluronic acid*. [JOO-veh-derm].

**Junovan** (Chemo). See *mifamritide*. [JOO-noh-van].

**K + 8, K + 10** (Uro). See *potassium*. [K plus 8].

**K + Care, K + Care ET** (Uro). See *potassium*. [K plus KAIR].

**Kadian** (Analges, Anes). See *morphine*. [KAY-dee-an].

**Kaletra** (Anti-infec) (generic *lopinavir, ritonavir*). Combination protease inhibitor antiviral drug used to treat HIV and AIDS. Capsule: 200 mg/50 mg. Oral liquid: 80 mg/20 mg per mL. Tablet: 100 mg/25 mg. [kah-LEE-trah].

**kanamycin** (Kantrex) (Anti-infec). Aminoglycoside antibiotic drug used to treat a variety of serious gram-negative infections; given orally preoperatively as a bowel prep before intra-abdominal surgery; given orally to treat hepatic coma by killing ammonia-producing bacteria in the intestines. Intramuscular or intravenous: 75 mg, 500 mg, 1 g. [KAN-ah-MY-sin].

**Kantrex** (Anti-infec). See *kanamycin*. [KAN-treks].

**Kaodene Non-Narcotic** (GI) (generic *bismuth, kaolin, pectin*). Over-the-counter combination anti-infective and absorbent drug used to treat diarrhea. Liquid. [KAY-oh-deen].

**Kaon, Kaon Cl-10, Kaon-Cl 20%** (Uro). See *potassium*. [KAY-awn].

**Kaopectate, Kaopectate Children's, Kaopectate Extra Strength** (GI). See *bismuth*. [KAY-oh-PEK-tayt].

**Kaopectate Maximum Strength** (GI). See *attapulgite*. [KAY-oh-PEK-tayt].

**Kapectolin** (GI) (generic *kaolin, pectin*). Combination over-the-counter absorbent drug used to treat diarrhea. Suspension: 90 g/2 g in 30 mL. [kay-PEK-toh-lin].

**Kariva** (OB/GYN) (generic *desogestrel, ethinyl estradiol*). Combination biphasic oral contraceptive drug. Pill pack, 28-day: (21 hormone tablets) 0.15 mg/20 mcg; (5 hormone tablets) 10 mcg; (2 inert tablets). [kah-REE-vah].

**Kay Ciel** (Uro). See *potassium*. [KAY see-EL].

**Kayexalate** (Hem). See *sodium polystyrene sulfonate*. [kay-EK-sah-layt].

**Kaylixir** (Uro). See *potassium*. [kay-LIK-zir].

**K-Dur 10, K-Dur 20** (Uro). See *potassium*. [KAY-dur].

**Keflex** (Anti-infec). See *cephalexin*. [KEH-fleks].

**Kelnor 1/35** (OB/GYN) (generic *ethynodiol, ethinyl estradiol*). Combination monophasic oral contraceptive drug. Pill pack, 28-day: (21 hormone tablets) 1 mg/35 mcg; (7 inert tablets). [KEL-nor].

**Kemstro** (GI, Neuro, Ortho). See *baclofen*. [KEM-stroh].

**Kenalog, Kenalog-10, Kenalog-40, Kenalog in Orabase** (Derm, ENT, Ortho, Pulm). See *triamcinolone*. [KEN-ah-lawg].

**Kenonel** (Derm). See *triamcinolone*. [KEN-oh-nel].

**Kepivance** (Chemo, ENT). See *palifermin*. [KEP-ih-vans].

**Keppra** (Analges, Neuro, Psych).   See *levetiracetam.* [KEP-prah].

**Kerafoam** (Derm).   See *urea.* [KAIR-ah-fohm].

**Keralac, Keralac Nailstik** (Derm).   See *urea.* [KAIR-ah-lak].

**KeriCort-10 Maximum Strength** (Derm).   See *hydrocortisone.* [KAIR-ee-kort].

**Kerlone** (Cardio).   See *betaxolol.* [KER-lohn].

**Ketalar** (Anes).   See *ketamine.* [KET-ah-lar].

**ketamine** (Ketalar) (Anes).   Schedule III drug used to induce and maintain general anesthesia. Intramuscular and intravenous: 10 mg/mL, 50 mg/mL, 100 mg/mL. [KET-ah-meen].

**Ketek** (Anti-infec).   See *telithromycin.* [KET-ek].

**KeriCort-10, Maximum Strength** (Derm).   See *hydrocortisone.* [KAIR-ee-cort-10].

**ketoconazole** (Extina, Nizoral, Nizoral A-D, Xolegel) (Anti-infec, Derm, ENT).   Over-the-counter and prescription antifungal and antiyeast drug; used to treat seborrheic dermatitis; used topically to treat tinea (ringworm) and other fungal skin infections; used to treat *Candida* yeast skin infections; used orally to treat treat systemic fungal and yeast infections of blastomycosis, coccidioidomycosis, histoplasmosis, and candidiasis; orphan drug used to prevent kidney toxicity in organ transplantation patients who receive cyclosporine. Cream: 2%. Foam: 2%. Gel: 2%. Shampoo: 1%, 2%. Tablet: 200 mg. [KEE-toh-KAWN-ah-zohl].

**Ketonex-1, Ketonex-2** (GI).   Infant formula for infants with maple syrup urine disease; nutritional supplement for adults with maple syrup urine disease. Powder (to be reconstituted). [KEE-toh-neks].

**ketoprofen** (Analges).   Nonsteroidal anti-inflammatory drug used to treat pain and inflammation; used to treat osteoarthritis, rheumatoid arthritis, and dysmenorrhea. Capsule: 50 mg, 75 mg. Extended-release capsule: 100 mg, 150 mg, 200 mg. [KEE-toh-PROH-fen].

**ketorolac** (Acular) (Analges, Ophth).   Nonsteroidal anti-inflammatory drug used to treat pain; used topically to treat pain and inflammation from eye allergies or after corneal surgery (Acular). Tablet: 10 mg. Intramuscular or intravenous: 15 mg/mL, 30 mg/mL. Ophthalmic solution: 0.09%. [kee-TOR-oh-lak].

**ketotifen** (Zaditor) (Ophth).   Over-the-counter and prescription antihistamine and mast cell stabilizer drug used to treat allergy symptoms in the eyes. Ophthalmic solution: 0.025%. [KEE-toh-TIF-en].

**Kindercal** (GI).   Lactose-free nutritional supplement. Liquid. [KIN-der-kal].

**Kineret** (Ortho).   See *anakinra.* [KIN-eh-ret].

**Kinrix** (Misc).   Combination drug used to prevent diphtheria, pertussis, tetanus, polio, and hepatitis B. Subcutaneous: Vaccine. [KIN-riks].

**Kionex** (Hem).   See *sodium polystyrene sulfonate.* [KY-oh-neks].

**Klonopin** (Neuro, Psych).   See *clonazepam.* [KLAWN-oh-pin].

**K-Lor** (Uro).   See *potassium.* [K-lohr].

**Klor-Con, Klor-Con 8, Klor-Con 10, Klor-Con/25, Klor-Con/EF, Klor-Con M10, Klor-Con M15, Klor-Con M20** (Uro).   See *potassium.* [KLOR-kawn].

**Klorvess** (Uro).   See *potassium.* [klor-VES].

**Klotrix** (Uro).   See *potassium.* [KLOH-triks].

**K-Lyte, K-Lyte/Cl, K-Lyte/Cl 50, K-Lyte DS** (Uro).   See *potassium.* [K-lite].

**Koate-DVI** (Hem).   See *factor VIII.* [KOH-ate D-V-I].

**Kogenate FS** (Hem).   See *factor VIII.* [KOH-jeh-nayt F-S].

**Kolum** (Uro).   See *potassium.* [KOH-lum].

**Kondremul Plain** (GI).   See *mineral oil.* [KAWN-dreh-mul].

**Konsyl, Konsyl-D** (GI).   See *psyllium.* [KAWN-sil].

**Konsyl Fiber** (GI).   See *polycarbophil.* [KAWN-sil FY-ber].

**K-Pek** (GI).   See *attapulgite.* [K-pek].

**K-Pek II** (GI).   See *loperamide.* [K-pek 2].

**K-Phos M.F., K-Phos Neutral, K-Phos No. 2** (Uro) (generic *potassium acid phosphate, sodium acid phosphate*).   Combination drug used to acidify the urine to prevent the formation of calcium kidney stones. Tablet: 155 mg/852 mg, 155 mg/350 mg, 305 mg/700 mg. [K-faws].

**K-Phos Original** (Uro).   See *potassium acid phosphate.* [K-faws].

**Kristalose** (GI).   See *lactulose.* [KRIS-tah-lohs].

**K-Tab** (Uro).   See *potassium.* [K-tab].

**kunecatechins** (Veregen) (Anti-infec, OB/GYN).   Antiviral drug used topically to treat condylomata acuminata (genital warts). Ointment: 15%. [KOO-nee-KAT-eh-chins].

**Kutrase** (GI) (generic *amylase, lipase, protease*).   Combination digestive enzyme drug used as replacement therapy. Capsule: 30,000 units/2400 units/30,000 units. [KOO-trays].

**Kuvan** (Misc).   See *sapropterin.* [KOO-van].

**Ku-Zyme, Ku-Zyme HP** (GI) (generic *amylase, lipase, protease*).   Combination digestive enzyme drug used as replacement therapy. Capsule: 15,000 units/1200 units/ 15,000 units, 30,000 units/8000 units/30,000 units. [KOO-zime].

**K-vescent** (Uro).   See *potassium.* [K-VES-sent].

**Kybernin P** (Hem).   See *antithrombin III.* [KY-ber-nin P].

**KY Plus** (OB/GYN).   See *nonoxynol-9.* [K-Y PLUS].

**Kytril** (Chemo, GI).   See *granisetron.* [KY-tril].

**labetalol** (Normodyne, Trandate) (Cardio, Endo).   Alpha-blocker and beta-blocker drug used to treat hypertension; used to treat hypertension caused by a pheochromocytoma of the adrenal gland. Tablet: 100 mg, 200 mg, 300 mg. Intravenous: 5 mg/mL. [lah-BAY-tah-lawl].

**Lacri-Lube NP, Lacri-Lube S.O.P.** (Ophth).   Lubricating ointment for dry eyes. Ophthalmic ointment. [LAK-rih-loob].

**Lacrisert** (Ophth).   Artificial tears used to treat dry eyes. Pellet (inserted in the conjunctival sac): 5 mg. [LAK-rih-sert].

**Lactaid Fast Act** (Misc).    See *lactase.* [LAK-tayd].

**lactase** (Dairy Ease, Lactaid Fast Act) (Misc).    Dietary enzyme supplement used when eating milk products. Capsule: 250 mg. Chewable tablet. [LAK-tays].

**lactated Ringer's** (LR) (I.V.).    Solution of dextrose, sodium, potassium, calcium, chloride, and lactate. Irrigating solution. Intravenous. [LAK-tay-ted RING-erz].

**lactic acid** (Aphthaid) (Anti-infec).    Used to treat aphthous stomatitis in AIDS patients. Orphan drug. [LAK-tic AS-id].

**LactiCare-HC** (Derm).    See *hydrocortisone.* [LAK-tih-kair-H-C].

**lactobin** (Anti-infec).    Used to treat diarrhea in AIDS patients. Orphan drug. [LAK-toh-bin].

**lactoferrin** (Hem).    Used to prevent graft-versus-host disease. Orphan drug. [LAK-toh-FAIR-rin].

**lactulose** (Cephulac, Cholac, Constulose, Enulose, Kristalose) (GI).    Osmotic laxative drug used to treat constipation; used to decrease blood ammonia in patients with liver disease and encephalopathy. Liquid: 10 g/15 mL. Crystals (to be reconstituted). [LAK-tyoo-lohs].

**Lamictal** (Neuro, Psych).    See *lamotrigine.* [lah-MIK-tawl].

**Lamisil, Lamisil AT** (Anti-infec).    See *terbinafine.* [LAM-ih-sil].

**lamivudine** (Epivir, Epivir-HBV) (Anti-infec, GI).    Nucleoside reverse transcriptase inhibitor antiviral drug used to treat HIV and AIDS; used to treat hepatitis B virus. Tablet: 100 mg, 150 mg, 300 mg. Oral liquid: 5 mg/mL, 10 mg/mL. [lah-MIV-yoo-deen].

**lamotrigine** (Lamictal) (Neuro, Psych).    Anticonvulsant drug used to treat complex partial and simple partial seizures; used to treat bipolar disorder; orphan drug used to treat Lennox-Gastaut syndrome. Chewable tablet: 2 mg, 5 mg, 25 mg. Tablet: 25 mg, 100 mg, 150 mg, 200 mg. [lah-MOH-trih-jeen].

**Lamprene** (Derm).    See *clofazimine.* [LAM-preen].

**Lanabiotic** (Derm) (generic *bacitracin, neomycin, polymyxin B, lidocaine*).    Combination over-the-counter antibiotic and anesthetic drug used topically on the skin. Ointment: 500 units/3.5 mg/10,000 units/40 mg per g. [LAN-ah-by-AW-tik].

**Lanacane** (Anes, Derm).    See *benzocaine.* [LAN-ah-kayn].

**Lanacort- 5 Creme, Lanacort-10 Creme** (Derm).    See *hydrocortisone.* [LAN-ah-kort].

**Lanophyllin** (Pulm).    See *theophylline.* [lan-AW-fih-lin].

**Lanoxicaps** (Cardio).    See *digoxin.* [lah-NAWK-see-kaps].

**Lanoxin** (Cardio).    See *digoxin.* [lan-AWK-sin].

**lanreotide** (Ipstyl, Somatuline Depot) (Endo).    Somatostatin-like hormone that decreases levels of growth hormone and insulin; used to treat acromegaly. Subcutaneous (prefilled syringe): 60 mg, 90 mg, 120 mg. [lan-REE-oh-tide]

**lansoprazole** (Prevacid, Prevacid I.V.) (GI).    Proton pump inhibitor drug used to treat heartburn, peptic ulcer, GERD, esophagitis, and *H. pylori* infection. Delayed-release capsule: 15 mg, 30 mg. Orally disintegrating tablet: 15 mg, 30 mg. Delayed-release tablet: 15 mg, 30 mg. Oral suspension granules: 15 mg. Intravenous: 30 mg/vial. [lan-SOH-prah-zohl].

**lantanoprost** (Xalatan) (Ophth).    Prostaglandin F receptor stimulator drug used topically to treat glaucoma. Ophthalmic solution: 0.005%. [lan-TAN-oh-prawst]

**lanthanum** (Fosrenol) (Uro).    Phosphate binder drug used to decrease blood levels of phosphate in patients with chronic kidney failure. Chewable tablet: 250 mg, 500 mg, 750 mg, 1000 mg. [LAN-thah-num].

**Lantus** (Endo).    See *insulin glargine.* [LAN-tus].

**lapatinib** (Tykerb) (Chemo).    Chemotherapy drug used to treat breast cancer. Tablet: 250 mg. [lah-PAT-ih-nib].

**Lariam** (Anti-infec).    See *mefloquine.* [LAIR-ee-am].

**laronidase** (Aldurazyme) (Misc).    Used to treat mucopolysaccharidosis. Intravenous: 2.9 mg/5 mL. [lah-RAWN-ih-days].

**Lasix** (Cardio, Uro).    See *furosemide.* [LAY-siks].

**L-asparaginase** (Chemo).    See *asparaginase.* [L-ah-SPAIR-ah-jih-nays].

**latanoprost** (Xalatan) (Ophth).    Prostaglandin F drug used topically in the eye to treat glaucoma. Ophthalmic solution: 0.005%. [lah-TAN-oh-prawst].

**L-baclofen** (Neuralgon) (Neuro, Ortho).    Skeletal muscle relaxant drug used to treat trigeminal neuralgia; used to treat severe muscle spasticity associated with multiple sclerosis, cerebral palsy, stroke, or spinal cord injury. Orphan drug. [L-BAK-loh-fen].

**Leena** (OB/GYN) (generic *norethindrone, ethinyl estradiol*).    Combination triphasic oral contraceptive drug. Pill pack, 28-day: (7 hormone tablets) 0.5 mg/35 mcg; (9 hormone tablets) 1 mg/35 mcg; (5 hormone tablets) 0.5 mg/35 mcg; (7 inert tablets). [LEE-nah].

**leflunomide** (Arava) (Cardio, GI, Ortho, Uro).    Immunomodulator drug used to treat rheumatoid arthritis; used to prevent rejection of a transplanted heart, liver, or kidney. Tablet: 10 mg, 20 mg. [leh-FLOO-noh-mide].

**Legatrin PM** (Neuro) (generic *acetaminophen, diphenhydramine*).    Combination over-the-counter analgesic and antihistamine drug used to relieve pain and induce sleep. Tablet: 500 mg/50 mg. [LEG-ah-trin P-M].

**lenalidomide** (Revlimid) (Chemo).    Immumodulator chemotherapy drug used to treat multiple myeloma and leukemia. Capsule: 5 mg, 10 mg, 15 mg, 25 mg. [LEN-ah-LID-oh-mide].

**lente insulin** (Lente Iletin II) (Endo).    Intermediate-acting insulin, derived from pig pancreas; used to treat type 1 diabetes mellitus. Subcutaneous: 100 units/mL. [LEN-tay IN-soo-lin].

**Lente Iletin II** (Endo).    See *lente insulin.* [LEN-tay EYE-leh-tin 2].

**lepirudin** (Refludan) (Hem).    Thrombin inhibitor anticoagulant drug used to treat heparin-induced thrombocytopenia. Intravenous (powder to be reconstituted): 50 mg. [leh-PEER-yoo-din].

**Lescol, Lescol XL** (Cardio). See *fluvastatin*. [LES-kawl].

**Lessina** (OB/GYN) (generic *levonorgestrel, ethinyl estradiol*). Combination monophasic oral contraceptive drug. Pill pack, 21-day: (21 hormone tablets) 0.1 mg/20 mcg. Pill pack, 28-day: (21 hormone tablets) 0.1 mg/20 mcg; (7 inert tablets). |leh-SEE-nah].

**lestaurtinib** (Chemo). Chemotherapy drug used to treat leukemia. Orphan drug. [les-TAR-tih-nib].

**Letairis** (Cardio). See *ambrisentan*. [leh-TAIR-is].

**letrozole** (Femara) (Chemo). Hormonal chemotherapy drug used to treat breast cancer. Tablet: 2.5 mg. [LEH-troh-zohl].

**Leucomax** (Anti-infec, Chemo, Hem). See *molgramostim*. [LOO-koh-maks].

**leucovorin** (Wellcovorin) (Chemo). Cytoprotective drug used to prevent toxicity in patients receiving methotrexate or fluorouracil chemotherapy. Tablet: 5 mg, 15 mg, 25 mg. Intravenous: 3 mg/mL, 10 mg/mL. [LOO-koh-VOR-in].

**Leukeran** (Chemo, Hem). See *chlorambucil*. [LOO-ker-an].

**Leukine** (Anti-infec, Chemo). See *sargramostim*. [LOO-keen].

**Leukotac** (Hem). See *inolimomab*. [LOO-koh-tak].

**leuprolide** (Eligard, Lupron, Lupron Depot, Lupron Depot-Ped, Lupron Depot-3 Months, Lupron Depot-4 Months, Lupron for Pediatric Use) (Chemo, Endo, OB/GYN). Hormonal chemotherapy drug used to treat cancer of the prostate gland, breast, and ovary; used to treat precocious puberty; used to treat endometrosis and uterine fibroids. Intramuscular or subcutaneous: 5 mg/mL. Microspheres for injection: 3.75 mg, 7.5 mg, 11.25 mg, 15 mg, 22.5 mg, 30 mg. [loo-PROH-lide].

**Leustatin** (Chemo). See *cladribine*. [loo-STAT-in].

**Leuvectin** (Chemo). Chemotherapy drug used to treat kidney cancer. Orphan drug. [loo-VEK-tin].

**levalbuterol** (Xopenex, Xopenex HFA) (Pulm). Bronchodilator drug used to prevent and treat asthma and bronchospasm. Nebulizer: 0.31 mg/3 mL, 0.63 mg/3 mL, 1.25 mg/3 mL. Aerosol: 45 mcg/puff. [LEE-val-BYOO-ter-awl].

**Levaquin** (Anti-infec). See *levofloxacin*. [LEV-ah-kwin].

**Levatol** (Cardio). See *penbutolol*. [LEE-vah-tawl].

**Levbid** (GI, Uro). See *L-hyoscyamine*. [LEV-bid].

**Levemir** (Endo). See *insulin detemir*. [LEV-eh-meer].

**levetiracetam** (Keppra) (Analges, Neuro, Psych). Anticonsultant drug used to treat simple partial seizures and myoclonic seizures; used to treat migraine headaches; used to treat bipolar disorder. Tablet: 250 mg, 500 mg, 750 mg, 1000 mg. Liquid: 100 mg/mL. Intravenous: 100 mg/mL. [LEE-veh-ty-RAY-seh-tam].

**Levitra** (Uro). See *vardenafil*. [leh-VEE-trah].

**Levlen** (OB/GYN) (generic *levonorgestrel, ethinyl estradiol*). Combination monophasic oral contraceptive drug. Pill pack, 21-day: (21 hormone tablets) 0.15 mg/30 mcg. Pill pack, 28-day: (21 hormone tablets) 0.15 mg/30 mcg; (7 inert tablets). [LEV-len].

**Levlite** (OB/GYN) (generic *levonorgestrel, ethinyl estradiol*). Combination monophasic oral contraceptive drug. Pill pack, 28-day: (21 hormone tablets) 0.1 mg/20 mcg; (7 inert tablets). [LEV-lite].

**levobetaxolol** (Betaxon) (Ophth). Beta-blocker drug used topically in the eye to treat glaucoma. Ophthalmic suspension: 0.5%. [LEE-voh beh-TAKS-oh-lawl].

**levobunolol** (Betagan Liquifilm) (Ophth). Beta-blocker drug used topically in the eye to treat glaucoma. Ophthalmic solution: 0.25%, 0.5%. [LEE-voh-BUN-oh-lawl].

**levocabastine** (Ophth). Used to treat keratoconjunctivitis. Ophthalmic suspension: 0.05%. [LEE-voh-KAB-ah-steen].

**levocarnitine** (Carnitor) (Anti-infec). Used to protect against toxicity in patients receiving zidovudine for AIDS. Orphan drug. [LEE-voh-KAR-nih-teen].

**levocetirizine** (Xyzal) (Derm, ENT). Antihistamine drug used to treat severe hives and urticaria; used to treat allergic rhinitis. Tablet: 5 mg. Oral liquid: 0.5 mg/mL. [LEE-voh-seh-TY-rah-zeen].

**Levo-Dromoran** (Analges, Anes). See *levorphanol*. [LEE-voh-DROH-mor-an].

**levofloxacin** (Levaquin, Quixin) (Anti-infec, Ophth). Fluoroquinolone antibiotic drug used to treat gram-negative and gram-positive bacterial infections; used to treat sinusitis, bronchitis, and pneumonia due to *S. pneumoniae* and *H. influenzae;* used to treat Legionnaire's disease of the lungs; used to treat staphylococcal and streptococcal skin infections; used to treat gonorrhea and nongonococcal urethritis; used to treat pelvic inflammatory disease and prostatitis; used to treat urinary tract infection due to *E. coli;* used topically to treat bacterial infection of the eyes (Quixin). Tablet: 250 mg, 500 mg, 750 mg. Oral liquid: 25 mg/mL. Intravenous: 250 mg/ 50 mL, 500 mg/ 20 mL, 500 mg/200 mL, 750 mg/150 mL. Ophthalmic solution: 0.5% (5 mg/mL). [LEE-voh-FLAWK-sah-sin].

**levoleucovorin** (Fusilev) (Chemo). Cytoprotective drug used to prevent toxicity in patients receiving methotrexate chemotherapy. Intravenous: 7.5 mg. [LEE-voh-LOO-koh-VOH-rin].

**levomethadyl** (ORLAAM) (Analges). Schedule II narcotic drug used to manage heroin and narcotic dependence and withdrawal. Orphan drug. Liquid: 10 mg/mL. [LEE-voh-METH-ah-dil].

**levonorgestrel** (Mirena, Plan B) (OB/GYN). Progestin hormone contraceptive drug used to prevent pregnancy (Mirena); used to prevent pregnancy after unprotected sexual intercourse (Plan B). Tablet: 0.75 mg. Intrauterine T-shaped implant (effective for 5 years): 52 mg. [LEE-voh-nor-JES-trel].

**Levophed** (Emerg). See *norepinephrine*. [LEE-voh-fed].

**Levora 0.15/30** (OB/GYN) (generic *levonorgestrel, ethinyl estradiol*). Combination monophasic oral contraceptive drug. Pill pack, 28-day: (21 hormone tablets) 0.15 mg/ 30 mcg; (7 inert tablets). [leh-VOR-ah].

**levorphanol** (Levo-Dromoran) (Analges, Anes).    Schedule II narcotic drug used to treat moderate-to-severe pain; used preoperatively to relieve pain and produce sedation. Tablet: 2 mg. Subcutaneous, intramuscular, intravenous: 2 mg/mL. [leh-VOR-fah-nawl].

**Levothroid** (Endo).    See *levothyroxine*. [LEE-voh-throyd].

**levothyroxine** (Levothroid, Levoxyl, Synthroid, Thyro-Tabs, Unithroid) (Endo).    Thyroid hormone $T_4$ replacement drug used to treat hypothyroidism; used to suppress pituitary gland secretion of TSH in Hashimoto's thyroiditis and thyroid cancer. Tablet: 0.025 mg, 0.05 mg, 0.075 mg, 0.088 mg, 0.1 mg, 0.112 mg, 0.125 mg, 0.137 mg, 0.15 mg, 0.175 mg, 0.2 mg, 0.3 mg. Intravenous (powder to be reconstituted): 200 mcg/10 mL, 500 mcg/10 mL. [LEE-voh-thy-RAWK-zeen].

**Levoxyl** (Endo).    See *levothyroxine*. [lee-VAWK-sil].

**Levsin, Levsin Drops, Levsin/SL** (GI, Uro).    See *L-hyoscyamine*. [LEV-sin].

**Levsinex Timecaps** (GI, Uro).    See *L-hyoscyamine*. [LEV-sih-neks].

**Levulan Kerastick** (Derm).    See *aminolevulinic acid*. [LEV-yoo-lan KAIR-ah-stik].

**Lexapro** (Psych).    See *escitalopram*. [LEK-sah-proh].

**Lexiscan** (Cardio).    See *regadenoson*. [LEK-sih-skan].

**Lexiva** (Anti-infec).    See *fosamprenavir*. [LEK-sih-vah].

**L-glutamine** (Hem).    Used to treat sickle cell disease. Orphan drug. [L-GLOO-tah-meen].

**L-hyoscyamine** (Anaspaz, Cystospaz, ED-SPAZ, IB-Stat, Levbid, Levsin, Levsin/SL, Levsin Drops, Levsinex Timecaps, Mar-Spas, Neosol, NuLev, Symax Duotab, Symax FasTab, Symax-SL, Symax-SR) (GI, Neuro, Uro).    Anticholinergic antispasmodic drug used to treat spasm of the smooth muscle of the stomach, intestines, and bladder; used in Parkinson's disease to decrease tremors and rigidity. Capsule: 0.375 mg. Timed-released capsule: 0.375 mg. Elixir: 0.125 mg/5 mL. Oral liquid: 0.125 mg/mL. Oral spray: 0.125 mg/mL (per spray). Tablet: 0.125 mg, 0.15 mg. Extended-release tablet: 0.375 mg. Orally disintegrating tablet: 0.125 mg, 0.25 mg. Sublingual tablet: 0.125 mg. Sustained-release tablet: 0.375 mg. Intravenous: 0.5 mg/mL. [L-HY-oh-SY-ah-meen].

**Lialda** (GI).    See *mesalamine*. [ly-AL-dah].

**Librax** (GI, Psych) (generic *chlordiazepoxide, clidinium*).    Combination antianxiety and antispasmodic drug used to treat stomach ulcers and irritable bowel syndrome. Capsule: 5 mg/2.5 mg. [LIB-raks].

**Librium** (Anes, GI, Psych).    See *chlordiazepoxide*. [LIB-ree-um].

**LidaMantle** (Anes, Derm, GI).    See *lidocaine*. [LY-dah-MAN-tal].

**Lidex, Lidex-E** (Derm).    See *fluocinonide*. [LY-deks].

**lidocaine** (Anestacon, Anestafoam, Dentipatch, Dermaflex, Dr. Scholl's Cracked Heel Relief, LidaMantle, Lidoderm Patch, LidoSite Topical System, Medi-Quik, Numby Stuff, Octocaine, Solarcaine Aloe Extra Burn Relief, TheraPatch Cold Sore, Unguentine Plus, Xylocaine, Xylocaine MPF, Xylocaine Viscous, Zilactin-L, Zingo) (Analges, Anes, Cardio, Derm, ENT, GI, Neuro, OB/GYN, Ortho, Uro).    Over-the-counter and prescription anesthetic drug used topically on the skin to treat the pain of herpes zoster lesions (shingles) and postherpetic neuralgia; used to treat the pain of abrasions, burns, cold sores, and sunburn, and eczema; used to numb the mucous membranes of the nose, mouth, and throat; used during endotracheal intubation; used to treat the pain of hemorrhoids; used during procedures on the urethra; used intranasally to treat migraine headaches; injected for local, regional, or spinal anesthesia; used for epidural anesthesia during labor and vaginal delivery or cesarean section; used to treat fibromyalgia with trigger point injections; used to treat cardiac arrhythmias. Cream: 0.5%, 3%, 4%. Foam: 4%. Gel: 0.5%, 2.5%. Jelly: 2%. Topical liquid: 2%, 2.5%, 4%. Lotion: 3%. Ointment: 5%. Patch: 4%, 5%, 10%, 10 x 14 cm, 23 mg/2 cm$^2$, 46.1 mg/2 cm$^2$ (patch can be cut into smaller pieces). Spray: 0.5%. Oral liquid: 2.5%. Viscous (thickened) solution: 2%. Powder intradermal injection: 0.5 mg/actuation. Intramuscular or intravenous: 0.5%, 0.5% with 1:200,000 epinephrine, 1%, 1% with 1:100,000 epinephrine, 1% with 1:200,000 epinephrine, 1.5%, 1.5% with 1:200,000 epinephrine, 2%, 2% with 1:50,000 epinephrine, 2% with 1:100,000 epinephrine, 2% with 1:200,000 epinephrine, 4%. [LY-doh-kayn].

**Lidoderm Patch** (Derm, Neuro).    See *lidocaine*. [LY-doh-derm].

**LidoSite Topical System** (Derm, Neuro).    See *lidocaine*. [LY-doh-site].

**Limbitrol, Limbitrol DS** (Psych) (generic *amitriptyline, chlordiazepoxide*).    Combination Schedule IV antidepressant and benzodiazepine antianxiety drug. Tablet: 12.5 mg/5 mg, 25 mg/10 mg. [LIM-bih-trawl].

**Lincocin** (Anti-infec).    See *lincomycin*. [LIN-koh-sin].

**lincomycin** (Lincocin) (Anti-infec).    Antibiotic drug used to treat serious gram-positive staphylococcal or streptococcal infections in patients who are allergic to penicillin; used to treat infections due to anaerobic bacteria. Capsule: 500 mg. Intravenous: 300 mg/2 mL. [LIN-koh-MY-sin].

**lindane** (Derm).    Scabicide and pediculocide drug used topically on the skin and hair to treat parasitic infection from scabies (mites) or pediculosis (lice). Lotion: 1%. Shampoo: 1%. [lin-DAYN].

**linezolid** (Zyvox) (Anti-infec).    Antibiotic drug used to treat gram-positive staphylococcal and streptococcal skin infections and pneumonia; used to treat methicillin-resistant staphylococcal pneumonia; used to treat vancomycin-resistant enterococcal infection. Tablet: 400 mg, 600 mg.

Intravenous (powder to be reconstituted): 100 mg/5 mL. [lih-NEZ-oh-lid].

**Linomide** (Chemo). See *roquinimex.* [LIN-oh-mide].

**lintuzumab** (Zamyl) (Chemo). Monoclonal antibody drug used to treat leukemia. Orphan drug. [lin-TOOZ-yoo-mab].

**Lioresal, Lioresal Intrathecal** (GI, Neuro, Ortho). See *baclofen.* [ly-OR-ch-sal].

**liothyronine** (Cytomel, Triostat) (Endo). Thyroid hormone $T_3$ replacement drug used to treat hypothyroidism; used to suppress pituitary gland TSH in Hashimoto's thyroiditis; orphan drug used to treat myxedema coma. Tablet: 5 mcg, 25 mcg, 50 mcg. Intravenous: 10 mcg/mL. [LY-oh-THY-roh-neen].

**liotrix** (Thyrolar) (Endo). Thyroid hormones $T_3$ and $T_4$ replacement drug used to treat hypothyroidism; used to suppress pituitary gland secretion of TSH in Hashimoto's thyroiditis and thyroid cancer. Tablet: 15 mg (¼ grain), 30 mg (½ grain), 60 mg (1 grain), 120 mg (2 grains), 180 mg (3 grains). [LY-oh-triks].

**lipids** (I.V.). See *intravenous lipids.* [LIP-ids].

**Lipisorb** (GI). Lactose-free nutritional supplement with MCT oil. Powder (to be reconstituted). [LIP-ih-sorb].

**Lipitor** (Cardio). See *atorvastatin.* [LIP-ih-tor].

**Lipofen** (Cardio). See *fenofibrate.* [LIH-poh-fen].

**Lipo-Niacin** (Cardio) (generic *niacin, vitamin B*). Combination vitamin B drug used to lower serum cholesterol and triglyceride levels. Tablet. [LIH-poh-NY-ah-sin].

**Lipo-PGE 1** (Cardio, Derm). Used to treat skin ulcers in patients with peripheral arterial disease. Orphan drug. [LIH-poh-P-G-E-1].

**liposomal ciprofloxacin** (Anti-infec, Pulm). Used to treat cystic fibrosis. Orphan drug. [LIH-poh-SOH-mal SIH-proh-FLAWK-sah-sin].

**liposomal cyclosporin A** (Cyclospire) (Hem). Used to treat bone marrow rejection. Orphan drug. [LIH-poh-SOH-mal SY-kloh-SPOR-in A].

**Liposyn II 10%, Liposyn II 20%, Liposyn III 10%, Liposyn III 20%, Liposyn III 30%** (I.V.). See *intravenous lipids.* [LIH-poh-sin].

**Lipram 4500, Lipram-PN10, Lipram-PN16, Lipram-PN20, Lipram-UL12, Lipram-UL18, Lipram-UL20** (GI) (generic *amylase, lipase, protease*). Combination digestive enzyme drug used as replacement therapy. Delayed-release capsule: 20,000 units/4500 units/25,000 units; 30,000 units/10,000 units/30,000 units; 39,000 units/ 12,000 units/39,000 units; 48,000 units/16,000 units/ 48,000 units; 58,500 units/18,000 units/58,500 units; 56,000 units/20,000 units/44,000 units; 65,000 units/ 20,000 units/65,000 units. [LIH-pram].

**Liquadd** (Psych). See *dextroamphetamine.* [LIH-kwih-add].

**Liquibid** (Pulm). See *guaifenesin.* [LIH-kwih-bid].

**Liquicet** (Analges) (generic *acetaminophen, hydrocodone*). Combination Schedule III nonnarcotic and narcotic analgesic drug for pain. Oral liquid: 500 mg/10 mg. [LIH-kwih-set].

**Liqui-Char** (Emerg, GI). See *activated charcoal.* [LIH-kwih-char].

**Liquid Pred** (Endo). See *prednisone.* [LIH-kwih PRED].

**Liquifilm Tears** (Ophth). Over-the-counter artificial tears for dry eyes. Ophthalmic solution. [LIH-kwih-film].

**LiquiVent** (Pulm). See *perflubron.* [LIH-kwih-vent].

**lisdexamfetamine** (Vyvanse) (Psych). Schedule II amphetamine stimulant drug used to treat attention-deficit/ hyperactivity disorder in children and adults. Capsule: 20 mg, 40 mg, 30 mg, 50 mg, 60 mg, 70 mg. [LIS-deks-am-FET-ah-meen].

**lisinopril** (Prinivil, Zestril) (Cardio). ACE inhibitor drug used to treat congestive heart failure and hypertension; used to improve survival rate after myocardial infarction. Tablet: 2.5 mg, 5 mg, 10 mg, 20 mg, 30 mg, 40 mg. [ly-SIN-oh-pril].

**lithium** (Lithobid) (Anti-infec, Chemo, Endo, Neuro, Psych). Antipsychotic drug used to treat the mania of manic-depressive disorder; used to treat bulimia and withdrawal from alcohol; used to treat postpartum psychosis and psychosis from corticosteroid drugs; used to treat tardive dyskinesia (side effect of antipsychotic drugs); used to prevent cluster headaches; used to treat SIADH; used to increase the neutrophil count in AIDS patients and patients receiving chemotherapy. Capsule: 150 mg, 300 mg, 600 mg. Tablet: 300 mg. Extended-release tablet: 300 mg, 450 mg. Syrup: 8 mEq/5 mL (300 mg/5 mL). [LITH-ee-um].

**Lithobid** (Anti-infec, Chemo, Endo, Psych). See *lithium.* [LITH-oh-bid].

**Lithostat** (Uro). See *acetohydroxamic acid.* [LITH-oh-stat].

**L-leucovorin** (Isovorin) (Chemo). Cytoprotective drug used to prevent toxicity in patients receiving fluorouracil or methotrexate chemotherapy. Orphan drug. [L-LOO-koh-VOR-in].

**Lobac** (Ortho) (generic *acetaminophen, salicylamide, phenyltoloxamine*). Combination analgesic, salicylate analgesic, and antihistamine drug used to treat pain, spasm, and stiffness associated with minor muscle injuries. Capsule: 300 mg/200 mg/20 mg. [LOH-bak].

**Locoid, Locoid Lipocream** (Derm). See *hydrocortisone.* [LOH-koyd].

**lodoxamide** (Alomide) (Ophth). Mast cell stabilizer drug used topically in the eyes to treat allergy symptoms. Ophthalmic solution: 0.1%. [loh-DAWK-sah-mide].

**Lodrane 24, Lodrane XR** (Derm, ENT). See *brompheniramine.* [LOH-drayn].

**Loestrin 21 1/20, Loestrin 1.5/30** (OB/GYN) (generic *norethindrone, ethinyl estradiol*). Combination monophasic oral contraceptive drug. Pill pack, 21-day: (21 hormone tablets): 1 mg/20 mcg. Pill pack, 28-day: (21 hormone tablets) 1.5 mg/30 mcg; (7 inert tablets). [loh-ES-trin].

**Loestrin 24 Fe** /GYN) (generic *norethindrone, ethinyl estradiol; ferrous fumarate*). Combination monophasic oral contraceptive drug with iron supplement. Pill pack, 28-day: (24 hormone tablets) 1 mg/20 mcg; (7 iron [Fe] tablets). [loh-ES-trin].

**Loestrin Fe 1/20, Loestrin Fe 1.5/30** (OB/GYN) (generic *norethindrone, ethinyl estradiol; ferrous fumarate*). Combination monophasic oral contraceptive drug with iron supplement. Pill pack, 28-day: (21 hormone tablets) 1 mg/20 mcg; (7 iron [Fe] tablets) 75 mg. Pill pack, 28-day: (21 hormone tablets) 1.5 mg/30 mcg, (7 iron [Fe] tablets) 75 mg. [loh-ES-trin].

**Lofibra** (Cardio).   See *fenofibrate*. [loh-FY-brah].

**Logen** (GI) (generic *atropine, diphenoxylate*).   Combination Schedule IV anticholinergic and narcotic drug used to decrease GI peristalsis and spasm; used to treat diarrhea. Tablet: 0.025 mg/2.5 mg. [LOH-jen].

**LoHist 12 Hour** (Derm, ENT).   See *brompheniramine*. [LOH-hist].

**LoKara** (Derm).   See *desonide*. [loh-KAIR-ah].

**Lomanate** (GI) (generic *atropine, diphenoxylate*). Combination Schedule IV anticholinergic and narcotic drug used to decrease GI peristalsis and spasm; used to treat diarrhea. Tablet: 0.025 mg/2.5 mg. [LOH-mah-nayt].

**lomefloxacin** (Maxaquin) (Anti-infec).   Fluoroquinolone antibiotic drug used to treat gram-negative and gram-positive bacterial infections; used to treat bronchitis and Legionnaire's disease of the lungs; used to treat urinary infections caused by *E. coli;* used to prevent infection after urethral or prostate surgery. Tablet: 400 mg. [LOH-mee-FLAWK-sah-sin].

**Lomotil** (GI) (generic *atropine, diphenoxylate*). Combination Schedule IV anticholinergic and narcotic drug used to decrease GI peristalsis and spasm; used to treat diarrhea. Tablet: 0.025 mg/2.5 mg. [loh-MOH-til].

**lomustine** (CeeNU) (Chemo).   Alkylating chemotherapy drug used to treat brain cancer and Hodgkin's lymphoma. Capsule: 10 mg, 40 mg, 100 mg. Dose pack: 100 mg (2 capsules), 40 mg (2 capsules), 10 mg (2 capsules). [loh-MUS-teen].

**Lonox** (GI) (generic *atropine, diphenoxylate*).   Combination Schedule IV anticholinergic and narcotic drug used to decrease GI peristalsis and spasm; used to treat diarrhea. Tablet: 0.025 mg/2.5 mg. [LOH-nawks].

**Lo/Ovral** (OB/GYN) (generic *norgestrel, ethinyl estradiol*). Combination monophasic oral contraceptive drug. Pill pack (Pilpak), 21-day: (21 hormone tablets) 0.3 mg/30 mcg. Pill pack (Pilpak), 28-day: (21 hormone tablets) 0.3 mg/30 mcg; (7 inert tablets). [loh-OV-rawl].

**loperamide** (Imodium A-D, K-Pek II) (GI).   Over-the-counter drug used to treat diarrhea. Capsule: 2 mg. Liquid: 1 mg/ 5 mL, 1 mg/7.5 mL.Tablet: 2 mg. [loh-PAIR-ah-mide].

**Lopid** (Cardio).   See *gemfibrozil*. [LOH-pid].

**Lopressor** (Analges, Cardio, GI).   See *metoprolol*. [loh-PRES-sor].

**Lopressor HCT 50/25, Lopressor HCT 100/25, Lopressor HCT 100/50** (Cardio) (generic *metoprolol, hydrochlorothiazide*).   Combination beta-blocker and diuretic drug used to treat hypertension. Tablet: 50 mg/25 mg, 100 mg/25 mg, 100 mg/50 mg. [loh-PRES-sor].

**Loprox** (Derm).   See *ciclopirox*. [LOH-prawks].

**loratadine** (Alavert, Alavert Children's, Claritin, Claritin Children's Allergy, Claritin Hives Relief, Claritin Reditabs, Claritin 24-Hour Allergy, Dimetapp Children's ND Non-Drowsy Allergy, Tavist ND, Triaminic Allerchews) (Derm, ENT).   Over-the-counter antihistamine drug used to treat allergic rhinitis and allergic skin reactions with itching. Tablet: 10 mg. Chewable tablet: 5 mg. Orally disintegrating tablet: 5 mg, 10 mg. Syrup: 5 mg/5 mL. Tablet: 10 mg. [lor-AH-tah-deen].

**lorazepam** (Ativan) (Anes, GI, Neuro, Psych).   Schedule IV benzodiazepine drug used to treat anxiety; used to treat status epilepticus; used as a preoperative drug for sedation; used to treat irritable bowel syndrome. Tablet: 0.5 mg, 1 mg, 2 mg. Liquid: 2 mg/mL. Intramuscular or intravenous: 2 mg/mL, 4 mg/mL. [lor-AZ-eh-pam].

**Lorcet, Lorcet-HD, Lorcet Plus** (Analges) (generic *acetaminophen, hydrocodone*).   Combination Schedule III nonsalicylate and narcotic analgesic drug for pain. Capsule: 500 mg/5 mg. Tablet: 650 mg/7.5 mg, 650 mg/10 mg. [LOR-set].

**Lortab** (Analges) (generic *acetaminophen, hydrocodone*). Combination Schedule III nonsalicylate and narcotic analgesic drug for pain. Oral liquid: 167 mg/2.5 mg. Tablet: 500 mg/2.5 mg, 500 mg/5 mg, 500 mg/7.5 mg, 500 mg/10 mg. [LOR-tab].

**Lortab ASA** (Analges) (generic *aspirin, hydrocodone*). Combination Schedule III salicylate and narcotic analgesic drug for pain. Tablet: 500 mg/5 mg. [LOR-tab].

**losartan** (Cozaar) (Cardio).   Angiotensin II receptor blocker drug used to treat hypertension; used to decrease the risk of stroke in patients with hypertension and left-sided heart failure. Tablet: 25 mg, 50 mg, 100 mg. [loh-SAR-tan].

**Lotemax** (Ophth).   See *loteprednol*. [LOH-teh-maks].

**Lotensin** (Cardio, Neuro).   See *benazepril*. [loh-TEN-sin].

**Lotensin HCT** (Cardio) (generic *benazepril, hydrochlorothiazide*).   Combination ACE inhibitor and diuretic drug used to treat hypertension. Tablet: 5 mg/ 6.25 mg, 10 mg/12.5 mg, 20 mg/12.5 mg, 20 mg/25 mg. [loh-TEN-sin H-C-T].

**loteprednol** (Alrex, Lotemax) (Ophth).   Corticosteroid drug used topically in the eyes to treat inflammation from infection or allergy. Ophthalmic suspension: 0.2%, 0.5%. [LOH-teh-PRED-nawl].

**Lotrel** (Cardio) (generic *amlodipine, benazepril*). Combination calcium channel blocker and ACE inhibitor drug used to treat hypertension. Capsule: 2.5 mg/10 mg, 5 mg/10 mg, 5 mg/20 mg, 5 mg/40 mg, 10 mg/20 mg, 10 mg/40 mg. [LOH-trel].

**Lotrenex** (GI).   See *alosetron*. [LOH-treh-neks].

**Lotrimin AF 1%** (Derm). See *clotrimazole*. [LOH-trih-min A-F 1%].

**Lotrimin AF 2%** (Derm). See *miconazole*. [LOH-trih-min A-F 2%].

**Lotrimin Ultra** (Derm). See *butenafine*. [LOH-trih-min UL-trah].

**Lotrisone** (Derm) (generic *betamethasone, clotrimazole*). Combination corticosteroid and antifungal drug used topically to treat inflammation and fungal infections of the skin. Lotion: 0.05%/1%. [LOH-trih-sohn].

**lovastatin** (Altoprev, Mevacor) (Cardio). HMG-CoA reductase inhibitor drug used to treat hypercholesterolemia and arteriosclerosis. Tablet: 10 mg, 20 mg, 40 mg. Extended-release tablet: 10 mg, 20 mg, 40 mg, 60 mg. [LOH-vah-STAT-in].

**Lovenox** (Cardio, Hem). See *enoxaparin*. [LUV-eh-nawks].

**Low-Ogestrel** (OB/GYN) (generic *norgestrel, ethinyl estradiol*). Combination monophasic oral contraceptive drug. Pill pack (Pilpak), 28-day: (21 hormone tablets) 0.3 mg/30 mcg; (7 inert tablets). [LOH-oh-JES-trel].

**loxapine** (Loxitane) (Psych). Dibenzapine antipsychotic drug used to treat schizophrenia. Capsule: 5 mg, 10 mg, 25 mg, 50 mg. [LAWK-sah-peen].

**Loxitane** (Psych). See *loxapine*. [LAWK-sih-tayn].

**Lozol** (Cardio, Uro). See *indapamide*. [LOH-zawl].

**L-threonin** (Threostat) (Neuro). Used to treat spasticity associated with amyotrophic lateral sclerosis. Orphan drug. [L-THREE-oh-nin].

**lubiprostone** (Amitiza) (GI). Chloride channel stimulator drug that increases fluid secretion in the intestines; used to treat chronic constipation and irritable bowel syndrome with constipation. Capsule: 8 mcg, 24 mcg. [LOO-bih-PRAWS-tohn].

**lucinactant** (Surfaxin) (Pulm). Used to treat meconium aspiration and respiratory distress syndrome in newborns. Orphan drug. [LOO-sih-NAK-tant].

**Lucentis** (Ophth). See *ranibizumab*. [loo-SEN-tis].

**Lufyllin** (Pulm). See *dyphylline*. [loo-FIL-in].

**Lufyllin-EPG** (Pulm) (generic *dyphylline, ephedrine, guaifenesin, phenobarbital*). Combination bronchodilator, expectorant, and barbiturate sedative drug. Elixir: 150 mg/24 mg/300 mg/24 mg. Tablet: 100 mg/16 mg/200 mg/16 mg. [loo-FIL-in-E-P-G].

**Lufyllin-GG** (Pulm) (generic *dyphylline, guaifenesin*). Combination bronchodilator and expectorant drug. Elixir liquid: 100 mg/100 mg. Tablet: 200 mg/200 mg. [loo-FIL-in-G-G].

**Lugol's solution** (Derm, Endo). See *iodine*. [LOO-gawlz soh LOO-shun].

**Lumigan** (Ophth). See *bimatoprost*. [LOO-mih-gan].

**Luminal** (Neuro). See *phenobarbital*. [LOO-mih-nawl].

**Lunesta** (Neuro). See *eszopiclone*. [loo-NES-tah].

**Lupron, Lupron Depot, Lupron Depot-Ped, Lupron Depot-3 Months, Lupron Depot-4 Months, Lupron for Pediatric Use** (Chemo, Endo, OB/GYN). See *leuprolide*. [LOO-prawn].

**Lustra, Lustra-AF** (Derm). See *hydroquinone*. [LUS-trah].

**Lutera** (OB/GYN) (generic *levonorgestrel, ethinyl estradiol*). Combination monophasic oral contraceptive drug. Pill pack, 28-day: (21 hormone tablets) 0.1 mg/20 mcg; (7 inert tablets). [loo-TAIR-ah].

**Lutrepulse** (OB/GYN). See *gonadorelin*. [LOO-treh-puls].

**lutropin alfa** (Luveris) (Endo, OB/GYN). Ovulation-stimulating drug used to stimulate ovulation in women with infertility. Subcutaneous (powder to be reconstituted): 82.5 units/vial. [loo-TROH-pin AL-fah].

**Luveris** (Endo, OB/GYN). See *lutropin alfa*. [loo-VAIR-is].

**Luvox** (Psych). See *fluvoxamine*. [LOO-vawks].

**Luxiq** (Derm). See *betamethasone*. [LUK-seek].

**Luxor CR** (Psych). See *fluvoxamine*. [LUK-sor].

**Lybrel** (OB/GYN) (generic *levonorgestrel, ethinyl estradiol*). Combination monophasic oral contraceptive drug that also eliminates monthly menstruation. Pill pack, 28-day: (28 hormone tablets) 0.09 mg/20 mcg. [LY-brel].

**LymphoCIDE** (Chemo). See *epratuzumab*. [LIM-foh-side].

**lymphocyte immune globulin** (Atgam) (Misc). Immunoglobulin drug used to treat rejection of a donor kidney after kidney transplantation; used to treat aplastic anemia. [LIM-foh-site im-MYOON GLAW-byoo-lin].

**Lyrica** (Derm, Endo, Neuro, Ortho). See *pregabalin*. [LEER-ih-kah].

**Lysodase** (Misc). Enzyme replacement drug used to treat Gaucher's disease. Orphan drug. [LY-soh-days].

**Lysodren** (Chemo, Endo). See *mitotane*. [LY-soh-dren].

**Maalox Antacid Barrier Maximum Strength** (GI). See *calcium carbonate*. [MAY-lawks].

**Maalox Extra Strength with Gas-X, Maalox Max Maximum Strength** (GI) (generic *calcium, simethicone*). Combination antacid and anti-gas drug used to treat heartburn and gas. Tablet: 500 mg/125 mg, 1000 mg/60 mg. [MAY-lawks].

**Maalox Regular Strength** (GI) (generic *aluminum, magnesium, simethicone*). Combination antacid and anti-gas drug used to treat heartburn and gas. Liquid: 200 mg/200 mg/20 mg. [MAY-lawks].

**Maalox Total Stomach Relief** (GI). See *bismuth*. [MAY-lawks].

**Macrobid** (Anti-infec, Uro). See *nitrofurantoin*. [MAK-roh-bid].

**Macrodantin** (Anti-infec, Uro). See *nitrofurantoin*. [MAK-roh-DAN-tin].

**Macrodex** (I.V.). See *dextran 70*. [MAK-roh-deks].

**Macugen** (Ophth). See *pegaptanib*. [MAK-yoo-jen].

**mafenide** (Sulfamylon) (Derm). Anti-infective drug used topically to treat severe burns. Cream. Liquid. [MAF-eh-nide].

**mafosfamide** (Chemo).    Used to treat cancerous meningitis. Orphan drug. [mah-FAWS-foh-mide].

**magnesium salicylate** (Doan's, Doan's Extra Strength, Novasal) (Analges).    Salicylate analgesic drug used to treat pain and inflammation of osteoarthritis and minor muscle injuries. Tablet: 377 mg, 404 mg, 580 mg, 600 mg. [mag-NEE-see-um sah-LIH-sih-layt].

**magnesium sulfate** (Neuro, OB/GYN, Uro).    Used to prevent seizures in pregnant women with preeclampsia; used to treat nephritis; used to treat preterm labor. Intramuscular or intravenous: 50% (4 mEq/mL). [mag-NEE-see-um SUL-fayt].

**Maitec** (Anti-infec).    See *gentamicin liposomal.* [MY-tek].

**Malarone** (Anti-infec) (generic *atrovaquone, proguanil*).    Combination anti-infective drug used to prevent and treat malaria. Tablet: 62.5 mg/25 mg, 250 mg/ 100 mg. [MAL-ah-rohn].

**malathion** (Ovide) (Derm).    Pediculocide drug used topically on the skin to treat parasitic infection from pediculosis (lice). Lotion: 0.5%. [MAL-ah-THY-awn].

**mannitol** (Bronchitol, Osmitrol, Resectisol) (Neuro, Ophth, Pulm, Uro).    Osmotic diuretic drug used to treat renal failure; used to decrease cerebral edema; used to decrease intraocular pressure and treat glaucoma; irrigating solution used during urologic surgery (Resectisol); orphan drug used to clear mucus in patients with cystic fibrosis (Bronchitol). Intravenous: 5%, 10%, 15%, 20%, 25%. Irrigating solution: 5 g/100 mL. [MAN-ih-tawl].

**manuka honey** (Medihoney) (Derm).    Absorbent dressing impregnated with honey and applied topically to the skin. Sterile dressing. [mah-NOO-kah HUN-ee].

**maprotiline** (Psych).    Tetracyclic antidepressant drug used to treat depression; used to treat manic-depressive disorder. Tablet: 25 mg, 50 mg, 75 mg. [mah-PROH-tih-leen].

**maraviroc** (Selzentry) (Anti-infec).    Antiviral drug used to treat a specific strain of HIV. Tablet: 150 mg, 300 mg. [MAIR-ah-VY-rawk].

**Marax** (Pulm) (generic *theophylline, ephedrine, hydroxyzine*).    Combination bronchodilator and antihistamine drug. Tablet: 130 mg/25 mg/10 mg. [MAIR-aks].

**Marax-DF** (Pulm) (generic *theophylline, ephedrine, hydroxyzine*).    Combination bronchodilator and antihistamine drug. Pediatric syrup: 97.5 mg/18.75 mg/7.5 mg. [MAIR-aks-D-F].

**Marcaine** (Anes, ENT, OB/GYN).    See *bupivacaine.* [MAR-kayn].

**Marezine** (GI).    See *cyclizine.* [MAIR-eh-zeen].

**Margesic** (Analges) (generic *acetaminophen, butalbital, caffeine*).    Combination nonsalicylate analgesic, barbiturate sedative, and stimulant drug for pain. Capsule: 325 mg/50 mg/40 mg. [mar-JEE-sik].

**Margesic H** (Analges) (generic *acetaminophen, hydrocodone*).    Combination Schedule III nonnarcotic and narcotic analgesic drug for pain. Capsule: 500 mg/5 mg. [mar-JEE-sik H].

**marijuana** (Chemo).    See *dronabinol.* [MAIR-ih-WAH-nah].

**Marinol** (Anti-infec, Chemo, GI).    See *dronabinol.* [MAIR-ih-nawl].

**Marogen** (Hem).    See *epoetin beta.* [MAIR-oh-jen].

**Marplan** (Psych).    See *isocarboxazid.* [MAR-plan].

**Mar-Spas** (GI, Uro).    See *L-hyoscyamine.* [MAR-spaz].

**MARstem** (Chemo).    Chemotherapy drug used to treat myelodysplastic syndrome. Orphan drug. [MAR-stem].

**Marten-Tab** (Analges) (generic *acetaminophen, butalbital, caffeine*).    Combination analgesic, barbiturate sedative, and stimulant drug for pain. Capsule: 325 mg/50 mg/ 40 mg. [MAR-ten-tab].

**Marthritic** (Analges).    See *salsalate.* [mar-THRIH-tik].

**Matulane** (Chemo).    See *procarbazine.* [MAH-tyoo-layn].

**Mavik** (Cardio).    See *trandolapril.* [MAV-ik].

**Maxair Autohaler** (Pulm).    See *pirbuterol.* [MAKS-air].

**Maxalt, Maxalt-MLT** (Analges).    See *rizatriptan.* [MAKS-alt].

**Maxamine** (Chemo).    See *histamine.* [MAK-sah-meen].

**Maxaquin** (Anti-infec).    See *lomefloxacin.* [MAK-sah-kwin].

**Maxidex** (Ophth).    See *dexamethasone.* [MAK-sih-deks].

**Maxidone** (Analges) (generic *acetaminophen, hydrocodone*).    Combination Schedule III nonnarcotic and narcotic analgesic drug for pain. Capsule: 750 mg/10 mg. [MAK-sih-dohn].

**Maxiflor** (Derm).    See *diflorasone.* [MAK-sih-floor].

**Maxipime** (Anti-infec).    See *cefepime.* [MAK-sih-peem].

**Maxitrol Ophthalmic** (Ophth) (generic *dexamethasone, neomycin, polymyxin B*).    Combination corticosteroid and antibiotic drug used topically in the eyes to treat inflammation and infection. Ophthalmic suspension or ointment: 0.1%/0.35%/10,000 units. [MAKS-ih-trawl of-THAL-mik].

**Maxivate** (Derm).    See *betamethasone.* [MAK-sih-vayt].

**Maxolon** (GI).    See *metoclopramide.* [MAK-soh-lawn].

**Maxzide, Maxzide-25MG** (Cardio, GI, Uro) (generic *hydrochlorothiazide, triamterene*).    Combination thiazide diuretic and potassium-sparing diuretic drug used to treat hypertension; used to treat edema from congestive heart failure, liver disease, or kidney disease. Tablet: 25 mg/ 37.5 mg, 50 mg/75 mg. [MAK-zide].

**mazindol** (Sanorex) (Ortho).    Used to treat Duchenne's muscular dystrophy. Orphan drug. [MAZ-in-dawl].

**M-Caps** (Derm, Uro).    See *methionine.* [M-kaps].

**MCT** (GI).    See *medium chain triglycerides.* [M-C-T].

**Mebaral** (Neuro).    See *mephobarbital.* [meh-BAIR-awl].

**mebendazole** (Vermox) (Misc).    Used to treat pinworms, roundworms, and hookworms. Chewable tablet: 100 mg. [meh-BEN-dah-zohl].

**mecamylamine** (Inversine) (Cardio, Psych).    Alpha-blocker drug used to treat malignant hypertension and severe hypertension; orphan drug used to treat Tourette's syndrome. Tablet: 2.5 mg. [MEK-ah-MIL-ah-meen].

**mecasermin** (Increlex, Iplex, Myotrophin (Endo, Neuro). Insulin-like growth factor used to treat growth failure in children; orphan drug used to treat amyotrophic lateral sclerosis (Myotrophin). Subcutaneous: 10 mg/mL, 36 mg/0.6 mL [meh-KAY-ser-min].

**mechlorethamine** (Mustargen) (Chemo, Hem). Alkylating chemotherapy drug used to treat leukemia, Hodgkin's lymphoma, mycosis fungoides, and cancer of the lung; used to treat polycythemia vera. Intraperitoneal, intracardiac, intrapleural, or intravenous (powder to be reconstituted): 10 mg. [MEH-klor-ETH-ah-meen].

**meclizine** (Antivert, Antivert/25, Antivert/50, Antrizine, Dramamine Less Drowsy Formula, Meni-D) (GI). Antiemetic drug used to treat nausea and vomiting associated with motion sickness and vertigo. Capsule: 25 mg. Chewable tablet: 25 mg. Tablet: 12.5 mg, 25 mg, 50 mg. [MEK-lih-zeen].

**meclofenamate** (Analges). Nonsteroidal anti-inflammatory drug used to treat pain and inflammation; used to treat osteoarthritis, rheumatoid arthritis, and dysmenorrhea. Capsule: 50 mg, 100 mg. [MEK-loh-FEN-ah-mayt].

**Medacote** (Derm) (generic *pyrilamine, zinc oxide*). Combination antihistamine and astringent drug used to treat skin itching. Lotion: 1%. [MED-ah-koht].

**Medigesic** (Analges) (generic *acetaminophen, butalbital, caffeine*). Combination analgesic, barbiturate sedative, and stimulant drug for pain. Capsule: 325 mg/50 mg/ 40 mg. [MED-ih-JEE-sik].

**Medihoney** (Derm). See *manuka honey*. [MED-ih-HUN-ee].

**Medi-Quik** (Anes, Derm). See *lidocaine*. [MED-ih-kwik].

**medium-chain triglyceride** (MCT) (GI). Nutritional supplement that provides extra calories in the form of an easily digested oil. Oil: 115 calories/15 mL. [MEE-dee-um CHAYN try-GLIS-eh-ride].

**Medotar** (Derm). See *coal tar*. [MED-oh-tar].

**Medrol** (Endo, Neuro). See *methylprednisolone*. [MED-rawl].

**medroxyprogesterone** (Depo-Provera, Depo-Sub Q Provera 104, Hematrol, Provera) (Chemo, Hem, OB/GYN). Progestin hormone drug used to treat amenorrhea, abnormal uterine bleeding, and endometrial hyperplasia; hormonal chemotherapy drug used to treat cancer of the breast, uterus, and kidney; used as a contraceptive drug to prevent pregnancy; orphan drug used to treat immune thrombocytopenia purpura. Tablet: 2.5 mg, 5 mg, 10 mg. Intramuscular or subcutaneous: 150 mg/mL, 160 mg/mL, 400 mg/mL. [meh-DRAWK-see-proh-JES-teh-rohn].

**mefenamic acid** (Ponstel) (Analges). Nonsteroidal anti-inflammatory drug used to treat pain; used to treat dysmenorrhea. Capsule: 250 mg. [MEH-feh-NAM-ik AS-id].

**mefloquine** (Lariam, Mephaquin) (Anti-infec). Used to prevent and treat malaria. Tablet: 250 mg. [MEH-floh-kwin].

**Mefoxin** (Anti-infec). See *cefoxitin*. [meh-FAWK-sin].

**Megace, Megace ES** (Anti-infec, Chemo). See *megestrol*. [MEG-ace].

**megestrol** (Megace, Megace ES) (Anti-infec, Chemo). Hormonal chemotherapy drug used to treat HIV wasting syndrome; used to treat cancer of the breast and uterus. Tablet: 20 mg, 40 mg. Oral liquid: 40 mg/mL, 125 mg/mL. [meh-JES-trawl].

**Melacine** (Chemo). Vaccine used to treat malignant melanoma. Orphan drug. [MEL-ah-seen].

**Melagesic PM** (Neuro) (generic *acetaminophen, melatonin*). Combination over-the-counter analgesic and sleep aid drug to relieve pain and regulate the wake-sleep cycle. Tablet: 500 mg/1.5 mg. [MEL-ah-JEE-sik P-M].

**Melanocid** (Chemo). Chemotherapy drug used to treat malignant melanoma. Orphan drug. [meh-LAN-oh-sid].

**melatonin** (Circadin) (Neuro). Used to treat sleep disorders. Orphan drug. [MEL-ah-TOH-nin].

**Melfiat-105** (GI). See *phendimetrazine*. [mel-FEE-at-105].

**Melimmune** (Chemo). Monoclonal antibody drug used to treat malignant melanoma. Orphan drug. [MEL-im-myoon].

**meloxicam** (Mobic) (Analges). Nonsteroidal anti-inflammatory drug used to treat pain and inflammation; used to treat osteoarthritis, rheumatoid arthritis, and ankylosing spondylitis. Tablet: 7.5 mg, 15 mg. Oral liquid: 7.5 mg/5 mL. [meh-LAWK-sih-kam].

**Melpaque HP** (Derm). See *hydroquinone*. [MEL-payk H-P].

**melphalan** (Alkeran) (Chemo). Alkylating chemotherapy drug used to treat multiple myeloma, malignant melanoma, and cancer of the breast, ovary, and testicle. Tablet: 2 mg. Intravenous (powder to be reconstituted): 50 mg. [MEL-fah-lan].

**Melquin-HP** (Derm). See *hydroquinone*. [MEL-kwin-H-P].

**memantine** (Namenda) (Neuro). NMDA receptor blocker drug used to treat moderate-to-severe Alzheimer's disease. Tablet: 5 mg, 10 mg. Liquid: 2 mg/mL. [meh-MAN-teen].

**Menactra** (Anti-infec, Neuro). Used to prevent meningococcal meningitis in children, teens, and adults. Subcutaneous: Vaccine. [meh-NAK-trah].

**Menest** (Chemo, OB/GYN). See *esterified estrogens*. [MEN-est].

**Meni-D** (GI). See *meclizine*. [MEN-ee-D].

**Menomune** (Anti-infec, Neuro). Used to prevent meningococcal meningitis in children. Subcutaneous: Vaccine. [MEN-oh-myoon].

**Menopur** (Endo, OB/GYN). See *menotropins*. [MEN-oh-pyoor].

**Menostar** (OB/GYN, Ortho). See *estradiol*. [MEN-oh-star].

**menotropins** (Menopur, Repronex) (Endo, OB/GYN). Ovulation-stimulating drug used to stimulate ovulation in women with infertility; used to treat male infertility. Intramuscular (powder to be reconstituted): 75 IU, 150 IU. [MEN-oh-TROH-pins].

**Mentax** (Derm). See *butenafine.* [MEN-taks].

**mepenzolate** (Cantil) (GI). Anticholinergic and antispasmodic drug used to decrease acid production and relieve spasm from peptic ulcer. Tablet: 25 mg [meh-PEN-zoh-layt].

**meperidine** (Demerol) (Analges, Anes). Schedule II narcotic drug used to treat moderate to severe pain; used to relieve pain during labor and delivery; used preoperatively to produce sedation and relieve pain and to help maintain general anesthesia. Tablet: 50 mg, 100 mg. Oral liquid: 50 mg/ 5 mL. Syrup: 50 mg/5 mL. Subcutaneous, intramuscular, intravenous: 10 mg/mL, 25 mg/mL, 50 mg/mL, 75 mg/mL, 100 mg/mL. [meh-PAIR-ih-deen].

**Mephaquin** (Anti-infec). See *mefloquine.* [MEF-ah-kwin].

**mephobarbital** (Mebaral) (Neuro). Schedule IV barbiturate drug used to treat tonic-clonic and petit mal seizures. Tablet: 32 mg, 50 mg, 100 mg. [MEH-foh-BAR-bih-tawl].

**Mephyton** (Hem). See *phytonadione.* [meh-FY-ton].

**mepivacaine** (Carbocaine, Polocaine, Polocaine MPF) (Anes, ENT, OB/GYN). Anesthetic drug used to produce regional, spinal, and epidural anesthesia; used for transvaginal and paracervical block anesthesia; used as a nerve block in pain management; used to produce local or nerve block anesthesia during dental procedures. Injection: 1%, 1.5%, 2%, 3%; 3% with 1:20,000 levonordefrin. [meh-PIV-ah-kayn].

**meprobamate** (Miltown) (Psych). Schedule IV drug used to treat anxiety and neurosis. Tablet: 200 mg, 400 mg. [MEP-roh-BAM-ate].

**Mepron** (Anti-infec). See *atovaquone.* [MEP-rawn].

**merbromin** (Mercurochrome) (Derm). Over-the-counter red antiseptic drug that contains mercury and is used topically as a staining agent in the laboratory. Liquid: 2%. [mer-BROH-min].

**mercaptopurine** (Purinethol) (Chemo). Antimetabolite chemotherapy drug used to treat leukemia. Tablet: 50 mg. [mer-KAP-toh-PYOOR-een].

**Mercurochrome** (Derm). See *merbromin.* [mer-KYOOR-oh-krohm].

**Meridia** (GI). See *sibutramine.* [meh-RID-ee-ah].

**Meritene** (GI). Nutritional supplement. Powder (to be reconstituted). [MAIR-ih-teen].

**meropenem** (Merrem I.V.) (Anti-infec). Carbapenem antibiotic drug used to treat gram-positive and gram-negative bacterial infections; used to treat staphylococcal and streptococcal skin infections; used to treat intra-abdominal infections, ruptured appendicitis, and peritonitis; used to treat meningitis; used to treat lung infections in patients with cystic fibrosis. Intravenous (powder to be reconstituted): 500 mg, 1 g. [MEER-oh-PEN-em].

**Merrem I.V.** (Anti-infec). See *meropenem.* [MEER-em I-V].

**Meruvax II** (Anti-infec). Used to prevent rubella in children. Subcutaneous: Vaccine. [MAIR-yoo-vaks 2].

**mesalamine** (Asacol, Canasa, Lialda, Pentasa, Rowasa) (GI). Anti-inflammatory, 5-ASA drug used to treat ulcerative colitis. Controlled-release capsule: 250 mg, 500 mg. Tablet: 1.2 g. Delayed-release tablet: 400 mg. Rectal enema: 4 g/60 mL. Suppository: 500 mg, 1000 mg. [meh-SAL-ah-meen].

**mesna** (Mesnex) (Chemo). Cytoprotective drug used to protect the bladder from toxicity in patients on ifosfamide chemotherapy. Tablet: 100 mg. Intravenous: 100 mg/mL. [MES-nah].

**Mesnex** (Chemo). See *mesna.* [MES-neks].

**Mersol** (Derm). See *thimerosal.* [MER-sawl].

**Mestinon** (Neuro). See *pyridostigmine.* [MES-tih-nawn].

**Metadate CD, Metadate ER** (Neuro, Psych). See *methylphenidate.* [MEH-tah-dayt].

**Metaglip** (Endo) (generic *glipizide, metformin*). Combination oral antidiabetic drug used to treat type 2 diabetes mellitus. Tablet: 2.5 mg/250 mg, 2.5 mg/500 mg, 5 mg/500 mg. [MET-ah-glip].

**Metamucil** (GI). See *psyllium.* [MET-ah-MYOO-sil].

**metaproterenol** (Alupent) (Pulm). Bronchodilator drug used to prevent and treat asthma and bronchospasm, particularly with bronchitis or emphysema. Syrup: 10 mg/5 mL. Aerosol inhaler: 0.65 mg/puff. Liquid for inhalation: 0.4%, 0.6%, 5%. Tablet: 10 mg, 20 mg. [MEH-tah-proh-TAIR-eh-nawl].

**metaraminol** (Aramine) (Anes). Vasopressor drug used to prevent and treat hypotension caused by spinal anesthesia or from blood loss during surgery. Subcutaneous, intramuscular, or intravenous: 10 mg/mL. [MET-ah-RAM-ih-nawl].

**Metaret** (Chemo). See *suramin.* [MET-ah-ret].

**Metastron** (Chemo). See *strontium-89.* [MET-ah-strawn].

**metaxalone** (Skelaxin) (Ortho). Skeletal muscle relaxant drug used to treat spasm and stiffness associated with minor muscle injuries. Tablet: 800 mg. [meh-TAK-sah-lohn].

**metformin** (Fortamet, Glucophage, Glucophage XR, Glumetza, Riomet) (Endo, OB/GYN). Biguanide oral antidiabetic drug used to treat type 2 diabetes mellitus; used to treat anovulation in women with polycystic ovaries. Tablet: 500 mg, 850 mg, 1000 mg. Extended-release tablet: 500 mg, 750 mg, 1000 mg. Oral liquid: 500 mg/5mL. [met-FOR-min].

**methacholine** (Provocholine) (Misc). Used to diagnose bronchial hyperreactivity and asthma. Powder (reconstituted to a liquid to be inhaled): 100 mg/5 mL. [METH-ah-KOH-leen].

**methadone** (Diskets, Dolophine, Methadone Intensol, Methadose) (Analges, Anes). Schedule II narcotic drug used to treat severe pain; used to treat dependence and withdrawal from heroin, cocaine and narcotic drugs. Tablet: 5mg, 10 mg. Dispersible tablet: 40 mg. Oral liquid: 5 mg/5 mL, 10 mg/ 5 mL, 10 mg/mL. Subcutaneous or intramuscular: 10 mg/mL. [METH-ah-dohn].

**Methadone Intensol** (Analges). See *methadone.* [METH-ah-dohn].

**Methadose** (Analges). See *methadone.* [METH-ah-dohs].

**methamphetamine** (Desoxyn) (GI, Psych). Schedule II amphetamine stimulant drug used to treat attention-deficit/hyperactivity disorder; used to treat obesity. Tablet: 5 mg. [METH-am-FET-ah-meen].

**methazolamide** (Ophth).   Carbonic anhydrase inhibitor drug used to treat glaucoma. Tablet: 25 mg, 50 mg. [METH-ah-ZOH-lah-mide].

**methenamine** (Hiprex, Urex) (Anti-infec, Uro).   Anti-infective drug used to treat urinary tract infections. Tablet: 1 g. [meth-EN-ah-meen].

**Methergine** (OB/GYN).   See *methylergonovine*. [METH-er-jeen]

**methimazole** (Tapazole) (Endo).   Antithyroid drug used to treat hyperthyroidism. Tablet: 5 mg, 10 mg. [meth-IM-ah-zohl].

**methionine** (M-Caps, Uracid) (Derm, Uro).   Acidifier drug that eliminates the ammonia in urine that causes odor and skin irritation in incontinent patients. Capsule: 200 mg. Tablet: 500 mg. [meh-THY-oh-neen].

**Methitest** (Chemo, Endo).   See *methyltestosterone*. [METH-ih-test].

**methocarbamol** (Robaxin, Robaxin-750) (Ortho).   Skeletal muscle relaxant drug used to treat spasm and stiffness associated with minor muscle injuries. Tablet: 500 mg, 750 mg. Intramuscular or intravenous: 100 mg/mL. [METH-oh-KAR-bah-mawl].

**methohexital** (Brevital) (Anes).   Schedule IV barbiturate drug used to induce and help maintain general anesthesia. Intravenous: 2.5 gm/20 mL. [METH-oh-HEK-sih-tawl].

**methotrexate** (Methotrexate LPF, Rheumatrex Dose Pack, Trexall) (Chemo, Derm, GI, Neuro, Ortho).   Antimetabolic chemotherapy drug used to treat cancer of the breast, ovary, head and neck, and lung; used to treat osteosarcoma, leukemia, lymphoma, and T-cell lymphoma (mycosis fungoides); used to treat severe psoriasis and dermatomyositis; used to treat rheumatoid arthritis and psoriatic arthritis; used to treat multiple sclerosis, ulcerative colitis, Crohn's disease, and lupus erythematosis; used to treat graft-versus-host disease. Tablet: 2.5 mg, 5 mg, 7.5 mg, 10 mg, 15 mg. Subcutaneous, intramuscular, intravenous: 25 mg/mL. [METH-oh-TREK-sayt].

**Methotrexate LPF** (Chemo, Derm, GI, Neuro, Ortho).   See *methotrexate*. [METH-oh-TREK-sayt L-P-F].

**methoxsalen** (8-MOP, Oxsoralen, Oxsoralen-Ultra, Uvadex) (Derm).   Psoralen drug that sensitizes the skin to the effects of ultraviolet light; used to treat severe, disabling psoriasis; causes repigmentation of skin in patients with vitiligo. Capsule: 10 mg. Gel capsule: 10 mg. Liquid: 20 mcg/mL. Lotion: 1% (10 mg/mL). [meth-AWK-sah-len].

**methscopolamine** (Pamine, Pamine Forte) (GI).   Anticholinergic antispasmodic drug used to decrease acid production and relieve spasm from peptic ulcer. Tablet: 2.5 mg, 5 mg. [METH-skoh-PAWL-ah-meen].

**methsuximide** (Celontin) (Neuro).   Anticonvulsant drug used to treat absence seizures. Capsule: 150 mg, 300 mg. [meth-SUK-sih-mide].

**methyclothiazide** (Enduron) (Cardio, GI, Uro).   Thiazide diuretic drug used to treat hypertension; used to treat edema from congestive heart failure, liver disease, or kidney disease. Tablet: 2.5 mg, 5 mg. [METH-ee-kloh-THY-ah-zide].

**methyl aminolevulinate** (Metvixia) (Derm).   Photosensitization drug used topically on the skin to treat actinic keratoses with a red-light lamp. Cream: 16.8%. [METH-il ah-MEE-noh-LEV-yoo-LIN-ate].

**methylbicyclone** (Pulm).   Used to treat cystic fibrosis. Orphan drug. [METH-il-by-SY-klohn].

**methylcellulose** (Citrucel, Citrucel Sugar Free) (GI).   Over-the-counter, bulk-producing laxative drug used to treat constipation. Tablet: 500 mg. Powder: 2 g/Tbsp. [METH-il-SEL-yoo-lohs].

**methyldopa** (Cardio).   Alpha$_2$ receptor stimulator drug used to dilate blood vessels in the extremities to treat hypertension. Tablet: 250 mg, 500 mg. Injection: 50 mg/mL. [METH-il-DOH-pah].

**methylene blue** (Urolene Blue) (Emerg, Uro).   Used to treat cyanide poisoning; used as a blue tissue dye diagnostic aid during surgery; antiseptic drug used in combination drugs to treat urinary tract infections. Tablet: 65 mg. Intravenous: 10 mg/mL. [METH-eh-leen BLOO].

**methylergonovine** (Methergine) (OB/GYN) Smooth muscle stimulant drug used to produce abortion; used to treat uterine bleeding after delivery.   Tablet: 0.2 mg. Intramuscular or intravenous: 0.2 mg/mL. [METH-il-AIR-goh-NOH-veen].

**Methylin, Methylin ER** (Neuro, Psych).   See *methylphenidate*. [METH-ih-lin].

**methylnaltrexone** (Relistor) (GI).   Narcotic antagonist drug used to treat severe constipation unresponsive to other laxative drugs in patients taking narcotic drugs for pain. Subcutaneous: 12 mg/0.6 mL. [METH-il-nal-TREK-sohn].

**methylphenidate** (Concerta, Daytrana, Metadate CD, Metadate ER, Methylin, Methylin ER, Ritalin, Ritalin LA, Ritalin-SR) (Neuro, Psych).   Schedule II stimulant drug used to treat attention-deficit disorder and attention-deficit/hyperactivity disorder in children and adults; used to treat narcolepsy; used to treat depression in elderly stroke patients; used to treat behavior after traumatic brain injury. Extended-release capsule: 10 mg, 20 mg, 30 mg, 40 mg, 50 mg, 60 mg. Tablet: 5 mg, 10 mg, 20 mg. Chewable tablet: 2.5 mg, 5 mg, 10 mg. Extended-release tablet: 10 mg, 18 mg, 20 mg, 27 mg, 36 mg, 54 mg. Liquid: 5 mg/5 mL, 10 mg/5 mL. Transdermal patch: 10 mg/9 hours, 15 mg/9 hours, 20 mg/9 hours, 30 mg/9 hours. [METH-il-FEN-ih-dayt].

**methylprednisolone** (A-Methapred, Depo-Medrol, Medrol, Solu-Medrol) (Derm, Endo, Neuro, Ortho, Pulm).   Corticosteroid anti-inflammatory drug used to treat severe inflammation in various body systems; used to treat multiple sclerosis; given after a spinal cord injury to improve neurologic functioning; used to treat adrenogenital syndrome; injected into joints to treat rheumatoid arthritis and osteoarthritis; injected near joints in the soft tissue to treat tendinitis and bursitis; injected into skin lesions; used to treat severe asthma. Tablet: 2 mg, 4 mg, 8 mg, 16 mg, 24 mg, 32 mg. Intramuscular or intravenous: 20 mg/mL, 40 mg/mL, 40 mg/3 mL, 80 mg/mL, 125 mg/2 mL,

125 mg/5 mL, 500 mg/mL, 500 mg/4 mL, 500 mg/8 mL, 500 mg/20 mL, 1000 mg/mL, 1000 mg/8 mL, 1000 mg/ 50 mL. [METH-il-pred-NIS-oh-lohn].

**methyltestosterone** (Android, Methitest, Testred, Virilon) (Chemo, Endo).   Schedule III male hormone used as male hormone replacement therapy in patients with cryptorchism or orchiectomy; used to treat delayed puberty in boys; hormonal chemotherapy drug used to treat breast cancer in women. Capsule: 10 mg. Tablet: 10 mg, 25 mg. Buccal tablet: 10 mg. [METH-il-tes-TAWS-teh-rohn].

**Meticorten** (Chemo, Endo, Ortho, Pulm, Neuro).   See *prednisone*. [MET-ee-KOHR-ten].

**Metimyd** (Ophth) (generic *prednisolone, sulfacetamide*).   Combination corticosteroid and sulfonamide anti-infective drug used topically in the eye to treat inflammation and infection. Ophthalmic solution: 0.5%/10%. [MET-ih-mid].

**metipranolol** (OptiPranolol) (Ophth).   Beta-blocker drug used topically in the eyes to treat glaucoma. Ophthalmic solution: 0.3%. [MET-ee-PRAN-oh-lawl].

**metoclopramide** (Maxolon, Octamide PFS, Reglan) (GI).   Gastric stimulant drug used to treat GERD and gastroparesis (delayed gastric emptying) in diabetic patients. Tablet: 5 mg, 10 mg. Syrup: 5 mg/5 mL. Intramuscular or intravenous: 5 mg/mL. [MEH-toh-KLOH-prah-mide].

**metolazone** (Zaroxolyn) (Cardio, Uro).   Thiazide diuretic drug used to treat hypertension; used to treat edema from congestive heart failure or kidney disease. Tablet: 2.5 mg, 5 mg, 10 mg. [meh-TOH-lah-zohn].

**metoprolol** (Lopressor, Toprol-XL) (Analges, Cardio, GI).   Cardioselective beta-blocker drug used to treat angina pectoris, hypertension, congestive heart failure, and myocardial infarction; used to prevent migraine headaches; used to treat bleeding varices in patients with portal hypertension; used to treat the side effect of muscle restlessness from antipsychotic drugs. Tablet: 25 mg, 50 mg, 100 mg. Extended-release tablet: 25 mg, 50 mg, 100 mg, 200 mg. Intravenous: 1 mg/mL. [meh-TOH-proh-lawl].

**metreleptin** (Misc).   Used to treat lipodystrophy. Orphan drug. [MEH-treh-LEP-tin].

**MetroCream** (Derm).   See *metronidazole*. [MEH-troh-kreem].

**Metrodin** (OB/GYN).   See *urofollitropin*. [MEH-troh-din].

**MetroGel** (Derm).   See *metronidazole*. [MEH-troh-jel].

**MetroGel-Vaginal** (OB/GYN).   See *metronidazole*. [MEH-troh-jel-VAJ-ih-nal].

**MetroLotion** (Derm).   See *metronidazole*. [MEH-troh-LOH-shun].

**metronidazole** (Flagyl, Flagyl ER, Flagyl 375, Flagyl IV, MetroCream, MetroGel, MetroGel-Vaginal, MetroLotion, Noritate, Vandazole) (Anti-infec, Derm, GI, OB/GYN).   Antibacterial and antiprotozoal drug used to treat infections, including *Helicobacter pylori* infection and Crohn's disease of the gastrointestinal tract and intestinal amebiasis; used to treat pelvic inflammatory disease, bacterial vaginosis, and *Trichomonas vaginalis* (MetroGel-Vaginal); used to treat hepatic encephalopathy; used to treat anaerobic bacterial infections of the abdomen, uterus, skin, bone, lungs, heart, and central nervous system; used topically to treat acne rosacea (MetroCream, MetroGel, MetroLotion) and infected decubitus ulcers. Capsule: 375 mg. Cream: 0.75%, 1%. Gel: 0.75%, 1%. Lotion: 0.75%. Tablet: 250 mg, 500 mg. Extended-release tablet: 750 mg. Intravenous: 5 mg/mL. Vaginal gel: 0.75%. [MEH-troh-NY-dah-zawl].

**Metvixia** (Derm).   See *methyl aminolevulinate*. [met-VIK-see-ah].

**metyrosine** (Demser) (Endo).   Blocks excessive production of hormones from the adrenal medulla to treat a pheochromocytoma. Capsule: 250 mg. [meh-TY-roh-seen].

**Mevacor** (Cardio).   See *lovastatin*. [MEV-ah-kor].

**mexiletine** (Mexitil) (Cardio).   Antiarrhythmic drug used to treat ventricular tachycardia. Capsule: 150 mg, 200 mg, 250 mg. [mek-SIL-eh-teen].

**Mexitil** (Cardio).   See *mexiletine*. [MEK-sih-til].

**Mexsana Medicated** (Derm) (generic *kaolin, zinc oxide*).   Combination over-the-counter protectant and astringent drug used topically to treat diaper rash and other skin irritations. Powder. [mek-SAN-ah].

**MG 217 Medicated Tar** (Derm).   See *coal tar*. [M-G 217].

**Miacalcin** (Ortho).   See *calcitonin-salmon*. [MEE-ah-KAL-sin].

**micafungin** (Mycamine) (Anti-infec).   Antifungal drug used to treat severe systemic yeast infections and esophageal candidiasis, particularly in immunocompromised patients. Intravenous: 50 mg, 100 mg. [MY-kah-FUN-jin].

**Micardis** (Cardio).   See *telmisartan*. [mih-KAR-dis].

**Micardis HCT** (Cardio) (generic *telmisartan, hydrochlorothiazide*).   Combination angiotensin II receptor blocker and diuretic drug used to treat hypertension. Tablet: 40 mg/12.5 mg, 80 mg/12.5 mg, 80 mg/25 mg. [my-KAR-dis H-C-T].

**Micatin** (Derm).   See *miconazole*. [MIK-ah-tin].

**miconazole** (Lotrimin AF 2%, Micatin, Monistat, Monistat-Derm, Monistat 3, Monistat 7, Monistat 1 Combination Pack, Monistat 3, Monistat 3 Combination Pack, Monistat 7, Monistat 7 Combination Pack, M-Zole 3 Combination Pack, M-Zole 7 Dual Pack, Neosporin AF, Prescription Strength Desenex, Ting 2%, Vagistat 3 Combination Pack, Zeasorb-AF) (Derm, OB/GYN).   Over-the-counter and prescription antifungal and antiyeast drug used topically to treat tinea (ringworm) of the skin and vaginal yeast infections. Cream: 2%. Gel: 2%. Liquid: 2%. Ointment: 2%. Powder: 2%. Spray liquid: 2%. Spray powder: 2%. Vaginal cream: 2%. Vaginal suppository: 100 mg, 200 mg, 1200 mg. Dual pack: Topical cream: 2%; vaginal suppository: 100 mg. Combination pack: Topical cream: 2%, vaginal suppository: 100 mg, 200 mg. [my-KAWN-ah-zohl].

**microfibrillar collagen hemostat** (Hemopad, Hemotene) (Hem). Collagen fiber drug used topically during surgery to control bleeding. Packet: 1 g. Pad: 2.5 × 5 cm, 5 × 8 cm, 8 × 10 cm. [MY-kroh-FIB-rih-lar KAWL-ah-jen HEE-moh-stat].

**Microgestin Fe 1/20** (OB/GYN) (generic *norethindrone, ethinyl estradiol; ferrous fumarate*). Combination monophasic oral contraceptive drug with iron supplement. Pill pack, 28-day: (21 hormone tablets) 1 mg/20 mcg; (7 iron [Fe] tablets) 75 mg. [MY-kroh-JES-tin].

**Microgestin Fe 1.5/30** (OB/GYN) (generic *norethindrone, ethinyl estradiol; ferrous fumarate*). Combination monophasic oral contraceptive drug with iron supplement. Pill pack, 28-day: (21 hormone tablets) 1.5 mg/30 mcg; (7 iron [Fe] tablets) 75 mg. [MY-kroh-JES-tin].

**MICRhoGAM** (Hem, OB/GYN). Immunoglobulin drug given to an Rh-negative mother after the birth of an Rh-positive infant; it prevents the mother from making antibodies during the next pregnancy and causing hemolytic disease if the next infant is Rh positive. Intramuscular: 5% gamma globulin. [MY-kroh-ROH-gam].

**Micro-K Extencaps, Micro-K 10 Extencaps, Micro-K LS** (Uro). See *potassium*. [MY-kroh-kay].

**Micronase** (Endo). See *glyburide*. [MY-kroh-nays].

**microNefrin** (Pulm). See *epinephrine*. [MY-kroh-NEH-frin].

**Microzide** (Cardio, Uro). See *hydrochlorothiazide*. [MY-kroh-zide].

**Midamor** (Cardio, Uro). See *amiloride*. [MID-ah-moor].

**midazolam** (Anes, Neuro). Schedule IV benzodiazepine drug used to relieve anxiety and produce sedation and amnesia prior to induction of general anesthesia; orphan drug used to treat seizures. Oral syrup: 2 mg/mL. Intramuscular and intravenous: 1 mg/mL, 5 mg/mL. [mih-DAZ-oh-lam].

**midodrine** (Amatine, ProAmatine) (Cardio). Alpha$_1$ receptor stimulator and vasopressor drug used to treat lightheadedness from orthostatic hypotension. Tablet: 2.5 mg, 5 mg, 10 mg. [MID-oh-dreen].

**Midol Extended Relief** (Analges). See *naproxen*. [MY-dawl].

**Midol Maximum Strength Cramp Formula** (Analges). See *ibuprofen*. [MY-dawl].

**Midol Maximum Strength Menstrual** (OB/GYN) (generic *acetaminophen, pyrilamine, caffeine*). Combination over-the-counter analgesic, antihistamine, and stimulant drug used to treat painful menstruation. Caplet/Gelcap: 500 mg/15 mg/60 mg. [MY-dawl].

**Midol Maximum Strength PMS** (OB/GYN) (generic *acetaminophen, pamabrom, pyrilamine*). Combination over-the-counter analgesic, diuretic, and antihistamine drug used to treat painful menstruation. Caplet/Gelcap: 500 mg/25 mg. [MY-dawl].

**Midol PM** (Neuro). See *diphenydramine*. [MY-dawl P-M].

**Midol Teen Maximum Strength** (OB/GYN) (generic *acetaminophen, pamabrom*). Combination analgesic and diuretic drug used to treat painful menstruation. Caplet: 500 mg/25 mg. [MY-dawl].

**Midrin** (Analges) (generic *acetaminophen, dichloralphenazone, isometheptene*). Combination analgesic, sedative, and vasoconstrictor drug used to treat migraine headaches. Capsule: 325 mg/100 mg/65 mg. [MID-rin].

**mifamuritide** (Junovan) (Chemo). Chemotherapy drug used to treat bone cancer. Orphan drug. [MIH-fah-MYOOR-ih-tide].

**Mifeprex** (OB/GYN). See *mifepristone*. [MIH-feh-preks].

**mifepristone** (Mifeprex) (Endo, OB/GYN). Antiprogesterone drug used to produce abortion; orphan drug used to treat Cushing's syndrome. Tablet: 200 mg. [MIH-feh-PRIS-tohn].

**miglitol** (Glyset) (Endo). Alpha-glucosidase inhibitor oral antidiabetic drug used to treat type 2 diabetes mellitus. Tablet: 25 mg, 50 mg, 100 mg. [MIG-lih-tawl].

**miglustat** (Zavesca) (Misc). Used to treat Gaucher disease. Capsule: 100 mg. [MIG-loo-stat].

**Migranal** (Analges). See *dihydroergotamine*. [MY-grah-nawl].

**Miles Nervine** (Neuro). See *diphenydramine*. [MY-els NER-veen].

**milk of magnesia** (MOM, Phillips' Milk of Magnesia, Phillips' Milk of Magnesia Concentrated) (GI). Over-the-counter magnesium-containing laxative drug used to treat constipation. Tablet: 500 mg. Suspension: 400 mg/5mL, 800 mg/5 mL. [MILK of mag-NEE-see-ah].

**Milophene** (OB/GYN). See *clomiphene*. [MY-loh-feen].

**milrinone** (Primacor) (Cardio). Used to treat congestive heart failure that has not responded to treatment with digoxin. Intravenous: 1 mg/mL. [MIL-rih-nohn].

**Miltown** (Psych). See *meprobamate*. [MIL-town].

**mineral oil** (Fleet Mineral Oil Enema, Kondremul Plain) (GI). Over-the-counter stool-softener laxative drug used to treat constipation. Oral liquid. Enema. [MIN-er-al OIL].

**Minetezol** (Misc). See *thiabendazole*. [mih-NEH-teh-zohl].

**Minidyne** (Derm). See *povidone iodine*. [MIN-ee-dine].

**Minipress** (Cardio). See *prazosin*. [MIN-ee-pres].

**Minirin** (Endo, Hem). See *desmopressin*. [MIN-ih-rin].

**Minitran** (Cardio). See *nitroglycerin*. [MIN-ih-tran].

**Minocin** (Anti-infec). See *minocycline*. [MIN-oh-sin].

**minocycline** (Arestin, Dynacin, Minocin, Myrac, Solodyn) (Anti-infec). Tetracycline antibiotic drug used to treat infections due to gram-negative and gram-positive bacteria; used to treat severe acne vulgaris; used to treat gonorrhea, syphilis, *Chlamydia,* and nongonococcal urethritis; used to treat pneumonia due to *S. pneumoniae, H. influenzae,* and *Mycoplasma;* used to treat Rocky Mountain spotted fever;

used to treat intestinal amebiasis; used to treat ulcerative gingivitis (trench mouth); used to treat rheumatoid arthritis; used to treat gallbladder infections due to *E. coli;* used topically as a powder to treat periodontal gum disease; orphan drug used to treat sarcoidosis. Capsule: 50 mg, 75 mg, 100 mg. Pellet-filled capsules: 50 mg, 100 mg. Dental powder: 1 mg. Extended-release tablet: 45 mg, 90 mg, 135 mg. Tablet: 50 mg, 75 mg, 100 mg. Liquid: 50 mg/5 mL. Intravenous (powder to be reconstituted): 100 mg. [MIN-oh-SY-kleen].

**minoxidil** (Rogaine, Rogaine Extra Strength for Men) (Cardio, Derm).    Over-the-counter and prescription vasodilator drug used orally to treat severe hypertension; used topically on the skin and hair to treat male and female pattern thinning hair and baldness (Rogaine). Topical liquid: 2%, 5%. Foam: 5%. Tablet: 2.5 mg, 10 mg. [mih-NAWK-sih-dil].

**Miochol-E** (Ophth).    See *acetylcholine.* [MY-oh-kawl-E].

**Miostat** (Ophth).    See *carbachol.* [MY-oh-stat].

**MiraLax** (GI).    See *polyethylene glycol.* [MEER-ah-laks].

**Mirapex** (Neuro).    See *pramipexole.* [MEER-ah-peks].

**Mircera** (Hem, Uro).    See *epoetin beta-methoxy polyethylene glycol.* [mir-SAIR-ah].

**Mircette** (OB/GYN) (generic *desogestrel, ethinyl estradiol*).    Combination biphasic oral contraceptive drug. Pill pack, 28-day: (21 hormone tablets, phase 1) 0.15 mg/20 mcg; (5 hormone tablets, phase 2) 10 mcg; (2 inert tablets). [meer-SET].

**Mirena** (OB/GYN).    See *levonorgestrel.* [mih-RAY-nah].

**mirtazapine** (Remeron, Remeron SolTab) (Psych).    Tetracyclic antidepressant drug used to treat depression. Tablet: 7.5 mg, 15 mg, 30 mg, 45 mg. Orally disintegrating tablet: 15 mg, 30 mg, 45 mg. [mir-TAZ-ah-peen].

**misoprostol** (Cytotec) (GI, OB/GYN).    Prostaglandin drug used to prevent gastric ulcers in patients taking aspirin or NSAID drugs; used to treat chronic constipation; used to induce labor in pregnant women; used to produce an abortion; used to control postpartum bleeding. Tablet: 100 mcg, 200 mcg. [MY-soh-PRAWS-tohl].

**mitoguazone** (Apep) (Chemo).    Chemotherapy drug used to treat non-Hodgkin's lymphoma. Orphan drug. [MIH-toh-GWAH-zohn].

**mitolactol** (Chemo).    Chemotherapy drug used to treat cancer of the brain and cervix. Orphan drug. [MIH-toh-LAK-tawl].

**mitomycin** (Mutamycin) (Chemo).    Chemotherapy antibiotic drug used to treat cancer of the head and neck, lung, stomach, colon, pancreas, breast, cervix, and bladder. Intravenous (powder to be reconstituted): 5 mg, 20 mg, 40 mg. Intravesical. [MIH-toh-MY-sin].

**mitotane** (Lysodren) (Chemo, Endo).    Chemotherapy drug used to treat cancer of the adrenal cortex; used to treat Cushing's syndrome. Tablet: 500 mg. [MIH-toh-tayn].

**mitoxantrone** (Novantrone) (Chemo, Neuro).    Mitosis inhibiting chemotherapy drug used to treat cancer of the breast and prostate gland; used to treat leukemia and non-Hodgkin's lymphoma; used to treat multiple sclerosis. Intravenous: 2 mg/mL. [mih-TAWK-san-trohn].

**Mivacron** (Anes, Pulm).    See *mivacurium.* [MIV-ah-krawn]

**mivacurium** (Mivacron) (Anes, Pulm).    Neuromuscular blocker drug used during surgery; used to treat patients who are intubated and on the ventilator. Intravenous. 2 mg/mL. [MIV-ah-KYOOR-ee-um].

**M-M-R II** (Anti-infec).    Combination drug used to prevent measles, mumps, and rubella in children. Subcutaneous: Vaccine. [M-M-R 2].

**Moban** (Psych).    See *molindone.* [MOH-ban].

**Mobic** (Analges).    See *meloxicam.* [MOH-bik].

**Mobigesic** (Analges) (generic *magnesium salicylate, phenyltoloxamine*).    Combination over-the-counter salicylate analgesic and sedative drug used to treat pain. Tablet: 325 mg/30 mg. [MOH-bih-JEE-sik].

**Moctanin** (GI).    See *monoctanoin.* [mawk-TAN-in].

**modafinil** (Provigil) (Neuro, Pulm).    Schedule IV stimulant drug used to treat narcolepsy; used to treat fatigue associated with sleep apnea and multiple sclerosis. Tablet: 100 mg, 200 mg. [moh-DAF-eh-nil].

**Modane** (GI).    See *bisacodyl.* [moh-DAYN].

**Modicon** (OB/GYN) (generic *norethindrone, ethinyl estradiol*).    Combination monophasic oral contraceptive drug. Pill pack (Dialpak), 28-day: (21 hormone tablets) 0.5 mg/35 mcg; (7 inert tablets). [MAWD-ih-kawn].

**Moduretic** (Cardio, Uro) (generic *amiloride, hydrochlorothiazide*).    Combination potassium-sparing diuretic and thiazide diuretic drug used to treat hypertension; used to treat edema from congestive heart failure, liver disease, or kidney disease. Tablet: 5 mg/ 50 mg. [MAW-dyoo-RET-ik].

**moexipril** (Univasc) (Cardio).    ACE inhibitor drug used to treat hypertension. Tablet: 7.5 mg, 15 mg. [moh-EK-sih-pril].

**molgramostim** (Leucomax) (Anti-infec, Chemo, Hem).    Granulocyte macrophage colony-stimulating factor drug used to increase the neutrophil count in AIDS patients or in patients after ganciclovir or zidovudine chemotherapy or bone marrow transplantation; used to increase the RBC count in patients with aplastic anemia. Orphan drug. [mol-GRAM-oh-stim].

**molindone** (Moban) (Psych).    Antipsychotic drug used to treat schizophrenia. Tablet: 5 mg, 10 mg, 25 mg, 50 mg. [moh-LIN-dohn].

**MOM** (GI).    See *milk of magnesia.* [M-O-M].

**mometasone** (Asmanex Twisthaler, Elocon, Nasonex) (Derm, ENT, Pulm).    Corticosteroid anti-inflammatory drug used topically to treat inflammation and itching from dermatitis, seborrhea, eczema, psoriasis, and yeast or fungal infections (Elocon); used intranasally to treat allergy symptoms in the nose (Nasonex); inhaled to prevent acute asthma attacks in adults and children (Asmanex Twisthaler). Cream: 0.1%. Liquid: 0.1%. Lotion: 0.1%. Ointment: 0.1%. Nasal spray:

0.05% (50 mcg/spray). AsthmaTwisthaler device (inhaled powder): 110 mcg/actuation, 220 mcg/actuation. [moh-MET-ah-zohn].

**Monarc-M** (Hem). See *factor VIII.* [MAWN-ark-M].

**monarsen** (Neuro). Used to treat myasthenia gravis. Orphan drug. [moh-NAR-sen].

**Monistat, Monistat 3, Monistat 7, Monistat 1 Combination Pack, Monistat 3 Combination Pack, Monistat 7 Combination Pack** (OB/GYN). See *miconazole.* [MAWN-ih-stat].

**Monistat 1** (OB/GYN). See *tioconazole.* [MAWN-ih-stat-1].

**Monistat-Derm** (Derm). See *miconazole.* [MAWN-ih-stat-derm].

**monobenzone** (Benoquin) (Derm). Used topically to darken depigmented areas of skin in patients with vitiligo. Cream: 20%. [MAW-noh-BEN-zohn].

**Mono-Chlor** (Derm). See *monochloroacetic acid.* [MAW-noh-klor].

**monochloroacetic acid** (Mono-Chlor) (Derm). Used topically on the skin to treat verrucae (common warts and plantar warts). Liquid: 80%. [MAW-noh-KLOR-oh-ah-SEE-tik AS-id].

**Monoclate-P** (Hem). See *factor VIII.* [MAWN-oh-klayt-P].

**monoctanoin** (Moctanin) (GI). Used to dissolve gallstones in patients who cannot undergo gallbladder surgery. Orphan drug. [mawn-AWK-tah-NOH-in].

**Monodox** (Anti-infec). See *doxycycline.* [MAWN-oh-dawks].

**Monoket** (Cardio). See *isosorbide mononitrate.* [MAWN-oh-ket].

**MonoNessa** (OB/GYN) (generic *norgestimate, ethinyl estradiol*). Combination monophasic oral contraceptive drug. Pill pack, 28-day: (21 hormone tablets): 0.25 mg/ 35 mcg; (7 inert tablets). [MAW-noh-NES-sah].

**Mononine** (Hem). See *factor IX.* [MAW-noh-neen].

**Monopril** (Cardio). See *fosinopril.* [MAW-noh-pril].

**Monopril HCT** (Cardio) (generic *fosinopril, hydrochlorothiazide*). Combination ACE inhibitor and diuretic drug used to treat hypertension. Tablet: 10 mg/ 12.5 mg, 20 mg/12.5 mg. [MAW-noh-pril H-C-T].

**montelukast** (Singulair) (Pulm). Leukotriene receptor blocker drug used to prevent and treat asthma. Chewable tablet: 4 mg, 5 mg. Tablet: 10 mg. Granules: 4 mg/packet. [MAWN-teh-LOO-kast].

**Monurol** (Uro). See *fosfomycin.* [mawn-YOOR-awl].

**moricizine** (Ethmozine) (Cardio). Antiarrhythmic drug used to treat ventricular arrhythmias. Tablet: 300 mg. [mor-IH-sih-zeen].

**morphine** (Astramorph PF, Avinza, DepoDur, Duramorph, Infumorph 200, Infumorph 500, Kadian, MS Contin, MSIR, Oramorph SR, RMS, Roxanol, Roxanol 100, Roxanol T) (Analges, Anes). Schedule II narcotic drug used to treat moderate-to-severe pain; used as a preoperative drug to relieve pain and provide sedation; used to induce general anesthesia. Extended-release capsule: 20 mg, 30 mg, 50 mg, 60 mg, 80 mg, 90 mg, 100 mg, 120 mg, 200 mg. Oral liquid: 10 mg/5 mL, 20 mg/mL, 20 mg/5 mL, 100 mg/5 mL. Tablet: 15 mg, 30 mg. Controlled-release tablet: 15 mg, 30 mg, 60 mg, 100 mg, 200 mg. Suppository: 5 mg, 10 mg, 20 mg, 30 mg. Subcutaneous, intramuscular, intravenous, epidural, intrathecal: 0.5 mg/mL, 1 mg/mL, 2 mg/mL, 4 mg/mL, 5 mg/mL, 8 mg/mL, 10 mg/mL, 15 mg/mL, 25 mg/mL, 50 mg/mL. [MOR-feen].

**morphine sulfate** (MS). See *morphine.* [MOR-feen SUL-fayt].

**morrhuate** (Scleromate) (Cardio). Sclerosing drug used to treat varicose veins. Injection (into the varicose vein): 50 mg/mL. [MOR-hyoo-ate].

**Motofen** (GI) (generic *atropine, difenoxin*). Combination Schedule IV anticholinergic and narcotic drug used to decrease GI peristalsis and spasm; used to treat diarrhea. Tablet: 0.025 mg/1 mg. [MOH-toh-fen].

**Motrin, Motrin IB, Motrin Migraine Pain, Children's Motrin, Infants' Motrin, Junior Strength Motrin** (Analges). See *ibuprofen.* [MOH-trin].

**Motrin Sinus Headache** (Analges, ENT) (generic *ibuprofen, pseudoephedrine*). Combination over-the-counter analgesic and decongestant drug. Tablet: 200 mg/30 mg. [MOH-trin].

**MoviPrep** (GI) (generic *polyethylene glycol, electrolyte solution*). Combination bowel evacuant and bowel prep. Oral liquid (powder to be reconstituted). [MOO-vee-prep].

**Moxatag** (Anti-infec). See *amoxicillin.* [MAWK-sah-tag].

**moxifloxacin** (Avelox, Avelox I.V., Vigamox) (Anti-infec, Ophth). Fluoroquinolone antibiotic drug used to treat gram-negative and gram-positive bacterial infections; used to treat sinusitis, bronchitis, Legionnaire's disease of the lungs, and pneumonia due to *S. pneumoniae* and *H. influenzae;* used to treat staphylococcal and streptococcal skin infections; used to treat intra-abdominal infections; used topically to treat bacterial infection of the eyes (Vigamox). Tablet: 400 mg. Intramuscular or intravenous: 400 mg/250 mL. Ophthalmic solution: 0.5% (5 mg/mL). [MAWK-sih-FLAWK-sah-sin].

**M-oxy** (Analges). See *oxycodone.* [m-AWK-see].

**MS Contin** (Analges). See *morphine.* [ M-S KAWN-tin].

**MSIR** (Analges). See *morphine.* [M-S-I-R].

**MTC-DOX** (Chemo) (generic *doxorubicin, iron particles*). Combination chemotherapy and iron particles drug used to treat liver cancer. Orphan drug. [M-T-C-DAWKS].

**Mucinex Children's, Mucinex Junior Strength** (Pulm). See *guaifenesin.* [MYOO-sih-neks].

**MucinexD** (ENT) (generic *guaifenesin, pseudoephedrine*). Combination over-the-counter expectorant and decongestant drug. Tablet: 600 mg/60 mg. [MYOO-sih-neks-D].

**Mucomyst** (Emerg, Pulm). See *acetylcysteine.* [MYOO-koh-mist].

**Mudrane** (Pulm) (generic *theophylline, ephedrine, potassium iodide, phenobarbital*). Combination bronchodilator, expectorant, and sedative drug. Tablet: 111 mg/16 mg/ 195 mg/8 mg. [MYOO-drayn].

**Mudrane GG** (Pulm) (generic *theophylline, ephedrine, guaifenesin, phenobarbital*). Combination bronchodilator, expectorant, and barbiturate sedative drug. Tablet: 111 mg/ 16 mg/195 mg/8 mg. [MYOO-drayn G-G].

**Mudrane GG-2** (Pulm) (generic *theophylline, guaifenesin*). Combination bronchodilator and expectorant drug. Tablet: 111 mg/100 mg. [MYOO-drayn G-G-2].

**Mumpsvax** (Anti-infec). Used to prevent mumps in children. Subcutaneous: Vaccine. [MUMPS-vaks].

**mupirocin** (Bactroban, Bactroban Nasal, Centany) (Derm, ENT). Antibiotic drug used topically on the skin to treat bacterial infections; used in the nose to treat methicillin-resistant *Staphylococcus aureus* (MRSA) colonization. Cream: 2%. Ointment: 2%. [myoo-PEER-oh-sin].

**Murine Ear** (ENT). See *carbamide*. [MYOOR-een].

**Murine Tears Plus** (Ophth). See *tetrahydrozoline*. [MYOOR-een].

**Muro 128** (Ophth). Over-the-counter drug used topically in the eye to reduce corneal edema after eye surgery. Ophthalmic ointment: 5%. Ophthalmic solution: 2%, 5%. [MYOOR-oh 128].

**Murocel** (Ophth). Over-the-counter artificial tears for dry eyes. Ophthalmic solution. [MYOOR-oh-sel].

**Murocoll-2** (Ophth) (generic *phenylephrine, scopolamine*). Combination mydriatic drug used topically to dilate the pupil before eye examinations or surgery. Ophthalmic solution: 10%/0.3%. [MYOOR-oh-kawl-2].

**muromonab-CD3** (Orthoclone OKT3) (Cardio, Chemo, GI, Uro). Immunosuppressant monoclonal antibody drug given after organ transplantation to prevent rejection of the donor heart, liver, or kidney; used to prevent or treat graft-versus-host disease following bone marrow transplantation. Intravenous: 5 mg/5 mL. [MYOOR-oh-MAWN-ab-C-D-3].

**Muse** (Uro). See *alprostadil*. [MYOOZ].

**Mustargen** (Chemo, Hem). See *mechlorethamine*. [MUS-tar-jen].

**Musterole Deep Strength Rub** (Ortho) (generic *methyl salicylate, menthol*). Combination over-the-counter analgesic drug used topically to treat the pain of osteoarthritis and minor muscle injuries. Liquid. [MUS-ter-awl].

**Mutamycin** (Chemo). See *mitomycin*. [MYOO-tah-MY-sin].

**M-Vax** (Chemo). Chemotherapy drug vaccine used to treat melanoma. Orphan drug. [M-vaks].

**M.V.I.-12** (I.V.). See *intravenous multivitamins*. [M-V-I-12].

**Myambutol** (Anti-infec, Pulm). See *ethambutol*. [my-AM-byoo-tawl].

**Mycamine** (Anti-infec). See *micafungin*. [MY-kah-meen].

**Mycelex** (Anti-infec, ENT). See *clotrimazole*. [MY-seh-leks].

**Mycelex-3** (Anti-infec, OB/GYN). See *butoconazole*. [MY-seh-leks-3].

**Mycelex-7** (Anti-infec, OB/GYN). See *clotrimazole*. [MY-seh-leks-7].

**Mycinettes** (ENT). See *benzocaine*. [MY-sih-NETZ].

**Myco-Biotic II** (Derm) (generic *neomycin, triamcinolone*). Combination antibiotic and corticosteroid drug used topically to treat inflammation and bacterial infections on the skin. Cream: 0.5%/0.1%. [MY-koh-by-AW-tik 2].

**Mycobutin** (Anti-infec). See *rifabutin*. [MY-koh-BYOO-tin].

**Mycogen II** (Derm) (generic *nystatin, triamcinolone*). Combination antiyeast and corticosteroid drug used topically to treat inflammation and yeast infections on the skin. Cream: 100,000 units/0.1%. Ointment: 100,000 units/0.1%. [MY-koh-jen 2].

**Mycograb** (Anti-infec). Used to treat systemic candidiasis. Orphan drug. [MY-koh-grab].

**Mycolog-II** (Derm) (generic *nystatin, triamcinolone*). Combination antiyeast and corticosteroid drug used topically to treat inflammation and yeast infections on the skin. Cream: 100,000 units/0.1%. Ointment: 100,000 units/0.1%. [MY-koh-lawg-2].

**mycophenolate** (CellCept, Myfortic) (Cardio, GI, Neuro, Uro). Immunosuppressant drug given after organ transplantation to prevent rejection of the donor heart, liver, or kidney; orphan drug used to treat myasthenia gravis. Capsule: 250 mg. Tablet: 500 mg. Delayed-release tablet: 180 mg, 360 mg. Oral suspension: 200 mg/mL. Intravenous (powder to be reconstituted): 500 mg/20 mL. [MY-koh-FEN-oh-layt].

**Mycostatin, Mycostatin Pastilles** (Derm, ENT). See *nystatin*. [MY-koh-STAT-in].

**Myco-Triacet II** (Derm) (generic *nystatin, triamcinolone*). Combination antiyeast and corticosteroid drug used topically on the skin to treat yeast infections. Cream: 100,000 units/0.1%. Ointment: 100,000 units/0.1%. [MY-koh-TRY-ah-set 2].

**Mydfrin** (Ophth). See *phenylephrine*. [MID-frin].

**Mydriacyl** (Ophth). See *tropicamide*. [mih-DRY-ah-sil].

**myelin** (Neuro). Used to treat multiple sclerosis. Orphan drug. [MY-eh-lin].

**Myfortic** (Uro). See *mycophenolate*. [my-FOR-tik].

**Mylanta, Mylanta Regular Strength, Mylanta Extra Strength** (GI) (generic *aluminum, magnesium, simethicone*). Combination antacid and anti-gas drug used to treat heartburn and gas. Liquid: 200 mg/200 mg/20 mg, 400 mg/400 mg/40 mg. [my-LAN-tah].

**Mylanta Antacid Gelcaps, Mylanta Ultra Tabs, Mylanta Supreme** (GI) (generic *calcium, magnesium*). Combination antacid drug used to treat heartburn. Gelcap: 550 mg/125 mg. Liquid: 400/135 mg. Tablet: 700 mg/ 300 mg. [my-LAN-tah].

**Mylanta Children's** (GI). See *calcium carbonate*. [my-LAN-tah].

**Mylanta Gas, Mylanta Gas Extra Strength** (GI). See *simethicone*. [my-LAN-tah].

**Myleran** (Chemo).    See *busulfan*. [MY-leh-ran].

**Mylicon** (GI).    See *simethicone*. [ [MY-lih-kawn].

**Mylinax** (Chemo).    See *cladribine*. [MY-lih-naks].

**Myobloc** (Ortho).    See *botulinum toxin type B*. [MY-oh-blawk].

**Myochrysine** (Ortho).    See *gold sodium thiomalate*. [MY-oh-KRIH-seen].

**Mylotarg** (Chemo).    See *gemtuzumab*. [MY-loh-targ]

**Myotrophin** (Neuro).    See *mecasermin*. [MY-oh-TROH-fin].

**Mylovenge** (Chemo).    Chemotherapy drug used to treat multiple myeloma. Orphan drug. [MY-loh-venj].

**Myozyme** (Misc).    See *alglucosidase alfa*. [MY-oh-zime].

**Myrac** (Anti-infec).    See *minocycline*. [MY-rak].

**Mysoline** (Neuro).    See *primidone*. [MY-soh-leen].

**Mytelase** (Neuro).    See *ambenonium*. [MY-teh-lays].

**M-Vax** (Chemo).    Used to treat malignant melanoma. Orphan drug. [M-vaks].

**M.V.I.-12, M.V.I. Pediatric** (I.V.).    Combination drug with 9 water-soluble and 3 fat-soluble vitamins. Intravenous. [M-V-I].

**M-Zole 3 Combination Pack, M-Zole 7 Dual Pack** (OB/GYN).    See *miconazole*. [M-zohl].

**Nabi-HB** (GI).    See *hepatitis B immunoglobulin*. [NAH-bee-H-B].

**nabilone** (Cesamet) (Chemo, GI).    Schedule II cannabinoid drug used to treat nausea and vomiting caused by chemotherapy. Capsule: 1 mg. [NAB-ih-lohn].

**nabumetone** (Analges).    Nonsteroidal anti-inflammatory drug used to treat the pain of osteoarthritis and rheumatoid arthritis. Tablet: 500 mg, 750 mg. [nah-BYOO-meh-tohn].

**nadolol** (Corgard) (Analges, Cardio, GI, Neuro).    Beta-blocker drug used to treat angina pectoris and hypertension; used to prevent migraine headaches; used to prevent bleeding varices in patients with portal hypertension; used to treat the tremors of Parkinson's disease. Tablet: 20 mg, 40 mg, 80 mg, 120 mg, 160 mg. [NAD-oh-lawl].

**nafarelin** (Synarel) (Endo, OB/GYN).    Hormonal drug used to treat precocious puberty; used to treat endometriosis. Nasal spray: 2 mg/mL. [NAF-ah-REL-in].

**nafcillin** (Anti-infec).    Penicillin-type antibiotic drug used to treat staphylococcal bacterial infections. Intravenous (powder to be reconstituted): 1 g, 2 g. [naf-SIL-in].

**naftifine** (Naftine) (Derm).    Antifungal drug used topically to treat tinea (ringworm) and other fungal skin infections. Cream: 1%. Gel: 1%. [NAF-tih-feen].

**Naftin** (Derm).    See *naftifine*. [NAF-tin].

**Naglazyme** (Misc).    See *galsulfase*. [NAG-lah-zime].

**nalbuphine** (Nubain) (Analges, Anes).    Narcotic analgesic drug used to treat moderate-to-severe pain; used to treat pain during labor and delivery; used as a preoperative drug and to maintain general anesthesia. Intravenous: 10 mg/mL, 20 mg/mL. [NAL-byoo-feen].

**Naldecon Senior EX** (Pulm).    See *guaifenesin*. [NAL-deh-kawn].

**Nalfon** (Analges).    See *fenoprofen*. [NAL-fawn].

**nalidixic acid** (NegGram) (Anti-infec).    Quinolone antibiotic drug used to treat gram-negative bacterial infections of the urinary tract. Tablet: 500 mg. [NAL-ih-DIK-sik AS-id].

**nalmefene** (Analges, Emerg).    Narcotic antagonist drug used to reverse the effects of narcotic overdose. Subcutaneous, intramuscular, intravenous: 100 mcg/mL, 1 mg/mL. [NAL-meh-feen]

**naloxone** (Narcan) (Analges, Anes, Emerg, Neuro, Psych).    Narcotic antagonist drug used to reverse the effects of narcotic drug overdose; used to reverse narcotic dependence in babies born to addicts; used to reverse the effects of narcotic drugs used during surgery; used to treat alcoholic coma. Endotracheal, intravenous: 0.02 mg/mL, 0.4 mg/mL. [nah-LAWK-sohn].

**naltrexone** (ReVia, Trexan, Vivitrol) (Psych).    Narcotic antagonist drug used to block the effect of narcotic drugs as ongoing treatment for former narcotic-dependent patients; used to treat alcohol dependence. Tablet: 50 mg. Intravenous, subcutaneous. [nal-TREK-sohn].

**Namenda** (Neuro).    See *memantine*. [nah-MEN-dah].

**Napa** (Cardio).    Used to alter the energy requirement for patients to have an implantable cardioverter defibrillator. Orphan drug. [NAP-ah].

**naphazoline** (Albalon, Privine) (ENT, Ophth).    Decongestant/vasoconstrictor drug used topically to treat irritation and allergy symptoms in the eyes; over-the-counter decongestant drug used topically to treat nasal stuffiness due to colds or allergies. Nasal drops: 0.05%. Nasal spray: 0.05%. Ophthalmic solution: 0.012%, 0.03%, 0.1%. [NAF-ah-ZOH-leen].

**Naprelan** (Analges).    See *naproxen*. [NAP-reh-lan].

**Naprosyn** (Analges).    See *naproxen*. [NAP-roh-sin].

**naproxen** (Aleve, Anaprox, Anaprox DS, Midol Extended Relief, Naprelan, Naprosyn) (Analges).    Prescription and over-the-counter nonsteroidal anti-inflammatory drug used to treat pain and inflammation; used to treat osteoarthritis, rheumatoid arthritis, ankylosing spondylitis, bursitis, tendinitis, and gout; used to treat dysmenorrhea (Midol). Tablet: 200 mg, 250 mg, 375 mg, 500 mg. Delayed-release tablet: 375 mg, 500 mg. Controlled-release tablet: 375 mg, 500 mg. Oral liquid: 125 mg/5 mL. [nah-PRAWK-sen].

**naratriptan** (Amerge) (Analges).    Serotonin receptor agonist drug used to treat migraine headaches. Tablet: 1 mg, 2.5 mg. [NAIR-ah-TRIP-tan].

**Narcan** (Analges, Anes, Emerg, Neuro, Psych).    See *naloxone*. [NAR-kan].

**Nardil** (Psych).    See *phenelzine*. [NAR-dil].

**Naropin** (Anes, OB/GYN).    See *ropivacaine*. [NAIR-oh-pin].

**Nasacort AQ, Nasacort HFA** (ENT).    See *triamcinolone*. [NAY-sah-kort].

**Nasalcrom** (ENT).    See *cromolyn*. [NAY-sal-krawm].

**Nasalide** (ENT).    See *flunisolide*. [NAY-sah-lide].

**Nascobal** (Hem).    See *cyanocobalamin*. [NAS-koh-bal].

**Nasonex** (ENT). See *mometasone*. [NAY-soh-neks].

**Natacyn** (Ophth). See *natamycin*. [NAT-ah-sin].

**natalizumab** (Tysabri) (GI, Neuro). Monoclonal antibody drug used to treat Crohn's disease; used to treat multiple sclerosis. Intravenous: 300 mg/15 mL. [NAY-tal-IZ-yoo-mab].

**natamycin** (Natacyn) (Ophth). Antifungal drug used topically to treat fungal infections of the eyes. Ophthalmic suspension: 5%. [nat-ah-MY-sin].

**nateglinide** (Starlix) (Endo). Meglitinide oral antidiabetic drug used to treat type 2 diabetes mellitus. Tablet: 60 mg, 120 mg. [nah-TEG-lih-nide].

**Natelle Plus DHA** (OB/GYN). Prenatal vitamin. Tablet. [nah-TEL PLUS D-H-A].

**Natrecor** (Cardio). See *nesiritide*. [NAY-treh-kor].

**Nature-Throid** (Endo). See *desiccated thyroid*. [NAY-chur-throid].

**Naturetin** (Cardio, Uro). See *bendroflumethiazide*. [NAH-tyoo-RAY-tin].

**Navane** (Neuro, Psych). See *thiothixene*. [NAH-vain].

**Navelbine** (Chemo). See *vinorelbine*. [NAY-vel-been].

**nebacumab** (Centoxin) (Anti-infec). Monoclonal antibody drug used to treat gram-negative bacteremia and shock. Orphan drug. [neh-BAK-yoo-mab].

**nebivolol** (Bystolic) (Cardio). Cardioselective beta-blocker drug used to treat hypertension. Tablet: 2.5 mg, 5 mg, 10 mg. [neh-BIV-oh-lawl].

**NebuPent** (Anti-infec). See *pentamidine*. [NEB-yoo-pent].

**Necon 0.5/35** (OB/GYN) (generic *norethindrone, ethinyl estradiol*). Combination monophasic oral contraceptive drug. Pill pack, 21-day: (21 hormone tablets) 0.5 mg/ 35 mcg. Pill pack, 28-day: (21 hormone tablets) 0.5 mg/ 35 mcg; (7 inert tablets). [NEE-kawn].

**Necon 1/35** (OB/GYN) (generic *norethindrone, ethinyl estradiol*). Combination monophasic oral contraceptive drug. Pill pack, 21-day: (21 hormone tablets) 1 mg/35 mcg. Pill pack, 28-day: (21 hormone tablets) 1 mg/35 mcg; (7 inert tablets). [NEE-kawn].

**Necon 1/50** (OB/GYN) (generic *norethindrone, mestranol*). Combination monophasic oral contraceptive drug. Pill pack, 21-day: (21 hormone tablets) 1 mg/50 mcg. Pill pack, 28-day: (21 hormone tablets) 1 mg/50 mcg; (7 inert tablets). [NEE-kawn].

**Necon 7/7/7** (OB/GYN) (generic *norethindrone, ethinyl estradiol*). Combination triphasic oral contraceptive drug. Pill pack, 28-day: (7 hormone tablets) 0.5 mg/35 mcg; (7 hormone tablets) 0.75 mg/35 mcg; (7 hormone tablets) 1 mg/35 mcg; (7 inert tablets). [NEE-kawn].

**Necon 10/11** (OB/GYN) (generic *norethindrone, ethinyl estradiol*). Combination biphasic combination oral contraceptive drug. Pill pack (Dialpak), 28-day: (10 hormone tablets) 0.5 mg/35 mcg; (11 hormone tablets) 1 mg/35 mcg; (7 inert tablets). [NEE-kawn].

**nedocromil** (Alocril) (Ophth). Mast cell stabilizer drug used topically to treat allergy symptoms in the eyes. Ophthalmic solution: 2%. [NEE-doh-KROH-mil].

**nefazodone** (Psych). Antidepressant drug used to treat depression. Tablet: 50 mg, 100 mg, 150 mg, 200 mg, 250 mg. [neh-FAZ-oh-dohn].

**Negaban** (Anti-infec). See *temocillin*. [NEG-ah-ban].

**NegGram** (Anti-infec). See *nalidixic acid*. [NEG-gram].

**nelarabine** (Arranon) (Chemo). Demethylating chemotherapy drug used to treat leukemia and lymphoma. Intravenous: 5 mg/mL. [neh-LAIR-ah-been].

**nelfinavir** (Viracept) (Anti-infec). Protease inhibitor antiviral drug used to treat HIV and AIDS. Tablet: 250 mg, 625 mg. Powder (to be reconstituted to an oral liquid as scoops or teaspoons): 50 mg. [nel-FIN-ah-veer].

**Neoasma** (Pulm) (generic *theophylline, guaifenesin*). Combination bronchodilator and expectorant drug. Tablet: 125 mg/100 mg. [NEE-oh-AS-mah].

**NeoDecadron Ophthalmic** (Ophth) (generic *dexamethasone, neomycin*). Combination corticosteroid and antibiotic drug used topically in the eyes to treat inflammation and bacterial infections. Ophthalmic solution: 0.1%/0.35%. [NEE-oh-DEK-ah-drawn of-THAL-mik].

**Neo-fradin** (Anti-infec). See *neomycin*. [NEE-oh-FRAY-din].

**Neofrin** (Ophth). See *phenylephrine*. [NEE-oh-frin].

**Neoloid** (GI). See *castor oil*. [NEE-oh-loyd].

**Neomark** (Chemo). See *broxuridine*. [NEE-oh-mark].

**neomycin** (Neo-fradin) (Anti-infec). Aminoglycoside antibiotic drug given orally as a bowel prep before intra-abdominal surgery; given orally to treat hepatic coma by killing ammonia-producing bacteria in the intestines. Tablet: 500 mg. Liquid: 125 mg/5 mL. [NEE-oh-MY-sin].

**Neoprofen** (Cardio). See *ibuprofen lysine*. [NEE-oh-PROH-fen].

**Neoral** (Cardio, Derm, GI, Hem, Ortho, Uro). See *cyclosporine*. [nee-OR-al].

**Neosar** (Chemo, Uro). See *cyclophosphamide*. [NEE-oh-sar].

**Neosol** (GI, Uro). See *L-hyoscyamine*. [NEE-oh-sawl].

**Neosporin AF** (Derm). See *miconazole*. [NEE-oh-SPOR-in A-F].

**Neosporin G.U. Irrigant** (Uro) (generic *neomycin, polymyxin B*). Combination antibiotic drug used to prevent urinary tract infection in patients with a urinary catheter. Irrigating solution: 40 mg/200,000 units. [NEE-oh-SPOR-in].

**Neosporin Ophthalmic Ointment** (Ophth) (generic *bacitracin, neosporin, polymyxin B*). Combination antibiotic drug used topically in the eyes. Ophthalmic ointment: 400 units/3.5 mg/10,000 units per g. [NEE-oh-SPOR-in].

**Neosporin Original** (Derm) (generic *bacitracin, neomycin, polymyxin B*). Combination over-the-counter antibiotic drug used topically on the skin. Ointment: 400 units/ 3.5 mg/5000 units per g. [NEE-oh-SPOR-in].

**Neosporin Plus Pain Relief Cream** (Derm) (generic *neomycin, polymyxin B, pramoxine*). Combination over-the-counter antibiotic and anesthetic drug used topically on the skin. Cream: 3.5 mg/10,000 units/10 mg per g. [NEE-oh-SPOR-in].

**Neosporin Plus Pain Relief Ointment** (Derm) (generic *bacitracin, neomycin, polymyxin B, pramoxine*). Combination over-the-counter antibiotic and anesthetic drug used topically on the skin. Ointment: 500 units/ 3.5 mg/10,000 units/10 mg. [NEE-oh-SPOR-in].

**neostigmine** (Prostigmin) (Neuro, Uro). Anticholinesterase drug used to treat myasthenia gravis; urinary antispasmodic drug used to prevent and treat postoperative urinary retention. Subcutaneous and intramuscular: 1:2000 solution (0.5 mg/mL), 1:4000 solution (0.25 mg/mL). [NEE-oh-STIG-meen].

**NeoStrata** (Derm). See *hydroquinone*. [NEE-oh-STRAH-tah].

**Neo-Synephrine** (Cardio, Emerg). See *phenylephrine*. [NEE-oh-sih-NEH-frin].

**Neo-Synephrine 4-Hour Mild Formula** (ENT). See *phenylephrine*. [NEE-oh-sih-NEF-rin].

**Neo-Synephrine 12-Hour** (ENT). See *oxymetazoline*. [NEE-oh-sih-NEF-rin].

**Neovastat** (Chemo). Chemotherapy drug used to treat cancer of the kidney. Orphan drug. [NEE-oh-VAS-stat].

**nepafenac** (Nevanac) (Ophth). Nonsteroidal anti-inflammatory drug used topically to treat pain and inflammation in the eye after corneal surgery. Ophthalmic suspension: 0.1%. [neh-PAF-en-nak].

**Nephro-Fer** (Hem). See *ferrous fumarate*. [NEH-froh-fair].

**Nepro** (GI). Lactose-free nutritional supplement. Liquid. [NEH-proh].

**Nesacaine, Nesacaine MPF** (Anes). See *chloroprocaine*. [NES-ah-kayn].

**nesiritide** (Natrecor) (Cardio). Human B-type natriuretic peptide drug used to treat severe congestive heart failure. Intravenous: 1.5 mg/mL. [neh-SEER-ih-tide].

**Nestle VHC 2.25** (GI). Lactose-free, gluten-free nutritional supplement. Liquid. [NEST-lee V-H-C].

**Neulasta** (Chemo). See *pegfilgrastim*. [noo-LAS-tah].

**Neumega** (Chemo, Hem). See *oprelvekin*. [noo-MAY-gah].

**Neupogen** (Anti-infec, Chemo, Hem). See *filgrastim*. [NOO-poh-jen].

**Neuprex** (Neuro). Used to treat meningococcal infection of the brain. Orphan drug. [NOO-preks].

**Neupro** (Neuro). See *rotigotine*. [NOO-proh].

**Neuralgon** (Neuro, Ortho). See *L-baclofen*. [nyoor-AL-gawn].

**Neurelan** (Neuro). See *fampridine*. [NYOOR-eh-lan].

**NeuroCell-PD** (Neuro). Fetal pig nerve cells that are surgically implanted in the brain to produce dopamine to treat Parkinson's disease. Orphan drug. [NYOOR-oh-sel-P-D].

**NeuroCell-HD** (Neuro). Fetal pig nerve cells that are surgically implanted in the brain to produce GABA, one of the chemical compounds lacking in patients with Huntington's chorea. Orphan drug. [NYOOR-oh-sel-H-D].

**NeuroendoMedix** (Chemo). See *indium 111*. [NYOOR-oh-EN-doh-MED-iks].

**Neurontin** (Analges, Neuro, Psych). See *gabapentin*. [nyoor-AWN-tin].

**Neurosolve** (Ophth). See *urea*. [NYOOR-oh-sawlv].

**Neutrexin** (Anti-infec, Chemo). See *trimetrexate*. [noo-TREK-sin].

**Neutra-Phos, Neutra-Phos K** (Misc). See *phosphorus*. [NOO-trah-faws].

**Neutrogena Clear Pore** (Derm). See *benzoyl peroxide*. [NOO-troh-JEE-nah].

**Neutrogena Oil-free Acne Wash** (Derm). See *salicylic acid*. [NOO-troh-JEE-nah].

**Neutrogena T/Gel Original** (Derm). See *coal tar*. [NOO-troh-JEE-nah T jel].

**Nevanac** (Ophth). See *nepafenac*. [NEV-ah-nak].

**nevirapine** (Viramune) (Anti-infec). Nonnucleoside reverse transcriptase inhibitor antiviral drug used to treat HIV and AIDS. Tablet: 200 mg. Oral liquid: 50 mg/5 mL. [neh-VEER-ah-peen].

**Nexavar** (GI, Uro). See *sorafenib*. [NEK-sah-var].

**Nexium, Nexium I.V.** (GI). See *esomeprazole*. [NEK-see-um].

**niacin** (Niacor, Niaspan) (Cardio). Vitamin B drug used to lower serum cholesterol and triglyceride levels. Extended-release and sustained-release capsule: 125 mg, 250 mg, 400 mg, 500 mg. Tablet: 100 mg, 250 mg, 500 mg. Controlled-release and timed-release tablet: 250 mg, 500 mg. Extended-release tablet: 500 mg, 750 mg, 1000 mg. [NY-ah-sin].

**Niacor** (Cardio). See *niacin*. [NY-ah-kor].

**Niaspan** (Cardio). See *niacin*. [NY-ah-span].

**nicardipine** (Cardene, Cardene I.V., Cardene SR) (Cardio). Calcium channel blocker drug used to treat angina pectoris and hypertension. Capsule: 20 mg, 30 mg. Sustained-release capsule: 30 mg, 45 mg, 60 mg. Intravenous: 2.5 mg/mL. [ny-KAR-dih-peen].

**Nicoderm CQ Step 1, Nicoderm CQ Step 2, Nicoderm CQ Step 3** (Pulm, Psych). See *nicotine*. [NIK-oh-derm C-Q].

**Nicorette** (Pulm, Psych). See *nicotine*. [NIK-oh-RET].

**nicotine** (Commit, Nicoderm CQ Step 1, Nicoderm CQ Step 2, Nicoderm CQ Step 3, Nicorette, Nicotrol Inhaler, Nicotrol NS, Nicotrol Step 1, Nicotrol Step 2, Nicotrol Step 3) (Pulm, Psych). Prescription and over-the-counter nicotine drug with nicotine in decreasing amounts to help persons to stop smoking. Chewing gum: 2 mg/piece, 4 mg/piece. Lozenge: 2 mg. Nasal spray: 0.5 mg/spray. Inhaler and cartridge: 4 mg/10 mg cartridge. Transdermal patch: 5 mg/ 4 hr, 7 mg/24 hr, 10 mg/24 hr, 14 mg/24 hr, 15 mg/24 hr, 21 mg/24 hr. [NIK-oh-teen].

**Nicotrol Inhaler, Nicotrol NS, Nicotrol Step 1, Nicotrol Step 2, Nicotrol Step 3** (Pulm, Psych).   See *nicotine*. [NIK-oh-trawl].

**Nifediac CC, Nifediac XL** (Cardio).   See *nifedipine*. [ny-FED-ee-ak].

**nifedipine** (Adalat CC, Afeditab CR, Nifediac CC, Nifediac XL, Procardia, Procardia XL) (Cardio, OB/GYN, Uro)   Calcium channel blocker drug used to prevent and treat angina pectoris, hypertension, and pulmonary arterial hypertension; used to treat Raynaud's disease; used to treat preterm labor; orphan drug used to treat interstitial cystitis. Capsule: 10 mg, 20 mg. Extended-release tablet: 30 mg, 60 mg, 90 mg. [ny-FED-ih-peen].

**Nilandron** (Chemo).   See *nilutamide*. [nil-AN-drohn].

**nilotinib** (Tasigna) (Chemo).   Chemotherapy drug used to treat leukemia. Capsule: 200 mg. [nih-LOH-tih-nib].

**Nilstat** (Derm, ENT).   See *nystatin*. [NIL-stat].

**nilutamide** (Nilandron) (Chemo).   Hormonal chemotherapy drug used to treat cancer of the prostate gland in men. Tablet: 50 mg, 150 mg. [nih-LOO-tah-mide].

**Nimbex** (Anes, Pulm).   See *cisatracurium*. [NIM-beks].

**nimodipine** (Nimotop) (Neuro).   Calcium channel blocker drug used to increase blood flow to improve neurologic deficits after subarachnoid hemorrhage. Capsule: 30 mg. [nih-MOH-dih-peen].

**Nimotop** (Neuro).   See *nimodipine*. [NIM-oh-top].

**nimotuzumab** (Chemo).   Monoclonal antibody drug used to treat brain cancer. Orphan drug. [NIH-moh-TOOZ-yoo-mab].

**Nipent** (Chemo).   See *pentostatin*. [NY-pent].

**niprisan** (Hemoxin) (Hem).   Used to treat sickle cell disease. Orphan drug. [NIP-rih-san].

**nisoldipine** (Sular, Sular ER) (Cardio).   Calcium channel blocker drug used to treat hypertension. Extended-release tablet: 8.5 mg, 10 mg, 17 mg, 20 mg, 25.5 mg, 30 mg, 34 mg, 40 mg. [ny-SOL-dih-peen].

**nitazoxanide** (Alinia, Cryptaz) (GI).   Antiprotozoal drug used to treat intestinal amebiasis, intestinal giardiasis, and diarrhea caused by protozoa. Tablet: 500 mg. Powder (to be reconstituted to oral liquid): 100 mg/5 mL. [NY-tah-ZAWK-sah-nide].

**nitisinone** (Orfadin) (Misc).   Used to treat tyrosinemia. Capsule: 2 mg, 5 mg, 10 mg. [ny-TIH-sih-nohn].

**Nitrek** (Cardio).   See *nitroglycerin*. [NY-trek].

**nitric oxide** (INOmax) (Pulm).   Used to treat persistent pulmonary hypertension and chronic lung disease in newborns; used to treat acute respiratory distress syndrome in adults on the ventilator; orphan drug used to diagnose sarcoidosis. Inhaled gas: 100 ppm, 800 ppm. [NY-trik AWK-side].

**Nitro-Bid** (Cardio).   See *nitroglycerin*. [NY-troh-bid].

**Nitro-Dur** (Cardio).   See *nitroglycerin*. [NY-troh-door].

**nitrofurantoin** (Furadantin, Macrobid, Macrodantin) (Anti-infec, Uro).   Antibiotic drug used to treat urinary tract infections. Capsule: 25 mg, 50 mg, 100 mg. Oral suspension: 25 mg/5 mL. [NY-troh-fyoor-AN-toh-in].

**nitrofurazone** (Furacin) (Derm).   Anti-infective drug used topically to treat severe burns. Cream: 0.2%. Liquid: 0.2%. Ointment: 0.2%. [NY-troh-FYOOR-ah-zohn].

**nitrogen mustard** (Chemo).   See *mechlorethamine*. [NY-troh-jen MUS-tard].

**nitroglycerin** (Minitran, Nitrek, Nitro-Bid, Nitro-Dur, Nitrolingual, NitroMist, NitroQuick, Nitrostat, NitroTab, Nitro-Time) (Cardio).   Nitrate drug used to prevent and treat angina pectoris; used to treat congestive heart failure after a myocardial infarction; used to induce intraoperative hypotension. Capsule: 2.5 mg, 6.5 mg, 9 mg. Sublingual tablet: 0.3 mg, 0.4 mg, 0.6 mg. Translingual spray: 0.4 mg/spray. Ointment: 2% (15 mg/1 inch). Transdermal patch: 9 mg, 18 mg, 20 mg, 22.4 mg, 36 mg, 40 mg, 44.8 mg, 54 mg, 60 mg, 67.2 mg, 80 mg, 120 mg, 160 mg. Intravenous: 5 mg/mL. [NY-troh-GLIH-sair-in].

**Nitrolingual** (Cardio).   See *nitroglycerin*. [NY-troh-LING-gwal].

**NitroMist** (Cardio).   See *nitroglycerin*. [NY-troh-mist].

**Nitropress** (Cardio).   See *nitroprusside*. [NY-troh-pres].

**nitroprusside** (Nitropress) (Cardio).   Peripheral vasodilator drug used to treat hypertensive crisis and acute congestive heart failure; orphan drug used to treat vasospasm after subarachnoid hemorrhage in the brain. Intravenous (powder to be reconstituted): 50 mg/5 mL. [NY-troh-PRUS-side].

**NitroQuick** (Cardio).   See *nitroglycerin*. [NY-troh-kwik].

**Nitrostat** (Cardio).   See *nitroglycerin*. [NY-troh-stat].

**NitroTab** (Cardio).   See *nitroglycerin*. [NY-troh-tab].

**Nitro-Time** (Cardio).   See *nitroglycerin*. [NY-troh-time].

**nizatidine** (Axid, Axid AR, Axid Pulvules) (GI).   Over-the-counter and prescription $H_2$ blocker drug used to treat heartburn, peptic ulcers, and *H. pylori* infection. Capsule: 150 mg, 300 mg. Tablet: 75 mg. Oral liquid: 15 mg/mL. [nih-ZAH-tih-deen].

**Nizoral, Nizoral A-D** (Derm).   See *ketoconazole*. [ny-ZOHR-al].

**Nolahist** (ENT, Ophth).   See *phenindamine*. [NOH-lah-hist].

**nonoxynol-9** (Advantage 24, Contraceptrol, Delfen, Gynol II, KY Plus, Semicid, Today Sponge, VCF) (OB/GYN).   Over-the-counter spermicide drug used to prevent pregnancy. Vaginal film: 28%. Vaginal foam: 12.5%. Vaginal gel: 2%, 2.2%, 3.5%, 4%. Vaginal jelly: 3%. Vaginal sponge: 1000 mg. Suppository: 100 mg. [nawn-AWK-sih-nawl-9].

**Nootropil** (Ortho).   See *piracetam*. [NOO-troh-pil].

**Nora-BE** (OB/GYN).   See *norethindrone*. [NOR-ah-B-E].

**Norco** (Analges) (generic *acetaminophen, hydrocodone*).   Combination Schedule III nonnarcotic and narcotic analgesic drug for pain. Tablet: 325 mg/5 mg, 325 mg/10 mg. [NOR-koh].

**Norcuron** (Anes, Pulm).   See *vecuronium*. [NOR-kyoor-awn].

**Nordette** (OB/GYN) (generic *levonorgestrel, ethinyl estradiol*).   Combination monophasic oral contraceptive drug. Pill pack, 21-day: (21 hormone tablets) 0.15 mg/ 30 mcg. Pill pack, 28-day: (21 hormone tablets) 0.15 mg/ 30 mcg; (7 inert tablets). [nor-DET].

**Norditropin** (Endo, OB/GYN).  See *somatropin*. [NOR-dih-TROH-pin].

**norepinephrine** (Levophed) (Emerg).  Vasopressor drug used to treat hypotension during cardiac arrest and resuscitation. Intravenous: 1 mg/mL. [NOR-ep-ih-NEH-frin].

**norethindrone** (Aygestin, Camila, Errin, Jolivette, Nora-BE, Nor-Q.D., Ortho Micronor) (OB/GYN).  Progestin hormone drug used to treat amenorrhea, abnormal uterine bleeding, and endometriosis (Aygestin); progestin-only oral contraceptive drug. Tablet: 5 mg. Pill pack, 28-day: (28 hormone tablets) 0.35 mg. [nor-ETH-in-drohn].

**Norflex** (Ortho).  See *orphenadrine*. [NOR-fleks].

**norfloxacin** (Noroxin) (Anti-infec).  Fluoroquinolone antibiotic drug used to treat gram-negative and gram-positive infections; used to treat urinary tract infections, prostatitis, and gonorrhea; used to treat Legionnaire's disease of the lungs. Tablet: 400 mg. [nor-FLAWK-sah-sin].

**Norgesic** (Ortho) (generic *aspirin, orphenadrine, caffeine*).  Combination analgesic, skeletal muscle relaxant and stimulant drug used to treat pain, spasm, and stiffness associated with minor muscle injuries. Tablet: 385 mg/25 mg/30 mg. [nor-JEE-sik].

**norgestrel** (Ovrette) (OB/GYN).  Progestin-only oral contraceptive drug. Pill pack, 28-day: (28 hormone tablets) 0.75 mg. [nor-JES-trel].

**Norinyl 1 + 35** (OB/GYN) (generic *norethindrone, ethinyl estradiol*).  Combination monophasic oral contraceptive drug. Pill pack (Wallette), 21-day: (21 hormone tablets) 1 mg/35 mcg. Pill pack, (Wallette), 28-day: (21 hormone tablets) 1 mg/35 mcg; (7 inert tablets). [NOR-ih-nil].

**Norinyl 1 + 50** (OB/GYN) (generic *norethindrone, mestranol*).  Combination monophasic oral contraceptive drug. Pill pack (Wallette), 21-day: (21 hormone tablets) 1 mg/50 mcg. Pill pack (Wallette), 28-day: (21 hormone tablets) 1 mg/50 mcg; (7 inert tablets). [NOR-ih-nil].

**Noritate** (Derm).  See *metronidazole*. [NOR-ih-tayt].

**normal saline** (NS) (0.9% NaCl) (I.V.).  Combination of sodium and water at the same concentration as tissue fluids. Intravenous fluid. [NOR-mal SAY-leen].

**Normix** (Neuro).  See *rifaximin*. [NOR-miks].

**Normocarb HF** (Hem).  See *biocarbonate infusate*. [NOR-moh-karb H-F].

**Normodyne** (Cardio, Endo).  See *labetalol*. [NOR-moh-dine].

**Normosang** (Chemo).  Chemotherapy drug used to treat myelodysplastic syndrome and acute porphyria. Orphan drug. [NOR-moh-sang].

**Noroxin** (Anti-infec).  See *norfloxacin*. [nor-AWK-sin].

**Norpace, Norpace CR** (Cardio).  See *disopyramide*. [NOR-pays].

**Norpramin** (Analges, Neuro, Psych, Uro).  See *desipramine*. [NOR-prah-min].

**Nor-Q.D.** (OB/GYN).  See *norethindrone*. [NOR-Q-D].

**Nortrel 0.5/35** (OB/GYN) (generic *norethindrone, ethinyl estradiol*).  Combination monophasic oral contraceptive drug. Pill pack, 21-day: (21 hormone tablets) 0.5 mg/35 mcg. Pill pack, 28-day (21 hormone tablets) 0.5 mg/35 mcg; (7 inert tablets). [nor-TREL].

**Nortrel 1/35** (OB/GYN) (generic *norethindrone, ethinyl estradiol*).  Combination monophasic oral contraceptive drug. Pill pack, 21-day: (21 hormone tablets) 1 mg/35 mcg. Pill pack, 28-day (21 hormone tablets) 1 mg/35 mcg; (7 inert tablets). [nor-TREL].

**Nortrel 7/7/7** (OB/GYN) (generic *norethindrone, ethinyl estradiol*).  Combination triphasic oral contraceptive drug. Pill pack, 28-day: (7 hormone tablets) 0.5 mg/35 mcg; (7 hormone tablets) 0.75 mg/35 mg; (7 hormone tablets) 1 mg/35 mcg; (7 inert tablets). [nor-TREL].

**nortriptyline** (Aventyl, Pamelor) (Analges, Neuro, Psych).  Tricyclic antidepressant drug used to treat depression; used to treat panic attacks; used to treat premenstrual dysphoric disorder; used to treat migraine headaches; used to treat nerve pain from phantom limb, diabetic neuropathy, peripheral neuropathy, and postherpetic neuralgia; used to treat tic douloureux. Capsule: 10 mg, 25 mg, 50 mg, 75 mg. Liquid: 10 mg/5 mL. [nor-TRIP-tih-leen].

**Norvasc** (Cardio).  See *amlodipine*. [NOR-vask].

**Norvir** (Anti-infec).  See *ritonavir*. [NOR-veer].

**Norwich Extra-Strength, Norwich Regular Strength** (Analges).  See *aspirin*. [NOR-wich].

**Novacet** (Derm) (generic *sodium sulfacetamide, sulfur*).  Combination anti-infective and keratolytic drug used topically on the skin to treat acne vulgaris. Lotion: 10%/5%. [NOH-vah-set].

**Novahistine DH** (ENT) (generic *chlorpheniramine, dihydrocodeine, phenylephrine*).  Combination Schedule III antihistamine, narcotic antitussive, and decongestant drug used to treat colds with severe coughs. Liquid: 2 mg/7.25 mg/5 mg. [NOH-vah-HIS-teen D-H].

**Novantrone** (Chemo, Neuro).  See *mitoxantrone*. [NOH-van-trohn].

**Novarel** (Endo, OB/GYN).  See *human chorioic gonadotropin*. [NOH-vah-rel].

**Novasal** (Analges).  See *magnesium salicylate*. [NOH-vah-sal].

**NovaSource Renal** (GI, Uro).  Nutritional supplement formulated for renal patients. Liquid. [NOH-vah-sors REE-nal].

**Novocain** (Anes, Ortho).  See *procaine*. [NOH-voh-kayn].

**Novolin N, Novolin N PenFill, Novolin N Prefilled** (Endo).  See *NPH insulin*. [NOH-voh-lin N].

**Novolin R, Novolin R PenFill, Novolin R Prefilled** (Endo).  See *regular insulin*. [NOH-voh-lin R].

**Novolin 70/30, Novolin 70/30 PenFill, Novolin 70/30 Prefilled** (Endo) (generic *NPH insulin, regular insulin*).  Combination intermediate-acting NPH and rapid-acting regular insulin drug used to treat type 1 diabetes mellitus. Subcutaneous: 100 units/mL. [NOH-voh-lin].

**NovoLog** (Endo). See *insulin aspart.* [NOH-voh-lawg].

**NovoLog Mix 70/30** (Endo) (generic *NPH insulin, regular insulin aspart*). Combination intermediate-acting NPH and rapid-acting regular insulin analog drug used to treat type 1 diabetes mellitus. Subcutaneous: 100 units/mL. [NOH-voh-lawg].

**NovoSeven, NovoSeven RT** (Hem). See *factor VIIa.* [NOH-voh-SEH-ven].

**Noxafil** (Anti-infec). See *posaconazole.* [NAWK-sah-fil].

**NPH insulin** (Humulin N, Novolin N, Novolin N PenFill, Novolin N Prefilled) (Endo). Intermediate-acting insulin, derived from recombinant DNA technology, used to treat type 1 diabetes mellitus. Subcutaneous: 100 units/mL. Novolin Pen or NovoPen cartridge [N-P-H IN-soo-lin].

**Nplate** (Hem). See *romiplostim.* [N-playt].

**Nubain** (Analges, Anes). See *nalbuphine.* [NOO-bayn].

**NuLev** (GI, Uro). See *L-hyoscyamine.* [NOO-lev].

**NuLytely** (GI) (generic *polyethylene glycol, electrolyte solution*). Combination bowel evacuant and bowel prep. Oral liquid (powder to be reconstituted). [noo-LITE-lee].

**Numby Stuff** (Anes, Derm). See *lidocaine.* [NUM-bee].

**Numorphan** (Analges, Anes). See *oxymorphone.* [noo-MOR-fan].

**Numzit Teething** (Anes, ENT). See *benzocaine.* [NUM-zit].

**Nupercainal** (Derm, GI). See *dibucaine.* [NOO-per-KAY-nawl].

**Nuquin HP** (Derm). See *hydroquinone.* [NOO-kwin H-P].

**Nursoy** (GI). Infant formula with soy protein. Liquid. Powder (to be reconstituted). [NUR-soy].

**Nutrament** (GI). Nutritional supplement. Liquid. [NOO-trah-ment].

**Nutramigen** (GI). Lactose-free, sucrose-free infant formula for infants with allergies. Liquid. Powder (to be reconstituted). [noo-TRAM-ih-jen].

**NutreStore** (GI). See *glutamine.* [NOO-treh-STOR].

**NutriFocus** (GI). Lactose-free, gluten-free nutritional supplement. Liquid. [NOO-trih-FOH-kuhs].

**NutriHeal** (GI). Nutritional supplement. Liquid. [NOO-trih-heel].

**Nutropin, Nutropin AQ, Nutropin Depot** (Endo). See *somatropin.* [noo-TROH-pin].

**NuvaRIng** (OB/GYN) (generic *etonogestrel, ethinyl estradiol*). Combination monophasic contraceptive drug. Vaginal ring, 3-inch (inserted for 3 weeks): 0.12 mcg/ 0.015 mg per 24 hours. [NOO-vah-ring].

**Nuvigil** (Neuro). See *armodanifil.* [noo-VIJ-il].

**Nydrazid** (Pulm). See *isoniazid.* [NY-drah-zid].

**Nyotran** (Anti-infec). See *nystatin.* [NY-oh-tran].

**nystatin** (Mycostatin, Mycostatin Pastilles, Nilstat, Nyotran, Nystop, Pedi-Dri) (Anti-infec, Derm, ENT, OB/GYN). Antiyeast drug used topically to treat yeast infections of the skin caused by *Candida albicans;* used topically to treat oral candidiasis (thrush); used topically to treat vaginal yeast infections; orphan drug used systemically to treat invasive fungal infections in the body (Nyotran). Cream: 100,000 units/g. Ointment: 100,000 units/g. Topical powder: 100,000 units/g. Oral liquid: 100,000 units/mL. Powder (to be reconstituted to an oral liquid): 100,000 units/g. Tablet: 500,000 units. Troche/Pastille: 200,000 units. Vaginal tablet: 100,000 units. [ny-STAT-in].

**Nystop** (Derm). See *nystatin.* [NY-stop].

**Nytol, Nytol Maximum Strength** (Neuro). See *diphenhydramine.* [NY-tawl].

**obatoclax** (Chemo). Used to treat leukemia. Orphan drug. [oh-BAH-toh-klaks].

**Ocean** (ENT). See *saline.* [OH-shun].

**OCL** (GI) (generic *polyethylene glycol, electrolyte solution*). Combination bowel evacuant and bowel prep. Oral liquid. [O-C-L].

**Octagam** (Anti-infec, Misc). See *human immune globulin.* [AWK-tah-gam].

**Octamide PFS** (GI). See *metoclopramide.* [AWK-tah-mide P-F-S].

**Octastatin** (GI). See *vapreotide.* [AWK-tah-STAT-in].

**Octicair** (ENT) (generic *hydrocortisone, neomycin, polymyxin B*). Combination corticosteroid and antibiotic drug used topically to treat ear infections. Ear drops: 1%/5 mg/ 10,000 units. [AWK-tih-kair].

**Octocaine** (Anes). See *lidocaine.* [AWK-toh-kayn].

**octoxynol-9** (Ortho-Gynol) (OB/GYN). Over-the-counter spermicide drug used to prevent pregnancy. Jelly: 1%. [awk-TAWK-sih-nawl-9].

**OctreoTher** (Chemo). See *edotreotide.* [awk-TREE-oh-thair].

**octreotide** (Sandostatin, Sandostatin LAR Depot) (Chemo, Endo, GI). Used to suppress the production of growth hormone in adults with acromegaly; used to treat severe diarrhea associated with carcinoid tumor, VIPoma, short bowel syndrome, irritable bowel syndrome, dumping syndrome, or AIDS; used to treat diarrhea caused by chemotherapy or radiation; used to decrease output in patients with a GI or pancreatic fistula. Subcutaneous or intravenous: 0.05 mg/mL, 0.1 mg/mL, 0.2 mg/mL, 0.5 mg/mL, 1 mg/mL, 10 mg/5 mL, 20 mg/5 mL, 30 mg/5 mL. [awk-TREE-oh-tide].

**OcuCoat, OcuCoat PF** (Ophth). See *hydroxypropyl methylcellulose.* [AW-kyoo-koht].

**Ocufen** (Ophth). See *flurbiprofen.* [AW-kyoo-fen].

**Ocuflox** (Anti-infec, Ophth). See *ofloxacin.* [AW-kyoo-flawks].

**Ocupress** (Ophth). See *carteolol.* [AW-kyoo-pres].

**Ocusulf-10** (Anti-infec, Ophth). See *sulfacetamide.* [AW-kyoo-sulf-10].

**ofloxacin** (Floxin, Floxin Otic, Ocuflox) (Anti-infec, ENT, Ophth). Fluoroquinolone antibiotic drug used to treat gram-negative and gram-positive bacterial infections; used to treat bronchitis, Legionnaire's disease of the lungs, and pneumonia due to *S. pneumoniae* and *H. influenzae;* used to treat staphylococcal and streptococcal skin infections; used to treat gonorrhea, nongonococcal urethritis, and pelvic inflammatory disease; used to treat urinary tract infections due to *E. coli;* used topically in the eye to treat bacterial infections (Ocuflox); used topically to treat infection of the external ear canal (otitis externa) and tympanic membrane (otitis media) (Floxin Otic). Tablet: 200 mg, 300 mg, 400 mg. Ophthalmic solution: 0.3% (3 mg/mL). Otic solution: 3 mg/mL. [oh-FLAWK-sah-sin].

**Ogen** (Chemo, OB/GYN). See *estropipate.* [OH-jen].

**Ogestrel 0.5/50** (OB/GYN) (generic *norgestrel, ethinyl estradiol*). Combination monophasic oral contraceptive drug. Pill pack, 28-day: (21 hormone tablets) 0.5 mg/50 mcg; (7 inert tablets). [oh-JES-trel].

**oglufamide** (Chemo). Chemotherapy drug used to treat cancer of the ovary. Orphan drug. [oh-GLOO-fah-mide].

**olanzapine** (Zyprexa, Zyprexa Zydis) (Neuro, Psych). Dibenzapine antipsychotic drug used to treat schizophrenia; used to treat mania in patients with manic-depressive disorder; used to treat psychosis and agitation in patients with Alzheimer's disease; used to treat obsessive-compulsive disorder. Tablet: 2.5 mg, 5 mg, 7.5 mg, 10 mg, 15 mg, 20 mg. Orally disintegrating tablet: 5 mg, 10 mg, 15 mg, 20 mg. Intramuscular: 10 mg. [oh-LAN-zah-peen].

**olmesartan** (Benicar) (Cardio). Angiotensin II receptor blocker drug used to treat hypertension. Tablet: 5 mg, 20 mg, 40 mg. [OL-meh-SAR-tan].

**olopatadine** (Pataday, Patanase, Patanol) (Ophth). Antihistamine drug used topically to treat allergy symptoms in the eyes; used to treat allergy symptoms in the nose (Patanase). Ophthalmic solution: 0.1%, 0.2%. Nasal spray. [OH-loh-PAT-ah-deen].

**olsalazine** (Dipentum) (GI). Anti-inflammatory, 5-ASA drug used to treat ulcerative colitis. Capsule: 250 mg. [ohl-SAL-ah-zeen].

**Olux, Olux-E** (Derm). See *clobetasol.* [OH-luks].

**Omacor** (Cardio). See *omega-3 fatty acids.* [OH-mah-kor].

**omalizumab** (Xolair) (Pulm). Monoclonal antibody drug used to treat moderate-to-severe asthma. Powder (to be reconstituted): 75 mg/0.6 mL, 250 mg/1.2 mL. [OH-mah-LIZ-yoo-mab].

**omega-3 fatty acids** (Animi-3, Omacor, Promega Pearls) (Cardio). Fish oil nutritional supplement used to lower serum cholesterol and triglyceride levels and increase HDL. Capsule/softgel: 500 mg, 600 mg, 900 mg. [oh-MAY-gah-3].

**omeprazole** (Prilosec, Prilosec OTC) (GI). Over-the-counter and prescription proton pump inhibitor drug used to treat heartburn, peptic ulcer, GERD, esophagitis, and *H. pylori*

infections. Delayed-release capsule: 10 mg, 20 mg, 40 mg. Delayed-release tablet: 20 mg. [oh-MEP-rah-zohl].

**Omnaris** (ENT). See *ciclesonide.* [awm-NAIR-is].

**Omnicef** (Anti-infec). See *cefdinir.* [AWM-nih-sef].

**Omnitrope, Omnitrope Pen 5, Omnitrope Pen 10** (Endo). See *somatropin.* [AWM-nih-trohp].

**Oncaspar** (Chemo). See *pegaspargase.* [AWN-kah-spar].

**Oncolym** (Chemo) (generic *iodine 131, murine MAb Lym-1*). Combination radioactive isotope iodine 131 and monoclonal antibody drug used to treat non-Hodgkin's lymphoma. Orphan drug. [AWN-koh-lim].

**Oncomun** (Chemo). Chemotherapy drug used to treat brain cancer. Orphan drug. [AWN-koh-myoon].

**Oncophage** (Chemo, Derm, Uro). Tumor-derived vaccine used to stimulate the immune system to fight kidney cancer and malignant melanoma. Orphan drug. [AWN-koh-fayj].

**Oncorad** (Chemo). Used to treat cancer of the ovary. Orphan drug. [AWN-koh-rad].

**ondansetron** (Zofran, Zofran ODT) (Chemo, GI). Serotonin blocker drug used to treat nausea and vomiting associated with surgery, chemotherapy, or radiation therapy. Tablet: 4 mg, 8 mg, 24 mg. Orally disintegrating tablet: 4 mg, 8 mg. Oral liquid: 4 mg/5 mL. Intravenous: 2 mg/mL, 32 mg/50 mL. [awn-DAN-seh-trawn].

**Onkolox** (Chemo). See *coumarin.* [AWN-koh-lawks].

**Ontak** (Chemo). See *denileukin.* [AWN-tak].

**Onxol** (Chemo). See *paclitaxel.* [AWN-zawl].

**Opana, Opana ER** (Analges, Anes). See *oxymorphone.* [oh-PAN-ah].

**Opcon-A** (Ophth) (generic *naphazoline, pheniramine*). Combination over-the-counter decongestant and antihistamine drug used topically in the eye to treat allergy symptoms. Eye drops: 0.05%/0.315%. [AWP-tih-kawn-A].

**Ophthetic** (Ophth). See *proparacaine.* [awf-THET-ik].

**Ophthocort** (Ophth) (generic *chloramphenicol, hydrocortisone, polymyxin B*). Combination corticosteroid and antibiotic drug used topically in the eyes to treat inflammation and bacterial infections. Ophthalmic ointment: 1%/0.5%/10,000 units. [AWF-thoh-kort].

**opium** (paregoric) (GI). Schedule III narcotic drug used to treat diarrhea. Liquid: 2 mg/5 mlL, 10 mg/ mL. [OH-pee-um].

**oprelvekin** (Neumega) (Chemo, Hem). Interleukin drug used to prevent thrombocytopenia following chemotherapy. Subcutaneous (powder to be reconstituted): 5 mg. [oh-PREL-veh-kin].

**Opticrom** (Ophth). See *cromolyn.* [AWP-tih-krawm].

**Optimental** (GI). Nutritional supplement. Liquid. [AWP-tih-MEN-tal].

**Optimmune** (Ophth). See *cyclosporine.* [AWP-tih-myoon].

**OptiPranolol** (Ophth). See *metipranolol.* [AWP-tih-PRAN-oh-lawl].

**Optivar** (Ophth). See *azelastine.* [AWP-tih-var].

**Orabase-B** (Anes, ENT). See *benzocaine*. [OR-ah-bays-B].

**Orabase HCA** (ENT). See *hydrocortisone*. [OR-ah-bays H-C-A].

**Oracea** (Anti-infec). See *doxycycline*. [OR-ah-SEE-ah].

**Oracit** (Hem) (generic *citric acid, sodium citrate*). Used to increase the alkalinity of body fluids. Oral liquid: 640 mg/490 mg. [OR-ah-sit]

**Orajel Mouth-Aid, Baby Orajel** (Anes, Dent, ENT). See *benzocaine*. [OR-ah-jel].

**Oralone** (ENT). See *triamcinolone*. [OR-ah-lohn].

**Oramorph SR** (Analges). See *morphine*. [OR-ah-morf S-R].

**Orap** (Psych). See *pimozide*. [OR-ap].

**Orapred, Orapred ODT** (Endo, Neuro, Pulm, Uro). See *prednisolone*. [OR-ah-pred].

**Orasone** (Chemo, Endo, Ortho, Pulm, Neuro). See *prednisone*. [OR-ah-sohn].

**Oraverse** (Anes). See *phentolamine*. [OR-ah-vers].

**Orencia** (Ortho). See *abatacept*. [oh-REN-see-ah].

**Orfadin** (Misc). See *nitisinone*. [or-FAD-in].

**Organidin NR** (Pulm). See *guaifenesin*. [or-GAN-ih-din N-R].

**Orinase** (Endo). See *tolbutamide*. [OR-ih-nays].

**ORLAAM** (Analges). See *levomethadyl*. [OR-laam].

**orlistat** (Alli, Xenical) (GI). Over-the-counter and prescription lipase inhibitor drug that blocks fat-digesting enzymes in the small intestine; used to treat obesity. Capsule: 60 mg, 120 mg. [OR-lih-stat].

**Ornidyl** (Anti-infec). See *eflornithine*. [OR-nih-dil].

**orphenadrine** (Banflex, Flexon, Norflex) (Ortho). Skeletal muscle relaxant drug used to treat spasm and stiffness associated with minor muscle injuries; used to treat nighttime leg cramps. Tablet: 100 mg. Sustained-release tablet: 100 mg. Intramuscular or intravenous: 30 mg/mL. [or-FEN-ah-dreen].

**Orphengesic, Orphengesic Forte** (Ortho) (generic *orphenadrine, aspirin, caffeine*). Combination skeletal muscle relaxant drug, analgesic, and stimulant drug used to treat the pain, spasm, and stiffness associated with minor muscle injuries. Tablet: 25 mg/385 mg/30 mg, 50 mg/770 mg/60 mg. [OR-fen-JEE-sik].

**Ortho-Cept** (OB/GYN) (generic *desogestrel, ethinyl estradiol*). Combination monophasic oral contraceptive drug. Pill pack, 28-day: (21 hormone tablets) 0.15 mg/30 mcg; (7 inert tablets). [OR-thoh-SEPT].

**Orthoclone OKT3** (Cardio, Chemo, GI, Uro). See *muromonab-CD3*. [OR-thoh-klohn O-K-T-3].

**Ortho-Cyclen** (OB/GYN) (generic *norgestimate, ethinyl estradiol*). Combination monophasic oral contraceptive drug. Pill pack (Dialpak), 28-day: (21 hormone tablets): 0.25 mg/35 mcg; (7 inert tablets). [OR-thoh-SY-klen].

**Ortho-Est** (Chemo, OB/GYN). See *estropipate*. [OR-thoh-est].

**Ortho Evra** (OB/GYN) (generic *norelgestromin, ethinyl estradiol*). Combination monophasic contraceptive drug. Transdermal patch (applied for 3 weeks): 0.15 mg/0.02 mg per 24 hours. [OR-thoh EV-rah].

**Ortho-Gynol** (OB/GYN). See *octoxynol-9*. [OR-thoh-GY-nawl].

**Ortho Micronor** (OB/GYN). See *norethindrone*. [OR-thoh MY-kroh-nor].

**Ortho-Novum 1/35, Ortho-Novum 1/50** (OB/GYN) (generic *norethindrone, ethinyl estradiol*). Combination monophasic oral contraceptive drug. Pill pack (Dialpak), 20-day: (21 hormone tablets) 1 mg/35 mcg; (7 inert tablets). Pill pack (Dialpak), 28-day: (21 hormone tablets) 1 mg/50 mcg; (7 inert tablets). [OR-thoh-NOH-vum].

**Ortho-Novum 7/7/7** (OB/GYN) (generic *norethindrone, ethinyl estradiol*). Combination triphasic oral contraceptive drug. Pill pack (Dialpak), 28-day: (7 hormone tablets) 0.5 mg/35 mcg; (7 hormone tablets) 0.75 mg/35 mcg; (7 hormone tablets) 1 mg/35 mcg; (7 inert tablets). [OR-thoh-NOH-vum].

**Ortho-Novum 10/11** (OB/GYN) (generic *norethindrone, ethinyl estradiol*). Combination biphasic oral contraceptive drug. Pill pack (Dialpak), 28-day: (10 hormone tablets) 0.5 mg/35 mcg; (11 hormone tablets) 1 mg/35 mcg; (7 inert tablets). [OR-thoh-NOH-vum].

**Ortho Tri-Cyclen, Ortho Tri-Cyclen Lo** (Derm, OB/GYN) (generic *norgestimate, ethinyl estradiol*). Combination triphasic oral contraceptive drug; used to treat acne. Pill pack (Dialpak), 28-day: (7 hormone tablets) 0.18 mg/35 mcg; (7 hormone tablets) 0.215 mg/35 mcg; (7 hormone tablets) 0.25 mg/35 mcg; (7 inert tablets). Pill pack (Dialpak), 28-day: (7 hormone tablets) 0.18 mg/25 mcg; (7 hormone tablets) 0.215 mg/25 mcg; (7 hormone tablets) 0.25 mg/25 mcg; (7 inert tablets). [OR-thoh try-SY-klen].

**Orthovisc** (Ortho). See *hyaluronic acid*. [OR-thoh-visk].

**Or-Tyl** (GI). See *dicyclomine*. [OR-til].

**Os-Cal 500** (Ortho). See *calcium carbonate*. [AWS-kal 500].

**oseltamivir** (Tamiflu) (Anti-infec, Pulm). Antiviral drug used to prevent and treat influenza virus infections. Capsule: 75 mg. Powder (to be reconstituted): 12 mg/mL. [OH-sel-TAM-ih-veer].

**Osmitrol** (Neuro, Ophth, Uro). See *mannitol*. [AWS-mih-trawl].

**Osmoglyn** (Ophth). See *glycerin*. [AWS-moh-glin].

**Osmolite, Osmolite HN** (GI). Lactose-free nutritional supplement. Liquid. [AWS-moh-lite].

**OsmoPrep** (GI). See *sodium phosphate*. [AWS-moh-prep].

**Osteo-D** (Ortho). See *secalciferol*. [AWS-tee-oh-D].

**Otosporin** (ENT) (generic *hydrocortisone, neomycin, polymyxin B*). Combination corticosteroid and antibiotic drug used topically in the ears to treat inflammation and bacterial infections. Ear drops: 1%/5 mg/10,000 units. [OH-toh-SPOR-in].

**Otrivin, Otrivin Pediatric Nasal** (ENT). See *xylometazoline*. [OH-trih-vin].

**Ovarex** (Chemo). Monoclonal antibody drug used to treat ovarian cancer. Orphan drug. [OH-vah-reks].

**Ovastat** (Chemo). See *treosulfan*. [OH-vah-stat].

**O-Vax** (Chemo). Chemotherapy vaccine used to treat ovarian cancer. Orphan drug. [OH-vaks].

**Ovcon-35, Ovcon-50** (OB/GYN) (generic *norethindrone, ethinyl estradiol*). Combination monophasic oral contraceptive drug. Pill pack, 28-day: (21 hormone tablets) 0.4 mg/35; (7 inert tablets). Pill pack, 28-day: (21 hormone tablets) 1 mg/50 mcg; (7 inert tablets). [AWV-kawn].

**Ovide** (Derm). See *malathion*. [OH-vide].

**Ovidrel** (Endo, OB/GYN). See *choriogonadotropin alfa*. [OH-vih-drel].

**Ovral** (OB/GYN) (generic *norgestrel, ethinyl estradiol*). Combination monophasic oral contraceptive drug. Pill pack (Pilpak), 21-day: (21 hormone tablets) 0.5 mg/50 mcg. Pill pack (Pilpak), 28-day: (21 hormone tablets) 0.5 mg/ 50 mcg; (7 inert tablets). [OV-rawl].

**Ovrette** (OB/GYN). See *norgestrel*. [OV-ret].

**oxacillin** (Anti-infec). Penicillin-type antibiotic drug used to treat staphylococcal bacterial infections. Liquid: 250 mg/ 5 mL. Intramuscular (powder to be reconstituted): 500 mg, 1 g, 2 g. [AWK-sah-SIL-in].

**oxaliplatin** (Eloxatin) (Chemo). Platinum chemotherapy drug used to treat cancer of the colon and ovary; used to treat non-Hodgkin's lymphoma. Intravenous: 50 mg, 100 mg. [AWK-sal-ih-PLAT-in].

**Oxandrin** (Anti-infec, Endo, Ortho). See *oxandrolone*. [awk-SAN-drin].

**oxandrolone** (Hepandrin, Oxandrin) (Anti-infec, Endo, GI, Ortho). Schedule III anabolic steroid drug used to promote weight gain following extensive surgery or trauma; used to treat bone pain in osteoporosis; used to treat wasting disease associated with HIV; used to treat short stature in patients with Turner's syndrome; used to treat delay of growth and puberty; orphan drug used to treat alcoholic hepatitis with malnutrition (Hepandrin); used to treat muscular dystrophy; used illegally by athletes. Tablet: 2.5 mg 10 mg. [awk-SAN-drah-lohn].

**oxaprozin** (Daypro, Daypro ALTA) (Analges). Nonsteroidal anti-inflammatory drug used to treat the pain and inflammation of osteoarthritis and rheumatoid arthritis. Caplet: 600 mg. Tablet: 600 mg. [AWK-sah-PROH-zin].

**oxazepam** (Serax) (GI, Psych). Schedule IV benzodiazepine drug used to treat anxiety and neurosis; used to treat alcohol withdrawal; used to treat irritable bowel syndrome. Capsule: 10 mg, 15 mg, 30 mg. Tablet: 15 mg. [awk-SAY-zeh-pam].

**oxcarbazepine** (Trileptal) (Neuro, Psych). Anticonvulsant drug used to treat simple partial seizures; used to treat diabetic neuropathy; used to treat bipolar disorder. Tablet: 150 mg, 300 mg, 600 mg. Liquid: 60 mg/mL. [AWKS-kar-BAZ-eh-peen].

**oxiconazole** (Oxistat) (Derm). Antifungal drug used topically to treat tinea (ringworm) and other fungal skin infections. Cream: 1%. Lotion: 1%. [AWK-see-KAWN-ah-zohl].

**oxidized cellulose** (Oxycel, Surgicel) (Hem). Topical cellulose applied during surgery or dental surgery to control bleeding. Pad: 3 × 3 inch. Pledget: 2 × 1 × 1 inch. Strip: ½ × 2 inch, 2 × 3 inch, 2 × 14 inch, 2 × 18 inch, 4 × 8 inch. Surgical Nu-knit: 1 × 1 inch, 3 × 4 inch, 6 × 9 inch. [AWK-sih-dized SEL-yoo-lohs].

**Oxipor VHC** (Derm). See *coal tar*. [AWK-see-por V-H-C].

**Oxistat** (Derm). See *oxiconazole*. [AWK-see-stat].

**Oxsodrol** (Cardio, GI, Uro). Used to treat the transplanted donor heart, liver, or kidney. Orphan drug. [AWK-soh-drohl].

**Oxsoralen, Oxsoralen-Ultra** (Derm). See *methoxsalen*. [AWK-soh-RAY-lin].

**oxybate** (Xyrem) (Neuro). Schedule III central nervous system stimulant drug used to treat narcolepsy. Liquid: 500 mg/mL. [AWK-see-bayt].

**oxybutynin** (Ditropan, Ditropan XL, Oxytrol) (Uro). Antispasmodic drug used to treat urinary urgency and frequency; used to treat overactive bladder associated with spina bifida. Syrup: 5 mg/5 mL. Tablet: 5 mg. Extended-release tablet: 10 mg, 15 mg. Transdermal patch: 3.9 mg/day. [AWK-see-BYOO-tih-nin].

**Oxycel** (Hem). See *oxidized cellulose*. [AWK-see-sel].

**oxychlorosene** (Clorpactin WCS-90) (Derm). Over-the-counter antibacterial, antifungal, and antiviral drug used topically to irrigate skin wounds. Powder (to be reconstituted to a solution). [AWK-see-KLOR-oh-seen].

**oxycodone** (M-oxy, OxyContin, OxyFast, OxyIR, Roxicodone, Roxicodone Intensol) (Analges). Schedule II narcotic analgesic drug used to treat moderate-to-severe pain. Capsule: 5 mg. Oral liquid: 5 mg/5 mL, 20 mg/mL. Tablet: 5 mg, 10 mg, 15 mg, 20 mg, 30 mg. Controlled-release tablet: 10 mg, 20 mg, 40 mg, 80 mg. [AWK-see-KOH-dohn].

**OxyContin** (Analges). See *oxycodone*. [AWK-see-KAWN-tin].

**OxyFAST** (Analges). See *oxycodone*. [AWK-see-FAST].

**OxyIR** (Analges). See *oxycodone*. [AWK-see-l-R].

**Oxy Medicated Cleanser Pads, Oxy Night Watch** (Derm). See *salicylic acid*. [AWK-see].

**Oxy Medicated Soap** (Derm). See *triclosan*. [AWK-see].

**oxymetazoline** (Afrin 12-Hour, Afrin Severe Congestion, Afrin Sinus, Dristan 12-Hr Nasal, Duration, Neo-Synephrine 12-Hour, Tyzine, Tyzine Pediatric, Vicks Sinex 12-Hour, Visine LR) (ENT, Ophth). Over-the-counter vasoconstrictor/decongestant drug used topically to treat nasal stuffiness due to colds and allergies; used topically to treat allergy symptoms in the eye (Visine). Ophthalmic solution: 0.025%. Intranasal solution: 0.5%, 0.1%. Nasal spray: 0.05%. [AWK-see-MET-ah-ZOH-leen].

**oxymetholone** (Anadrol-50) (Anti-infec, Chemo, Endo, Hem). Schedule III anabolic steroid drug used to treat many different types of anemia, including anemia caused by chemotherapy drugs; used to treat wasting disease associated with HIV; used illegally by athletes. Tablet: 50 mg. [AWK-see-METH-oh-lohn].

**oxymorphone** (Numorphan, Opana, Opana ER) (Analges, Anes).   Schedule II narcotic analgesic drug used to treat moderate-to-severe pain; used preoperatively to provide sedation; used to induce and help maintain general anesthesia; used to relieve anxiety in patients with dyspnea from pulmonary edema. Tablet: 5 mg, 10 mg. Extended-release tablet: 5 mg, 7.5 mg, 10 mg, 15 mg, 20 mg, 30 mg, 40 mg. Subcutaneous, intramuscular, intravenous: 1 mg/mL. [AWK-see-MOR-fohn].

**Oxy Oil-Free Maximum Strength Acne Wash** (Derm).   See *benzoyl peroxide.* [AWK-see].

**oxypurinol** (Uro).   Used to treat hyperuricemia in patients who cannot take allopurinol. Orphan drug. [AWK-see-PYOOR-ih-nawl].

**oxytocin** (Pitocin) (OB/GYN).   Hormone drug used to stimulate weak uterine contractions during labor; used to treat postpartum uterine bleeding; used to treat incomplete abortion. Intramuscular or intravenous: 10 units/mL. [AWK-see-TOH-sin].

**Oxytrol** (Uro).   See *oxybutynin.* [AWK-see-trawl].

**P₁E₁, P₂E₁, P₄E₁, P₆E₁** (Ophth) (generic *pilocarpine, epinephrine*).   Combination miotic and epinephrine drug used topically in the eyes to treat glaucoma. Ophthalmic solution: 1%/1%, 2%/1%, 4%/1%, 6%/1%. [P-1-E-1].

**Pacerone** (Cardio).   See *amiodarone.* [PAY-seh-rohn].

**packed red blood cells** (PRBCs) (I.V.).   Cellular blood product. Intravenous. [PAKD RED BLUD SELZ].

**Packer's Pine Tar** (Derm).   See *coal tar.* [PAK-erz PINE TAR].

**paclitaxel** (Abraxane, Onxol, Taxol) (Chemo).   Mitosis inhibitor taxoid-type chemotherapy drug used to treat cancer of the head and neck, breast, esophagus, stomach, lung, ovary, uterus, prostate gland, testicle, and bladder; used to treat leukemia, Wilm's tumor, and Kaposi's sarcoma. Intravenous: 6 mg/mL. [PAK-lih-TAK-sel].

**Palcaps 10, Palcaps 20** (GI) (generic *amylase, lipase, protease*).   Combination digestive enzyme drug used as replacement therapy. Delayed-release capsule: 33,200 units/10,000 units/37,500 units; 66,400 units/20,000 units/75,000 units. [PAL-kaps].

**Palgic** (Derm, ENT, Ophth).   See *carbinoxamine.* [PAL-jik].

**palifermin** (Kepivance) (Chemo, ENT).   Recombinant DNA technology drug used to increase the production of epithelial cells to treat severe erosions of the oral mucous membranes in patients receiving chemotherapy. Intravenous (powder for injection): 6.25 mg. [PAL-ee-FAIR-min].

**paliperidone** (Invega) (Psych).   Antipsychotic drug used to treat schizophrenia. Extended-release tablet: 3 mg, 6 mg, 9 mg. [PAL-ee-PAIR-ih-dohn].

**palivizumab** (Synagis) (Anti-infec, Pulm).   Monoclonal antibody drug used to treat respiratory synctial virus infection. Intramuscular (powder to be reconstituted): 50 mg/0.5 mL, 100 mg/mL. [PAL-ih-VIZ-yoo-mab].

**palonosetron** (Aloxi) (Chemo, GI).    Antiemetic drug used to treat postoperative nausea and vomiting caused by chemotherapy drugs. Capsule: 0.5 mg. Intravenous: 0.25 mg, 0.75 mg. [PAL-oh-NOH-seh-trawn].

**pamabrom** (Maximum Strength Aqua-Ban) (Uro).   Over-the-counter diuretic drug used to treat edema from menstruation. Tablet: 50 mg. [PAM-ah-brohm].

**Pamelor** (Analges, Neuro, Psych).   See *nortriptyline* [PAM-eh-lor].

**pamidronate** (Aredia) (Chemo, OB/GYN, Ortho).   Bone resorption inhibitor drug used to treat osteoporosis in postmenopausal women; used to treat osteoporosis caused by corticosteroid drugs; used to treat hypercalcemia caused by cancer; used to treat the metastatic bone lesions of breast cancer and multiple myeloma; used to treat Paget's disease of the bones. Intravenous: 3 mg/mL, 6 mg/mL, 9 mg/mL. [PAM-ih-DROH-nayt].

**Pamine, Pamine Forte** (GI).   See *methscopolamine.* [PAM-een].

**Pamisyl** (GI).   See *4-aminosalicylic acid.* [PAM-ih-sil].

**Pamprin Maximum Pain Relief** (OB/GYN) (generic *acetaminophen, magneium salicylate, pamabrom*).   Combination over-the-counter analgesic and diuretic drug used to treat painful menstruation. Caplet: 250 mg/250 mg/25 mg. [PAM-prin].

**Pamprin Multi-Symptom Maximum Strength** (OB/GYN) (generic *acetaminophen, pamabrom, pyrilamine*).   Combination over-the-counter analgesic, diuretic, and antihistamine drug used to treat painful menstruation. Caplet/Tablet: 500 mg/25 mg/15 mg. [PAM-prin].

**Panacet** (Analges) (generic *acetaminophen, hydrocodone*).   Combination Schedule III nonnarcotic and narcotic analgesic drug for pain. Tablet: 500 mg/5 mg. [PAN-ah-set].

**Panadol Extra Strength, Children's Panadol, Infants' Drops Panadol, Junior Strength Panadol** (Analges).   See *acetaminophen.* [PAN-ah-dawl].

**Panafil** (Derm).   See *papain.* [PAN-ah-fil].

**Panasol** (Analges) (generic *aspirin, hydrocodone*).   Combination Schedule III salicylate and narcotic analgesic drug for pain. Tablet: 500 mg/5 mg. [PAN-ah-sawl].

**Panasol-S** (Chemo, Endo, Ortho, Pulm, Neuro).   See *prednisone.* [PAN-ah-sawl-S].

**PAN-Cide** (Chemo).   Used to treat pancreatic cancer. Orphan drug. [PAN-side],

**Pancrease, Pancrease MT4, Pancrease MT 10, Pancrease MT 16, Pancrease MT 20** (GI) (generic *amylase, lipase, protease*).   Combination digestive enzyme drug used as replacement therapy. Capsule, tablet: 12,000 units/4000 units/12,000 units; 30,000 units/10,000 units/30,000 units; 48,000 units/16,000 units/48,000 units; 56,000 units/20,000 units/44,000 units. [PAN-kree-ace].

**Pancrecarb MS-4, Pancrecarb MS-8, Pancrecarb MS-16** (GI) (generic *amylase, lipase, protease*).   Combination digestive enzyme drug used as replacement therapy.

Delayed-release capsule: 25,000 units/4000 units/ 25,000 units; 40,000 units/8000 units/45,000 units; 52,000 units/16,000 units/52,000 units. [PAN-kree-karb].

**pancuronium** (Anes, Pulm). Neuromuscular blocker drug used during surgery; used to treat patients who are intubated and on the ventilator. Intravenous: 1 mg/mL, 2 mg/mL. [PAN-kyoor-OH-nee-um].

**Pandel** (Derm). See *hydrocortisone*. [pan-DEL].

**Panfil G** (Pulm) (generic *dyphylline, guaifenesin*). Combination bronchodilator and expectorant drug used to treat asthma and bronchitis with a productive cough. Liquid: 300 mg/150 mg. [PAN-fil].

**Pangestyme CN-10, Pangestyme CN-20, Pangestyme EG, Pangestyme MT 16, Pangestyme UL 12, Pangestyme UL 18, Pangestyme UL 20** (GI) (generic *amylase, lipase, protease*). Combination digestive enzyme drug used as replacement therapy. Delayed-release capsule: 20,000 units/4500 units/25,000 units; 33,200 units/ 10,000 units/37,500 units; 39,000 units/12,000 units/ 39,000 units; 48,000 units/16,000 units/48,000 units; 58,500 units/18,000 units/58,500 units; 65,000 units/ 20,000 units/65,000 units; 66,400 units/20,000 units/ 75,000 units. [pan-JES-time].

**Panhematin** (Hem). See *hemin*. [pan-HEE-mah-tin].

**panitumumab** (Vectibix) (Chemo). Monoclonal antibody drug used to treat colorectal cancer. Intravenous: 20 mg/mL. [PAN-ih-TOOM-yoo-mab].

**Panlor DC, Panlor SS** (Analges) (generic *acetaminophen, caffeine, dihydrocodeine*). Combination Schedule III nonnarcotic analgesic, stimulant, and narcotic analgesic drug for pain. Tablet: 356 mg/30 mg/16 mg, 712 mg/ 60 mg/32 mg. [PAN-lor].

**Panocaps, Panocaps MT 16, Panocaps MT 20** (GI) (generic *amylase, lipase, protease*). Combination digestive enzyme drug used as replacement therapy. Delayed-release capsule: 20,000 units/4500 units/25,000 units; 48,000 units/16,000 units/48,000 units; 56,000 units/ 20,000 units/44,000 units. [PAN-oh-kaps].

**Panokase** (GI) (generic *amylase, lipase, protease*). Combination digestive enzyme drug used as replacement therapy. Tablet: 30,000 units/8000 units/30,000 units. [PAN-oh-kays].

**Panorex** (Chemo). Monoclonal antibody drug used to treat pancreatic cancer. Orphan drug. [PAN-oh-reks].

**PanOxyl, PanOxyl 5, PanOxyl 10, PanOxyl AQ 2½, PanOxyl AQ 5, PanOxyl AQ 10** (Derm). See *benzoyl peroxide*. [pan-AWK-sil].

**Panretin** (Chemo, Derm). See *alitretinoin*. [pan-RET-in].

**Panthoderm** (Derm). See *dexpanthenol*. [PAN-thoh-derm].

**pantoprazole** (Protonix, Protonix I.V.) (GI). Proton pump inhibitor drug used to treat GERD and esophagitis. Delayed-release tablet: 20 mg, 40 mg. Delayed release oral suspension (granules to be sprinkled on food): 40 mg packet. Intravenous: 40 mg. [pan-TOH-prah-zohl].

**Panzem** (Chemo). Angiogenesis inhibiting drug used to treat cancer of the brain and ovary; used to treat multiple myeloma. Orphan drug. [PAN-zem].

**papain** (Accuzyme, Ethezyme, Ethezyme 830, Gladase, Gladase-C, Panafil) (Derm). Enzyme drug used topically to debride burns and wounds. Ointment:. Spray. [PAH-payn].

**papaverine** (Cardio, Neuro, Uro). Peripheral vasodilator drug used to treat spasm in the cerebral arteries; used to treat peripheral vascular disease; orphan drug used topically to treat sexual dysfunction in patients with spinal cord injury. Extended-release capsule: 150 mg. Topical gel. Intravenous: 30 mg/mL. [pah-PAV-eh-reen].

**Paracaine** (Ophth). See *proparacaine*. [PAIR-ah-kayn].

**Paraflex** (Ortho). See *chlorzoxazone*. [PAIR-ah-fleks].

**Parafon Forte DSC** (Ortho). See *chlorzoxazone*. [PAIR-ah-fawn FOR-tay D-S-C].

**Paraplatin** (Chemo). See *carboplatin*. [PAIR-ah-PLAT-in].

**Parcopa** (Neuro) (generic *carbidopa, levodopa*). Combination drug used to treat Parkinson's disease. Orally disintegrating tablet: 10 mg/100 mg, 25 mg/100 mg, 25 mg/250 mg. [par-KOH-pah].

**paregoric** (GI). See *opium*. [PAIR-eh-GOR-ik].

**Paremyd** (Ophth) (generic *hydroxyamphetamine, tropicamide*). Combination mydriatic drug used topically to dilate the pupil before eye examinations or surgery. Ophthalmic solution: 1%/0.25%. [PAIR-eh-mid].

**Parepectolin** (GI). See *attapulgite*. [PAIR-eh-PEK-toh-lin].

**paricalcitol** (Zemplar) (Endo). Used to treat hyperparathyroidism in patients with kidney disease. Capsule: 1 mcg, 2 mcg, 4 mcg. Injection (during hemodialysis): 2 mcg/mL, 5 mcg/mL. [PAIR-ih-KAL-sih-tawl].

**Parlodel, Parlodel Snap Tabs** (Endo, Neuro). See *bromocriptine*. [PAR-loh-del].

**Parnate** (Psych). See *tranylcypromine*. [PAR-nayt].

**paromomycin** (Humatin) (Anti-infec). Aminoglycoside antibiotic and amebicide drug used to treat intestintal amebiasis; used to treat hepatic coma by killing ammonia-producing bacteria in the intestines. Capsule: 250 mg. [PAIR-oh-moh-MY-sin].

**paroxetine** (Paxil, Paxil CR) (Neuro, OB/GYN, Psych). Selective serotonin reuptake inhibitor (SSRI) drug used to treat depression, anxiety, obsessive-compulsive disorder, social anxiety disorder, panic disorder, posttraumatic stress disorder, and premenstrual dysphoric disorder; used to treat the hot flashes of menopause; used to treat diabetic neuropathy. Oral liquid: 10 mg/5 mL. Tablet: 10 mg, 20 mg, 30 mg, 40 mg. Controlled-release tablet: 12.5 mg, 25 mg, 37.5 mg. [pah-RAWK-seh-teen].

**Partaject** (Chemo). See *busulfan*. [PAR-tah-jekt].

**Paser** (GI, Pulm). See *4-aminosalicylic acid*. [PAY-ser].

**Pataday** (Ophth). See *olopatadine*. [PAT-ah-day].

**Patanase** (ENT). See *olopatadine*. [PAT-ah-nays].

**Patanol** (Ophth). See *olopatadine*. [PAT-ah-nawl].

**patupilone** (Chemo). Chemotherapy drug used to treat ovarian cancer. Orphan drug. [pah-TOO-pih-lohn].

**Paxil, Paxil CR** (Neuro, OB/GYN, Psych). See *paroxetine*. [PAK-sil].

**PCE Dispertab** (Anti-infec). See *erythromycin*. [P-C-E DIS-per-tab].

**PC-Tar** (Derm). See *coal tar*. [P-C-TAR].

**PediaCare Children's Cold & Allergy** (ENT) (generic *chlorpheniramine, pseudoephedrine*). Combination over-the-counter antihistamine and decongestant drug. Liquid: 1 mg/15 mg. [PEE-dee-ah-kair].

**PediaCare Children's Decongestant** (ENT). See *phenylephrine*. [PEE-dee-ah-kair].

**PediaCare Children's Nighttime Cough** (ENT). See *diphenhydramine*. [PEE-dee-ah-kair].

**PediaCare Fever** (Analges). See *ibuprofen*. [PEE-dee-ah-kair].

**PediaCare Infants' Cold and Cough** (ENT) (generic *dextromethorphan, pseudoephedrine*). Combination over-the-counter nonnarcotic antitussive and decongestant drug used to treat colds and coughs. Oral drops: 2.5 mg/7.5 mg. [PEE-dee-ah-kair].

**PediaCare Infants' Cough** (ENT). See *dextromethorphan*. [PEE-dee-ah-kair].

**PediaCare Infants' Decongestant** (ENT). See *pseudoephedrine*. [PEE-dee-ah-kair].

**Pedialyte Solution, Pedialyte Freezer Pops** (GI). Electrolyte solution given to children to replace water and electrolytes lost from vomiting and diarrhea. Oral liquid. Frozen pop. [PEE-dee-ah-lite].

**Pediapred** (Endo, Pulm, Uro). See *prednisolone*. [PEE-dee-ah-pred].

**Pediarix** (Misc). Combination drug used to prevent diphtheria, pertussis, tetanus, polio, and hepatitis B. Subcutaneous: Vaccine. [PEE-dee-ah-riks].

**PediaSure** (GI). Infant formula. Liquid. [PEE-dee-ah-shoor].

**PediaSure with Fiber** (GI). Lactose-free infant nutritional supplement. Liquid. [PEE-dee-ah-shoor].

**Pediatex, Pediatex 12** (Derm, ENT, Ophth). See *carbinoxamine*. [PEE-dee-ah-teks].

**Pediazole** (Anti-infec) (generic *erythromycin, sulfisoxazole*). Combination antibiotic and sulfonamide drug used to treat otitis media. Liquid (granules to be reconstituted): 200 mg/600 mg per 5 mL. [PEE-dee-ah-zohl].

**Pedi-Boro** (Derm). See *aluminum acetate*. [PEE-dee-BUR-oh].

**Pedi-Dri** (Derm). See *nystatin*. [PEE-dee-dry].

**Pediotic** (ENT) (generic *hydrocortisone, neomycin, polymyxin B*). Combination corticosteroid and antibiotic drug used topically to treat ear infections. Ear drops: 1%/5 mg/10,000 units. [PEE-dee-OH-tik].

**Pedi-Pro** (Derm). See *benzalkonium*. [PEE-dee-proh].

**PedvaxHIB** (Misc). Used to prevent *H. influenzae* infection in children. Subcutaneous: Vaccine. [PEED-vaks-H-I-B].

**PEG** (GI). See *polyethylene glycol*. [P-E-G].

**pegademase bovine** (Adagen) (Anti-infec). Enzyme replacement therapy used to treat ADA deficiency in patients with AIDS. Intramuscular: 250 units/mL. [peg-AD-eh-mays BOH-vine].

**pegaptanib** (Macugen) (Ophth). Vascular endothelial growth factor blocker drug used to treat wet macular degeneration of the retina. Ophthalmic injection into the vitreous humor: 0.3 mg/mL. [peg-AP-tah-nib].

**pegaspargase** (Oncaspar) (Chemo). Chemotherapy enzyme drug used to treat leukemia. Intramuscular or intravenous: 750 IU/mL. [peg-AS-par-jays].

**Pegasys** (Chemo). See *peginterferon alfa-2a*. [PEG-ah-sis].

**pegfilgrastim** (Neulasta) (Chemo). Granulocyte colony-stimulating factor drug used to increase the neutrophil count in patients after chemotherapy. Subcutaneous: 10 mg/mL. [PEG-fil-GRAH-stim].

**peginterferon alfa-2a** (Pegasys) (Chemo, GI). Immunomodulator drug used to treat hepatitis B virus and hepatitis C virus; used to treat cancer of the kidney and leukemia. Subcutaneous: 180 mcg. [PEG-in-ter-FEER-awn AL-fah-2-a].

**peginterferon alfa-2b** (PEG-Intron) (Chemo, GI). Immunomodulator drug used to treat hepatitis C virus; used to treat cancer of the kidney; used to treat leukemia and malignant melanoma. Subcutaneous: 50 mcg/0.5 mL, 80 mcg/0.5 mL, 120 mcg/0.5 mL, 150 mcg/0.5 mL. Redipen. [PEG-in-ter-FEER-awn AL-fah-2-b].

**PEG-Intron** (Chemo, GI). See *peginterferon alfa-2b*. [peg-IN-trawn].

**pegvisomant** (Somavert) (Endo). Antagonist drug that blocks growth hormone at the receptors on the cell membrane; orphan drug used to treat acromegaly. Subcutaneous (powder to be reconstituted): 10 mg, 15 mg, 20 mg. [peg-VY-soh-mant].

**peldesine** (Chemo). Chemotherapy drug used to treat mycosis fungoides. Orphan drug. [PEL-deh-seen].

**pemetrexed** (Alimta) (Chemo). Antimetabolite chemotherapy drug used to treat non-small cell lung cancer and malignant pleural mesothelioma. Intravenous: 500 mg. [PEM-eh-TREK-sed].

**pemirolast** (Alamast) (Ophth). Mast cell stabilizer drug used topically to treat allergy symptoms in the eyes. Ophthalmic solution: 0.1%. [peh-MEER-oh-last].

**penbutolol** (Levatol) (Cardio). Beta-blocker drug used to treat hypertension. Tablet: 20 mg. [pen-BYOO-toh-lawl].

**penciclovir** (Denavir) (Anti-infec, Derm). Antiviral drug used topically to treat herpes simplex virus type 1 lesions (cold sores). Cream: 1%. [pen-SY-kloh-veer].

**Penecort** (Derm). See *hydrocortisone*. [PEN-eh-kort].

**penicillamine** (Cuprimine, Depen) (Ortho, Uro). Used to treat cystinuria; used to treat severe rheumatoid arthritis; used to treat Wilson's disease. Capsule: 125 mg, 250 mg. Tablet: 250 mg. [PEN-ih-SIL-ah-meen].

**penicillin G** (Pfizerpen) (Anti-infec). Penicillin antibiotic drug used to treat various types of bacterial infections, including gonorrhea, syphilis, endocarditis, Lyme disease, botulism, pneumonia from *S. pneumoniae,* and meningococcal meningitis. Intramuscular or intravenous (powder to be reconstituted): 1,00,000 units/50 mL. [PEN-ih-SIL-in G].

**penicillin G benzathine** (Bicillin L-A, Permapen) (Anti-infec).   Penicillin antibiotic drug used to treat various types of bacterial infections, including syphilis, streptococcal pharyngitis, pneumonia due to *S. pneumoniae;* used prophylactically to prevent subacute bacterial endocarditis in at risk patients undergoing dental or surgical procedures. Intramuscular: 600,000 units/mL. [PEN-ih-SIL-in G BEN-zah-theen].

**penicillin G procaine** (Anti-infec).   Penicillin antibiotic drug used to treat various types of bacterial infections, including syphilis, endocarditis, streptococcal infections, pneumonia due to *S. pneumoniae,* pericarditis, meningitis, peritonitis; used to treat staphylococcal infections of the skin; used to treat inhaled anthrax from bioterrorism. Intramuscular or intravenous: 600,000 unit/mL. [PEN-ih-SIL-in G PRO-kayn].

**penicillin V** (Penicillin VK, Veetids) (Anti-infec).   Penicillin antibiotic drug used to treat a variety of bacterial infections, including otitis media, streptococcal pharyngitis, pneumonia due to *S. pneumoniae,* pericarditis, meningitis, staphylococcal infection of the skin, and Lyme disease; used to treat anthrax exposure from bioterrorism. Tablet: 250 mg, 500 mg. Liquid: 125 mg/5 mL, 250 mg/5 mL. [PEN-ih-SIL-in V].

**Penicillin VK** (Anti-infec).   See *penicillin V.* [PEN-ih-SIL-in V-K].

**Penlac Nail Lacquer** (Derm).   See *ciclopirox.* [PEN-lak].

**Pentacea** (Chemo).   Chemotherapy drug used to treat lung cancer. Orphan drug. [PEN-tah-SEE-ah].

**Pentacel** (Misc).   Combination drug used to prevent diphtheria, pertussis, tetanus, polio, and *Hemophilus influenzae.* Subcutaneous: Vaccine. [PEN-tah-sel].

**Pentam 300** (Anti-infec).   See *pentamidine.* [PEN-tam 300].

**pentamidine** (NebuPent, Pentam 300, Pneumopent) (Anti-infec).   Antiprotozoal drug used to prevent and treat *Pneumocystis carinii* pneumonia in AIDS patients; used to treat leishmaniasis. Intramuscular or intravenous (powder to be reconstituted): 300 mg. Aerosol: 300 mg. [pen-TAM-ih-deen].

**Pentasa** (GI).   See *mesalamine.* [pen-TAH-sah].

**pentazocine** (Talwin) (Analges, Anes).   Schedule IV narcotic analgesic drug used to treat moderate-to-severe pain; used preoperatively to relieve pain and maintain general anesthesia. Subcutaneous, intramuscular, or intravenous: 30 mg/mL. [pen-TAZ-oh-seen].

**pentetate zinc trisodium** (Emerg).   Chelating drug used to treat accidental contamination with plutonium, americium, or curium. Intravenous: 200 mg/mL. [PEN-teh-tayt ZINK try-SOH-dee-um].

**pentobarbital** (Anes, Neuro).   Schedule II barbiturate drug used for short-term treatment of insomnia; anticonvulsant drug used to treat status epilepticus; used preoperatively to provide sedation. Intramuscular: 50 mg/mL. [PEN-toh-BAR-bih-tawl].

**Pentolair** (Ophth).   See *cyclopentolate.* [PEN-toh-lair].

**pentosan** (Elmiron) (Uro).   Urinary tract analgesic drug; orphan drug used to treat interstitial cystitis. Capsule: 100 mg. [PEN-toh-san].

**pentostatin** (Nipent) (Chemo).   Antimetabolite chemotherapy drug used to treat leukemia; used to treat mycosis fungoides. Intravenous (powder to be reconstituted): 10 mg. [PEN-toh-STAT-in].

**Pentothal** (Anes).   See *thiopental.* [PEN-toh-thawl].

**pentoxifylline** (Trental) (Cardio, Hem).   Decreases the viscosity of the blood and increases the flexibility of red blood cells to improve blood flow in patients with intermittent claudication and prevent blood clots in patients with peripheral vascular disease. Controlled-release tablet: 400 mg. Extended-release tablet: 400 mg. [PEN-tawk-SIF-ih-leen].

**Pentrax** (Derm).   See *coal tar.* [PEN-traks].

**Pepcid, Pepcid AC, Pepcid AC Maximum Strength, Pepcid RPD** (GI).   See *famotidine.* [PEP-sid].

**Pepcid Complete** (GI) (generic *famotidine, calcium, magnesium*).   Over-the-counter combination H$_2$ blocker and antacid drug used to treat heartburn, peptic ulcer, GERD, or esophagitis. Chewable tablet: 10 mg/800 mg/165 mg. [PEP-sid].

**Peptamen** (GI).   Nutritional supplement formulated for patients with GI problems. Liquid. [PEP-tah-men].

**Peptinex, Peptinex DT** (GI).   Lactose-free, gluten-free nutritional supplement formulated for patients with GI disease. Liquid. [PEP-tih-neks].

**Pepto-Bismol, Pepto-Bismol Maximum Strength** (GI).   See *bismuth.* [PEP-toh-BIZ-mawl].

**Percocet** (Analges) (generic *acetaminophen, oxycodone*).   Combination Schedule II nonsalicylate and narcotic analgesic drug for pain. Tablet: 325 mg/2.5 mg, 325 mg/5 mg, 325 mg/7.5 mg, 325 mg/10 mg, 500 mg/7.5 mg, 650 mg/10 mg. [PER-koh-set].

**Percodan** (Analges) (generic *aspirin, oxycodone*).   Combination Schedule II salicylate and narcotic analgesic drug for pain. Tablet: 325 mg/4.5 mg. [PER-koh-dan].

**Percogesic** (ENT) (generic *acetaminophen, phenyltoloxamine*).   Combination over-the-counter analgesic and antihistamine drug. Tablet: 325 mg/30 mg. [PER-koh-JEE-sik].

**Percogesic Extra Strength** (ENT) (generic *acetaminophen, diphenhydramine*).   Combination over-the-counter analgesic and antihistamine drug. Tablet: 500 mg/12.5 mg. [PER-koh-JEE-sik].

**Perdiem Fiber Therapy** (GI).   See *psyllium.* [per-DEE-um].

**Perdiem Overnight Relief** (GI) (generic *psyllium, senna*).   Combination over-the-counter bulk-producing and irritant/stimulant laxative drug used to treat constipation. Granules. [per-DEE-um].

**perflubron** (LiquiVent) (Pulm).   Used to treat acute respiratory distress syndrome. Orphan drug. [PER-floo-brawn].

**perfosfamide** (Pergamid) (Chemo). Used during bone marrow transplantation. Orphan drug. [per-FAWS-fah-mide].

**Pergamid** (Chemo). See *perfosfamide*. [PER-gah-mid].

**Peri-Colace** (GI) (generic *docusate, senna*). Combination over-the-counter stool softener and irritant/stimulant laxative drug used to treat constipation. Tablet: 50 mg/8.6 mg. [PAIR-ee-KOH-lays].

**Peridex** (ENT). See *chlorhexidine*. [PAIR-ih-deks]

**perindopril** (Aceon) (Cardio, Neuro). ACE inhibitor drug used to treat hypertension; used to decrease the risk of stroke; used to decrease the risk of myocardial infarction in patients with coronary artery disease. Tablet: 2 mg, 4 mg, 8 mg. [per-IN-doh-pril].

**PerioChip** (ENT). See *chlorhexidine*. [PAIR-ee-oh-chip].

**PerioGard** (ENT). See *chlorhexidine*. [PAIR-ee-oh-gard]].

**Periostat** (Anti-infec). See *doxycycline*. [PAIR-ee-oh-stat].

**Perloxx** (Analges) (generic *acetaminophen, oxycodone*). Combination Schedule II nonnarcotic and narcotic analgesic drug for pain. Tablet: 300 mg/2.5 mg, 300 mg/5 mg, 300 mg/7.5 mg, 300 mg/10 mg. [PER-lawks].

**Permapen** (Anti-infec). See *penicillin G benzathine*. [PER-mah-pen].

**permethrin** (Acticin, Elimite) (Derm). Scabicide and pediculocide drug used topically on the skin to treat parasitic infection from scabies (mites) or pediculosis (lice). Cream: 5%. Lotion: 1%. [per-METH-rin].

**Pernox Lathering Abradant Scrub, Pernox Scrub for Oily Skin** (Derm) (generic *salicylic acid, sulfur*). Combination over-the-counter keratolytic drug used topically on the skin to treat acne vulgaris. [PER-nawks].

**Peroxyl** (ENT). See *hydrogen peroxide*. [per-AWK-sil].

**perphenazine** (GI, Psych). Phenothiazine antipsychotic drug used to treat psychosis and schizophrenia; used to treat nausea and vomiting. Oral liquid: 16 mg/5 mL. Tablet: 2 mg, 4 mg, 8 mg, 16 mg. [per-FEN-ah-zeen].

**Persantine** (Cardio, Hem). See *dipyridamole*. [per-SAN-teen].

**Pfizerpen** (Anti-infec). See *penicillin G*. [FY-zer-pen].

**Phazyme, Phazyme 95, Phazyme 125** (GI). See *simethicone*. [FAY-zime].

**Phenadoz** (Anes, Emerg, GI). See *promethazine*. [FEN-ah-dohz].

**phenazopyridine** (Azo-Standard, Baridium, Geridium, Prodium, Pyridium, Urogesic, UTI Relief) (Uro). Urinary tract analgesic drug. Tablet: 95 mg, 97.2 mg, 100 mg, 200 mg. [fen-AZ-oh-PY-rih-deen].

**phendimetrazine** (Bontril, Bontril PDM, Melfiat-105, Prelu-2) (GI). Schedule III appetite suppressant drug used to treat obesity. Sustained-release capsule: 105 mg. Tablet: 35 mg. [FEN-dih-MEH-trah-zeen].

**phenelzine** (Nardil) (Psych). MAO inhibitor drug used to treat depression. Tablet: 15 mg. [FEN-el-zeen].

**Phenergan** (Anes, Derm, Emerg, ENT, GI, Ophth). See *promethazine*. [FEN-er-gan].

**Phenergan VC** (ENT) (generic *phenylephrine, promethazine*). Combination decongestant and antihistamine drug. Syrup: 5 mg/6.25 mg. [FEN-er-gan V-C].

**Phenex-1, Phenex-2** (GI). Infant formula for infants and adults with PKU. Powder (to be reconstituted). [FEE-neks].

**phenindamine** (Nolahist) (ENT, Ophth). Over-the-counter antihistamine drug used to treat allergic rhinitis and allergic conjunctivitis. Tablet: 25 mg. [feh-NIN-dah-meen].

**phenobarbital** (Luminal, Solfoton) (Neuro). Schedule IV barbiturate drug used to treat tonic-clonic, complex partial, and simple partial seizures; used to provide sedation; used for short-term treatment of insomnia. Tablet: 15 mg, 16 mg, 30 mg, 60 mg, 90 mg, 100 mg. Capsule: 16 mg. Liquid: 15 mg/5 mL, 20 mg/5 mL. Intramuscular: 30 mg/mL, 60 mg/mL, 65 mg/mL, 130 mg/mL. [FEE-noh-BAR-bih-tawl].

**phenoxybenzamine** (Endo). Used to treat hypertension and sweating associated with pheochromocytoma of the adrenal medulla. Capsule: 10 mg. [fen-AWK-see-BEN-zah-meen].

**phentermine** (Adipex-P, Ionamin, Pro-Fast HS, Pro-Fast SA, Pro-Fast-SR) (GI). Schedule IV appetite suppressant drug used to treat obesity. Capsule: 15 mg, 18.75 mg, 30 mg, 37.5 mg. Tablet: 8 mg, 37.5 mg. [FEN-ter-meen].

**phentolamine** (Oraverse) (Anes, Cardio, Endo). Antihypertensive drug used to treat hypertension caused by a pheochromocytoma of the adrenal medulla; used as a test to diagnose pheochromocytoma; used to treat hypertensive crisis or rebound hypertension after discontinuation of another antihypertensive drug; used to reverse anesthesia after a dental procedure (Oraverse). Intramuscular or intravenous (powder to be reconstituted): 5 mg/2 mL. [fen-TOHL-ah-meen].

**phenylbutyrate** (Chemo). Chemotherapy drug used to treat leukemia. Orphan drug. [FEN-il-BYOO-tih-rate].

**phenylephrine** (Afrin Children's Pump Mist, AK-Dilate, Altafrin, Formulation R, 4-Way Fast Acting, Hem-Prep, Mydfrin 2.5%, Neofrin, Neo-Synephrine, Neo-Synephrine 4-Hour, Pediacare Children's Decongestant, Preparation H Cooling Gel, Rhinall, Sudafed PE, Vicks Sinex) (Cardio, Emerg, ENT, GI, Ophth). Vasopressor drug used to treat hypotension during shock and cardiac resuscitation; vasoconstrictor and decongestant drug used topically to treat allergy symptoms in the eye; over-the-counter drug used to relieve nasal stuffiness due to colds and allergies; mydriatic drug used to dilate the pupil during eye surgery; used topically to treat hemorrhoids. Subcutaneous, intramuscular, intravenous: 1% (10 mg/mL). Tablet: 10 mg. Chewable tablet: 10 mg. Orally disintegrating tablet or strip: 10 mg. Oral liquid: 2.5 mg/mL, 2.5 mg/5 mL, 7.5 mg/5 mL. Nasal spray: 0.125%, 0.25%, 0.5%, 1%. Ophthalmic solution: 0.12%, 2.5%, 10%. Topical gel. [FEN-il-EF-rin].

**Phenyl-Free** (GI). Infant formula with iron for infants with PKU. Liquid. Powder (to be reconstituted). [FEN-il-free].

**Phenytek** (Neuro). See *phenytoin*. [FEN-ih-tek].

**phenytoin** (Dilantin Infatab, Dilantin Kapseals, Dilantin-125, Phenytek) (Neuro).   Anticonvulsant drug used to treat tonic-clonic and complex partial seizures; used to prevent seizures during brain surgery; used to prevent seizures due to toxemia in pregnant women. Capsule: 100 mg. Extended-release capsule: 30 mg, 100 mg, 200 mg, 300 mg. Chewable tablet: 50 mg. Liquid: 125 mg/5 mL. Intravenous or intramuscular: 50 mg/mL. [FEN ih TOH in].

**Phillips' Milk of Magnesia, Concentrated Phillips' Milk of Magnesia** (GI).   See *milk of magnesia.* [FIL-ips]

**Phillips' Liqui-Gels** (GI).   See *docusate.* [FIL-ips].

**pHisoHex** (Derm).   See *hexachlorophene.* [FY-soh-heks].

**Phos-Lo** (Uro).   See *calcium acetate.* [FAWS-loh].

**Phosphocol 32** (Chemo).   Radioactive phosphate drug used to treat pleural and peritoneal effusions caused by metastases in cancer patients. Intrapleural or intraperitoneal: 5 mCi/mL. [FAW-foh-kawl 32].

**Phospholine Iodide** (Ophth).   See *echothiophate.* [FAWS-foh-leen EYE-oh-dide].

**phosphorated carbohydrate solution** (Emetrol) (GI).   Over-the-counter antiemetic drug used to treat nausea and vomiting and motion sickness. Oral liquid: 21.5 mg/5 mL. [FAWS-for-aa-ted KAR-boh-HY-drayt].

**phosphorus** (Neutra-Phos, Neutra-Phos K) (Misc).   Phosphorus dietary supplement. Powder: 250 mg. [FAWS-foh-rus].

**Photofrin** (Chemo).   See *porfimer.* [FOH-toh-frin].

**Phrenilin Forte** (Analges) (generic *acetaminophen, butalbital*).   Combination nonsalicylate and barbiturate analgesic and sedative drug for pain. Capsule: 650 mg/ 50 mg. [FREN-ih-lin FOR-tay].

**physostigmine** (Antilirium) (Emerg, Psych).   Antagonist drug used as an antidote to reverse an overdose of a tricyclic antidepressant drug. Intramuscular or intravenous: 1 mg/mL. [FY-soh-STIG-meen].

**phytonadione** (Mephyton) (Hem).   Vitamin K drug given to newborns to prevent hemorrhagic disease of the newborn; given to adults with a vitamin K deficiency. Tablet: 5 mg. Intramuscular: 2 mg/mL, 10 mg/mL. [FY-toh-nah-DY-ohn].

**Pilocar** (Ophth).   See *pilocarpine.* [PY-loh-kar].

**pilocarpine** (Akarpine, Isopto Carpine, Pilocar, Pilopine HS, Salagen) (ENT, Ophth).   Miotic drug used to constrict the pupil to treat glaucoma; used to treat dry mouth due to salivary gland dysfunction after radiation for head and neck cancer or due to Sjögren's syndrome. Tablet: 5 mg, 7.5 mg. Ophthalmic gel: 4%. Ophthalmic solution: 0.25%, 0.5%, 1%, 2%, 3%, 4%, 5%, 6%, 8%, 10%. Tablet: 5 mg, 7.5 mg. [PY-loh-KAR-peen].

**Pilopine HS** (Ophth).   See *pilocarpine.* [PY-loh-peen H-S].

**Pima** (Pulm).   See *potassium iodide.* [PEE-mah].

**pimecrolimus** (Elidel) (Derm).   Immunmodulator drug used topically on the skin to treat atopic dermatitis (eczema). Cream: 1%. [PIM-eh-KROH-lih-mus].

**pimozide** (Orap) (Neuro).   Antipsychotic drug used to treat Tourette's syndrome. Tablet: 1 mg, 2 mg. [PIM-oh-zide].

**pindolol** (Visken) (Cardio).   Beta-blocker drug used to treat hypertension. Tablet: 5 mg, 10 mg. [PIN-doh-lawl].

**Pin-Rid** (GI).   See *pyrantel.* [PIN-rid].

**Pin-X** (GI).   See *pyrantel.* [PIN-X].

**pioglitazone** (Actos) (Endo).   Thiazolidinedione oral antidiabetic drug used to treat type 2 diabetes mellitus. Tablet: 15 mg, 30 mg, 45 mg. [PY-oh-GLIT ah-zohn].

**piperacillin** (Anti-infec).   Penicillin-type antibiotic drug used to treat various types of bacterial infections, including gonorrhea, endometritis, pelvic inflammatory disease, pneumonia caused by *H. influenzae* or *S. pneumoniae,* urinary and intra-abdominal infections caused by *E. coli,* and septicemia; used prophylactically before abdominal and vaginal surgery to prevent infection. Intramuscular and intravenous (powder to be reconstituted). [PIP-er-ah-SIL-in].

**piracetam** (Nootropil) (Ortho).   Used to treat myoclonus. Orphan drug. [pih-RAY-seh-tam].

**pirbuterol** (Maxair Autohaler) (Pulm).   Bronchodilator drug used to prevent and treat asthma and bronchospasm, particularly with bronchitis or emphysema. Aerosol inhaler: 0.2 mg/puff. [peer-BYOO-ter-awl].

**pirfenidone** (Pulm).   Used to treat pulmonary fibrosis. Orphan drug. [peer-FEN-ih-dohn].

**piritrexim** (Anti-infec).   Used to treat *Pneumocystis carinii* pneumonia, *Mycobacterium avium-intracellulare,* and *Toxoplasma gondii* infection in AIDS patients. Orphan drug. [PEER-ih-TREK-sim].

**piroxicam** (Feldene) (Analges).   Nonsteroidal anti-inflammatory drug used to treat the pain of osteoarthritis, rheumatoid arthritis, and dysmenorrhea. Capsule: 10 mg, 20 mg. [pih-RAWK-sih-kam].

**Pitocin** (OB/GYN).   See *oxytocin.* [pih-TOH-sin].

**Pitressin** (Endo, GI).   See *vasopressin.* [pih-TRES-in].

**Plan B** (OB/GYN).   See *levonorgestrel.* [PLAN B].

**Plaquase** (Uro).   See *collagenase.* [PLAH-kways].

**Plaquenil** (Anti-Infec, Derm, Ortho).   See *hydroxychloroquine.* [PLAH-kwih-nil].

**Plaretase 8000** (GI) (generic *amylase, lipase, protease*).   Combination digestive enzyme drug used as replacement therapy. Tablet: 30,000 units/8000 units/30,000 units. [PLAIR-tays].

**Plasbumin-5, Plasmbumin-20, Plasbumin-25** (I.V.).   See *albumin.* [plas-BYOO-min].

**plasma** (I.V.).   Blood product that contains no cellular components and is given intravenously to replace plasma proteins (albumin) and clotting factors. Intravenous. [PLAS-mah].

**Plasmanate** (I.V.).   See *plasma protein fraction.* [PLAS-mah-nayt].

**Plasma-Plex** (I.V.).   See *plasma protein fraction.* [PLAS-mah-pleks].

**plasma protein fraction** (PPF) (Plasmanate, Plasma-Plex, Protenate) (I.V.).   Blood product that contains no cellular components and is transfused to replace plasma proteins. Intravenous: 5%. [PLAZ-mah PROH-teen FRAK-shun].

**platelets** (I.V.).    Blood cellular product. Intravenous. [PLAYT-lets].

**Plavix** (Cardio, Hem, Neuro).    See *clopidogrel*. [PLAV-iks].

**Plegisol** (Cardio).    See *cardioplegic solution*. [PLEJ-ih-sawl].

**Plenaxis** (Chemo).    See *abarelix*. [pleh-NAK-sis].

**Plendil** (Cardio).    See *felodipine*. [PLEN-dil].

**Pletal** (Cardio, Hem).    See *cilostazol*. [PLEH-tal].

**Plexion, Plexion SCT, Plexion TS** (Derm) (generic *sodium sulfacetamide, sulfur*).    Combination anti-infective and keratolytic drug used topically on the skin to treat acne vulgaris. Cream, cleanser, suspension, or pads: 10%/5%. [PLEKS-ee-awn].

**plitidepsin** (Aplidin) (Chemo).    Chemotherapy drug used to treat leukemia and multiple myeloma. Orphan drug. [PLIH-tih-DEP-sin].

**pneumococcal vaccine** (Pneumovax 23, Prevnar) (Pulm).    Vaccine used to protect infants against pneumonia due to *Streptococcus pneumoniae* (Prevnar); used to protect the elderly and other at-risk patients against pneumococcal pneumonia (Pneumovax 23). Intramuscular: 2-4 mcg of each of 7 different strains/0.5 mL. Subcutaneous or intramuscular: 25 mcg of each of 23 different strains/0.5 mL. [NOO-moh-KAW-kawl vak-SEEN].

**Pneumopent** (Anti-infec).    See *pentamidine*. [NOO-moh-pent].

**Pneumovax 23** (Pulm).    See *pneumococcal vaccine*. [NOO-moh-vaks 23].

**Podocon-25** (Derm, OB/GYN).    See *podophyllum*. [POH-doh-kawn-25].

**podofilox** (Condylox) (Derm, OB/GYN).    Used topically on the skin to treat condylomata acuminata (genital warts). Gel: 0.5%. Liquid: 0.5%. [POH-doh-FIL-awks].

**Podofin** (Derm, OB/GYN).    See *podophyllum*. [POH-doh-fin].

**podophyllum** (Podocon-25, Podofin) (Derm, OB/GYN). Used topically on the skin to treat condylomata acuminata (genital warts). Liquid: 25%. [POH-doh-FIL-um].

**Polaramine Expectorant** (ENT) (generic *dexchlorpheniramine, guaifenesin, pseudoephedrine*).    Combination antihistamine, expectorant, and decongestant drug used to treat colds and allergies with a productive cough. Liquid: 2 mg/100 mg/ 20 mg. [poh-LAIR-ah-meen eks-PEK-toh-rant].

**Polocaine, Polocaine MPF** (Anes, ENT, OB/GYN).    See *mepivacaine*. [POH-loh-kayn].

**polaxamer 188** (Flocor) (Derm, Hem, Neuro).    Used to treat severe burns; used to treat sickle cell crisis; used to treat vasospasm after a subarachnoid hemorrhage in the brain. Orphan drug. [poh-LAWK-sah-mer 188].

**poloxamer 331** (Protox) (Anti-infec).    Used to treat toxoplasmosis in AIDS patients. Orphan drug. [poh-LAWK-sah-mer 331].

**polycarbophil** (Equalactin, FiberCon, Fiber-Lax, Konsyl Fiber) (GI).    Over-the-counter, bulk-producing laxative drug used to treat constipation. Chewable tablet: 625 mg. Tablet: 500 mg, 625 mg. [PAWL-ee-KAR-boh-fil].

**Polycitra, Polycitra-K, Polycitra-LC** (Uro) (generic *potassium citrate, sodium citrate, citric acid*).    Combination drug used to prevent the formation of calcium oxalate and uric acid kidney stones. Liquid: 550 mg/500 mg/334 mg. Syrup: 550 mg/500 mg/334 mg. Crystals (to be reconstituted in water). [PAWL-ee-SIH-trah].

**polydimethylsiloxane** (AdatoSil 5000) (Ophth).    Silicone oil injected into the posterior chamber during eye surgery to treat retinal detachment. Silicone oil. [PAWL-ee-dy-METH-il-sih-LAWK-sayn].

**polyethylene glycol** (GlycoLax, MiraLax, PEG) (GI). Osmotic laxative drug used to treat constipation. Powder (to be reconstituted to a liquid). [PAWL-ee-ETH-ih-leen GLY-kawl].

**Polygam S/D** (Anti-infec, Misc).    See *human immune globulin*. [PAWL-ee-gam S-D].

**poly-L-lactic acid** (Sculptra) (Derm).    Synthetic filler drug used to fill areas of fat loss in the face. Injection. [PAWL-ee-L-LAK-tik AS-id].

**polymyxin B** (Anti-infec, Derm, Ophth).    Antibiotic drug used to treat serious infections including *E. coli, H. influenzae, Pseudomonas,* and *Klebsiella;* used topically to treat *Pseudomonas* eye infections; included in many combination topical antibiotic drugs to treat skin infections. Intramuscular and intrathecal (powder to be reconstituted): 500,000 units. Ophthalmic solution (powder to be reconstituted): 500,000 units/20 mL. [PAWL-ee-MIK-sin B].

**Polysporin** (Derm) (generic *bacitracin, polymyxin B*). Combination over-the-counter antibiotic drug used topically on the skin to treat bacterial infections. Ointment: 500 units/10,000 units per g. [PAWL-ee-SPOR-in].

**Polysporin Ophthalmic Ointment** (Ophth) (generic *bacitracin, polymyxin B*).    Combination antibiotic drug used topically in the eyes to treat bacterial infections. Ointment: 500 units/10,000 units per g. [PAWL-ee-SPOR-in of-THAL-mik].

**Polytar** (Derm).    See *coal tar*. [PAWL-ee-tar].

**Ponstel** (Analges).    See *mefenamic acid*. [pawn-STEL].

**Pontocaine** (Anes).    See *tetracaine*. [PAWN-toh-kayn].

**poractant alfa** (Curosurf) (Pulm).    Surfactant drug used to prevent and treat respiratory distress syndrome in newborn infants and adults. Liquid (via endotracheal tube): 80 mg/1.5 mL, 80 mg/3 mL. [por-AK-tant AL-fah].

**porfimer** (Photofrin) (Chemo).    Chemotherapy photosensitizing drug used to treat cancer of the skin, esophagus, lung, and bladder. Intravenous (powder to be reconstituted): 75 mg. [POHR-fih-mer].

**porfiromycin** (Promycin) (Chemo).    Chemotherapy drug used to treat cancer of the head and neck and cervix of the uterus. Orphan drug. [por-FEER-oh-MY-sin].

**Porphozyme** (Uro).    Used to treat intermittent porphyria. Orphan drug. [POR-foh-zime].

**Portagen** (GI).   Lactose-free nutritional supplement. Powder (to be reconstituted). [POR-tah-jen].

**Portia** (OB/GYN) (generic *levonorgestrel, ethinyl estradiol*). Combination monophasic oral contraceptive drug. Pill pack, 21-day: (21 hormone tablets) 0.15 mg/30 mcg. Pill pack, 28-day: (21 hormone tablets) 0.15 mg/30 mcg; (7 inert tablets). [POR-shee-ah].

**posaconazole** (Noxafil) (Anti-infec).   Antifungal drug used to treat severe systemic fungal and yeast infections such as aspergillosis and candidiasis in immunocompromised patients. Oral suspension: 40 mg/mL. [POH-sah-KAWN-ah-zohl].

**Posurdex** (Ophth).   See *dexamethasone*. [PAWS-yoor-deks].

**Potasalan** (Uro).   See *potassium*. [poh-TAS-ah-lan].

**potassium** (Cena-K, Effer-K, Gen-K, K + 8, K + 10, K + Care, K + Care ET, Kaon, Kaon Cl-10, Kaon-Cl-20%, Kay Ciel, Kaylixir, K-Dur 10, K-Dur 20, K-Lor, Klor-Con, Klor-Con 8, Klor-Con 10, Klor-Con/25, Klor-Con/EF, Klor-Con M10, Klor-Con M15, Klor-Con M20, Klorvess, Klotrix, K-Lyte, K-Lyte/Cl, K-Lyte/Cl 50, K-Lyte DS, Kolyum, K-Tab, K-vescent, Micro-K Extencaps, Micro-K 10 Extencaps, Micro-K LS, Potasalan, Twin-K) (Uro).   Used to replace potassium loss caused by diuretic drugs. Controlled-release capsule: 8 mEq (600 mg), 10 mEq (750 mg). Tablet: 99 mg, 500 mg, 595 mg. Controlled-release tablet: 8 mEq (600 mg), 10 mEq (750 mg), 15 mEq (1125 mg), 20 mEq (1500 mg). Effervescent tablet: 20 mEq, 25 mEq, 50 mEq. Extended-release tablet: 8 mEq (600 mg), 10 mEq (750 mg). Liquid: 20 mEq/15 mL, 40 mEq/15 mL. Powder (to be reconstituted: 15 mEq, 20 mEq, 25 mEq. [poh-TAS-see-um].

**potassium acid phosphate** (K-Phos Original) (Uro).   Used to acidify the urine to prevent the formation of calcium kidney stones. Tablet: 500 mg. [poh-TAS-ee-um AS-id FAWS-fayt].

**potassium citrate** (Urocit-K) (Ortho, Uro).   Used to prevent the formation of calcium oxalate or uric acid kidney stones, particularly in patients with gout. Tablet: 5 mEq, 10 mEq. [poh-TAS-ee-um SIH-trayt].

**potassium iodide** (Pima, SSKI) (Pulm).   Expectorant drug used to thin mucus in the lungs. Liquid: 1 g/mL. Syrup: 325 mg/5 mL. [poh-TAS-ee-um EYE-oh-dide].

**povidone iodine** (Betadine, Minidyne) (Derm, Ophth).   Over-the-counter and prescription iodine-containing topical antibacterial, antiviral, antifungal, and antiyeast drug used in wounds, ulcers, and incisions to prevent infection; used as a surgical skin scrub; used as a topical eye irrigating solution prior to surgery. Aerosol: 5%. Foam: 7.5%. Liquid: 10%. Ointment: 1%, 10%. Ophthalmic solution: 5%. Spray: 10%. Surgical scrub: 7.5%. Swabstick: 10%. Topical solution: 1%, 10%. Vaginal gel: 10%. [POH-vih-dohn EYE-oh-dine].

**pralatrexate** (Chemo).   Chemotherapy drug used to treat mycosis fungoides. Orphan drug. [PRAL-ah-TREK-sayt].

**pralidoxime** (Protopam) (Emerg, Neuro).   Used to reverse the effect of pesticide (organophosphate) poisoning; used to reverse the effect of an overdose of an anticholinergic drug;

used to treat myasthenia gravis. Intravenous: 1 g/20 mL. [PRAL-ih-DAWK-zeem].

**pramipexole** (Mirapex) (Neuro).   Dopamine receptor stimulant drug used to treat Parkinson's disease and restless legs syndrome. Tablet: 0.125 mg, 0.25 mg, 0.5 mg, 0.75 mg, 1 mg, 1.5 mg. [PRAM-ih-PEK-sohl].

**pramiracetam** (Psych).   Used to treat symptoms of mental dysfunction following electroshock therapy. Orphan drug. [PRAM-ih-RAY-seh-tam].

**pramlintide** (Symlin) (Endo).   Amylin analog antidiabetic drug used to treat type 1 and type 2 diabetes mellitus. Subcutaneous: 0.6 mg/mL. SimlinPen 60 prefilled injector pen: 60 mcg. SymlinPen 120 prefilled injector pen: 120 mcg. [PRAM-lin-tide].

**pramoxine** (ProctoFoam NS, Tronothane, Tuks) (Anes, Derm, GI).   Over-the-counter anesthetic drug used topically to treat the pain of abrasions, burns, sunburn, insect bites, poison ivy, and dry, itchy skin; used to treat cold sores; used to treat the pain and itching of hemorrhoids. Cream: 1%. Foam: 1%. Gel: 1%. Lotion: 1%. Ointment: 1%. Spray: 1%. [prah-MAWK-seen].

**PrandiMet** (Endo) (generic *metformin, repaglinide*). Combination oral antidiabetic drug used to treat type 2 diabetes mellitus. Tablet: 500 mg/1 mg, 500 mg/2 mg. [PRAN-dih-met].

**Prandin** (Endo).   See *repaglinide*. [PRAN-din].

**Pravachol** (Cardio).   See *pravastatin*. [PRAH-vah-kawl].

**pravastatin** (Pravachol) (Cardio).   HMG-CoA reductase inhibitor drug used to treat hypercholesterolemia and arteriosclerosis. Tablet: 10 mg, 20 mg, 40 mg, 80 mg. [PRAH-vah-STAT-in].

**praziquantel** (Biltricide) (Misc).   Used to treat worm infestations. Tablet: 600 mg. [prah-ZIH-kwan-tel].

**prazosin** (Minipress) (Cardio).   Alpha-blocker drug used to treat hypertension. Capsule: 1 mg, 2 mg, 5 mg. [PRAY-zoh-sin].

**Precedex** (Anes, Pulm).   See *dexmedetomidine*. [PRES-eh-deks].

**Precose** (Endo).   See *acarbose*. [PREE-kohs].

**Predcor** (Derm, Endo, Neuro, Ortho).   See *prednisolone*. [PRED-kor].

**Pred Forte, Pred Mild** (Ophth).   See *prednisolone*. [PRED FOR-tay].

**Pred-G Ophthalmic** (Ophth) (generic *gentamicin, prednisolone*).   Combination antibiotic and corticosteroid drug used topically in the eyes. Ophthalmic suspension: 0.3%/1%. Ophthalmic ointment: 0.3%0.6%. [pred-G of-THAL-mik].

**prednicarbate** (Dermatop E) (Derm).   Corticosteroid drug used topically to treat inflammation and itching from dermatitis, seborrhea, eczema, psoriasis, and yeast or fungal infections. Cream: 0.1%. Ointment: 0.1%. [PRED-nih-KAR-bayt].

**Prednicen-M** (Chemo, Endo, Ortho, Pulm, Neuro). See *prednisone*. [PRED-nih-sen- M].

**prednimustine** (Sterecyt) (Chemo). Chemotherapy drug used to treat non-Hodgkin's lymphoma. Orphan drug. [PRED-nih-MUS-teen].

**Prednisol** (Ophth). See *prednisolone*. [PRED nih sawl].

**prednisolone** (Econopred Plus, Flo-Pred, Orapred, Orapred ODT, Pediapred, Prelone, Pred Forte, Pred Mild, Prednisol, Prelone) (Chemo, Derm, Endo, GI, Neuro, Ophth, Ortho, Pulm, Uro). Corticosteroid anti-inflammatory drug used to treat severe inflammation in various body systems; used to treat multiple sclerosis and lupus erythematosus; used to treat severe psoriasis, dermatitis, and mycosis fungoides; used to treat the inflammation of osteoarthritis, rheumatoid arthritis, bursitis, and tenosynovitis; used to treat nephrotic syndrome; used to treat severe asthma and pleurisy from tuberculosis; used to treat flareups of ulcerative colitis and Crohn's disease; used to treat leukemia and lymphoma; used topically to treat inflammation of the eyes and corneal injury (Econopred Plus, Pred Forte, Pred Mild, Prednisol). Oral liquid: 5 mg/5 mL, 15 mg/5 mL. Tablet: 5 mg. Orally disintegrating tablet: 10 mg, 15 mg, 30 mg. Syrup: 15 mg/5 mL. Ophthalmic suspension: 0.12%, 1%. Ophthalmic solution: 1%. [pred-NIS-oh-lohn].

**prednisone** (Deltasone, Liquid Pred, Meticorten, Orasone, Panasol-S, Prednicen-M, Prednisone Intensol Concentrate, Sterapred, Sterapred DS) (Chemo, Endo, Ortho, Pulm, Neuro). Corticosteroid anti-inflammatory drug used to treat severe inflammation in various body systems; used to treat the inflammation of osteoarthritis and rheumatoid arthritis; used to treat severe asthma; used in chemotherapy protocols to decrease inflammation; used to treat multiple sclerosis. Tablet: 1 mg, 2.5 mg, 5 mg, 10 mg, 20 mg, 50 mg. Oral liquid: 5 mg/mL, 5 mg/5 mL. Syrup: 5 mg/5 mL. [PRED-nih-sohn].

**Prednisone Intensol Concentrate** (Chemo, Endo, Ortho, Pulm, Neuro). See *prednisone*. [PRED-nih-sohn in-TEN-sawl].

**Prefest** (OB/GYN, Ortho) (generic *norgestimate, estradiol*). Combination hormone drug used to treat the symptoms of menopause; used to prevent postmenopausal osteoporosis. Tablet: 0.09 mg/1 mg. [PREE-fest].

**pregabalin** (Lyrica) (Derm, Endo, Neuro, Ortho). Anticonvulsant drug used to treat partial onset seizures; used to treat the pain of fibromyalgia, diabetic peripheral neuropathy, and herpes zoster infection (shingles). Capsule: 25 mg, 50 mg, 75 mg, 100 mg, 150 mg, 200 mg, 225 mg, 300 mg. [pree-GAB-ah-lin].

**Pregestimil** (GI). Infant formula for infants with GI malabsorption disorders. Powder (to be reconstituted). [pree-JES-tih-mil].

**Pregnyl** (Endo, OB/GYN). See *human chorioic gonadotropin*. [PREG-nil].

**Prelone** (Endo). See *prednisolone*. [PREE-lohn].

**Prelu-2** (GI). See *phendimetrazine*. [PRAY-loo-2].

**Premarin, Premarin Intravenous, Premarin Vaginal** (Chemo, OB/GYN, Ortho). See *conjugated estrogens*. [PREM-ah-rin].

**Premphase** (OB/GYN, Ortho) (generic *medroxyprogesterone, conjugated estrogens*). Combination hormone drug used to treat the symptoms of menopause; used to prevent postmenopausal osteoporosis. Tablet: 5 mg/0.625 mg. [PREM-fays].

**Prempro** (OB/GYN, Ortho) (generic *medroxyprogesterone, conjugated estrogens*). Combination hormone drug used to treat the symptoms of menopause; used to prevent postmenopausal osteoporosis. Tablet: 1.5 mg/0.3 mg, 1.5 mg/0.45 mg, 2.5 mg/0.625 mg, 5 mg/0.625 mg. [PREM-proh].

**Premsyn PMS** (OB/GYN) (generic *acetaminophen, pamabrom, pyrilamine*). Combination over-the-counter analgesic, diuretic, and antihistamine drug used to treat painful menstruation. Caplet: 500 mg/25 mg/15 mg. [PREM-sin P-M-S].

**Prenilin** (Analges) (generic *acetaminophen, butalbital*). Combination nonsalicylate analgesic and barbiturate sedative drug for pain. Tablet: 325 mg/50 mg. [PREN-ih-lin].

**Preparation H** (GI). See *phenylephrine*. [PREP-ah-RAY-shun H].

**Prepidil** (OB/GYN). See *dinoprostone*. [PREP-ih-dil].

**Prevacid, Prevacid I.V.** (GI). See *lansoprazole*. [PREV-ah-sid].

**Prevacid NapraPAC** (Analges, GI) (generic *lansoprazole, naproxen*). Combination proton pump inhibitor drug and nonsteroidal anti-inflammatory drug used to treat heartburn and GI ulcers in patients who take a nonsteroidal anti-inflammatory drug for arthritis. NapraPAC 375: Tablet: 375 mg, delayed-release capsule: 15 mg. NapraPAC 500: Tablet: 500 mg, delayed-release capsule: 15 mg. [PREV-ah-sid].

**Prevalite** (Cardio, Emerg, Endo, GI). See *cholestyramine*. [PREV-ah-lyte].

**Preven** (OB/GYN) (generic *levonorgestrel, ethinyl estradiol*). Combination hormone drug taken after unprotected sexual intercourse to prevent pregnancy. Tablet: 0.25 mg/0.05 mg. [pree-VEN].

**Previfem** (OB/GYN) (generic *norgestimate, ethinyl estradiol*). Combination monophasic oral contraceptive drug. Pill pack, 28-day: (21 hormone tablets) 0.25 mg/35 mcg; (7 inert tablets). [PREV-ih-fem].

**Prevnar** (Pulm). See *pneumococcal vaccine*. [PREV-nar].

**Prevpac** (GI) (generic *amoxicillin, clarithromycin, lansoprazole*). Combination antibiotic and proton pump inhibitor drug used to treat peptic ulcers caused by *H. pylori*. Daily packet: Amoxicillin capsule: 500 mg; clarithromycin tablet: 500 mg; lansoprazole capsule: 30 mg. [PREV-pak].

**Prezista** (Anti-infec). See *darunavir*. [preh-ZIS-tah].

**Prialt** (Analges).   See *ziconotide*. [PREE-alt].

**Priftin** (Anti-infec, Pulm).   See *rifapentine*. [PRIF-tin].

**prilocaine** (Citanest) (Anes, ENT).   Anesthetic drug used to produce local and regional anesthesia during dental procedures. Injection: 4%, 4% with 1:200,000 epinephrine. [PRY-loh-kayn].

**Prilosec, Prilosec OTC** (GI).   See *omeprazole*. [PRY-loh-sek].

**PrimaCare Advantage** (OB/GYN) (generic *vitamins, minerals, omega-3 fatty acids, DHA, EPA, ALA, docusate*).   Combination prenatal vitamin supplement and stool softener drug. [PRY-mah-KAIR].

**Primacor** (Cardio).   See *milrinone*. [PRY-mah-kor].

**primaquine** (Anti-infec).   Used to treat *Pneumocystis carinii* pneumonia in AIDS patients. Orphan drug. [PRY-mah-kwin].

**Primatene** (ENT, Pulm) (generic *ephedrine, guaifenesin*).   Combination over-the-counter decongestant and expectorant drug used to treat a productive cough. Tablet: 12.5 mg/200 mg. [PRY-mah-teen].

**Primatene Dual Action** (Pulm) (generic *theophylline, ephedrine, guaifenesin*).   Combination bronchodilator and expectorant drug used to treat asthma, bronchitis, and productive cough. Tablet: 60 mg/12.5 mg/100 mg. [PRY-mah-teen].

**Primatene Mist** (Pulm).   See *epinephrine*. [PRY-mah-teen MIST].

**Primaxin I.M., Primaxin I.V.** (Anti-infec) (generic *imipenem, cilastatin*).   Combination carbapenem antibiotic drug and a drug that inhibits an enzyme that breaks down carbapenem; used to treat infections of the skin, lungs, urinary tract, bone, and gynecologic infections; used to treat endocarditis, intra-abdominal infections, and septicemia. Intramuscular or intravenous (powder to be reconstituted): 250 mg/250 mg, 500 mg/500 mg, 750 mg/750 mg. [pry-MAK-sin].

**primidone** (Mysoline) (Neuro).   Anticonvulsant drug used to treat tonic-clonic and simple partial and complex partial seizures; used to treat benign familial tremor. Tablet: 50 mg, 250 mg. [PRIM-ih-dohn].

**Primsol** (Anti-infec, Uro).   See *trimethoprim*. [PRIM-ih-sawl].

**Principen** (Anti-infec).   See *ampicillin*. [PRIN-sih-pen].

**Prinivil** (Cardio).   See *lisinopril*. [PRIN-ih-vil].

**Prinzide** (Cardio) (generic *lisinopril, hydrochlorothiazide*).   Combination ACE inhibitor and diuretic drug used to treat hypertension. Tablet: 10 mg/12.5 mg, 20 mg/12.5 mg, 20 mg/25 mg. [PRIN-zide].

**Pristiq** (Psych).   See *desvenlafaxine*. [pris-TEEK].

**Privine** (ENT).   See *naphazoline*. [PRIH-veen].

**ProAir HFA** (Pulm).   See *albuterol*. [PROH-air].

**ProAmatine** (Cardio).   See *midodrine*. [proh-AM-ah-teen].

**Pro-Banthine** (GI).   See *propantheline*. [proh-BAN-theen].

**probenecid** (Anti-infec, Ortho).   Used to decrease uric acid levels to treat gout and gouty arthritis; used to prolong the therapeutic blood level of certain antibiotic drugs. Tablet: 0.5 g. [proh-BEN-eh-sid].

**Probenecid and Colchicine** (GI) (generic *probenecid, cholchicine*).   Combination drug that decreases uric acid levels; used to treat gout and gouty arthritis. Tablet: 500 mg/0.5 mg. [proh-BEN-eh-sid and KOHL-chih-seen].

**procainamide** (Pronestyl) (Cardio).   Antiarrhythmic drug used to treat ventricular tachycardia. Capsule: 250 mg, 375 mg, 500 mg. Tablet: 375 mg. Extended-release tablet: 250 mg, 500 mg, 750 mg, 1000 mg. Intramuscular or intravenous: 500 mg/mL. [proh-KAY-nah-mide].

**procaine** (Novocain) (Anes, Ortho).   Local, regional nerve block, and spinal anesthetic drug; used to treat fibromyalgia with trigger point injections. Injection: 1%, 2%, 10%. [PROH-kayn].

**procarbazine** (Matulane) (Chemo).   Chemotherapy drug used to treat cancer of the brain and lung; used to treat malignant melanoma, Hodgkin's lymphoma, non-Hodgkin's lymphoma, mycosis fungoides, and multiple myeloma. Capsule: 50 mg. [proh-KAR-bah-zeen].

**Procardia, Procardia XL** (Cardio).   See *nifedipine*. [proh-KAR-dee-ah].

**Prochieve** (OB/GYN).   See *progesterone*. [PROH-cheev].

**prochlorperazine** (Compazine, Compro) (Analges, GI, Psych).   Phenothiazine antipsychotic drug used to treat schizophrenia; used to treat anxiety; used to treat nausea and vomiting; used to treat migraine headaches. Tablet: 5 mg, 10 mg. Spansules: 10 mg, 15 mg. Syrup: 5 mg/5mL. Suppository: 2.5 mg, 5 mg, 25 mg. Intramuscular: 5 mg/mL. [PROH-klor-PAIR-ah-zeen].

**prochymal** (Hem).   Used to treat graft-versus-host disease. Orphan drug. [proh-KY-mal].

**Procort** (Derm).   See *hydrocortisone*. [PROH-kort].

**Procrit** (Hem).   See *epoetin alfa*. [PROH-krit].

**Proctocort** (GI).   See *hydrocortisone*. [PRAWK-toh-kort].

**ProctoCream-HC** (Derm, GI) (generic *hydrocortisone, pramoxine*).   Combination corticosteroid and anesthetic drug used topically to treat inflammation and itching from perianal dermatitis and hemorrhoids. [PRAWK-toh-kreem-H-C].

**Proctofoam-HC** (GI) (generic *hydrocortisone, pramoxine*).   Combination corticosteroid anti-inflammatory and anesthetic drug used topically to treat ulcerative colitis. Foam: 1%/1%. [PRAWK-toh-fohm-H-C].

**ProctoFoam NS** (Anes, GI).   See *pramoxine*. [PRAWK-toh-fohm N-S].

**procyclidine** (Neuro).   Anticholinergic drug used to treat Parkinson's disease. Tablet: 5 mg. [proh-SY-klih-deen].

**Procysteine** (Pulm, Neuro).   Used to treat adult respiratory distress syndrome; used to treat amyotrophic lateral sclerosis. Orphan drug. [proh-SIS-teen].

**Prodium** (Uro).   See *phenazopyridine*. [PROH-dee-um].

**Profasi** (Endo, OB/GYN).   See *human chorioic gonadotropin*. [proh-FAW-see].

**Pro-Fast HS, Pro-Fast SA, Pro-Fast SR** (GI).   See *phentermine*. [PROH-fast].

**Profilnine SD** (Hem).    See *factor IX*. [PROH-fil-NINE S-D].

**Progestasert** (OB/GYN).    See *progesterone*. [proh-JES-tah-sert].

**progesterone** (Crinone, Endometrin, Prochieve, Progestasert, Prometrium) (OB/GYN).    Progesterone hormone drug used to treat amenorrhea; used during assisted reproductive technology to treat infertility; hormone contraceptive implant drug that is effective for one year (Progestasert). Capsule: 100 mg. Intramuscular: 50 mg/mL. Vaginal gel: 4%, 8%. Vaginal insert: 100 mg. Intrauterine T-shaped implant: 38 mg. [proh-JES-teh-rohn].

**Proglycem** (Endo).    See *diazoxide*. [proh-GLY-sem].

**Prograf** (Cardio, GI, Uro).    See *tacrolimus*. [PROH-graf].

**Prolastin** (Pulm).    See *alpha₁-proteinase inhibitor*. [proh-LAS-tin].

**Proleukin** (Chemo).    See *aldesleukin*. [proh-LOO-kin].

**Proloprim** (Anti-infec, Uro).    See *trimethoprim*. [PROH-loh-prim].

**Promacet** (Analges) (generic *acetaminophen, butalbital*).    Combination nonsalicylate analgesic and barbiturate sedative drug for pain. Tablet: 650 mg/50 mg. [PROH-mah-set].

**Promega Pearls** (Cardio).    See *omega-3 fatty acids*. [proh-MAY-gah].

**promethazine** (Phenadoz, Phenergan) (Anes, Derm, Emerg, ENT, GI, Ophth).    Antihistamine drug used to treat allergic skin reactions and itching; used to treat the symptoms of seasonal and perennial allergies, allergic rhinitis, and allergic conjunctivitis; used to treat allergic reactions from foods and other allergens; used to control the severity of an allergic reaction to blood products; used to prevent or treat nausea, vomiting, and motion sickness; used to provide preoperative sedation. Syrup: 6.25 mg/5 mL. Tablet: 12.5 mg, 25 mg, 50 mg. Suppository: 12.5 mg, 25 mg, 50 mg. Intramuscular or intravenous: 25 mg/mL, 50 mg/mL. [proh-METH-ah-zeen].

**Prometrium** (OB/GYN).    See *progesterone*. [proh-MEE-tree-um].

**Promit** (I.V.).    See *dextran 1*. [PROH-mit].

**Promycin** (Chemo).    See *porfiromycin*. [proh-MY-sin].

**Pronestyl** (Cardio).    See *procainamide*. [proh-NES-til].

**propafenone** (Rythmol) (Cardio).    Antiarrhythmic drug used to treat atrial flutter, atrial fibrillation, and ventricular tachycardia. Tablet: 150 mg, 225 mg, 300 mg. Extended-release capsule: 225 mg, 325 mg, 425 mg. [PROH-pah-FEE-nohn].

**propantheline** (Pro-Banthine) (GI).    Anticholinergic antispasmodic drug used to decrease acid production and treat spasm from peptic ulcer. Tablet: 7.5 mg, 15 mg. [proh-PAN-theh-leen].

**PROPApH Acne Maximum Strength, PROPApH Astringent Cleanser Maximum Strength, PROPApH Cleansing for Oily Skin, PROPApH Foaming Face Wash, PROPApH Peel-off Acne Mask** (Derm).    See *salicylic acid*. [PRAW-pah-P-H].

**proparacaine** (Alcaine, Ophthetic, Paracaine) (Ophth).    Anesthetic drug used topically to numb the eyes. Ophthalmic solution: 0.5%. [proh-PAIR-ah-kayn].

**Propecia** (Derm).    See *finasteride*. [proh-PEE-shee-ah].

**Propine** (Ophth).    See *dipivefrin*. [PROH-peen].

**Proplex T** (Hem).    See *factor IX*. [PROH-pleks T].

**propofol** (Diprivan) (Anes, Pulm).    Sedative drug used to induce and maintain general anesthesia; used to sedate patients who are intubated and on the ventilator. Intravenous: 10 mg/mL. [PROH-poh-fawl].

**propoxyphene** (Darvon-N, Darvon Pulvules) (Analges).    Schedule IV narcotic analgesic drug used to treat pain. Capsule: 65 mg. Tablet: 100 mg. [proh-PAWK-see-feen].

**propranolol** (Inderal, Inderal LA, InnoPran XL, Propranolol Intensol) (Analges, Cardio, Endo, GI, Neuro, Psych).    Beta-blocker drug used to treat angina pectoris, hypertension, atrial flutter, atrial fibrillation, ventricular tachycardia, premature ventricular contractions, and myocardial infarction; used to treat hypertrophic subaortic stenosis; used to treat hypertension caused by a pheochromocytoma of the adrenal medulla; used to prevent migraine headaches; used to treat the tremors of Parkinson's disease and essential familial tremor; used to treat anxiety disorder and performance anxiety; used to treat muscle restlessness caused by antipsychotic drugs; used to prevent bleeding GI varices in patients with portal hypertension. Extended-release capsule: 60 mg, 80 mg, 120 mg, 160 mg. Oral liquid: 4 mg/mL, 8 mg/mL. Concentrated oral liquid: 80 mg/mL. Tablet: 10 mg, 20 mg, 40 mg, 60 mg, 80 mg, 90 mg. Intravenous: 1 mg/mL. [proh-PRAN-oh-lawl].

**Propranolol Intensol** (Analges, Cardio, Endo, GI, Neuro, Psych).    See *propranolol*. [proh-PRAN-oh-lawl in-TEN-sawl].

**propylthiouracil** (Endo).    Antithyroid drug used to treat hyperthyroidism. Tablet: 50 mg. [PROH-pil-THY-oh-YOOR-ah-sil].

**ProQuad** (Anti-infec).    Combination drug used to prevent measles, mumps, rubella, and varicella in children. Subcutaneous: Vaccine. [PROH-kwad].

**Proquin XR** (Anti-infec).    See *ciprofloxacin*. [PROH-quin X-R].

**Proscar** (Uro).    See *finasteride*. [PROH-skar].

**Prosed/DS** (Uro) (generic *atropine, hyoscyamine, methenamine, methylene blue, phenyl salicylate*).    Combination urinary tract antispasmodic, anti-infective, antiseptic, and analgesic drug; used to treat urinary tract infections with pain and spasms. Tablet: 0.06 mg/ 0.06 mg/81.6 mg/10.8 mg/36.2 mg. [PROH-sed D-S].

**ProSobee** (GI).    Lactose-free, sucrose-free infant formula with soy protein for infants with allergies. Liquid. Powder (to be reconstituted). [proh-SOH-bee].

**ProSom** (Neuro).    See *estazolam*. [PROH-sawm].

**prostaglandin E1** (Cardio).    See *alprostadil*. [PRAWS-tah-GLAN-din E-1].

**Prostigmin** (Neuro, Uro).    See *neostigmine*.
   [proh-STIG-min].

**Prostin E2** (OB/GYN).    See *dinoprostone*. [PRAWS-tin E-2].

**Prostin VR Pediatric** (Cardio).    See *alprostadil*.
   [PRAWS-tin V-R].

**protamine sulfate** (Hem).    Heparin antagonist drug used to
   treat heparin overdose or reverse the effect of heparin
   administered during surgery. Intravenous: 10 mg/mL.
   [PROH-tah-meen SUL-fayt].

**protaxel** (Chemo).    Chemotherapy drug used to treat ovarian
   cancer. Orphan drug. [proh-TAK-sel].

**protein C concentrate** (Ceprotin) (Hem).    Recombinant
   DNA activated protein C-type thrombolytic drug used to
   treat patients with congenital protein C deficiency.
   Intravenous (powder to be reconstituted): 500 units,
   1000 units. [PROH-teen C].

**Protenate** (I.V.).    See *plasma protein fraction*.
   [PROH-teh-nayt].

**protirelin** (Neuro, Pulm).    Used to treat amyotrophic lateral
   sclerosis; used to prevent respiratory distress syndrome in
   premature infants. Orphan drug. [proh-TY-reh-lin].

**Protonix, Protonix I.V.** (GI).    See *pantoprazole*.
   [proh-TAWN-iks].

**Protopam** (Emerg, Neuro).    See *pralidoxime*.
   [PROH-toh-pam].

**Protopic** (Derm).    See *tacrolimus*. [proh-TAWP-ik].

**Protox** (Anti-infec).    See *poloxamer 331*. [PROH-tawks].

**protirelin** (Neuro).    Used to treat amyotrophic lateral
   sclerosis. Orphan drug. [PROH-teh-REL-in].

**protriptyline** (Vivactil) (Analges, Neuro, OB/GYN,
   Psych).    Tricyclic antidepressant drug used to treat
   depression and premenstrual dysphoric disorder; used to
   treat migraine headaches; used to treat nerve pain from
   phantom limb, diabetic neuropathy, peripheral neuropathy,
   and postherpetic neuralgia; used to treat tic douloureux.
   Tablet: 5 mg, 10 mg. [proh-TRIP-tih-leen].

**Protropin** (Endo).    See *somatrem*. [pro-TROH-pin].

**Proventil, Proventil HFA** (Pulm).    See *albuterol*.
   [proh-VEN-til].

**Provera** (Chemo, OB/GYN).    See *medroxyprotesterone*.
   [proh-VAIR-ah].

**Provigil** (Neuro, Pulm).    See *modafinil*. [proh-VIJ-il].

**Provocholine** (Misc).    See *methacholine*.
   [PROH-voh-KOH-leen].

**Proxinium** (Chemo).    Chemotherapy drug used to treat cancer of the head and neck. Orphan drug. [prawk-SIN-ee-um].

**Prozac, Prozac Weekly** (Analges, Cardio, Psych).    See
   *fluoxetine*. [PROH-zak].

**prussian blue** (Radiogardase) (Emerg).    Chelating drug used
   to treat radioactive cesium or thallium overdose. Capsule:
   0.5 g. [PRUS-shun BLOO].

**pseudoephedrine** (Dimetapp Decongestant Pediatric,
   Dimetapp Maximum Strength Non-Drowsy, Drixoral 12
   Hour Non-Drowsy Formula, PediaCare Infants'
   Decongestant, Sudafed Children's Non-Drowsy, Sudafed
   Non-Drowsy, Triaminic Allergy Congestion) (ENT).
   Over-the-counter decongestant drug used to treat nasal
   stuffiness due to colds and allergies. Capsule: 60 mg. Gel
   capsule: 30 mg. Drops: 7.5 mg/0.8 mL. Syrup: 15 mg/5 mL.
   Oral liquid: 15 mg/5 mL, 30 mg/5 mL. Tablet: 30 mg,
   60 mg. Extended-release tablet: 120 mg, 240 mg. Chewable
   tablet: 15 mg. [soo-doh-eh-FEH-drin].

**Psorcon E** (Derm).    See *diflorasone*. [SOR-kawn E].

**Psorent** (Derm).    See *coal tar*. [SOR-ent].

**Psorian** (Derm).    See *betamethasone*. [SOR-ee-an].

**Psoriatec** (Derm).    See *anthralin*. [soh-RY-ah-tek].

**psyllium** (Fiberall, Genfiber, Hydrocil Instant, Konsyl,
   Konsyl-D, Metamucil, Perdiem Fiber Therapy, Reguloid,
   Syllact) (GI).    Over-the-counter, bulk-producing laxative
   drug used to treat constipation. Capsule. Granules. Powder.
   Wafer. [SIL-ee-um].

**PulmaDex** (Pulm).    Used to treat cystic fibrosis. Orphan
   drug. [PUL-mah-deks].

**Pulmicort Respules, PulmicortTurbuhaler** (Pulm).    See
   *budesonide*. [PUL-moh-kort].

**Pulmocare** (GI, Pulm).    Nutritional supplement used to meet
   the nutritional needs of patients with pulmonary disease.
   Liquid. [PUL-moh-kair].

**PulmoLAR** (Pulm).    Used to treat pulmonary arterial
   hypertension. Orphan drug. [PUL-moh-lar].

**Pulmozyme** (Pulm).    See *dornase alfa*. [PUL-moh-zime].

**Purinethol** (Chemo).    See *mercaptopurine*.
   [pyoor-RIN-eh-thawl].

**PUVA** (Derm) (generic *psoralen, ultraviolet light wavelength A*).
   Combination light-sensitizing drug and light therapy used
   to treat severe psoriasis. [POO-vah].

**pyrantel** (Antiminth, Pin-Rid, Pin-X) (GI).    Over-the-
   counter drug used to treat pinworms and roundworms.
   Capsule: 180 mg. Tablet: 180 mg. Liquid: 50 mg/mL.
   [py-RAN-tel].

**pyrazinamide** (Pulm).    Antitubercular antibiotic drug used
   only to treat tuberculosis. Tablet: 500 mg.
   [PY-rah-ZIN-ah-mide].

**Pyridium** (Uro).    See *phenazopyridine*. [py-RID-ee-um].

**Pyridium Plus** (Uro) (generic *butabarbital, hyoscyamine,
   phenazopyridine*).    Combination sedative, urinary tract
   antispasmodic, and urinary tract analgesic drug. Tablet:
   15 mg/0.3 mg/150 mg. [py-RID-ee-um PLUS].

**pyridostigmine** (Mestinon) (Neuro).    Anticholinesterase drug
   used to treat myasthenia gravis. Liquid: 60 mg/5 mL.
   Tablet: 60 mg. Extended-release tablet: 180 mg.
   Intravenous: 5 mg/mL. [py-RID-oh-STIG-meen].

**pyridoxine** (Aminoxin, Vitelle Nestrex) (OB/GYN,
   Pulm).    Vitamin $B_6$ drug used to treat vitamin $B_6$
   deficiency caused by the drug isoniazid (used to treat
   tuberculosis) or oral contraceptive drugs. Tablet: 25 mg,
   50 mg, 100 mg, 250 mg, 500 mg. Enteric-coated tablet:
   20 mg. [PEER-ih-DAWK-seen].

**pyrimethamine** (Daraprim) (Anti-infec). Used to treat toxoplasmosis; used to prevent and treat malaria. [PY-rih-METH-ah-meen].

**pyrithione zinc** (Denorex Everyday Dandruff, Dermazinc, DHS Zinc, Head & Shoulders, Head & Shoulders Dry Scalp, Zincon, ZNP Bar (Derm). Over-the-counter drug used topically to treat psoriasis, seborrheic dermatitis, and eczema. Shampoo: 0.25%, 1%, 2%. Soap: 2%. [py-RITH-ee-own ZINK].

**pyruvate** (Pulm). Used to treat interstitial lung disease. Orphan drug. [py-ROO-vayt].

**Quadramet** (Analges, Chemo). See *samarium-153*. [KWAH-drah-met].

**Quadrinal** (Pulm) (generic *theophylline, ephedrine, potassium iodide, phenobarbital*). Combination bronchodilator, expectorant, and sedative drug. Tablet: 65 mg/24 mg/320 mg/24 mg. [KWAH-drih-nal].

**Qualaquin** (Anti-infec). See *quinine*. [KWAL-ah-kwin.]

**Quasense** (OB/GYN) (generic *levonorgestrel, ethinyl estradiol*). Combination monophasic oral contraceptive drug. Pill pack, 28-day: (21 hormone tablets) 0.15 mg/30 mcg; (7 inert tablets). [KWAH-sens].

**quazepam** (Doral) (Neuro). Schedule IV benzodiazepine drug used to treat insomnia. Tablet: 7.5 mg, 15 mg. [KWAH-zeh-pam].

**Quelicin** (Anes, Pulm). See *succinylcholine*. [KWEL-ih-sin].

**Questran, Questran Light** (Cardio, Emerg, Endo, GI). See *cholestyramine*. [KWES-tran].

**quetiapine** (Seroquel, Seroquel XR) (Neuro, Psych). Dibenzapine antipsychotic drug used to treat schizophrenia; used to treat both the mania and depression of manic-depressive disorder; used to treat psychosis and agitation in patients with Alzheimer's disease or Parkinson's disease. Tablet: 25 mg, 50 mg, 100 mg, 200 mg, 300 mg, 400 mg. Extended-release tablet: 200 mg, 300 mg. Sustained-release tablet: 400 mg. [kweh-TY-ah-peen].

**Quibron, Quibron-300** (Pulm) (generic *theophylline, guaifenesin*). Combination bronchodilator and expectorant drug. Capsule: 150 mg/90 mg, 300 mg/180 mg. [KWIH-brawn].

**quinacrine** (Pulm). Used to prevent recurrence of pneumothorax. Orphan drug. [KWIN-ah-krin].

**quinapril** (Accupril) (Cardio). ACE inhibitor drug used to treat congestive heart failure and hypertension. Tablet: 5 mg, 10 mg, 20 mg, 40 mg. [KWIN-ah-pril].

**Quinaretic** (Cardio) (generic *quinapril, hydrochlorothiazide*). Combination ACE inhibitor and diuretic drug used to treat hypertension. Tablet: 10 mg/12.5 mg, 20 mg/12.5 mg, 20 mg/25 mg. [KWIN-ah-RET-ik].

**quinidine** (Cardio). Antiarrhythmic drug used to treat atrial flutter, atrial fibrillation, atrial tachycardia, and ventricular tachycardia. Tablet: 200 mg, 300 mg, 324 mg. Sustained-release tablet: 300 mg. Intramuscular or intravenous: 80 mg/mL. [KWIN-ih-deen].

**quinine** (Qualaquin) (Anti-infec). Used to treat malaria. Capsule: 200 mg, 260 mg, 325 mg. Tablet: 260 mg. [KWY-nine].

**Quixin** (Ophth). See *levofloxacin*. [KWIK-sin].

**QVAR** (Pulm). See *beclomethasone*. [KVAR-var]

**rabeprazole** (AcipHex) (GI). Proton pump inhibitor drug used to treat GERD and esophagitis. Delayed-release tablet: 20 mg. [rah-BEP-rah-zohl].

**Radiogardase** (Emerg). See *prussian blue*. [RAY-dee-oh-GAR-days].

**raloxifene** (Evista) (Chemo, OB/GYN, Ortho). Selective estrogen receptor modulator (SERM) drug used to prevent and treat osteoporosis in postmenopausal women; used to treat osteoporosis in men; used to treat uterine fibroids; used to prevent breast cancer; used to treat gynecomastia in men. Tablet: 60 mg. [rah-LAWK-sih-feen].

**raltegravir** (Isentress) (Anti-infec). Integrase inhibitor antiviral drug used to treat HIV and AIDS. Tablet: 400 mg. [ral-TEG-rah-veer].

**ramelteon** (Rozerem) (Neuro). Nonbarbiturate sedative drug used to treat insomnia. Tablet: 8 mg. [rah-MEL-tee-awn].

**ramipril** (Altace) (Cardio). ACE inhibitor drug used to treat hypertension and congestive heart failure; used to decrease the risk of a myocardial infarction or stroke in patients with coronary artery disease. Capsule: 1.25 mg, 2.5 mg, 5 mg, 10 mg. [RAM-ih-pril].

**Ranexa** (Cardio). See *ranolazine*. [rah-NEK-sah].

**ranibizumab** (Lucentis) (Ophth). Monoclonal antibody drug used to treat wet macular degeneration. Injection (into the vitreous humor): 10 mg/mL. [RAN-ih-BIZ-yoo-mab].

**Raniclor** (Anti-infec). See *cefaclor*. [RAN-ih-klor].

**ranitidine** (Zantac, Zantac 75, Zantac 150 Maximum Strength, Zantac EFFERdose) (GI). Over-the-counter and prescription $H_2$ blocker drug used to treat heartburn, peptic ulcer, GERD, esophagitis, and *H. pylori* infection. Capsule: 150 mg, 300 mg. Effervescent tablet: 25 mg. Tablet: 75 mg, 150 mg, 300 mg. Syrup: 15 mg/mL. Intramuscular or intravenous: 1 mg/mL, 25 mg/mL. [rah-NIT-ih-deen].

**ranolazine** (Ranexa) (Cardio). Drug used to treat angina pectoris. Extended-release tablet: 500 mg, 1000 mg. [rah-NOL-ah-zeen].

**Rapamune** (Derm, Uro). See *sirolimus*. [RAP-ah-myoon].

**rapamycin** (Chemo). Chemotherapy drug used to treat bone cancer. Orphan drug. [RAP-ah-MY-sin].

**Raptiva** (Derm). See *efalizumab*. [rap-TEE-vah].

**rasagiline** (Azilect) (Neuro). MAO inhibitor drug used to treat Parkinson's disease. Tablet: 0.5 mg, 1 mg. [rah-SAJ-ih-leen].

**rasburicase** (Elitek) (Chemo). Used to treat elevated uric acid levels in patients receiving chemotherapy. Intravenous: 1.5 mg. [ras-BYOOR-ih-kays].

**Razadyne, Razadyne ER, Razadyne Oral Solution** (Neuro). See *galantamine*. [RAY-zah-dine].

**RCF** (GI). Infant formula with soy protein. Liquid. [R-C-F].

**Rebetol** (Anti-infec, GI). See *ribavirin*. [REE-beh-tawl].

**Rebif** (Anti-infec, Neuro). See *interferon beta-1a*. [REE-bif].

**Receptin** (Anti-infec). See *recombinant human soluble CD4*. [ree-SEP-tin].

**Reclast** (Chemo, Ortho). See *zoledronic acid*. [REE-klast].

**Reclipsin** (OB/GYN) (generic *desogestrel, ethinyl estradiol*). Combination monophasic oral contraceptive drug. Pill pack, 28-day: (21 hormone tablets) 0.15 mg/ 30 mcg; (7 inert tablets). [reh-KLIP-sin].

**recombinant human soluble CD4** (Receptin) (Anti-infec). Antiviral drug used to treat HIV and AIDS. Orphan drug. [ree-KAWM-bih-nant HYOO-man SAWL-yoo-bl C-D-4].

**Recombinate** (Hem). See *factor VIII*. [ree-COM-bih-nayt].

**Recombivax HB** (GI). See *hepatitis B vaccine*. [ree-KAWM-bih-vaks H-B].

**Recothrom** (Hem). See *thrombin*. [REE-koh-thrawm].

**Rectagene II** (GI) (generic *bismuth, zinc oxide*). Combination anti-infective and astringent drug used topically to treat hemorrhoids. Suppository. [REK-tah-jeen 2].

**ReFacto** (Hem). See *factor VIII*. [ree-FAK-toh].

**Refludan** (Hem). See *lepirudin*. [reh-FLOO-dan].

**regadenoson** (Lexiscan) (Cardio). Vasodilator drug used during myocardial perfusion scan for patients who cannot undergo exercise stress testing. Intravenous. [REE-gah-DEN-oh-son].

**Reglan** (GI). See *metoclopramide*. [REG-lan].

**Regranex** (Derm). See *becaplermin*. [ree-GRAN-eks].

**Regular Iletin II** (Endo). See *regular insulin*. [REG-yoo-lar EYE-leh-tin 2].

**regular insulin** (Humulin R, Humulin R Regular U-500, Novolin R, Novolin R PenFill, Novolin R Prefilled, Regular Iletin II) (Endo). Rapid-acting insulin, derived from pig pancreas or DNA recombinant technology, used to treat type 1 diabetes mellitus. Subcutaneous: 100 units/mL, 500 units/mL. Prefilled syringe: 100 units/mL. NovoPen and Novolin Pen cartridges: 100 units/mL. [REG-yoo-lar IN-soo-lin].

**Reguloid** (GI). See *psyllium*. [REG-yoo-loyd].

**Relenza** (Anti-infec, Pulm). See *zanamivir*. [reh-LEN-zah].

**Relistor** (GI). See *methylnaltrexone*. [REL-is-tor].

**Relpax** (Analges). See *eletriptan*. [REL-paks].

**remacemide** (Ecovia) (Neuro). Used to treat Huntington's chorea. Orphan drug. [reh-MAY-seh-mide].

**Remeron, Remeron SolTab** (Psych). See *mirtazapine*. [REM-er-awn].

**Remicade** (Derm, GI, Ortho). See *infliximab*. [REM-ih-kayd].

**Remifemin** (OB/GYN). See *black cohosh*. [REM-ee-FEM-in].

**remifentanil** (Ultiva) (Anes). Schedule II narcotic drug used to relieve pain and induce and maintain general anesthesia. Intravenous: 1 mg/3 mL, 2 mg/5 mL, 5 mg/10 mL. [REM-ee-FEN-tah-nil].

**Remitogen** (Chemo). Chemotherapy drug used to treat non-Hodgkin's lymphoma. Orphan drug. [reh-MIT-oh-jen].

**Remodulin** (Pulm). See *treprostinil*. [ree-MAW-dyoo-lin].

**Removab** (Chemo). See *catumazomab*. [REM-oh-vab].

**Remular S** (Ortho). See *chlorzoxazone*. [REM-yoo-lar-S].

**Renacidin** (Uro) (generic *citric acid, lactone, magnesium acid citrate, magnesium hydroxycarbonate*). Combination drug used to dissolve calcium and magnesium kidney stones in patients who cannot have surgery; used to dissolve kidney stone fragments after surgery. Powder (to be reconstituted) or liquid irrigating solution (given via nephrostomy tube and/or catheter). [REN-ah-SY-din].

**Renagel** (Uro). See *sevelamer*. [REH-nah-jel].

**Renova** (Derm). See *tretinoin*. [reh-NOH-vah].

**Renvela** (Uro). See *sevelamer*. [ren-VEL-ah].

**ReoPro** (Cardio, Hem). See *abciximab*. [REE-oh-proh].

**repaglinide** (Prandin) (Endo). Meglidinide oral antidiabetic drug used to treat type 2 diabetes mellitus. Tablet: 0.5 mg, 1 mg, 2 mg. [reh-PAG-lih-nide].

**Repan CF** (Analges) (generic *acetaminophen, butalbital*). Combination nonsalicylate and barbiturate analgesic and sedative drug for pain. Tablet: 650 mg/50 mg. [REE-pan C-F].

**Replagal** (Misc). See *alpha-galactosidase A*. [REP-lah-gal].

**repository corticotropin** (H.P. Acthar Gel) (Endo). Corticosteroid drug used in diagnostic testing to assess adrenal cortex function. Intramuscular or subcutaneous: 80 units/mL. [ree-PAW-sih-toh-ree KOR-tih-koh-TROH-pin].

**Reprexain** (Analges) (generic *hydrocodone, ibuprofen*). Combination Schedule III narcotic and nonsteroidal anti-inflammatory analgesic drug for pain. Tablet: 5 mg/200 mg. [ree-PREK-sayn].

**Repronex** (Endo, OB/GYN). See *menotropins*. [REE-proh-neks].

**Requip, Requip XL** (Neuro). See *ropinirole*. [REE-kwhip].

**Rescriptor** (Anti-infec). See *delavirdine*. [reh-SKRIP-tor].

**Resectisol** (Uro). See *mannitol*. [reh-SEK-tih-sawl].

**reserpine** (Cardio, Psych). Used to treat hypertension; used to treat agitation in patients with psychosis; used to treat tardive dyskinesia side effect of antipsychotic drugs. Tablet: 0.1 mg, 0.25 mg. [reh-SIR-peen].

**resiniferatoxin** (Analges). Used to treat severe pain. Orphan drug. [reh-SIN-ih-FAIR-ah-TAWK-sin].

**Resol** (GI). Electrolyte solution given to replace water and electrolytes lost due to vomiting or diarrhea. Oral liquid: 240 mL. [REE-sawl].

**Resource, ReSource Diabetic, ReSource Fruit Beverage, ReSource Just for Kids, Resource Plus** (GI). Lactose-free and/or gluten-free nutritional supplement. Liquid. [REE-sors].

**Respalor** (GI, Pulm).    Lactose-free nutritional supplement formulated for patients with pulmonary disease. Liquid. [RES-pah-lohr].

**RespiGam** (Anti-infec, Pulm).    See *respiratory syncytial virus immunoglobulin*. [RES-pih-gam].

**respiratory syncytial virus immunoglobulin** (Hypermune RSV, Respigam) (Anti-infec, Pulm).    Immunoglobulin drug used to treat respiratory syncytial virus infection in pediatric patients. 50 mg/mL. [sin-SIH-shal VY-rus IM-myoo-noh-GLAW-byoo-lin].

**Restasis** (Ophth).    See *cyclosporine*. [reh-STAY-sis].

**Restoril** (Neuro).    See *temazepam*. [RES-toh-ril].

**Restylane** (Derm).    See *hyaluronic acid*. [RES-tih-layn].

**retapamulin** (Altabax) (Derm, ENT).    Pleuromutilins antibiotic drug used topically to treat impetigo infection of the skin; used to treat methicillin-resistant *Staphylococcus aureus* colonization in the nose. Ointment: 1%. [RET-ah-PAM-yoo-lin].

**Retavase** (Cardio, Hem).    See *reteplase*. [REH-tah-vays].

**reteplase** (Retavase) (Cardio, Hem).    Tissue plasminogen activator drug used to dissolve blood clots that caused a myocardial infarction. Intravenous (powder to be reconstituted): 18.1 mg (10.4 units/10 mL). [REH-teh-plays].

**Retin-A, Retin-A Micro** (Derm).    See *tretinoin*. [REH-tin-A].

**Retisert** (Ophth).    See *fluocinolone*. [RET-ih-sert].

**Retrovir** (Anti-infec).    See *zidovudine*. [REH-troh-veer].

**Revatio** (Pulm).    See *sildenafil*. [reh-VAH-tee-oh].

**Reversol** (Anes).    See *edrophonium*. [ree-VER-sawl].

**Rev-Eyes** (Ophth).    See *dapiprazole*. [REV-eyez].

**ReVia** (Psych).    See *naltrexone*. [reh-VEE-ah].

**reviparin** (Clivarine) (Hem).    Used to treat deep venous thrombosis. Orphan drug. [REV-ih-PAIR-in].

**Revlimid** (Chemo).    See *lenalidomide*. [REV-lih-mid].

**Rexin-G** (Chemo).    Retroviral vector drug used to treat pancreatic cancer. Orphan drug. [REK-sin-G].

**Reyataz** (Anti-infec).    See *atazanavir*. [RAY-ah-taz].

**Rezipas** (GI).    See *4-aminosalicylic acid*. [REZ-ih-pas].

**Rheomacrodex** (I.V.).    See *dextran 40*. [REE-oh-MAK-roh-deks].

**Rheumatrex Dose Pack** (Chemo, Derm, GI, Neuro, Ortho).    See *methotrexate*. [ROO-mah-treks].

**Rhinall** (ENT).    See *phenylephrine*. [RY-nawl].

**Rhinocort Aqua** (ENT).    See *budesonide*. [RY-noh-kort AW-kwah].

**RhoGAM** (Hem, OB/GYN).    Immunoglobulin drug given to an Rh-negative mother after the birth of an Rh-positive infant; it prevents the mother from making antibodies during the next pregnancy and causing hemolytic disease if the next infant is Rh positive. Intramuscular: 5% gamma globulin. [ROH-gam].

**Rhophylac** (Hem, OB/GYN).    Immunoglobulin drug used to treat immune thrombocytopenia purpura; used after abortion, amniocentesis, or chorionic villus sampling to treat an Rh-negative mother with an Rh-positive baby to prevent hemorrhagic disease of the newborn in a subsequent pregnancy. Intramuscular or intravenous (powder to be reconstituted): 600 units (120 mcg), 1500 units (300 mcg), 2500 units (500 mcg), 5000 units (1000 mcg), 15,000 units (3000 mcg). [ROH-fih-lak].

**RibaPak** (Anti-infec, GI).    See *ribavirin*. [RY-bah-pak].

**Ribasphere** (Anti-infec, GI).    See *ribavirin*. [RY-bah-sfeer].

**Ribatab** (Anti-infec, GI).    See *ribavirin*. [RY-bah-tab].

**ribavirin** (Copegus, Rebetol, RibaPak, Ribasphere, Ribatab, Virazole) (Anti-infec, GI, Pulm).    Antiviral drug used to treat respiratory syncytial virus; used to treat hepatitis C virus infection. Powder for inhalation: 6 g/100 mL. Capsule: 200 mg. Tablet: 200 mg, 400 mg, 600 mg. Oral liquid: 40 mg/mL. [RY-bah-VY-rin].

**RID** (Derm) (generic *piperonyl, pyrethrin*).    Combination over-the-counter drug used topically on the skin and hair to treat parasitic infection from pediculosis (lice). Mousse: 4%/0.33%. Shampoo: 4%/0.33%. [RID].

**Ridaura** (Ortho).    See *auranofin*. [ry-DAW-rah].

**rifabutin** (Mycobutin) (Anti-infec).    Used to prevent *Mycobacterium avium-intracellulare* infection in AIDS patients. Capsule: 150 mg. [RY-fah-BYOO-tin].

**Rifadin** (Derm, ENT, Pulm).    See *rifampin*. [RY-fah-din].

**rifalazil** (Pulm).    Used to treat tuberculosis. Orphan drug. [ry-FAL-ah-zil].

**Rifamate** (Pulm) (generic *isoniazid, rifampin*).    Combination antitubercular antibiotic drug used to treat tuberculosis. Capsule: 150 mg/300 mg. [RY-fah-mayt].

**rifampin** (Rifadin, Rimactane) (Derm, ENT, Pulm).    Antitubercular antibiotic drug used to treat tuberculosis; used to prevent *Mycobacterium avium-intracellulare* infection in AIDS patients; used to treat persons who carry *Neisseria meningitides* in the nose; used to treat leprosy. Capsule: 150 mg, 300 mg. Intravenous (powder to be reconstituted): 600 mg. [ry-FAM-pin].

**rifapentine** (Priftin) (Anti-infec, Pulm).    Antitubercular antibiotic drug used to treat tuberculosis; orphan drug used to prevent *Mycobacterium avium-intracellulare* in AIDS patients. Tablet: 150 mg. [RIF-ah-PEN-teen].

**Rifater** (Pulm) (generic *isoniazid, pyrazinamide, rifampin*).    Combination antitubercular antibiotic drug used to treat tuberculosis. Tablet: 50 mg/300 mg/120 mg. [ry-FAT-er].

**rifaximin** (Normix, Xifaxan) (Anti-infec, Neuro).    Antibiotic drug used to treat traveler's diarrhea due to *E. coli;* used to treat encephalopathy caused by liver disease. Tablet: 200 mg. Orphan drug. [rih-FAK-sih-min].

**rilonacept** (Arcalyst) (Misc).    Interleukin-1 inhibitor drug used to treat cryopyrin-associated periodic syndrome (CAPS). Subcutaneous: 160 mg/2 mL. [rih-LAWN-ah-sept].

**Rilutek** (Neuro).    See *riluzole*. [RIL-yoo-tek].

**riluzole** (Rilutek) (Neuro).    Used to treat amyotrophic lateral sclerosis and Huntington's chorea. Tablet: 50 mg. [RIL-yoo-zohl].

**Rimactane** (Derm, ENT, Pulm).    See *rifampin*. [rih-MAK-tayn].

**rimantadine** (Flumadine) (Anti-infec, Pulm).    Antiviral drug used to prevent and treat influenza A virus infection. Tablet: 100 mg. Syrup: 50 mg/5 mL. [rih-MAN-teh-deen].

**rimexolone** (Vexol) (Ophth).    Corticosteroid drug used topically in the eyes to treat inflammation. Ophthalmic suspension: 1%. [rih-MEK-soh-lohn].

**Rimso-50** (Uro).    See *dimethyl sulfoxide*. [RIM-soh-50].

**Ringer's lactate** (RL) (I.V.).    Fluid of dextrose, sodium, potassium, calcium, chloride, and lactate. Intravenous. Irrigating solution. [RING-erz LAK-tayt].

**Riomet** (Endo).    See *metformin*. [RY-oh-met].

**Riopan** (GI) (generic *aluminum, magnesium*).    Combination antacid drug used to treat heartburn. Oral suspension: 540 mg/5 mL. [RY-oh-pan].

**Riopan Plus, Riopan Plus Double Strength** (GI) (generic *aluminum, magnesium, simethicone*).    Combination antacid and anti-gas drug used to treat heartburn and gas. Tablet: 480 mg/20 mg, 1080 mg/20 mg. [RY-oh-pan PLUS].

**risedronate** (Actonel) (OB/GYN, Ortho).    Bone resorption inhibitor drug used to prevent bone loss and treat osteoporosis in men and postmenopausal women; used to treat Paget's disease of the bone; used to prevent and treat osteoporosis caused by corticosteroid drugs. Tablet: 5 mg, 30 mg, 35 mg, 75 mg, 150 mg (once monthly). [rih-SED-roh-nayt].

**Risperdal, Risperdal M-Tab** (Neuro, Psych).    See *risperidone*. [RIS-per-dawl].

**risperidone** (Risperdal, Risperdal M-Tab) (Neuro, Psych).    Antipsychotic drug used to treat schizophrenia; used to treat mania in patients with manic-depressive disorder; used to treat self-injury and aggressive behavior in children with autism; used to treat psychosis and agitation in patients with Alzheimer's disease and Parkinson's disease; used to treat obsessive-compulsive disorder; used to treat Tourette'syndrome. Tablet: 0.25 mg, 0.5 mg, 1 mg, 2 mg, 3 mg, 4 mg. Orally disintegrating tablets: 0.5 mg, 1 mg, 2 mg, 3 mg, 4 mg. Liquid: 1 mg/mL.Intramuscular: 12.5 mg/2 mL, 25 mg/2 mL, 37.5 mg/2 mL, 50 mg/2 mL. [ris-PAIR-ih-dohn].

**Ritalin, Ritalin LA, Ritalin-SR** (Neuro, Psych).    See *methylphenidate*. [RIT-ah-lin].

**ritonavir** (Norvir) (Anti-infec).    Protease inhibitor antiviral drug used to treat HIV and AIDS. Capsule: 100 mg. Oral liquid: 80 mg/mL. [rih-TOH-nah-veer].

**Rituxan** (Chemo, Ortho).    See *rituximab*. [rih-TUK-san].

**rituximab** (Rituxan) (Chemo, Ortho).    Monoclonal antibody drug used to treat non-Hodgkin's lymphoma and leukemia; used to treat rheumatoid arthritis. Intravenous: 10 mg/mL. [rih-TUK-sih-mab].

**rivastigmine** (Exelon, Exelon Oral Solution, Exelon Patch) (Neuro).    Cholinesterase inhibitor drug used to treat mild-to-moderate Alzheimer's disease; used to treat dementia associated with Parkinson's disease. Capsule: 1.5 mg, 3 mg, 4.5 mg, 6 mg. Liquid: 2 mg/mL. Transdermal patch: 4.6 mg/24 hr, 9.5 mg/24 hr. [RIH-vah-STIG-meen].

**Rizaben** (Chemo).    See *tranilast*. [RY-zah-ben].

**rizatriptan** (Maxalt, Maxalt-MLT) (Analges).    Serotonin receptor agonist drug used to treat migraine headaches. Tablet: 5 mg, 10 mg. Orally disintegrating tablet: 5 mg, 10 mg. [RY-zah-TRIP-tan].

**RMS** (Analges).    See *morphine*. [R-M-S].

**Robaxin, Robaxin-750** (Ortho).    See *methocarbamol*. [roh-BAK-sin].

**Robinul, Robinul Forte** (GI).    See *glycopyrrolate*. [ROH-bih-nul].

**Robitussin** (Pulm).    See *guaifenesin*. [ROH-bih-TUS-sin].

**Robitussin Allergy & Cough** (ENT) (generic *brompheniramine, dextromethorphan, pseudoephedrine*).    Combination over-the-counter antihistamine, nonnarcotic antitussive, and decongestant drug. Liquid: 2 mg/10 mg/30 mg. [ROH-bih-TUS-sin].

**Robitussin Cold & Cough** (ENT) (generic *dextromethorphan, pseudoephedrine*).    Combination over-the-counter antitussive and decongestant drug. Liquid: 10 mg/20 mg. [ROH-bih-TUS-sin].

**Robitussin Cold Sinus & Congestion, Robitussin PE, Robitussin Severe Congestion** (ENT) (generic *guaifenesin, pseudoephedrine*).    Combination over-the-counter expectorant and decongestant drug. Liqui-Gel: 200 mg/30 mg. Syrup: 100 mg/30 mg. Tablet: 200 mg/30 mg. [ROH-bih-TUS-sin].

**Robitussin CoughGels, Robitussin Pediatric Cough** (ENT).    See *dextromethorphan*. [ROH-bih-TUS-sin].

**Robitussin Flu** (ENT) (generic *acetaminophen, chlorpheniramine, dextromethorphan, pseudoephedrine*).    Combination over-the-counter analgesic, antihistamine, nonnarcotic antitussive, and decongestant drug for colds, flu, and coughs. Liquid: 160 mg/1 mg/5 mg/15 mg. [ROH-bih-TUS-sin].

**Robitussin Flu Nighttime** (ENT) (generic *acetaminophen, chlorpheniramine, dextromethorphan, pseudoephedrine*).    Combination over-the-counter analgesic, antihistamine, nonnarcotic antitussive, and decongestant drug for colds and flu and coughs. Syrup: 500 mg/4 mg/20 mg/60 mg. [ROH-bih-TUS-sin].

**Robitussin Flu Non-Drowsy** (ENT) (generic *acetaminophen, dextromethorphan, pseudoephedrine*).    Combination over-the-counter analgesic, nonnarcotic antitussive, and decongestant drug for colds and coughs. Syrup: 500 mg/20 mg/60 mg. [ROH-bih-TUS-sin].

**Robitussin-DM** (ENT) (generic *dextromethorphan, guaifenesin*).    Combination over-the-counter nonnarcotic antitussive and expectorant drug for productive coughs. Liquid: 10 mg/100 mg. [ROH-bih-TUS-sin].

**Robitussin Maximum Strength Cough & Cold, Robitussin Pediatric Cough & Cold** (ENT) (generic *dextromethorphan,* *pseudoephedrine*). Combination over-the-counter nonnarcotic antitussive and decongestant drug for colds and coughs. Syrup: 15 mg/30 mg. [ROH-bih-TUS-sin].

**Robitussin Pediatric Cough & Cold** (ENT) (generic *chlorpheniramine, dextromethorphan*). Combination over-the-counter antihistamine and nonnarcotic antitussive drug for colds and coughs. Liquid: 1 mg/7.5 mg [ROH-bih-TUS-sin].

**Robitussin PM Cough & Cold** (ENT) (generic *chlorpheniramine, dextromethorphan, pseudoephedrine*). Combination over-the-counter antihistamine, nonnarcotic antitussive, and decongestant drug for colds and coughs. Liquid: 2 mg/10 mg/15 mg. [ROH-bih-TUS-sin].

**Rocaltrol** (Uro). See *calcitriol*. [roh-KAL-trawl].

**Rocephin** (Anti-infec). See *ceftriaxone*. [roh-SEF-in].

**rocuronium** (Zemuron) (Anes, Pulm). Neuromuscular blocker drug used during surgery; used to treat patients who are intubated and on the ventilator. Intravenous: 10 mg/mL. [ROH-kyoor-OH-nee-um].

**Rogaine, Rogaine Extra Strength for Men** (Derm). See *minoxidil*. [ROH-gayn].

**Rohypnol** (Psych). See *flunitrazepam*. [roh-HIP-nawl].

**Rolaids, Rolaids Calcium Rich, Rolaids Multisymptom** (GI) (generic *calcium, magnesium*). Combination antacid drug used to treat heartburn. Tablet: 412 mg/80 mg, 550 mg/110 mg, 675 mg/135 mg. [ROH-laydz].

**Rolaids Extra Strength** (GI). See *calcium carbonate*. [ROH-laydz].

**Romazicon** (Emerg, Psych). See *flumazenil*. [roh-MAY-zih-kawn].

**romiplostim** (Nplate) (Hem). Used to treat thrombocytopenia purpura. Intravenous. [roh-MIP-loh-stim].

**Rondec** (ENT) (generic *chlorpheniramine, phenylephrine*). Combination antihistamine and decongestant drug. Syrup: 4 mg/12.5 mg. [RAWN-dek].

**Rondec-DM** (ENT) (generic *chlorpheniramine, dextromethorphan, phenylephrine*). Combination antihistamine, nonnarcotic antitussive, and antihistamine drug. Oral drops: 1 mg/3 mg/3.5 mg. [RAWN-dek-D-M].

**Rondec TR** (ENT) (generic *carbinoxamine, pseudoephedrine*). Combination antihistamine and decongestant drug. Tablet: 8 mg/120 mg. [RAWN-dek T-R].

**ropinirole** (Requip, Requip XL) (Neuro). Dopamine receptor stimulant drug used to treat Parkinson's disease; used to treat restless legs syndrome. Tablet: 0.25 mg, 0.5 mg, 1 mg, 2 mg, 3 mg, 4 mg, 5 mg. Extended-release tablet: 2 mg, 4 mg, 8 mg. [roh-PIN-ih-rohl].

**ropivacaine** (Naropin) (Anes, OB/GYN). Anesthetic drug used to produce local and regional anesthesia during surgery; used for epidural anesthesia during labor and vaginal delivery or cesarean section. Injection: 0.2%, 0.5, 0.75%, 1%. [roh-PIV-ah-kayn].

**roquinimex** (Linomide) (Chemo). Used to prolong remission in leukemia patients after bone marrow transplantation. Orphan drug. [roh-KWIN-ih-meks].

**Rosac** (Derm) (generic *sodium sulfacetamide, sulfur*) Combination anti-infective and keratolytic drug used topically to treat acne vulgaris and acne rosacea on the skin. Cream: 10%/5% [ROH-sak].

**Rosanil** (Derm) (generic *sodium sulfacetamide, sulfur*). Combination anti-infective and keratolytic drug used topically to treat acne vulgaris and acne rosacea on the skin. Cleanser: 10%/5%. [ROH-sah-nil].

**rose bengal** (Rosets) (Ophth). Drug used topically to reveal corneal abrasions. Dye strips. [ROHS BEN-gal].

**Rosets** (Ophth). See *rose bengal*. [roh-SETS].

**rosiglitazone** (Avandia) (Endo, OB/GYN). Thiazolidinedione oral antidiabetic drug used to treat type 2 diabetes mellitus; used to treat anovulation in women with polycystic ovaries. Tablet: 2 mg, 4 mg, 8 mg. [ROH-sih-GLIT-ah-zohn].

**Rosula, Rosula CLK, Rosula NS** (Derm) (generic *sodium sulfacetamide, sulfur or urea*). Combination anti-infective and keratolytic drug used topically on the skin to treat acne vulgaris and acne rosacea. Gel or pad: 10%/10%. [roh-SOO-lah].

**rosuvastatin** (Crestor) (Cardio). HMG-CoA reductase inhibitor drug used to treat hypercholesterolemia and arteriosclerosis. Tablet: 5 mg, 10 mg, 20 mg, 40 mg. [roh-SOO-vah-STAT-in].

**Rotarix** (GI). Used to prevent rotavirus gastroenteritis in children. Subcutaneous: Vaccine. [ROH-tah-riks].

**RotaTeq** (Anti-infec). Used to prevent rotavirus gastroenteritis in children. Subcutaneous: Vaccine. [ROH-tah-tek].

**rotigotine** (Neupro) (Neuro). Dopamine receptor stimulant drug used to treat Parkinson's disease. Transdermal patch: 2 mg/24 hr., 4 mg/24 hr., 6 mg/24 hr. [roh-TIG-oh-teen].

**Rovamycine** (Anti-infec). See *spiramycin*. [ROH-vah-MY-seen].

**Rowasa** (GI). See *mesalamine*. [roh-WAH-sah].

**Roxanol, Roxanol 100, Roxanol T** (Analges). See *morphine*. [RAWK-sah-nawl].

**Roxicet** (Analges) (generic *acetaminophen, oxycodone*). Combination Schedule II nonsalicylate and narcotic analgesic drug for pain. Tablet: 325 mg/5 mg. Oral liquid: 325 mg/5 mg. [RAWK-sih-set].

**Roxicodone, Roxicodone Intensol** (Analges). See *oxycodone*. [RAWK-sih-KOH-dohn].

**Roxilox** (Analges) (generic *acetaminophen, oxycodone*). Combination Schedule II nonsalicylate and narcotic analgesic drug for pain. Capsule: 500 mg/5 mg. [RAWK-sih-lawks].

**Roxiprin** (Analges) (generic *aspirin, oxycodone*). Combination Schedule II salicylate and narcotic analgesic drug for pain. Tablet: 325 mg/4.5 mg. [RAWK-sih-prin].

**Rozerem** (Neuro).   See *ramelteon*. [roh-ZAIR-em].

**Rubesol-1000** (Hem).   See *cyanocobalamin*. [ROO-beh-sawl-1000].

**rubitecan** (Anti-infec).   Used to treat pediatric HIV and AIDS. Orphan drug. [roo-BIH-teh-kan].

**rufinamide** (Misc).   Used to treat Lennox-Gastaut syndrome. Orphan drug. [roo-FIN-ah-mide].

**Rythmol** (Cardio).   See *propafenone*. [RITH-mawl].

**S2** (Pulm).   See *epinephrine*. [S-2].

**sacrosidase** (Sucraid) (Misc).   Dietary enzyme supplement used to treat sucrase deficiency. Solution: 8500 IU/mL. [SAH-kroh-SY-days].

**Saizen** (Derm, Endo).   See *somatropin*. [SAY-zen].

**Salagen** (ENT).   See *pilocarpine*. [SAL-ah-jen].

**Salex** (Derm).   See *salicylic acid*. [SAY-leks].

**Salflex** (Analges).   See *salsalate*. [SAL-fleks].

**salicylic acid** (Clearasil Acne-Fighting Pads, Clearasil Clearstick, Clearasil Double Clear, Clearasil Medicated Deep Cleanser, Compound W, Compound W for Kids, Dr. Scholl's Clear Away OneStep, Dr. Scholl's Corn/Callus Remover, Dr. Scholl's Wart Remover Kit, DuoFilm, DuoPlant, Fostex Acne Cleansing, Fostex Acne Medication Cleansing, Freezone, Neutrogena Oil-free Acne Wash, Oxy Medicated Cleanser Pads, Oxy Night Watch, PROPApH Acne Maximum Strength, PROPApH Astringent Cleanser Maximum Strength, PROPHApH Cleansing for Oily Skin, PROPApH Foaming Face Wash, PROPApH Peel-off Acne Mask, Salex, Stri-Dex Clear, Stri-Dex Pads, Wart-Off) (Derm).   Over-the-counter and prescription keratolytic drug used topically on the skin to treat acne vulgaris; used (in a stronger concentration) to remove verrucae (common warts, plantar warts), corns, and calluses; used to remove psoriasis plaques. Bar: 2%. Cream: 2%. Gel: 2%. Liquid or wash/foaming wash: 0.5%, 2%. Lotion: 0.5%, 0.6%. Mask: 2%. Cleansing pad: 0.5%, 1.25%, 2%. Stick: 1.25%, 2%. Strips: 40%. Corn and callus removal cream: 6%. Corn and callus removal lotion: 6%. Transdermal patch for warts: 40%. Wart removal disk/pad: 40%. Wart removal gel: 17%. Wart removal liquid: 12.6%, 13.6%, 17%. Wart removal strips: 40%. [SAL-ih-SIL-ik AS-id].

**saline** (Afrin Saline, Ayr Saline, Ocean) (ENT).   Over-the-counter moisturizing salt water drug used topically in the nose. Nasal spray: 0.4%, 0.65%. [SAY-leen].

**salmeterol** (Serevent Diskus) (Pulm).   Bronchodilator drug used to prevent and treat asthma, exercise-induced bronchospasm, and chronic obstructive pulmonary disease. Diskus (inhaled powder): 50 mcg. [sal-MEE-ter-awl].

**Salonpas Pain Relief Patch** (Analges) (generic *menthol, methyl salicylate*).   Combination over-the-counter analgesic drug used topically on the skin to relieve pain from injury and muscle spasm. Patch. [sah-LAWN-pas].

**Salprofen** (Analges).   See *ibuprofen*. (sal-PROH-fen).

**salsalate** (Amigesic, Arthra-G, Marthritic, Salflex, Salsitab) (Analges).   Salicylate analgesic drug used to treat the pain and inflammation of osteoarthritis. Tablet: 500 mg, 750 mg. [SAL-sah-layt].

**Salsitab** (Analges).   See *salsalate*. [SAL-sih-tab].

**Sal-Tropine** (GI, Neuro, Uro).   See *atropine*. [sal-TROH-peen].

**samarium 153** (Quadramet) (Analges, Chemo).   Radioactive drug used to treat bone pain in cancer patients with bone metastases from cancer. Intravenous: 50 mCi/mL. [sah-MAIR-ee-um-153].

**Sanctura, Sanctura XR** (Uro).   See *trospium*. [SANK-toor-ah].

**Sandimmune** (Cardio, GI, Hem, Uro).   See *cyclosporine*. [SAND-ih-myoon].

**Sandostatin, Sandostatin LAR Depot** (Chemo, Endo, GI).   See *octreotide*. [SAN-doh-STAT-in].

**Sanorex** (Ortho).   See *mazindol*. [SAN-oh-reks].

**Santyl** (Derm).   See *collagenase*. [SAN-til].

**Sanvar** (Endo).   See *vapreotide*. [SAN-var].

**sapropterin** (Kuvan) (Misc).   Used to treat elevated blood levels of phenylalanine and phenylketonuria (PKU). Tablet: 100 mg. [SAH-prawp-TAIR-in].

**saquinavir** (Fortovase, Invirase) (Anti-infec).   Protease inhibitor antiviral drug used to treat HIV and AIDS; orphan drug (Fortovase) used to treat pediatric HIV. Capsule: 200 mg. Tablet: 500 mg. [sah-KWIN-ah-veer].

**Sarafem** (Psych).   See *fluoxetine*. [SAIR-ah-fem].

**sargramostim** (Leukine) (Anti-infec, Chemo).   Granulocyte macrophage colony-stimulating factor used to increase the neutrophil count in AIDS patients and in cancer patients after chemotherapy or bone marrow transplantation. Intravenous (powder to be reconstituted): 250 mcg/mL, 500 mcg/mL. [sar-GRAM-oh-stim].

**Sarmustine** (Chemo).   Alkylating chemotherapy drug used to treat brain cancer. Orphan drug. [sar-MUS-teen].

**sarsasapogentin** (Neuro).   Used to treat amyotrophic lateral sclerosis. Orphan drug. [sar-SAS-ah-poh-JEN-tin].

**saw palmetto** (Uro).   Over-the-counter dietary supplement used to treat benign prostatic hypertrophy. [SAW pal-MEH-toh].

**Scalpicin** (Derm).   See *hydrocortisone*. [SKAL-pih-sin]

**Scleromate** (Cardio).   See *morrhuate*. [SKLER-oh-mayt].

**Sclerosol** (Chemo, Pulm).   See *talc*. [SKLER-oh-sawl].

**Scopace** (GI, Neuro).   See *scopolamine*. [SKOH-pays].

**scopolamine** (Isopto Hyoscine, Scopace, Transderm-Scōp) (Anes, GI, Neuro, Ophth).   Anticholinergic drug used as a sedative and to decrease secretions before surgery; used to treat delirium tremens; used to treat irritable bowel syndrome and diverticulitis (Scopace); used to treat nausea and vomiting after surgery or chemotherapy; used topically as a patch to prevent motion sickness (Transderm-Scōp); mydriatic drug used topically to dilate the pupil to treat eye inflammation; used topically to produce mydriasis of the eye prior to examination or surgery. Ophthalmic solution:

0.25%. Tablet: 0.4 mg. Transdermal patch: 1.5 mg. Subcutaneous: 0.3 mg/mL, 0.4 mg/mL, 0.86 mg/mL, 1 mg/mL. [skoh-PAWL-ah-meen].

**Scot-Tussin Allergy Relief Formula Clear** (ENT). See *diphenhydramine*. [skawt-TUS-sin].

**Sculptra** (Derm). See *poly-L-lactic acid*. [SKULP-trah].

**Seasonale** (OB/GYN) (generic *levonorgestrel, ethinyl estradiol*). Combination monophasic oral contraceptive drug. Pill pack, 91-day, extended regimen: (84 hormone tablets) 0.15 mg/30 mcg; (7 inert tablets). [SEE-son-AL].

**Seasonique** (OB/GYN) (generic *levonorgestrel, ethinyl estradiol*). Combination biphasic oral contraceptive drug. Pill pack, 91-day, extended-regimen: (84 hormone tablets) 0.15 mg/30 mcg; (7 hormone tablets) 10 mcg. [SEE-son-EEK].

**secalciferol** (Osteo-D) (Ortho). Used to treat familial rickets. Orphan drug. [SEH-kal-SIF-eh-rawl].

**secobarbital** (Seconal Sodium Pulvules) (Neuro). Schedule II barbiturate drug used preoperatively to provide sedation; used for short-term treatment of insomnia. Capsule: 100 mg. [SEK-oh-BAR-bih-tawl].

**Seconal Sodium Pulvules** (Neuro). See *secobarbital*. [SEK-oh-nawl].

**SecreFlo** (Misc). See *secretin*. [SEE-kreh-floh].

**secretin** (SecreFlo) (Misc). Used to diagnose pancreatic function. Intravenous: 16 mcg/8 mL. [seh-KREE-tin].

**Sectral** (Cardio). See *acebutolol*. [SEK-trawl].

**Sedapap** (Analges) (generic *acetaminophen, butalbital*). Combination nonsalicylate analgesic and barbiturate sedative drug for pain. Tablet: 650 mg/50 mg. [SEE-dah-pap].

**selegiline** (Eldepryl, Emsam, Zelapar) (Neuro). MAO inhibitor drug used to treat Parkinson's disease. Capsule: 5 mg. Tablet: 5 mg. Orally disintegrating tablet: 1.25 mg. Transdermal patch: 6 mg/24 hr, 9 mg/24 hr, 12 mg/24 hr. [seh-LEJ-ih-leen].

**selenium sulfide** (Head & Shoulders Intensive Treatment, Selsun, Selsun Blue) (Derm). Over-the-counter drug used topically on the scalp to treat seborrheic dermatitis. Lotion: 1%, 2.5%. Shampoo: 1%. [seh-LEE-nee-um SUL-fide].

**Selfemra** (Psych). See *fluoxetine*. [sel-FEM-rah].

**Selsun, Selsun Blue** (Derm). See *selenium sulfide*. [SEL-sun].

**Selzentry** (Anti-infec). See *maraviroc*. [sel-ZEN-tree].

**Semicid** (OB/GYN). See *nonoxynol-9*. [SEM-ih-sid].

**Senexon** (GI). See *sennosides*. [seh-NEK-sawn].

**senna** (GI). See *sennosides*. [SEN-nah].

**sennosides** (Black Draught, Evac-u-gen, ex•lax, ex•lax chocolated, Fletcher's Castoria, Maximum Relief ex•lax, Senexon, Senna, Senokot, SenokotXTRA, X-Prep Liquid) (GI). Over-the-counter irritant/stimulant laxative drug used to treat constipation. Granules: 15 mg/5 mL, 20 mg/ 5 mL. Liquid: 8.8 mg/5mL, 33 mg/5 mL. Oral drops: 8.8 mg/mL. Chewable tablet: 10 mg. Tablet: 6 mg, 8.6 mg, 15 mg, 17 mg, 25 mg. Syrup: 8.8 mg/5 mL. [SEN-oh-sides].

**Senokot, SenokotXTRA** (GI). See *sennosides*. [SEN-oh-kawt].

**Senokot-S** (GI) (generic *docusate, senna*). Combination over-the-counter stool softener and irritant/stimulant laxative drug used to treat constipation. Tablet: 50 mg/ 8.6 mg. [SEN-oh-kawt-S].

**Sensipar** (Chemo, Endo). See *cinacalcet*. [SEN-sih-par].

**Sensorcaine, Sensorcaine MPF, Sensorcaine MPF Spinal** (Anes, ENT, OB/GYN). See *bupivacaine*. [SEN-sor-kayn].

**Septocaine** (Septocaine) (Anes, ENT). See *articaine*. [SEP-toh-kayn].

**Septopal** (Anti-infec). See *gentamicin*. [SEP-toh-pawl].

**Septra, Septra DS, Septra IV** (Anti-infec) (generic *sulfamethoxazole, trimethoprim*). Combination antibiotic and sulfonamide anti-infective drug used to treat bronchitis, otitis media, traveler's diarrhea, urinary tract infection, and prostatitis; used to treat *Pneumocystis carinii* pneumonia in AIDS patients. Oral suspension: 200 mg/40 mg per 5 mL. Tablet: 400 mg/80 mg, 800 mg/160 mg. Intravenous: 80 mg/16 mg per 5 mL, 400 mg/80 mg per 5 mL. [SEP-trah].

**Serax** (GI, Psych). See *oxazepam*. [SEER-aks].

**Serevent Diskus** (Pulm). See *salmeterol*. [SAIR-eh-vent DIS-kus].

**sermorelin** (Geref) (Endo). Used to treat growth hormone deficiency in children; used to evaluate the ability of the anterior pituitary gland to secrete growth hormone; orphan drug used to treat wasting syndrome in AIDS patients; orphan drug used to treat infertility due to failure to ovulate. Subcutaneous injection (powder to be reconstituted): 50 mcg/2 mL. [SER-moh-REL-in].

**Seromycin Pulvules** (Pulm). See *cycloserine*. [SAIR-oh-MY-sin].

**Serophene** (OB/GYN). See *clomiphene*. [SAIR-oh-feen].

**Seroquel, Seroquel XR** (Neuro, Psych). See *quetiapine*. [SAIR-oh-kwel].

**Serostim, Serostim LQ** (Anti-infec, Endo). See *somatropin*. [SAIR-oh-stim].

**sertaconazole** (Ertaczo) (Derm). Antifungal drug used topically to treat tinea (ringworm) and other fungal skin infections. Cream: 2%. [SER-tah-KAWN-ah-zohl].

**sertraline** (Zoloft) (Psych). Selective serotonin reuptake inhibitor (SSRI) drug used to treat depression, panic attacks, obsessive-compulsive disorder, social anxiety, posttraumatic stress disorder, and premenstrual dysphoric disorder. Tablet: 25 mg, 50 mg, 100 mg. Liquid: 20 mg/mL. [SER-trah-leen].

**sevelamer** (Renagel, Renvela) (Uro). Phosphate binder drug used to decrease serum phosphorus levels in patients on hemodialysis. Tablet: 400 mg, 800 mg. [seh-VEL-ah-mer].

**sevoflurane** (Ultane) (Anes). Anesthetic drug used to induce and maintain general anesthesia. Inhaled gas. [SEE-voh-FLOOR-ayn].

**Shellgel** (Ophth).   See *sodium hyaluronate*. [SHEL-jel].

**Shur-Clens** (Derm).   Over-the-counter drug used topically on the skin to absorb drainage from burns, skin ulcers, and wounds. Gauze dressing containing 20% solution. [SHOOR-klens].

**Sibelium** (Neuro).   See *flunarizine*. [sih-BEL-ee-um].

**sibutramine** (Meridia) (GI).   Schedule IV appetite suppressant drug used to treat obesity. Capsule: 5 mg, 10 mg, 15 mg. [sih-BYOO-trah meen].

**Silace** (GI).   See *docusate*. [SY-lays].

**Siladryl** (Derm, ENT).   See *diphenhydramine*. [SIL-ah-dril].

**sildenafil** (Revatio, Viagra) (Pulm, Uro).   PDE5 inhibitor drug used to treat pulmonary arterial hypertension (Revatio); used to treat male impotence due to erectile dysfunction (Viagra). Tablet: 20, 25 mg, 50 mg, 100 mg. [sil-DEN-ah-fil].

**Silphen Cough** (ENT).   See *diphenhydramine*. [SIL-fen CAWF].

**Silvadene** (Derm).   See *silver sulfadiazine*. [SIL-vah-deen].

**silver nitrate** (chemical formula $AgNO_3$) (Derm, ENT, OB/GYN, Ophth).   Used topically to cauterize skin lesions (warts, granulation tissue); used to cauterize small blood vessels to stop nosebleeds and oozing from the umbilical cord in a newborn; used topically in the eye to prevent gonorrhea-caused blindness in newborns. Liquid: 10%, 25%, 50%. Ointment: 10%. Topical ophthalmic solution: 1%. [SIL-ver NY-trayt].

**silver sulfadiazine** (Silvadene) (Derm).   Anti-infective drug used topically on the skin to treat severe burns. Cream. [SIL-ver SUL-fah-DY-ah-zeen].

**Simcor** (Cardio) (generic *niacin, simvastatin*).   Combination B vitamin and HMG-CoA reductase inhibitor drug used to lower serum cholesterol levels. Tablet: 500 mg/20 mg, 750 mg/20 mg. [SIM-kor].

**simethicone** (Degas, Gas Relief, Gas-X, Gas-X Extra Strength, Genasyme, Mylanta Gas, Mylanta Gas Maximum Strength, Mylicon, Phazyme, Phazyme 95, Phazyme 125) (GI).   Antiflatulent drug for intestinal gas. Capsule: 125 mg, 180 mg. Chewable tablet: 80 mg, 125 mg. Orally disintegrating strip: 62.5 mg. Oral drops: 40 mg/0.6 mL. Tablet: 60 mg, 95 mg. [sy-METH-ih-kohn].

**Similac Human Milk Fortifier, Similac Low-Iron, Similac with Iron, Similac PM 60/40 Low-Iron** (GI).   Infant formula. Liquid. Powder (to be reconstituted). [SIM-ih-lak].

**Simulect** (GI, Uro).   See *basiliximab*. [SIM-yoo-lekt].

**simvastatin** (Zocor) (Cardio).   HMG-CoA reductase inhibitor drug used to treat hypercholesterolemia and arteriosclerosis. Tablet: 5 mg, 10 mg, 20 mg, 40 mg, 80 mg. [SIM-vah-STAT-in].

**sinecatechins** (Derm).   See *kunecatrechins*. [SIN-ee-KAT-eh-chins].

**Sinemet-10/100, Sinemet-25/100, Sinemet-25/250, Sinemet CR** (Neuro) (generic *carbidopa, levodopa*).   Combination dopamine precursor drug used to treat Parkinson's disease.

Tablet: 10 mg/100 mg, 25 mg/100 mg, 25 mg/250 mg, 50 mg/200 mg. Extended-release tablet: 25 mg/100 mg, 50 mg/200 mg. [SIN-eh-met].

**Sinequan** (Analges, Neuro, Psych).   See *doxepin*. [SIN-eh-kwan].

**Singulair** (Pulm).   See *montelukast*. [SING-gyoo-lair].

**siplizumab** (Chemo).   Chemotherapy drug used to treat mycosis fungoides. Orphan drug. [sip LIZ-yoo-mab].

**sirolimus** (Rapamune) (Derm, Uro).   Immunosuppressant drug given after kidney transplant to prevent rejection of the donor kidney; used to treat severe psoriasis. Oral liquid: 1 mg/mL. Tablet: 1 mg, 2 mg. [sir-OH-lih-mus].

**sitagliptin** (Januvia) (Endo).   DPP-4 inhibitor antidiabetic drug used to treat type 2 diabetes mellitus. Tablet: 25 mg, 50 mg, 100 mg. [SIH-tah-GLIP-tin].

**sitaxsentan** (Cardio, Pulm).   Used to treat pulmonary arterial hypertension. Orphan drug. [sih-TAK-sen-tan].

**Skelaxin** (Ortho).   See *metaxalone*. [skeh-LAK-sin].

**Skelid** (Ortho).   See *tiludronate*. [SKEL-id].

**Slow FE** (Hem).   See *ferrous sulfate*. [SLOH F-E].

**SMA Iron Fortified, SMA Lo-Iron** (GI).   Infant formula with iron. Liquid. Powder (to be reconstituted). [S-M-A].

**sodium bicarbonate** (Emerg, Endo, GI, Uro).   Used to treat metabolic acidosis during cardiac arrest and resuscitation; used to treat metabolic acidosis due to kidney disease, uncontrolled diabetes mellitus, severe dehydration, or severe diarrhea. Subcutaneous, intravenous: 4.2% (0.5 mEq/mL), 5% (0.6 mEq/mL), 7.5% (0.9 mEq/mL), 8.4% (1 mEq/mL). [SOH-dee-um by-KAR-boh-nayt].

**sodium citrate** (Citra pH) (GI).   Antacid drug used to treat heartburn. Oral solution: 450 mg. [SOH-dee-um SIH-trayt].

**sodium ferric gluconate** (Ferrlecit) (Hem, Uro).   Iron compound used to treat iron deficiency anemia in patients undergoing hemodialysis. Intravenous: 12.5 mg/mL. [SOH-dee-um FAIR-ik GLOO-koh-nayt].

**sodium hyaluronate** (AMO Vitrax, Amvisc, Amvisc Plus, Coease, Healon, Healon GV, Shellgel) (Ophth).   Ophthalmic solution injected into the anterior segment during eye surgery. Intraocular injection: 10 mg/mL, 12 mg/mL, 14 mg/mL, 16 mg/mL, 30 mg/mL. [SOH-dee-um HY-al-yoo-RAW-nayt].

**sodium iodide 123, sodium iodide 131** (Iodotope) (Chem, Endo).   Radioactive drug used in the radioactive iodide (RAI) uptake test to diagnose thyroid gland function; used to treat hyperthyroidism and thyroid cancer. Radioactive capsule. Radioactive oral liquid. [SOH-dee-um EYE-oh-dide].

**sodium nitrite** (Emerg).   Used to treat cyanide poisoning. Intravenous: 30 mg/mL. [SOH-dee-um NY-trite].

**sodium phenylbutyrate** (Buphenyl) (Uro).   Used to treat urea cycle disorder. Tablet: 500 mg. [SOH-dee-um FEN-il-BYOO-tih-rayt].

**sodium phosphate** (Fleet Enema, Fleet Phospho-soda, OsmoPrep, Visicol) (GI).   Over-the-counter and prescription osmotic enema and laxative drug used to treat constipation;

bowel evacuant. Tablet. Enema. Oral solution. [SOH-dee-um FAWS-fayt].

**sodium phosphate 32** (Chemo). Radioactive drug used to treat polycythemia vera and leukemia. Intravenous: 0.67 mCi/mL [SOH-dee-um FAWS-fayt 32].

**sodium polystyrene sulfonate** (Kayexalate, Kionex, SPS) (Hem). Used to decrease elevated blood levels of potassium. Oral liquid: 15 g/60 mL. Powder (to be reconstituted): 15 g/4 tsp. [SOH-dee-um PAWL-ee-STY-reen sul-FAW-nayt].

**sodium tetradecyl** (Sotradecol) (Cardio, GI). Sclerosing drug used to treat varicose veins; used to stop bleeding from esophageal varices. Injection into the varicose vein or esophageal varix: 10 mg/mL, 30 mg/mL. [SOH-dee-um TET-rah-DEK-il].

**sodium thiosalicylate** (Ortho). Salicylate non-aspirin drug used to treat gout; used to treat rheumatic fever. Intramuscular: 50 mg/mL. [SOH-dee-um THY-oh-sah-LIH-sih-layt].

**sodium thiosulfate** (Chemo, Emerg). Used to treat cyanide poisoning; used to treat nephrotoxicity caused by the chemotherapy drug cisplatin. Intravenous: 100 mg/mL (10%), 250 mg/mL (25%). [SOH-dee-um THY-oh-SUL-fayt].

**Sodol** (Ortho) (generic *aspirin, carisoprodol*). Combination analgesic and skeletal muscle relaxant drug used to treat pain, spasm, and stiffness associated with minor muscle injuries. Tablet: 325 mg/200 mg. [SOH-dawl].

**Solaquin, Solaquin Forte** (Derm). See *hydroquinone*. [SOL-ah-kwin].

**Solaraze** (Derm). See *diclofenac*. [SOH-lar-ayz].

**Solarcaine, Solarcaine Medicated First Aid** (Anes, Derm). See *benzocaine*. [SOH-lar-kayn].

**Solarcaine Aloe Extra Burn Relief** (Anes, Derm). See *lidocaine*. [SOH-lar-kayn].

**Solfoton** (Neuro). See *phenobarbital*. [sawl-FOH-ton].

**Solganal** (Ortho). See *aurothioglucose*. [SOL-gah-nawl].

**Solia** (OB/GYN) (generic *desogestrel, ethinyl estradiol*). Combination monophasic oral contraceptive drug. Pill pack, 28-day: (21 hormone tablets): 0.15 mg/30 mcg; (7 inert tablets). [SOH-lee-ah].

**solifenacin** (Vesicare) (Uro). Anticholinergic drug used to treat urgency and frequency of overactive bladder. Tablet: 5 mg, 10 mg. [SOHL-ih-FEN-ah-sin].

**Soliris** (Hem). See *eculizumab*. [soh-LIR-is].

**Solodyn** (Anti-infec). See *minocycline*. [SOH-loh-dine].

**Soltamox** (Chemo). See *tamoxifen*. [SOL-tah-mawks].

**Solu-Cortef** (Endo). See *hydrocortisone*. [SAWL-yoo-KOR-tef].

**Solu-Medrol** (Endo, Neuro). See *methylprednisolone*. [SAWL-yoo-MED-rawl].

**Soma** (Ortho). See *carisoprodol*. [SOH-mah].

**Soma Compound** (Ortho) (generic *aspirin, carisoprodol*). Combination analgesic and skeletal muscle relaxant drug used to treat pain, spasm, and stiffness associated with minor muscle injuries. Tablet: 325 mg/200 mg. [SOH-mah KAWM-pownd].

**Soma Compound with Codeine** (Ortho) (generic *aspirin, carisoprodol, codeine*). Combination Schedule III analgesic, skeletal muscle relaxant, and narcotic analgesic drug used to treat pain, spasm, and stiffness associated with muscle injuries. Tablet: 325 mg/200 mg/16 mg. [SOH-mah KAWM-pownd with KOH deen].

**SomatoKine** (Endo). Insulin-like growth hormone drug used to treat growth failure in children with insulin resistance syndrome. Orphan drug. [soh-MAT-oh-kine].

**Somatoline Depot** (Endo). See *lanreotide*. [soh-MAH-toh-line DEE-poh].

**somatostatin** (Zecnil) (GI). Used to treat bleeding esophageal varices and fistula of the stomach and intestines. Orphan drug. [soh-MAH-toh-STAT-in].

**SomatoTher** (Chemo). See *indium 111*. [soh-MAH-toh-thair].

**Somatrel** (Endo). Used to diagnose the ability of the pituitary gland to release growth hormone. Orphan drug. [SOH-mah-trel].

**somatrem** (Protropin) (Endo). Growth hormone replacement drug for adults and children with growth failure; used to treat short stature in patients with Turner syndrome. Injection. Orphan drug. [SOH-mah-trem].

**somatropin** (Accretropin, Biotropin, Genotropin, Genotropin Miniquick, Humatrope, Norditropin, Nutropin, Nutropin AQ, Nutropin Depot, Omnitrope, Omnitrope Pen 5, Omnitrope Pen 10, Saizen, Serostim, Serostim LQ, Tev-Tropin, Zorbtive) (Anti-infec, Endo, OB/GYN). Growth hormone replacement drug for adults with growth hormone deficiency and for children with growth failure; used to treat children with short stature due to Turner syndrome; used to treat growth failure of infants born small for gestational age; used to treat AIDS wasting syndrome (Biotropin, Serostim); orphan drug used to treat women undergoing induction of ovulation for infertility (Norditropin); orphan drug used to treat patients with severe burns (Saizen); used to treat short bowel syndrome (Zorbtive). Subcutaneous or intramuscular: 5 mg/1.5 mL, 6 mg/05 mL, 10 mg/1.5 mL, 15 mg/1.5 mL, (powder to be reconstituted): 8.8 mg/10 mL, 0.2 mg/vial, 0.4 mg/vial, 0.6 mg/vial, 0.8 mg/vial, 1 mg/vial, 1.2 mg/vial, 1.4 mg/vial, 1.6 mg/vial, 1.8 mg/vial, 2 mg/vial, 4 mg/vial, 5 mg/vial, 5.8 mg/vial, 6 mg/vial, 8 mg/vial, 10 mg/vial, 12 mg/vial, 13.8 mg/vial, 24 mg/vial. Easypod injection device. Click.easy cartridge. [SOH-mah-TROH-pin].

**Somatuline Depot** (Endo). See *lanreotide*. [soh-MAH-tyoo-line DEE-poh].

**Somavert** (Endo). See *pegvisomant*. [SOH-mah-vert].

**Sominex** (Neuro). See *diphenydramine*. [SAW-mih-neks].

**Sominex Pain Relief** (Analges, ENT) (generic *acetaminophen, diphenhydramine*). Over-the-counter combination analgesic and antihistamine drug used to relieve pain and induce sleep. Tablet: 500 mg/25 mg. [SAW-mih-neks].

**Sonata** (Neuro). See *zaleplon*. [soh-NAW-tah].

**sorafenib** (Nexavar) (GI, Uro). Chemotherapy drug used to treat cancer of the liver and kidney. Tablet: 200 mg. [soh-RAF-eh-nib].

**sorbitol** (Uro). Irrigating solution used during urologic surgery. Solution: 3%. [SOR-bih-tawl].

**Sorbsan** (Derm). Over-the-counter drug used topically on the skin to absorb drainage from burns, skin ulcers, and wounds. Gauze dressing containing calcium fibers. [SORB-san].

**Soriatane** (Derm). See *acitretin*. [soh-RY-ah-tayn].

**sorivudine** (Bravavir) (Anti-infec). Used to treat herpes zoster infection (shingles) in immunocompromised patients. Orphan drug. [soh-RIV-yoo-deen].

**sotalol** (Betapace, Betapace AF) (Cardio). Beta-blocker drug used to treat ventricular tachycardia. Tablet: 80 mg, 120 mg, 160 mg, 240 mg. [SOH-tah-lawl].

**Sotradecol** (Cardio, GI). See *sodium tetradecyl*. [SOH-trah-DEH-kawl].

**Sotret** (Derm). See *isotretinoin*. [soh-TRET].

**Soyalac** (GI). Lactose-free infant formula with soy protein. Liquid. Powder (to be reconstituted). [SOY-ah-lak].

**Spanidin** (Hem). See *gusperimus*. [SPAN-ih-din].

**Spartaject** (Chemo). See *busulfan*. [SPAR-tah-jekt].

**Spasmolin** (GI) (generic *atropine, hyoscyamine, scopolamine, phenobarbital*). Combination anticholinergic and barbiturate sedative drug used to decrease spasm and provide sedation; used to treat GI spasm associated with irritable bowel syndrome, spastic colon, diverticulitis, and peptic ulcer. Tablet: 0.0194mg/0.1037 mg/0.0065 mg/16.2 mg. [SPAZ-moh-lin].

**Spectazole** (Derm). See *econazole*. [SPEK-tah-zohl].

**spectinomycin** (Trobicin) (Anti-infec). Antibiotic drug used to treat gonorrhea. Intramuscular: 400 mg/mL. [spek-TIN-oh-MY-sin].

**Spectracef** (Anti-infec). See *cefditoren*. [SPEK-trah-sef].

**Spheramine** (Neuro). Human retinal cells surgically implanted in the brain to produce dopamine to treat Parkinson's disease. Orphan drug. [SFEER-ah-meen].

**spiramycin** (Rovamycine) (Anti-infec). Used to treat parasite infections in AIDS patients. Orphan drug. [SPY-rah-MY-sin].

**Spiriva** (Pulm). See *tiotropium*. [spy-REE-vah].

**spironolactone** (Aldactone) (Cardio, Uro). Potassium-sparing diuretic drug used to treat hypertension; used to treat edema from congestive heart failure, liver disease, or kidney disease; used to treat hyperaldosteronism. Tablet: 25 mg, 50 mg, 100 mg. [spih-RAWN-oh-LAK-tohn].

**Sporanox** (Anti-infec). See *itraconazole*. [SPOR-ah-nawks].

**Sporidin-G** (Anti-infec). See *bovine immunoglobulin*. [SPOR-ih-din-G].

**Sportscreme** (Ortho) (generic *trolamine, alcohol*). Combination over-the-counter salicylate analgesic drug used topically to treat the pain of osteoarthritis and minor muscle injuries. Cream: 10%. [SPORTS-kreem].

**Sprintec** (OB/GYN) (generic *norgestimate, ethinyl estradiol*). Combination monophasic oral contraceptive drug. Pill pack, 28-day: (21 hormone tablets): 0.25 mg/35 mcg; (7 inert tablets). [SPRIN-tek].

**Sprycel** (Chemo). See *dasatinib*. [SPRY-sel].

**SPS** (Hem). See *sodium polystyrene sulfonate*. [S-P-S].

**squalamine** (Chemo). Used to treat cancer of the ovary. Orphan drug. [SKWAL-ah-meen].

**Sronyx** (OB/GYN) (generic *levonorgestrel, ethinyl estradiol*). Combination monophasic oral contraceptive drug. Pill pack, 28-day: (21 hormone tablets) 0.1 mg/ 20 mcg; (7 inert tablets). [SRAWN-eks].

**SSKI** (Pulm). See *potassium iodide*. [S-S-K-I].

**Stadol** (Analges, Anes). See *butorphanol*. [STAY-dawl].

**Stagesic** (Analges) (generic *acetaminophen, hydrocodone*). Combination Schedule III nonnarcotic and narcotic analgesic drug for pain. Capsule: 500 mg/5 mg. [stay-JEE-sik].

**Stalevo 50, Stalevo 100, Stalevo 150** (Neuro) (generic *carbidopa, entacapone, levodopa*). Combination drug used to treat Parkinson's disease. Tablet: 12.5 mg/ 200 mg/50 mg; 25 mg/200 mg/100 mg; 37.5 mg/ 200 mg/150 mg. [stah-LEE-voh].

**Starlix** (Endo). See *nateglinide*. [STAR-liks].

**stavudine** (Zerit) (Anti-infec). Nucleoside reverse transcriptase inhibitor antiviral drug used to treat HIV and AIDS. Capsule: 15 mg, 20 mg, 30 mg, 40 mg. Oral liquid (powder to be reconstituted): 1 mg/mL. [STAV-yoo-deen].

**Stavzor** (GI, Neuro, Psych). See *valproic acid*. [STAV-zohr].

**StemEx** (Hem). Used to treat cancer of the blood. Orphan drug. [STEM-eks].

**Stenorol** (Derm). See *halofuginone*. [STEN-oh-rawl].

**Sterapred, Sterapred DS** (Endo, Ortho). See *prednisone*. [STAIR-ah-pred].

**Sterecyt** (Chemo). See *prednimustine*. [STAIR-eh-sit].

**SteriNail** (Derm) (generic *sodium propionate, tolnaftate, undecylenic acid*). Over-the-counter antifungal drug used topically to treat fungal infections of the skin and nails (onychomycosis). Liquid. [STAIR-ee-nayl].

**Steritalc** (Chemo, Pulm). See *talc*. [STAIR-ih-talc].

**Stimate** (Endo). See *desmopressin*. [STIM-ate].

**Sting-Eze** (Derm) (generic *benzocaine, diphenhydramine*). Combination over-the-counter anesthetic and antihistamine drug used topically to numb the skin and stop itching. Concentrated liquid. [STING-eez].

**St. Joseph Adult Chewable Aspirin** (Analges, Cardio, Hem, Neuro). See *aspirin*. [SAYNT JOH-sef].

**Storz Sulf** (Anti-infec, Ophth). See *sulfacetamide*. [STORS SULF].

**Strattera** (Psych). See *atomoxetine*. [strah-TAIR-ah].

**Streptase** (Cardio, Hem, Ophth, Pulm). See *streptokinase*. [STREP-tays].

**streptokinase** (Streptase) (Cardio, Hem, Ophth, Pulm). Thrombolytic enzyme drug used to dissolve blood clots;

given at the time of a myocardial infarction; used to treat pulmonary embolism, deep venous thrombosis, arterial thrombosis, and retinal artery thrombosis. Intravenous (powder to be reconstituted): 250,000 units/6 mL; 750,000 units/6 mL; 1,500,000 units/6 mL. [STREP-toh-KY-nays].

**streptomycin** (Pulm). Aminoglycoside antibiotic drug used to treat *Mycobacterium avium-intracellulare* in AIDS patients; used to treat tuberculosis. Intramuscular: 400 mg/mL. [STREP-toh-MY-sin].

**streptozocin** (Zanosar) (Chemo). Alkylating chemotherapy drug used to treat cancer of the pancreas and colon; used to treat Hodgkin's lymphoma and pheochromocytoma. Intravenous (powder to be reconstituted): 100 mg/mL. [STREP-toh-ZOH-sin]

**Striant** (Endo). See *testosterone*. [STRY-ant].

**Stri-Dex Anti-Bacterial Foaming Wash, Stri-Dex Cleansing Bar, Stri-Dex Face Wash** (Derm). See *triclosan*. [STRY-deks].

**Stri-Dex Clear, Stri-Dex Pads** (Derm). See *salicylic acid*. [STRY-deks].

**Stromectol** (Misc). See *ivermectin*. [stroh-MEK-tawl].

**strontium-89** (Metastron) (Chemo). Radioactive drug used to treat bone pain in cancer patients with bone metastases. Intravenous: 4 mCi/mL. [STRAWN-shee-um-89].

**Sublimaze** (Anes). See *fentanyl*. [SUB-lih-mays].

**Suboxone** (Analges) (generic *buprenorphine, naloxone*). Combination narcotic and narcotic antagonist drug used to treat narcotic addiction. Orphan drug. [sub-AWK-sohn].

**Suby's Solution G** (Uro) (generic *citric acid, sodium carbonate, magnesium oxide*). Used to dissolve phosphate kidney stones. Irrigating solution (via catheter). [SOO-beez soh-LOO-shun G].

**Suboxone** (Psych) (generic *buprenorphine, naloxone*). Combination Schedule III narcotic drug and narcotic antagonist drug used to treat narcotic addiction. Orphan drug. Sublingual tablet: 2 mg/0.5 mg, 8 mg/2 mg. [soo-BAWK-sohn].

**Subutex** (Psych). See *buprenorphine*. [SOO-byoo-treks].

**succimer** (Chemet) (Emerg, Uro). Chelating drug used to treat lead, mercury, or arsenic poisoning; used to prevent cystine kidney stones in patients with cystinuria. Capsule: 100 mg. [SUK-sih-mer].

**succinylcholine** (Anectine, Anectine Flo-Pack, Quelicin) (Anes, Pulm). Neuromuscular blocker drug used during surgery; used to treat patients who are intubated and on the ventilator. Intravenous: 20 mg/mL, 50 mg/mL. [SUK-sih-nil-KOH-leen]

**Sucraid** (Misc). See *sacrosidase*. [SOO-krayd].

**sucralfate** (Carafate) (Chemo, GI). Used to treat oral ulcers or GI ulcers caused by excess acid, infection, radiation, or chemotherapy. Suspension: 1 g/10 mL. Tablet: 1 g. [soo-KRAL-fayt].

**Sucrets Children's Sore Throat** (ENT). See *dyclonine*. [soo-KRETZ].

**Sudafed Children's Non-Drowsy, Sudafed Non-Drowsy** (ENT). See *pseudoephedrine*. [SOO-dah-fed].

**Sudafed Children's Non-Drowsy Cold & Cough** (ENT) (generic *dextromethorphan, pseudoephedrine*). Combination over-the-counter nonnarcotic antitussive and decongestant drug. Liquid, 5 mg/15 mg. [SOO-dah-fed].

**Sudafed Maximum Strength Sinus Nighttime Plus Pain Relief** (ENT) (generic *acetaminophen, diphenhydramine, pseudoephedrine*). Combination over-the-counter analgesic, antihistamine, and decongestant drug. Tablet: 500 mg/25 mg/30 mg. [SOO-dah-fed].

**Sudafed Non-Drowsy Severe Cold** (ENT) (generic *acetaminophen, dextromethorphan, pseudoephedrine*). Combination over-the-counter analgesic, nonnarcotic antitussive, and decongestant drug. Tablet: 500 mg/ 15 mg/30 mg. [SOO-dah-fed].

**Sudafed Non-Drowsy Sinus** (ENT) (generic *guaifenesin, pseudoephedrine*). Combination over-the-counter expectorant and decongestant drug. LiquiCap: 120 mg/ 30 mg. [SOO-dah-fed].

**Sudafed PE** (ENT). See *phenylephrine*. [SOO-dah-fed].

**Sudafed PE Multi-Symptom Severe Cold, Sudafed PE Nighttime Cold** (ENT) (generic *acetaminophen, diphenhydramine, phenylephrine*). Combination over-the-counter analgesic, antihistamine, and decongestant drug. Tablet: 325 mg/12.5 mg/5 mg, 325 mg/25 mg/5 mg. [SOO-dah-fed].

**Sulfacet-R** (Derm) (generic *sodium sulfacetamide, sulfur*). Combination anti-infective and keratolytic drug used topically on the skin to treat acne vulgaris. Lotion: 10%/5%. [SUL-fah-set-R].

**Sufenta** (Anes, OB/GYN, Pulm). See *sufentanil*. [soo-FEN-tah].

**sufentanil** (Sufenta) (Anes, OB/GYN, Pulm). Schedule II narcotic drug used to induce and maintain general anesthesia; used to provide epidural pain relief during labor and delivery; used to sedate patients who are intubated and on the ventilator. Epidural, intravenous: 50 mcg/mL. [soo-FEN-tah-nil].

**Sular, Sular ER** (Cardio). See *nisoldipine*. [SOO-lar].

**sulconazole** (Exelderm) (Derm). Antifungal drug used topically to treat tinea (ringworm) and other fungal skin infections. Cream: 1%. Liquid: 1%. [sul-KAWN-ah-zohl].

**sulfacetamide** (AK-Sulf, Bleph-10, Carmol Scalp Treatment, Cetamide, Ocusulf-10, Storz Sulf, Sulster) (Anti-infec, Derm, Ophth). Sulfonamide anti-infective drug used topically to treat seborrheic dermatitis; used topically in the eye to treat bacterial infections. Lotion: 10%. Ophthalmic solution: 1%, 10%, 30%. Ophthalmic ointment: 10%. [SUL-fah-SEE-tah-mide].

**sulfadiazine** (Anti-infec, ENT, Neuro, Uro).   Sulfonamide drug used to treat a variety of bacterial infections, including urinary tract infections, otitis media, meningitis, rheumatic fever, and toxoplasmosis; orphan drug used to treat *Toxoplasma gondii* encephalitis in AIDS patients. Tablet: 500 mg. [SUL-fah-DY-ah-zeen].

**sulfadoxine** (Fansidar) (Anti-infec).   Used to prevent and treat malaria. Tablet: 500 mg. [SUL-fah-DAWK-seen].

**Sulfamylon** (Derm).   See *mafonido.* [SUL-fah-MY-lawn].

**sulfanilamide** (AVC) (OB/GYN).   Used topically to treat vaginal yeast infections caused by *Candida albicans.* Vaginal cream: 15%. [SUL-fah-NIL-ah-mide].

**sulfasalazine** (Azulfidine, Azulfidine EN-tabs) (GI, Ortho).   Anti-inflammatory drug used to treat ulcerative colitis and Crohn's disease; used to treat ankylosing spondylitis. Tablet: 500 mg. Delayed-release tablet: 500 mg. [SUL-fah-SAL-ah-zeen].

**Sulfatrim** (Anti-infec) (generic *sulfamethoxazole, trimethoprim*).   Combination antibiotic and sulfonamide anti-infective drug used to treat bronchitis, otitis media, traveler's diarrhea, urinary tract infection, and prostatitis; used to treat *Pneumocystis carinii* pneumonia in AIDS patients. Oral suspension: 200 mg/40 mg per 5 mL. Tablet: 400 mg/80 mg, 800 mg/160 mg. Intravenous: 80 mg/16 mg per 5 mL, 400 mg/80 mg per 5 mL. [SUL-fah-trim].

**sulfinpyrazone** (Anturane) (Ortho).   Used to decrease uric acid levels to treat gout and gouty arthritis. Capsule: 200 mg. Tablet: 100 mg. [SUL-fin-PEER-ah-zohn].

**sulfisoxazole** (Gantrisin Pediatric) (Anti-infec).   Sulfonamide drug used to treat a variety of bacterial infections, including urinary tract infections, otitis media, and meningitis; used to treat toxoplasmosis. Oral suspension: 500 mg/5 mL. Tablet: 500 mg. [SUL-fih-SAWK-sih-zohl].

**Sulfoxyl** (Derm) (generic *benzoyl peroxide, sulfur*).   Combination antibiotic and keratolytic drug used topically on the skin to treat acne vulgaris. Lotion: 5%/2%, 10%, 5%. [sul-FAWK-sil].

**sulindac** (Clinoril) (Analges).   Nonsteroidal anti-inflammatory drug used to treat the pain and inflammation of bursitis, tendinitis, osteoarthritis, rheumatoid arthritis, gout, and ankylosing spondylitis. Tablet: 150 mg, 200 mg. [soo-LIN-dak].

**Sulster** (Anti-infec, Ophth).   See *sulfacetamide.* [SUL-ster].

**Sulster Solution** (Ophth) (generic *prednisolone, sulfacetamide*).   Combination corticosteroid and sulfonamide anti-infective drug used topically in the eyes to treat inflammation and infection. Ophthalmic solution: 0.25%/10%. [SUL-ster soh-LOO-shun].

**sumatriptan** (Imitrex) (Analges).   Serotonin receptor agonist drug used to treat migraine headaches. Tablet: 25 mg, 50 mg, 100 mg. Nasal spray: 5 mg, 20 mg. Subcutaneous: 4 mg/0.5 mL, 6 mg/0.5 mL. [soo-mah-TRIP-tan].

**Sumycin 250, Sumycin 500, Symycin Syrup** (Anti-infec).   See *tetracycline.* [soo-MY-sin].

**sunitinib** (Sutent) (Chemo).   Chemotherapy drug used to treat cancer of the stomach and kidney. Capsule: 12.5 mg, 25 mg, 50 mg. [soo-NIT-ih-nib].

**Supartz** (Ortho).   See *hyaluronic acid.* [SOO-partz].

**Supervent** (Pulm).   See *tyloxapol.* [SOO-per-vent].

**Suplena** (GI, Uro) Nutritional supplement formulated for patients with renal disease.   Liquid. [soo-PLEH-nah].

**Supprelin, Supprelin LA** (Endo).   See *histrelin.* [suh-PRELL-in].

**Suprane** (Anes).   See *desflurane.* [SOO-prayn].

**Suprax** (Anti-infec).   See *cefixime.* [SOO-praks].

**suramin** (Metaret) (Chemo).   Chemotherapy drug used to treat prostate cancer. Orphan drug. [SIR-ah-min].

**Surfak Liquigels** (GI).   See *docusate.* [SIR-fak].

**Surfaxin** (Pulm).   See *lucinactant.* [sir-FAK-sin].

**Surgicel** (Hem).   See *oxidized cellulose.* [SIR-jih-sel].

**Surmontil** (Psych).   See *trimipramine.* [sir-MAWN-til].

**Survanta** (Pulm).   See *beractant.* [sir-VAN-tah].

**Sustacal** (GI).   Milk-based or lactose-free nutritional supplement. Liquid. Pudding. [SUS-tah-kal].

**Sustiva** (Anti-infec).   See *efavirenz.* [sus-TEE-vah].

**Sutent** (Chemo).   See *sunitinib.* [SOO-tent].

**Syllact** (GI).   See *psyllium.* [SIL-akt].

**Symax Duotab, Symax FasTab, Symax-SL, Symax-SR** (GI, Uro).   See *L-hyoscyamine.* [SY-maks].

**Symbicort** (Pulm) (generic *budesonide, formoterol*).   Combination corticosteroid anti-inflammatory and bronchodilator drug used to treat asthma. Aerosol canister for inhalation: 80 mcg/4.5 mcg per actuation, 160 mcg/4.5 mcg per actuation. [SIM-bih-kort].

**Symbyax** (Psych) (generic *olanzapine, fluoxetine*).   Combination benzodiazepine and selective serotonin reuptake inhibitor (SSRI) drug used to treat manic-depressive disorder. Capsule: 6 mg/25 mg, 6 mg/50 mg, 12 mg/25 mg, 12 mg/50 mg. [SIM-by-aks].

**Symlin** (Endo).   See *pramlintide.* [SIM-lin].

**Symmetrel** (Anti-infec, Neuro, Pulm).   See *amantadine.* [SIM-eh-trel].

**Synacort** (Derm).   See *hydrocortisone.* [SIN-ah-kort].

**Synagis** (Anti-infec, Pulm).   See *palivizumab.* [SIN-ah-jis].

**Synalar** (Derm).   See *fluocinolone.* [SIN-ah-lar].

**Synalgos-DC** (Analges) (generic *aspirin, dihydrocodeine, caffeine*).   Combination Schedule III salicylate, narcotic, and caffeine drug. Capsule: 356.4 mg/16 mg/30 mg. [sin-AL-gohs D-C].

**Synarel** (Endo, OB/GYN).   See *nafarelin.* [SIN-ah-rel].

**Synera** (Anes, Derm) (generic *lidocaine, tetracaine*).   Combination anesthetic drug used topically to prevent pain during excision of skin lesions or biopsy. Patch: 70 mg/70 mg. [sih-NAIR-ah].

**Synercid** (Anti-infec) (generic *dalfopristin, quinupristin*).   Combination antibiotic drug used to treat staphylococcal and streptococcal skin infections; used to treat severe bacterial infections from methicillin-resistant and vancomycin-resistant bacteria. Intravenous: 350 mg/500 mg per 10 mL. [SIN-er-sid].

**Synophylate-GG** (Pulm) (generic *theophylline, guaifenesin*). Combination bronchodilator and expectorant drug used to treat asthma and bronchitis with productive coughs. Syrup: 150 mg/100 mg. [sih-NAW-fih-layt-G-G].

**Synovir** (Anti-infec, Chemo, GI). See *thalidomide*. [SIN-oh-veer].

**Syntest H.S., Syntest D.S.** (OB/GYN) (generic *methyl-testosterone, esterified estrogens*). Combination hormone drug used to treat the symptoms of menopause. Tablet: 1.25 mg/0.625 mg, 2.5 mg/1.25 mg. [SIN-test].

**Synthroid** (Endo). See *levothyroxine*. [SIN-throyd].

**Synvisc** (Ortho). See *hyaluronic acid*. [SIN-visk].

**Syprine** (GI). See *trientine*. [SIP-reen].

**3HT** (Anti-infec). See *lamivudine*. [3-H-T].

**Tabloid** (Chemo, Derm, GI). See *thioguanine*. [TAB-loyd].

**Taclonex, Taclonex Scalp** (Derm) (generic *betamethasone, calcipotriene*). Combination corticosteroid and vitamin D-type drug used topically on the skin and scalp to treat psoriasis. Gel: 0.064%/0.005%. Ointment: 0.064%/0.005%. Topical liquid: 0.064%/0.005%. [TAK-loh-neks].

**tacrine** (Cognex) (Neuro). Cholinesterase inhibitor drug used to treat mild-to-moderate Alzheimer's disease. Capsule: 10 mg, 20 mg, 30 mg, 40 mg. [TAK-reen].

**tacrolimus** (Prograf, Protopic) (Cardio, Chemo, Derm, GI, Ortho, Uro). Immunosuppressant drug given to organ transplantation patients to prevent rejection of the donor heart, liver, or kidney; used to prevent and treat graft-versus-host disease following stem cell transplantation; used to treat rheumatoid arthritis; used to treat Crohn's disease; used topically to treat atopic dermatitis (eczema), vitiligo, and psoriasis. Ointment: 0.03%, 0.1%. Capsule: 0.5 mg, 1 mg, 5 mg. Intravenous: 5 mg/mL. [tah-KROH-lih-mus].

**tadalafil** (Cialis) (Uro). PDE5 inhibitor drug used to treat male impotence caused by erectile dysfunction. Tablet: 2.5 mg (for daily use), 5 mg, 10 mg, 20 mg. [tah-DAL-ah-fil].

**Tagamet, Tagamet HB 200** (GI). See *cimetidine*. [TAG-ah-met].

**Talacen** (Analges) (generic *acetaminophen, pentazocine*). Combination Schedule IV nonsalicylate and narcotic analgesic drug used to treat moderate-to-severe pain. Tablet: 650 mg/25 mg. [TAL-ah-sen].

**talc** (Sclerosol, Steritalc) (Chemo, Pulm). Sclerosing drug administered via chest tube into the lung to treat malignant pleural effusion and pneumothorax. Aerosol. Powder. [TALC].

**talotrexin** (Chemo). Used to treat leukemia. Orphan drug. [TAL-oh-TREK-sin].

**Talwin** (Analges, Anes). See *pentozocine*. [TAL-win].

**Talwin Compound** (Analges) (generic *aspirin, pentozocine*). Combination Schedule IV salicylate and narcotic analgesic drug used to treat moderate-to-severe pain. Tablet: 325 mg/12.5 mg. [TAWL-win KAWM-pownd].

**Talwin NX** (Analges) (generic *naloxone, pentazocine*). Combination Schedule IV narcotic antagonist and narcotic analgesic drug used to treat moderate-to-severe pain. Tablet: 0.5 mg/50 mg. [TAWL-win N-X].

**Tambocor** (Cardio). See *flecainide*. [TAM-boh-kor].

**Tamiflu** (Anti-infec, Pulm). See *oseltamivir*. [TAM-ih-floo].

**tamoxifen** (Soltamox) (Chemo). Hormonal chemotherapy drug used to treat breast cancer and malignant melanoma; used to decrease the risk of breast cancer in high-risk women; used to treat carcinoid syndrome; used to treat gynecomastia in men. Tablet: 10 mg, 20 mg. Oral liquid: 10 mg/5 mL. [tah-MAWK-sih-fen].

**tamsulosin** (Flomax) (Uro). Alpha$_1$ receptor blocker drug used to treat benign prostatic hypertrophy. Capsule: 0.4 mg. [tam-SOO-loh-sin].

**Tantum** (Chemo). See *benzydamine*. [TAN-tum].

**Tapazole** (Endo). See *methimazole*. [TAP-eh-zohl].

**Tarabine PFS** (Chemo). See *cytarabine*. [TAIR-ah-been P-F-S].

**Taraphilic** (Derm). See *coal tar*. [TAR-ah-FIL-ik].

**Tarceva** (Chemo). See *erlotinib*. [tar-SEE-vah].

**Targretin** (Chemo, Derm). See *bexarotene*. [TAR-greh-tin].

**Tarka** (Cardio) (generic *trandolapril, verapamil*). Combination ACE inhibitor and calcium channel blocker drug used to treat hypertension. Tablet: 1 mg/240 mg, 2 mg/180 mg, 2 mg/240 mg, 4 mg/240 mg. [TAR-kah].

**Tasigna** (Chemo). See *nilotinib*. [tah-SIG-nah].

**Tasmar** (Neuro). See *tolcapone*. [TAZ-mar].

**Tavist Allergy** (Derm, ENT). See *clemastine*. [TAV-ist].

**Tavist Allergy/Sinus/Headache** (ENT) (generic *acetaminophen, clemastine, pseudoephedrine*). Combination over-the-counter analgesic, antihistamine, and decongestant drug used to treat allergies and sinus congestion. Tablet: 500 mg/0.335 mg/30 mg. [TAV-ist].

**Tavist ND** (Derm, ENT). See *loratadine*. [TAV-ist N-D].

**Tavist Sinus Maximum Strength** (ENT) (generic *acetaminophen, pseudoepinephrine*). Combination over-the-counter analgesic and decongestant drug used to treat sinus congestion. Tablet: 500 mg/30 mg. [TAV-ist].

**Taxol** (Chemo). See *paclitaxel*. [TAK-sawl].

**Taxoprexin** (Chemo) (generic *docosahexanoic acid [DHA], paclitaxel*). Combination chemotherapy drug used to treat cancer of the esophagus, stomach, pancreas, and prostate gland; used to treat malignant melanoma. Orphan drug. [TAK-soh-PREK-sin].

**Taxotere** (Chemo). See *docetaxel*. [TAKS-oh-teer].

**tazarotene** (Avage, Tazorac) (Derm). Vitamin A-type (retinoid) drug used topically on the skin to treat acne vulgaris and psoriasis. Cream: 0.05%, 0.1%. Gel: 0.05%, 0.1%. [tah-ZAIR-oh-teen].

**Tazicef** (Anti-infec). See *ceftazidime*. [TAZ-ih-sef].

**Tazidime** (Anti-infec). See *ceftazidime*. [TAZ-ih-dime].

**Tazorac** (Derm). See *tazarotene.* [TAZ-oh-rak].

**Taztia XT** (Analges, Cardio). See *diltiazem.* [taz-TY-ah X-T].

**Tearisol** (Ophth). Over-the-counter artificial tears for dry eyes. Ophthalmic solution. [TEER-ih-sawl].

**Tears Naturale, Tears Naturale Free, Tears Naturale II, Tears Natural Forte** (Ophth). Over-the-counter artificial tears for dry eyes. Ophthalmic solution. [TEERZ nah-tyoor-AL].

**Tebamide** (GI). See *trimethobenzamide.* [TEB-ah-mide].

**Teceleukin** (Chemo). See *aldesleukin.* [TEK-ee-LOO-kin].

**Tedrigen** (Pulm) (generic *theophylline, ephedrine, phenobarbital*). Combination over-the-counter bronchodilator and barbiturate sedative drug. Tablet: 120 mg/22.5 mg/7.5 mg. [TED-rih-jen].

**Tegretol, Tegretol-XR** (Neuro). See *carbamazepine.* [TEG-reh-tawl].

**Tegrin-HC** (Derm). See *hydrocortisone.* [TEG-rin-H-C].

**Tekturna** (Cardio). See *aliskiren.* [tek-TER-nah].

**Tekturna HCT** (Cardio) (generic *aliskiren, hydrochlorothiazide*). Combination renin inhibitor and diuretic drug used to treat hypertension. Tablet: 150 mg/12.5 mg, 150 mg/25 mg, 300 mg/12.5 mg, 300 mg/25 mg. [tek-TER-nah H-C-T].

**Teladar** (Derm). See *betamethasone.* [TEL-ah-dar].

**telbivudine** (Tyzeka) (Anti-infec, GI). Nucleoside reverse transcriptase inhibitor antiviral drug used to treat chronic hepatitis B. Tablet: 600 mg. [tel-BY-vyoo-deen].

**telithromycin** (Ketek) (Anti-infec). Ketolide antibiotic drug used to treat pneumonia due to *S. pneumoniae, H. influenzae,* and *Mycoplasma.* Tablet: 300 mg, 400 mg. [teh-LITH-roh-MY-sin].

**telmisartan** (Micardis) (Cardio). Angiotensin II receptor blocker drug used to treat hypertension. Tablet: 20 mg, 40 mg, 80 mg. [TEL-mih-SAR-tan].

**temazepam** (Restoril) (Neuro). Schedule IV benzodiazepine drug used to treat insomnia. Capsule: 7.5 mg, 15 mg, 22.5 mg, 30 mg. [teh-MAZ-eh-pam].

**temocillin** (Negaban) (Anti-infec). Used to treat lung infection caused by *Burkholderia cepacia.* Orphan drug. [TEM-oh-SIL-lin].

**Temodar** (Chemo). See *temozolomide.* [TEM-oh-dar].

**temoporfin** (Foscan) (Chemo). Chemotherapy drug used to treat head and neck cancer. Orphan drug. [TEE-moh-POR-fin].

**Temovate** (Derm). See *clobetasol.* [TEM-oh-vayt].

**temozolomide** (Temodar) (Chemo). Alkylating chemotherapy drug used to treat cancer of the brain and malignant melanoma. Capsule: 5 mg, 20 mg, 100 mg, 140 mg, 180 mg, 250 mg. [TEM-oh-ZOHL-oh-mide].

**Tempra 1, Tempra 2, Tempra 3** (Analges). See *acetaminophen.* [TEM-prah].

**temsirolimus** (Torisel) (Chemo). Protein-tyrosine kinase inhibitor chemotherapy drug used to treat kidney cancer. Intravenous: 25 mg/mL. [TEM-sir-OH-lih-mus].

**Tencon** (Analges) (generic *acetaminophen, butalbital*). Combination nonsalicylate analgesic and barbiturate sedative drug for pain. Tablet: 650 mg/50 mg. [TEN-con].

**tenecteplase** (TNKase) (Cardio, Hem). Tissue plasminogen activator drug given at the time of a myocardial infarction to dissolve a blood clot. Intravenous (powder to be reconstituted): 50 mg/10mL. [teh-NEK-teh-plays].

**Tenex** (Cardio, Psych). See *guanfacine.* [TEN-eks].

**teniposide** (Vumon) (Chemo). Mitosis inhibitor chemotherapy drug used to treat leukemia and non-Hodgkin's lymphoma. Intravenous: 10 mg/mL. [teh-NIP-oh-side].

**tenofovir** (Viread) (Anti-infec, GI). Nucleotide analog reverse transcriptase inhibitor antiviral drug used to treat HIV and AIDS; used to treat chronic hepatitis B. Tablet: 300 mg. [teh-NOH-foh-veer].

**Tenoretic 50, Tenoretic 100** (Cardio) (generic *atenolol, chlorthalidone*). Combination beta-blocker and diuretic drug used to treat hypertension. Tablet: 50 mg/25 mg, 100 mg/25 mg. [TEN-oh-REH-tik].

**Tenormin** (Analges, Cardio, GI). See *atenolol.* [teh-NOR-min].

**Tensilon** (Anes, Neuro). See *edrophonium.* [TEN-sih-lawn].

**Tera-Gel** (Derm). See *coal tar.* [TAIR-ah-jel].

**Terazol 3, Terazol 7** (OB/GYN). See *terconazole.* [TAIR-ah-zohl].

**terazosin** (Hytrin) (Cardio, Uro). Alpha-blocker drug used to treat hypertension; used to treat benign prostatic hypertrophy. Capsule: 1 mg, 2 mg, 5 mg, 10 mg. Tablet: 1 mg, 2 mg, 5 mg, 10 mg. [ter-AZ-oh-sin].

**terbinafine** (DesenexMyax, Lamisil, Lamisil AT) (Derm). Over-the-counter antifungal drug used topically to treat tinea (ringworm) and other fungal skin infections and nails (onychomycosis). Cream: 1%. Gel: 1%. Spray: 1%. Tablet: 250 mg. Oral granules (to be sprinkled on food): 125 mg/packet. [ter-BIN-ah-feen].

**terbutaline** (Brethine) (OB/GYN, Pulm). Bronchodilator drug used to prevent and treat asthma and bronchospasm; used to treat preterm labor in women. Tablet: 2.5 mg, 5 mg. Subcutaneous: 1 mg/mL. [ter-BYOO-tah-leen].

**terconazole** (Terazol 3, Terazol 7, Zazole) (OB/GYN). Used topically to treat vaginal yeast infections. Vaginal cream: 0.4%, 0.6%. Vaginal suppository: 80 mg. [ter-KAWN-ah-zohl].

**teriparatide** (Forteo) (Endo, Ortho). Parathyroid hormone used to stimulate new bone growth in men and postmenopausal women at high risk for fracture from osteoporosis. Subcutaneous: 250 mcg/mL. [TAIR-ee-PAIR-ah-tide].

**terlipressin** (Glypressin) (GI). Used to treat bleeding esophageal ulcers and hepatorenal syndrome. Orphan drug. [TER-lih-PRES-sin].

**Terrell** (Anes). See *isoflurane.* [teh-REL].

**Tessalon** (ENT). See *benzonatate.* [TES-ah-lawn].

**Testim** (Endo). See *testosterone.* [TES-tim].

**testolactone** (Chemo).   Schedule III hormonal chemotherapy drug used to treat breast cancer. Tablet: 50 mg. [TES-toh-LAK-tohn].

**Testopel** (Endo).   See *testosterone.* [TES-toh-pel].

**testosterone** (Androderm, AndroGel, Delatestryl, Depo-Testosterone, Striant, Testim, Testopel, TheraDerm Testosterone Transdermal System) (Chemo, Endo). Schedule III male hormone used to treat the lack of testosterone due to absence, injury, or malfunction of the testes or malfunction of the pituitary gland; used to treat delayed puberty in boys; hormonal chemotherapy drug used to treat breast cancer in women; orphan drug used to treat weight loss in AIDS patients. Buccal system (curved adhesive tablet): 30 mg. Gel: 1%. Intramuscular: 100 mg/mL, 200 mg/mL. Sublingual: (orphan drug). Transdermal patch: 2.5 mg/24 hr, 5 mg/24 hr. Subcutaneous pellet: 75 mg. [tes-TAWS-teh-rohn].

**Testred** (Chemo, Endo).   See *methyltestosterone.* [TES-tred].

**Tetcaine** (Ophth).   See *tetracaine.* [TET-kayn].

**tetrabenazine** (Xenazine) (Neuro, Psych).   Used to treat Huntington's disease and chorea; orphan drug used to treat tardive dyskinesia side effects of antipsychotic drugs. Tablet: 12.5 mg, 25 mg. [TEH-trah-BEN-ah-zeen].

**tetracaine** (Altacaine, Pontocaine, Tetcaine) (Anes, Ophth).   Anesthetic drug used to produce spinal anesthesia; anesthetic drug used topically to numb the eye. Injection: 0.2%, 0.3%, 1%. Ophthalmic solution: 0.5%. [TEH-trah-kayn].

**tetracycline** (Sumycin 250, Sumycin 500, Sumycin Syrup) (Anti-infec).   Tetracycline antibiotic drug used to treat infection due to gram-negative and gram-positive bacteria; used to treat severe acne vulgaris; used to treat gonorrhea, syphilis, *Chlamydia,* and nongonococcal urethritis; used to treat pneumonia due to *S. pneumoniae, H. influenzae,* and *Mycoplasma;* used to treat Rocky Mountain spotted fever; used to treat intestinal amebiasis; used to treat ulcerative gingivitis (trench mouth); used with metronidazole to treat stomach ulcers caused by *H. pylori.* Capsule: 250 mg, 500 mg. Oral suspension: 125 mg/5 mL. [TEH-trah-SY-kleen].

**tetrahydrozoline** (Murine Tears Plus, Tyzine, Tyzine Pediatric, Visine, Visine Advanced Relief) (Ophth).   Over-the-counter and prescription decongestant/vasoconstrictor drug used topically to treat irritation and allergy symptoms in the eyes; used topically to treat nasal stuffiness due to colds and allergies. Ophthalmic solution: 0.05%. Nasal drops/spray: 0.05%, 0.1%. [TEH-trah-hy-DRAW-zoh-leen].

**tetraiodothyroacetic acid** (Endo).   Used to suppress thyroid-stimulating hormone in patients with thyroid cancer. Orphan drug. [TEH-trah-eye-OH-do-THY-roh-ah-SEE-tik AS-id].

**Teveten** (Cardio).   See *eprosartan.* [TEV-eh-ten].

**Teveten HCT** (Cardio) (generic *eprosartan, hydrochlorothiazide*).   Combination angiotensin II receptor blocker and diuretic drug used to treat hypertension. Tablet: 600 mg/12.5 mg, 600 mg/25 mg. [TEV-eh-ten H-C-T].

**Tev-Tropin** (Endo).   See *somatropin.* [tev-TROH-pin].

**Texacort** (Derm).   See *hydrocortisone.* [TEKS-ah-kort].

**tezacitabine** (Chemo).   Chemotherapy drug used to treat cancer of the esophagus and stomach. Orphan drug. [TEZ-ah-SIT-ah-been].

**T-Gen** (GI).   See *trimethobenzamide.* [T-jen].

**Thalagen** (Hem).   Used to treat beta-thalassemia. Orphan drug. [THAL-ah-jen].

**thalidomide** (Synovir, Thalomid) (Anti-Infec, Chemo, GI).   Immunomodulator drug used to treat multiple myeloma, cancer of the brain and prostate gland, aphthous stomatitis in AIDS patients, and leprosy; used to prevent graft-versus-host disease after bone marrow transplantation; orphan drug used to treat Kaposi's sarcoma, wasting syndrome associated with AIDS, and Crohn's disease. Capsule: 50 mg, 100 mg, 200 mg. [thah-LID-oh-mide].

**Thalomid** (Anti-infec, Chemo, GI).   See *thalidomide.* [THAL-oh-mid].

**Tham** (Emerg).   See *tromethamine.* [THAM].

**Theo-24** (Pulm).   See *theophylline.* [THEE-oh-24].

**Theochron** (Pulm).   See *theophylline.* [THEE-oh-krawn].

**Theodrine** (Pulm) (generic *theophylline, ephedrine, phenobarbital*).   Combination over-the-counter bronchodilator and sedative drug. [THEE-oh-dreen].

**Theolate** (Pulm) (generic *theophylline, guaifenesin*).   Combination bronchodilator and expectorant drug. Liquid: 150 mg/90 mg. [THEE-oh-layt].

**Theomax DF** (Pulm) (generic *theophylline, ephedrine, hydroxyzine*).   Combination bronchodilator and antihistamine drug. Pediatric syrup: 97.5 mg/18.75 mg/7.5 mg. [THEE-oh-maks D-F].

**theophylline** (Asmalix, Bronkodyl, Elixophyllin, Lanophyllin, Theo-24, Theochron, Uniphyl) (Pulm).   Bronchodilator drug used to treat bronchospasm associated with asthma, chronic bronchitis, and emphysema; stimulant drug used to treat apnea in premature infants. Capsule: 100 mg, 200 mg. Extended-release capsule: 100 mg, 125 mg, 200 mg, 300 mg, 400 mg. Liquid elixir: 80 mg/15 mL. Tablet: 300 mg. Extended-release tablet: 100 mg, 200 mg, 300 mg, 400 mg, 450 mg, 600 mg. Timed-release tablet: 100 mg, 200 mg, 300 mg, 400 mg, 600 mg. [thee-AW-fih-lin].

**TheraCys** (Chemo).   See *BCG.* [THAIR-ah-sis].

**Theraderm Testosterone Transdermal System** (Endo).   See *testosterone.* [THAIR-ah-derm tes-TAWS-teh-rohn].

**Theraflu Cold & Cough** (ENT) (generic *dextromethorphan, pheniramine, phenylephrine*).   Combination over-the-counter nonnarcotic antitussive, antihistamine, and decongestant drug used to treat colds and flu with coughs. Powder (to be mixed with water): 20 mg/20 mg/10 mg. [THAIR-ah-floo].

**Theraflu Daytime Severe Cold** (ENT) (generic *acetaminophen, phenylephrine*).   Combination over-the-counter analgesic and decongestant drug used to treat colds. Powder (to be mixed with water): 650 mg/10 mg. [THAIR-ah-floo].

**Theraflu Cold & Sore Throat, Theraflu Flu & Sore Throat** (ENT) (generic *acetaminophen, pheniramine, phenylephrine*). Combination over-the-counter analgesic, antihistamine, and decongestant drug used to treat colds and flu with sore throat. Powder (to be mixed with water): 325 mg/20 mg/10 mg, 650 mg/20 mg/10 mg. [THAIR-ah-floo].

**Theraflu Flu & Cold** (ENT) (generic *acetaminophen, chlorpheniramine, pseudoephedrine*). Combination over-the-counter analgesic, antihistamine, and decongestant drug used to treat colds and flu. Powder (to be mixed with water): 1000 mg/4 mg/60 mg. [THAIR-ah-floo].

**Theraflu Non-Drowsy Flu, Cold & Cough, Theraflu Severe Cold Non-Drowsy, Theraflu Severe Cold & Congestion Non-Drowsy** (ENT) (generic *acetaminophen, dextromethorphan, pseudoephedrine*). Combination over-the-counter analgesic, nonnarcotic antitussive, and decongestant drug used to treat colds with coughs. Powder (to be mixed with water): 1000 mg/20 mg/60 mg. [THAIR-ah-floo].

**Theraflu Severe Cold & Congestion Nighttime** (ENT) (generic *acetaminophen, chlorpheniramine, dextromethorphan, pseudoephedrine*). Combination over-the-counter analgesic, antihistamine, nonnarcotic antitussive, and decongestant drug used to treat colds with coughs. Powder (to be mixed with water): 1000 mg/4 mg/30 mg/60 mg. [THAIR-ah-floo].

**Theragyn** (Chemo). Monoclonal antibody drug used to treat ovarian cancer. Orphan drug. [THAIR-ah-jin].

**Therapatch Cold Sore** (Anes, ENT). See *lidocaine*. [THAIR-ah-patch].

**Therapeutic Mineral Ice, Therapeutic Mineral Ice Exercise Formula** (Ortho) (generic *methyl salicylate, menthol*). Combination over-the-counter analgesic drug used topically on the skin to treat the pain of osteoarthritis and minor muscle injuries. Gel. [THAIR-ah-PYOO-tik MIN-er-al].

**TheraCys** (Chemo). See *BCG*. [THAIR-ah-sis].

**Therevac-SB, Therevac-Plus** (GI) (generic *docusate, glycerin, benzocaine*). Over-the-counter stool softener and analgesic drug used to treat constipation. Enema. [THAIR-ee-vak].

**thiabendazole** (Minetezol) (Misc). Used to treat infestations of worms. Chewable tablet: 500 mg. Oral liquid: 500 mg/5 mL. [THY-ah-BEN-dah-zohl].

**thimerosal** (Mersol) (Derm). Over-the-counter mercury-containing skin antiseptic drug. Solution. Tincture. [thy-MAIR-oh-sawl].

**thioguanine** (Tabloid) (Chemo, Derm, GI). Antimetabolite chemotherapy drug used to treat leukemia; used to treat psoriasis, ulcerative colitis, and Crohn's disease. Tablet: 40 mg. [THY-oh-GWAH-neen].

**Thiola** (Uro). See *tiopronin*. [THY-oh-lah].

**thiopental** (Pentothal) (Anes). Schedule III barbiturate drug used to induce and maintain general anesthesia.

Intravenous: 20 mg/mL (2%), 25 mg/mL (2.5%). [THY-oh-PEN-tawl].

**Thioplex** (Chemo). See *thiotepa*. [THY-oh-pleks].

**thioridazine** (Psych). Phenothiazine antipsychotic drug used to treat schizophrenia; used to treat psychosis with agitation in patients with Alzheimer's disease. Tablet: 10 mg, 15 mg, 25 mg, 50 mg, 100 mg, 150 mg, 200 mg. [THY-oh-RID-ah-zeen].

**thiotepa** (Thioplex) (Chemo). Alkylating chemotherapy drug used to treat cancer of the breast, ovary, and bladder; used to treat Hodgkin's lymphoma. Intravenous, intracavitary, or intravesical (powder to be reconstituted): 15 mg. [THY-oh-TEP-ah].

**thiothixene** (Navane) (Neuro, Psych). Antipsychotic drug used to treat schizophrenia; used to treat psychosis and agitation in patients with Alzheimer's disease. Capsule: 1 mg, 2 mg, 5 mg, 10 mg, 20 mg. [THY-oh-THIK-seen].

**Thorazine** (Analges, Anes, GI, Psych). See *chlorpromazine*. [THOR-ah-zeen].

**Threostat** (Neuro). See *L-threonin*. [THREE-oh-stat].

**Thrombate III** (Hem). See *antithrombin III*. [THRAWM-bayt 3].

**thrombin** (Evithrom, Recothrom, Thrombin-JMI, Thrombogen, Thrombostat) (Hem). Hemostatic drug used topically to control bleeding. Liquid. Powder. [THRAWM-bin].

**Thrombin-JMI** (Hem). See *thrombin*. [THRAWM-bin-J-M-I].

**Thrombogen** (Hem). See *thrombin*. [THRAWM-boh-jen].

**Thrombostat** (Hem). See *thrombin*. [THRAWM-boh-stat].

**thymalfasin** (Zadaxin) (Chemo, GI). Chemotherapy drug used to treat liver cancer and malignant melanoma; used to treat hepatitis C. Orphan drug. [thy-MAL-fah-sin].

**Thymoglobulin** (Chemo, Hem). See *antithymocyte globulin*. [THY-moh-GLAW-byoo-lin].

**Thyrogen** (Endo). See *thyrotropin alfa*. [THY-roh-jen].

**Thyrolar** (Endo). See *liotrix*. [THY-roh-lar].

**ThyroShield** (Endo). See *iodine*. [THY-roh-sheeld].

**Thyro-Tabs** (Endo). See *levothyroxine*. [THY-roh-tabs].

**thyrotropin alfa** (Thyrogen) (Endo). Recombinant DNA thyroid-stimulating hormone drug used to diagnose serum levels of thyroglobulin; used with radioactive iodine to treat thyroid cancer. Intramuscular: 1.1 mg (4 IU)/10 mL. [THY-roh-TROH-pin AL-fah].

**tiagabine** (Gabitril Filmtabs) (Neuro). Anticonvulsant drug used to treat complex partial and simple partial seizures. Tablet (Filmtabs): 2 mg, 4 mg, 12 mg, 16 mg. [ty-AG-ah-been].

**tiapride** (Psych). Used to treat Tourette's syndrome. Orphan drug. [TEE-ah-pride].

**Tiazac** (Analges, Cardio). See *diltiazem*. [TY-ah-zak].

**tiazofurin** (Chemo). Chemotherapy drug used to treat leukemia. Orphan drug. [ty-AZ-oh-FYOOR-in].

**Ticar** (Anti-infec). See *ticarcillin*. [TY-kar].

**ticarcillin** (Ticar) (Anti-infec). Penicillin-type antibiotic drug used to treat a variety of bacterial infections, including endocarditis, peritonitis, endometritis, pelvic inflammatory disease, skin and soft tissue infections, urinary tract infection due to *E. coli,* and septicemia. Intramuscular or intravenous (powder to be reconstituted): 3 g. [TY-kar-SIL-in].

**TICE BCG** (Chemo). See *BCG.* [TICE B-C-G].

**Ticlid** (Hem, Neuro). See *ticlopidine.* [TY-klid].

**ticlopidine** (Ticlid) (Hem, Neuro). Platelet aggregation inhibitor drug used to prevent a second stroke. Tablet: 250 mg. [ty-KLOH-pih-deen].

**Tigan** (GI). See *trimethobenzamide.* [TY-gan].

**Tikosyn** (Cardio). See *dofetilide.* [TEE-koh-sin].

**tilarginine** (Cardio). Used to treat cardiogenic shock. Orphan drug. [ty-LAR-jih-neen].

**Tilia Fe** (OB/GYN) (generic *norethindrone, ethinyl estradiol; ferrous sulfate*). Combination triphasic oral contraceptive drug with iron supplement. Pill pack, 28-day: (5 hormone tablets) 1 mg/20 mcg; (7 hormone tablets) 1 mg/30 mcg; (9 hormone tablets) 1 mg/35 mcg; (7 iron [Fe] tablets) 75 mg. [TIL-ee-ah F-E].

**tiludronate** (Skelid) (Ortho). Bone resorption inhibitor drug used to treat Paget's disease of the bones. Tablet: 240 mg. [ty-LOO-droh-nayt].

**Timentin** (Anti-infec) (generic *ticarcillin, clavulanic acid*). Combination penicillin-type antibiotoic and penicillinase inhibitor drug used to treat penicillin-resistant bacterial infections. Intravenous (powder to be reconstituted): 3 g/0.1 mg per 100 mL. [tih-MEN-tin].

**Timolide 10-25** (Cardio) (generic *timolol, hydrochlorothiazide*). Combination beta-blocker and diuretic drug used to treat hypertension. Tablet: 10 mg/25 mg. [TIM-oh-lide].

**timolol** (Betimol, Blocadren, Istalol, Timoptic, Timoptic GFS, Timoptic-XE) (Analges, Cardio, Ophth). Beta-blocker drug used to treat hypertension and myocardial infarction; used to treat migraine headaches; used topically to treat glaucoma. Tablet: 5 mg, 10 mg, 20 mg. Ophthalmic gel: 0.25%, 0.5%. Ophthalmic solution: 0.25%, 0.5%. [TIM-oh-lawl].

**Timoptic, Timoptic GFS, Timoptic-XE** (Ophth). See *timolol.* [tim-AWP-tik].

**Tinactin, Tinactin for Jock Itch** (Derm). See *tolnaftate.* [tih-NAK-tin].

**Tindamax** (GI, OB/GYN). See *tinidazole.* [TIN-dah-maks].

**Ting 1%** (Derm). See *tolnaftate.* [TING].

**Ting 2%** (Derm). See *miconazole.* [TING].

**tinidazole** (Tindamax) (GI, OB/GYN). Antiprotozoal drug used to treat the sexually transmitted disease trichomoniasis; used to treat intestinal infections from amoebas and *Giardiasis.* Tablet: 250 mg, 500 mg. [ty-NID-ah-zohl].

**tinzaparin** (Innohep) (Cardio, Hem). Low molecular weight heparin anticoagulant drug used to prevent or treat deep venous thrombosis and pulmonary embolus. Subcutaneous: 20,000 units/mL. [tin-ZAH-pah-rin].

**tioconazole** (Monistat 1, Vagistat-1) (OB/GYN). Over-the-counter antiyeast drug used topically to treat vaginal yeast infections. Vaginal ointment: 6.5%. [TY-oh-KAWN-ah-zohl].

**tiopronin** (Thiola) (Uro). Used to prevent the formation of cystine kidney stones in patients with cystinuria. Tablet: 100 mg. [TY-oh-PROH-nin].

**tiotropium** (Spiriva) (Pulm). Bronchodilator drug used to treat bronchospasm from chronic obstructive pulmonary disease and emphysema. Powder for inhalation: 1mg/capule. [TEE-oh-TROH-pee-um].

**tipifarnib** (Zarnestra) (Chemo). Chemotherapy drug used to treat leukemia. Orphan drug. [tih-PIF-ar-nib].

**tipranavir** (Aptivus) (Anti-infec). Protease inhibitor antiviral drug used to treat HIV and AIDS. Capsule: 250 mg. Oral liquid: 100 mg/mL. [tih-PRAY-nah-veer].

**tirapazamine** (Chemo). Chemotherapy drug used to treat head and neck cancer. Orphan drug. [TY-rah-PAZ-ah-meen].

**tiratricol** (Triacana) (Endo). Antithyroid drug used to suppress thyroid-stimulating hormone from the pituitary gland in patients with thyroid cancer who cannot tolerate levothyroxine. Orphan drug. [TEER-ah-TRY-kawl].

**tirofiban** (Aggrastat) (Cardio, Hem). Platelet aggregation inhibitor drug used to treat acute coronary syndrome; used to treat patients who are undergoing angioplasty or stent placement. Intravenous: 50 mcg/mL, 250 mcg/mL. [TY-roh-FY-ban].

**Tisit** (Derm) (generic *piperonyl, pyrethrin*). Combination over-the-counter pediculocide drug used topically on the skin and scalp to treat parasitic infection from pediculosis (lice). Gel: 3%/0.3%. Lotion: 2%/0.3%. Shampoo: 4%/0.33%. [TIS-it].

**Titralac, Titralac Extra Strength** (GI). Calcium-containing antacid drug used to treat heartburn. Chewable tablet: 420 mg, 750 mg. [TIH-trah-lak].

**Titralac Plus** (GI) (generic *calcium, simethicone*). Combination antacid and anti-gas drug used to treat heartburn and gas. Tablet: 420 mg/20 mg. Liquid: 500 mg/20 mg. [TIH-trah-lak PLUS].

**tizanidine** (Zanaflex) (Neuro, Ortho). Skeletal muscle relaxant drug used to treat severe muscle spasticity associated with multiple sclerosis, cerebral palsy, stroke, or spinal cord injury. Capsule: 2 mg, 4 mg, 6 mg. Tablet: 2 mg, 4 mg. [ty-ZAN-ih-deen].

**TNKase** (Cardio, Hem). See *tenecteplase.* [T-N-K-ays].

**TOBI** (Anti-infec). See *tobramycin.* [TOH-bee].

**TobraDex Ophthalmic** (Ophth) (generic *dexamethasone, tobramycin*). Combination corticosteroid and antibiotic drug used topically in the eyes to treat inflammation and bacterial infections. Ophthalmic suspension or ointment: 0.1%/0.3%. [TOH-brah-deks of-THAL-mik].

**tobramycin** (AK-TOB, Defy, TOBI, Tobrex) (Anti-infec, Ophth).    Aminoglycoside antibiotic drug used to treat serious infections due to gram-negative bacteria, such as pneumonia, peritonitis, meningitis, and septicemia; inhaled to treat cystic fibrosis patients with *Pseudomonas* infections of the lungs; used topically in the eye to treat bacterial infections. Intramuscular or intravenous: 0.8 mg/mL, 1.2 mg/mL, 10 mg/mL. Nebulizer solution: 300 mg/5 mL. Ophthalmic solution: 0.3%. Ophthalmic ointment: 3 mg/g. [TOH-brah-MY-sin].

**Tobrex** (Anti-infec).    See *tobramycin.* [TOH-breks].

**Today Sponge** (OB/GYN).    See *nonoxynol-9.* [too-DAY].

**Tofranil, Tofranil-PM** (Analges, Neuro, Psych, Uro).    See *imipramine.* [TOH-frah-nil].

**tolazamide** (Endo).    Sulfonylurea oral antidiabetic drug used to treat type 2 diabetes mellitus. Tablet: 100 mg, 250 mg, 500 mg. [tol-AZ-ah-mide].

**tolbutamide** (Orinase) (Endo).    Sulfonylurea oral antidiabetic drug used to treat type 2 diabetes mellitus. Tablet: 500 mg. [tol-BYOO-tah-mide].

**tolcapone** (Tasmar) (Neuro).    COMT inhibitor drug used to treat Parkinson's disease. Tablet: 100 mg, 200 mg. [TOL-kah-pohn].

**tolmetin** (Analges, Ortho).    Nonsteroidal anti-inflammatory drug used to treat the pain and inflammation of osteoarthritis and rheumatoid arthritis. Capsule: 400 mg. Tablet: 200 mg, 600 mg. [TOL-meh-tin].

**tolnaftate** (Absorbine Athlete's Foot, Absorbine Footcare, Aftate for Athlete's Foot, Aftate for Jock Itch, Tinactin, Tinactin for Jock Itch, Ting 1%) (Derm).    Over-the-counter antifungal drug used topically on the skin to treat tinea (ringworm), onychomycosis, and other fungal infections of the skin. Cream: 1%. Gel: 1%. Liquid: 1%. Powder: 1%. Spray liquid: 1%. Spray powder: 1%. [tol-NAF-tayt].

**tolterodine** (Detrol, Detrol LA) (Uro).    Anticholinergic drug used to treat the urgency and frequency of overactive bladder. Extended-release capsule: 2 mg, 4 mg. Tablet: 1 mg, 2 mg. [tohl-TAIR-oh-deen].

**Topamax** (Neuro, Psych).    See *topiramate.* [TOH-pah-maks].

**Topicort, Topicort LP** (Derm).    See *desoximetasone.* [TOP-ih-kort].

**topiramate** (Topamax) (Analges, Neuro, Psych).    Anticonvulsant drug used to treat tonic-clonic seizures and simple and complex partial seizures; used to treat migraine headaches; used to treat bipolar disorder; used to treat alcohol and cocaine dependence; used to treat bulimia; used to aid in weight loss and stopping smoking; orphan drug used to treat Lennox-Gastaut syndrome. Sprinkle capsule: 15 mg, 25 mg. Tablet: 25 mg, 50 mg, 100 mg. [toh-PEER-ah-mayt].

**Toposar** (Chemo).    See *etoposide.* [TOH-poh-sar].

**topotecan** (Hycamtin) (Chemo).    Mitosis inhibitor chemotherapy drug used to treat cancer of the lung, ovary, and cervix. Capsule: 0.25 mg, 1 mg. Intravenous (powder to be reconstituted): 4 mg. [TOH-poh-TEE-kan].

**Toprol-XL** (Analges, Cardio, GI).    See *metoprolol.* [TOH-prawl-X-L].

**toralizumab** (Hem).    Used to treat thrombocytopenia purpura. Orphan drug. [TOR-ah- LIZ-yoo-mab].

**toremifene** (Fareston) (Chemo).    Hormonal chemotherapy drug used to treat breast cancer; orphan drug used to treat desmoid tumors. Tablet: 60 mg. [toh-REM-ih-feen].

**Torisel** (Chemo).    See *temsirolimus.* [TOR-ih-sel].

**Tornalate** (Pulm).    See *bitolterol.* [TOR-nah-layt].

**torsemide** (Demadex) (Cardio, Uro).    Loop diuretic drug used to treat hypertension; used to treat edema from congestive heart failure, liver disease, or kidney disease. Tablet: 5 mg, 10 mg, 20 mg, 100 mg. Intravenous: 10 mg/mL. [TOR-seh-mide].

**Total Block VL** (Derm).    Used to prevent skin sensitivity in patients undergoing photodynamic therapy. Orphan drug. [TOH-tal BLAWK V-L].

**total parenteral nutrition (TPN)** (I.V.).    Fluid of amino acids, electrolytes, vitamins, and minerals. Intravenous. [TOH-tal pah-REN-ter-al noo-TRIH-shun].

**trabectedin** (Yondelis) (Chemo).    Chemotherapy drug used to treat ovarian cancer and sarcoma. Orphan drug. [trah-BEK-teh-din].

**Tracleer** (Pulm).    See *bosentan.* [TRAK-leer].

**Tracrium** (Anes, Pulm).    See *atracurium.* [TRAK-ree-um].

**tramadol** (Ultram, Ultram ER) (Analges).    Nonnarcotic analgesic drug used to treat moderate-to-severe pain and chronic pain. Tablet: 50 mg. Extended-release tablets: 100 mg, 200 mg, 300 mg. [TRAM-ah-dawl].

**Trandate** (Endo).    See *labetalol.* [TRAN-dayt].

**trandolapril** (Mavik) (Cardio).    ACE inhibitor drug used to treat hypertension; used to treat congestive heart failure and left ventricular failure after a myocardial infarction. Tablet: 1 mg, 2 mg, 4 mg. [tran-DOH-lah-pril].

**tranexamic acid** (Cyklokapron) (Hem).    Hemostatic drug used to prevent or treat hemorrhage in patients with hemophilia during or after surgery or tooth extraction. Tablet: 500 mg. Intravenous: 100 mg/mL. [TRAN-ek-SAM-ik AS-id].

**tranilast** (Rizaben) (Chemo).    Chemotherapy drug used to treat brain cancer. Orphan drug. [TRAN-ih-last].

**Transderm-Scōp** (GI).    See *scopolamine.* [TRANS-derm SKOHP].

**TransMID** (Chemo).    Chemotherapy drug used to treat brain cancer. Orphan drug. [trans- MID].

**Tranxene, Tranxene-SD, Tranxene-SD Half Strength, Tranxene T-tab** (GI, Psych).    See *clorazepate.* [TRAN-zeen].

**tranylcypromine** (Parnate) (Psych).    MAO inhibitor drug used to treat depression. Tablet: 10 mg. [TRAN-il-SIP-roh-meen].

**trastuzumab** (Herceptin) (Chemo).    Monoclonal antibody drug used to treat breast and pancreatic cancer. Intravenous (powder to be reconstituted): 440 mg/20 mL. [tras-TOOZ-yoo-mab].

**TraumaCal** (GI).   Lactose-free nutrional supplement formulated for patients with severe stress from disease or trauma. Liquid. [TRAW-mah-KAL].

**Travatan. Travatan Z** (Ophth).   See *travoprost.* [TRAV-oh-tan].

**travoprost (Travatan, Travatan Z)** (Ophth).   Prostaglandin F drug used topically in the eye to treat glaucoma. Ophthalmic solution: 0.004%. [TRAV-oh-prawst].

**trazodone** (Psych).   Antidepressant drug used to treat depression; used to treat withdrawal from cocaine addiction. Tablet: 50 mg, 100 mg, 150 mg, 300 mg. [TRAZ-oh-dohn].

**Treanda** (Chemo).   See *bendamustine.* [tree-AN-dah].

**Trecator-SC** (Pulm).   See *ethionamide.* [TREK-ah-tor-S-C].

**Trellium Plus** (Uro) (generic *butabarbital, hyoscyamine, phenazopyridine, butabarbital*).   Combination barbiturate sedative, urinary tract antispasmodic, and urinary tract analgesic drug used to treat spasms of the urinary tract from infection or stones. Tablet: 15 mg/0.3 mg/150 mg, [TREL-ee-um PLUS].

**Trelstar Depot, Trelstar LA** (Chemo, Endo).   See *triptorelin.* [TREL-star].

**Trental** (Cardio, Hem).   See *pentoxifylline.* [TREN-tawl].

**treosulfan** (Ovastat) (Chemo).   Chemotherapy drug used to treat ovarian cancer. Orphan drug. [TREE-oh-SUL-fan].

**treprostinil** (Remodulin) (Pulm).   Vasodilator drug used to treat pumonary arterial hypertension. Subcutaneous catheter or central venous line: 1 mg/mL, 2.5 mg/mL, 5 mg/mL, 10 mg/mL. [treh-PRAWS-tih-nil].

**tretinoin** (Altinac, Atrilin, Avita, Renova, Retin-A, Retin-A Micro, Vesanoid) (Chemo, Derm, Ophth).   Vitamin A-type (retinoid) drug used topically on the skin to treat acne vulgaris (Atrilin, Retin-A); used to treat facial wrinkles and areas of hyperpigmentation (Renova); oral chemotherapy drug used to treat leukemia (Vesanoid); orphan drug used to treat squamous metaplasia of the cornea. Capsule: 10 mg. Cream: 0.02%, 0.025%, 0.05%, 0.1%. Gel: 0.01%, 0.025%, 0.04, 0.05%, 0.1%. Liquid: 0.05%. [TREE-tih-NOH-in].

**Trexall** (Chemo, Derm, GI, Neuro, Ortho).   See *methotrexate.* [TREKS-awl].

**Trexan** (Psych).   See *naltrexone.* [TREK-san].

**Treximet** (Analges) (generic *naproxen, sumatriptan*).   Combination nonsteroidal anti-inflammatory and serotonin receptor agonist drug used to treat migraine headaches. Tablet: 500 mg/85 mg. [TREK-sih-met].

**Triacana** (Endo).   See *tiratricol.* [TRY-ah-KAN-ah].

**triacetin** (Fungoid, Fungoid Crème, Fungoid Tincture) (Derm).   Antifungal drug used topically to treat tinea (ringworm), onychomycosis, and other fungal skin infections; used to treat *Candida* skin infections. Aerosol spray. Cream. Liquid. [try-AS-eh-tin].

**Triad** (Analges) (generic *acetaminophen, butalbital, caffeine*).   Combination nonsalicylate, barbiturate, and stimulant analgesic and sedative drug for pain. Capsule: 325 mg/50 mg/40 mg. [TRY-ad].

**triamcinolone** (Aristospan Intra-articular, Aristospan Intralesional, Azmacort, Delta-Tritex, Flutex, Kenalog, Kenalog 10, Kenalog 40, Kenalog in Orabase, Kenonel, Nasacort AQ, Nasacort HFA, Oralone, Triderm, Triesence, Tri-Kort, Trilog, Trivaris, Zytopic) (Chemo, Derm, Endo, ENT, Hem, Ophth, Ortho, Pulm).   Corticosteroid anti-inflammatory drug used to treat severe inflammation in various body systems; injected into a joint to treat osteoarthritis and rheumatoid arthritis; injected into skin lesions; inhaled to prevent acute asthma attacks; used to treat inflammation from aspiration pneumonitis; used to treat edema; used to treat leukemia and lymphoma; used to treat thyroiditis; used topically to treat dermatitis, eczema, and skin inflammation; injected into the vitreous humor to treat uveitis (Trivaris, Zytopic); used topically in the nose to treat allergy symptoms (Nasacort); used to treat inflammation and ulcers in the mouth (Kenalog in Orabase, Oralone). Aerosol inhaler (plus spacer mouthpiece): 75 mcg/activation, 100 mcg/activation. Aerosol topical spray: 0.147 mg/g. Cream: 0.025%, 0.1%, 0.5%. Lotion: 0.025%, 0.1%. Ointment: 0.025%, 0.1%, 0.5%. Skin aerosol spray: 2 seconds/actuation. Intra-articular or intradermal: 5 mg/mL, 10 mg/mL, 20 mg/mL, 40 mg/mL. Intramuscular: 10 mg/mL, 40 mg/mL. Aerosol nasal inhaler: 55 mcg/spray. Nasal spray: 55 mcg/spray. Oral paste: 0.1%. Intraocular injection: 40 mg/mL, 80 mg/mL. [TRY-am-SIN-oh-lohn].

**Triaminic Allerchews** (Derm, ENT).   See *loratadine.* [TRY-ah-MIN-ik].

**Triaminic Allergy Congestion** (ENT).   See *pseudoepherine.* [TRY-ah-MIN-ik].

**Triaminic Cold & Allergy** (ENT) (generic *chlorpheniramine, pseudoephedrine*).   Combination over-the-counter antihistamine and decongestant drug for colds and allergies. Liquid: 1 mg/15 mg. Softchew tablet: 1 mg/15 mg. [TRY-ah-MIN-ik].

**Triaminic Cough** (ENT) (generic *dextromethorphan, pseudoephedrine*).   Combination over-the-counter nonnarcotic antitussive and decongestant drug for coughs and congestion. Liquid: 5 mg/15 mg. [TRY-ah-MIN-ik].

**Triaminic Cough & Runny Nose, Triaminic Multisymptom** (ENT).   See *diphenhydramine.* [TRY-ah-MIN-ik].

**triamterene** (Dyrenium) (Cardio, GI, Uro).   Potassium-sparing diuretic drug used to treat edema from congestive heart failure, liver disease, or kidney disease. Capsule: 50 mg, 100 mg. [try-AM-teh-reen].

**Triaz, Triaz Cleanser** (Derm).   See *benzoyl peroxide.* [TRY-az].

**triazolam** (Halcion) (Neuro).   Schedule IV benzodiazepine drug used to treat insomnia. Tablet: 0.125 mg, 0.25 mg. [try-AZ-oh-lam].

**Triban** (GI).    See *trimethobenzamide*. [TRY-ban].

**Tri-Chlor** (Derm).    See *tricholoroacetic acid*. [TRY-klor].

**trichloroacetic acid** (Tri-Chlor) (Derm).    Used topically on the skin to treat condylomata acuminata (genital warts). Liquid: 80%. [try-KLOR-oh-ah-SEE-tik AS-id].

**triclosan** (Clearasil Antibacterial Soap, Clearasil Daily Face Wash, Oxy Medicated Soap, Stri-Dex Anti-Bacterial Foaming Wash, Stri Dex Cleansing Bar, Stri Dex Face Wash (Anti-Infec, Derm).    Over-the-counter antibiotic drug used topically on the skin to treat acne vulgaris. Bar of soap: 1%. Foaming liquid: 1%. Liquid: 0.3%, 1%. [TRIK-loh-san].

**Tricor** (Cardio).    See *fenofibrate*. [TRY-kor].

**Triderm** (Derm).    See *triamcinolone*. [TRY-derm].

**trientine** (Syprine) (GI).    Chelating drug used to treat Wilson's disease and decrease elevated copper levels. Capsule: 250 mg. [TRY-en-teen].

**Triesence** (Derm).    See *triamcinolone*. [try-EH-sens].

**trifluoperazine** (Psych).    Phenothiazine antipsychotic drug used to treat schizophrenia; used to treat anxiety. Tablet: 1 mg, 2 mg, 5 mg, 10 mg. [try-FLOO-oh-PAIR-ah-zeen].

**trifluridine** (Viroptic) (Ophth).    Antiviral drug used topically to treat viral infections of the eye. Ophthalmic solution: 1%. [try-FLOOR-eh-deen].

**Triglide** (Cardio).    See *fenofibrate*. [TRY-glide].

**Trihexy-2, Trihexy-5** (Neuro).    See *trihexyphenidyl*. [try-HEK-see].

**trihexyphenidyl** (Trihexy-2, Trihexy-5) (Neuro).    Anti-cholinergic drug used to treat Parkinson's disease. Tablet: 2 mg, 5 mg. Liquid: 2 mg/5 mL. [try-HEK-see-FEN-ah-dil].

**Tri-Kort** (Derm, Endo, Ortho).    See *triamcinolone*. [TRY-kort].

**Tri-Legest 21** (OB/GYN) (generic *norethindrone, ethinyl estradiol*).    Combination triphasic oral contraceptive drug. Pill pack, 21-day: (5 hormone tablets) 1 mg/20 mcg; (7 hormone tablets) 1 mg/30 mcg; (9 hormone tablets) 1 mg/35 mcg. [TRY-leh-jest 21].

**Tri-Legest Fe** (OB/GYN) (generic *norethindrone, ethinyl estradiol*).    Combination triphasic oral contraceptive drug. Pill pack, 28-day: (5 hormone tablets) 1 mg/20 mcg; (7 hormone tablets) 1 mg/30 mcg; (9 hormone tablets) 1 mg/35 mcg; (7 iron [Fe] tablets) 75 mg. [TRY-leh-jest F-E].

**Trileptal** (Neuro, Psych).    See *oxcarbazepine*. [try-LEP-tal].

**Tri-Levlen** (OB/GYN) (generic *levonorgestrel, ethinyl estradiol*).    Combination triphasic oral contraceptive drug. Pill pack, 21-day: (6 hormone tablets) 0.05 mg/30 mcg; (5 hormone tablets) 0.075 mg/40 mcg; (10 hormone tablets) 0.125 mg/30 mcg. Pill pack, 28-day: (6 hormone tablets) 0.05 mg/30 mcg; (5 hormone tablets) 0.075 mg/40 mcg; (10 hormone tablets) 0.125 mg/30 mcg; (7 inert tablets). [try-LEV-len].

**Trilog** (Derm).    See *triamcinolone*. (TRY-lawg].

**TriLyte** (GI) (generic *polyethylene glycol, electrolyte solution*).    Combination bowel evacuant and bowel prep. Oral liquid (powder to be reconstituted). [try-LITE].

**trimethobenzamide** (Tebamide, T-Gen, Tigan, Triban) (GI).    Anticholinergic antiemetic drug used to treat nausea and vomiting. Capsule: 300 mg Suppository: 100 mg, 200 mg. Intramuscular: 100 mg/mL. [try-METH-oh-BEN-zah-mide].

**trimethoprim** (Primsol, Proloprim, TMP) (Anti-infec, Uro).    Antibiotic drug used to treat urinary tract infections; combined with sulfa drugs to treat other types of infections. Tablet: 100 mg, 200 mg. Oral liquid: 50 mg/5 mL. [try-METH-oh-prim].

**trimetrexate** (Neutrexin) (Anti-infec, Chemo).    Folate antagonist drug used to treat *Pneumocystis carinii* pneumonia in AIDS patients; chemotherapy drug used to treat cancer of the head and neck, lung, pancreas, colon, rectum, bone, muscle, and prostate gland. Intravenous (powder to be reconstituted): 25 mg. [TRY-meh-TREK-sayt].

**trimipramine** (Surmontil) (GI, Psych).    Tricyclic antidepressant drug used to treat depression; used to treat peptic ulcer disease. Capsule: 25 mg, 50 mg, 100 mg. [try-MIP-rah-meen].

**Trimox** (Anti-infec).    See *amoxicillin*. [TRY-mawks].

**Trinam** (Cardio) (generic *vascular endothelial growth factor gene*).    Used to prevent intimal hyperplasia in blood vessels that have been surgically anastomosed. Biodegradable device with drug reservoir. Orphan drug. [TRY-nam].

**TriNessa** (OB/GYN) (generic *norgestimate, ethinyl estradiol*).    Combination triphasic oral contraceptive drug. Pill pack, 28-day: (7 hormone tablets) 0.18 mg/35 mcg; (7 hormone tablets) 0.215 mg/35 mcg; (7 hormone tablets) 0.25 mg/35 mcg; (7 inert tablets). [try-NES-sah].

**Tri-Norinyl** (OB/GYN) (generic *norethindrone, ethinyl estradiol*).    Combination triphasic oral contraceptive drug. Pill pack (Wallette), 21-day: (7 hormone tablets) 0.5 mg/35 mcg; (9 hormone tablets) 1 mg/35 mcg; (5 hormone tablets) 0.5 mg/35 mcg. Pill pack, 28-day: (7 hormone tablets) 0.5 mg/35 mcg; (9 hormone tablets) 1 mg/35 mcg; (5 hormone tablets) 0.5 mg/35 mcg; (7 inert tablets). [try-NOR-ih-nil].

**Triostat** (Endo).    See *liothyronine*. [TREE-oh-stat].

**Tripedia** (Misc).    Combination drug used to prevent diphtheria, pertussis, and tetanus. Subcutaneous: Vaccine. [try-PEE-dee-ah].

**Triphasil** (OB/GYN) (generic *levonorgestrel, ethinyl estradiol*).    Combination triphasic oral contraceptive drug. Pill pack, 21-day: (6 hormone tablets) 0.05 mg/30 mcg; (5 hormone tablets) 0.075 mg/40 mcg; (10 hormone tablets) 0.125 mg/30 mcg. Pill pack, 28-day: (6 hormone tablets) 0.05 mg/30 mcg; (5 hormone tablets) 0.075 mg/40 mcg; (10 hormone tablets) 0.125 mg/30 mcg; (7 inert tablets). [try-FAY-sil].

**Triple Antibiotic** (Derm) (generic *bacitracin, neomycin, polymyxin B*).    Combination over-the-counter antibiotic drug used topically on the skin to treat bacterial infections. Ointment: 400 units/3.5 mg/5000 units per g. [TRIH-pul AN-tih-by-AW-tik].

**Tri-Previfem** (OB/GYN) (generic *norgestimate, ethinyl estradiol*).   Combination triphasic oral contraceptive drug. Pill pack, 28-day: (7 hormone tablets) 0.18 mg/35 mcg; (7 hormone tablets) 0.215 mg/35 mcg; (7 hormone tablets) 0.25 mg/35 mcg; (7 inert tablets). [try-PREV-ih-fem].

**triprolidine** (Zymine) (Derm, ENT, Ophth).   Antihistamine drug used to treat symptoms of seasonal and perennial allergies, allergic rhinitis, allergic conjunctivitis, and skin allergies and itching. Oral liquid: 1.25 mg/5 mL. [try-PROH-lih-deen].

**triptorelin** (Decapeptyl, Trelstar Depot, Trelstar LA) (Chemo, Endo).   Hormonal chemotherapy drug used to treat cancer of the prostate gland, ovary, and pancreas; used to treat endometriosis and leiomyomata; used to treat growth hormone deficiency. Intramuscular (microgranules): 3.75 mg, 11.25 mg. [TRIP-toh-REL-in].

**Trisenox** (Chemo).   See *arsenic trioxide*. [TRY-seh-nawks].

**Tri-Sprintec** (OB/GYN) (generic *norgestimate, ethinyl estradiol*).   Combination triphasic oral contraceptive drug. Pill pack, 28-day: (7 hormone tablets) 0.18 mg/35 mcg; (7 hormone tablets) 0.215 mg/35 mcg); (7 hormone tablets) 0.25 mg/35 mcg; (7 inert tablets). [try-SPRIN-tek].

**Tri-Statin II** (Derm) (generic *nystatin, triamcinolone*).   Combination antiyeast and corticosteroid drug used topically to treat yeast infections and inflammation of the skin. Cream: 100,000 units/0.1%. [try-STAT-in 2].

**Trivaris** (Ophth).   See *triamcinolone*. [try-VAIR-is].

**Trivora** (OB/GYN) (generic *levonorgestrel, ethinyl estradiol*).   Combination triphasic oral contraceptive drug. Pill pack, 28-day: (6 hormone tablets) 0.05 mg/30 mcg; (5 hormone tablets) 0.075 mg/40 mcg; (10 hormone tablets) 0.125 mg/30 mcg; (7 inert tablets). [try-VOR-ah].

**Trizivir** (Anti-infec) (generic *abacavir, lamivudine, zidovudine*).   Combination nucleoside reverse transcriptase inhibitor antiviral drug used to treat HIV and AIDS. Tablet: 300 mg/150 mg/300 mg. [TRY-zih-veer].

**Trobicin** (Anti-infec).   See *spectinomycin*. [TROH-bih-sin].

**tromethamine** (Tham) (Emerg).   Used to treat metabolic acidosis during cardiac arrest and resuscitation. Intravenous: 150 mEq/500 mL. [troh-METH-ah-meen].

**Tronolane** (Anes, GI) (generic *pramoxine, zinc oxide*).   Combination over-the-counter anesthetic and astringent drug used topically to treat pain and irritation in the perianal area and hemorrhoids. Cream: 1%. [TRAW-noh-layn].

**Tronolane Suppository** (GI).   See *zinc oxide*. [TRAW-noh-layn].

**Tronothane** (Anes, Derm).   See *pramoxine*. [TRAWN-oh-thayn].

**tropicamide** (Mydriacyl) (Ophth).   Mydriatic drug used topically to dilate the pupil prior to eye examination or surgery. Ophthalmic solution: 0.5%, 1%. [troh-PIK-ah-mide].

**trospium** (Sanctura, Sanctura XR) (Uro).   Anticholinergic drug used to treat the urgency and frequency of overactive bladder. Tablet: 20 mg. [TROHS-pee-um].

**troxacitabine** (Troxatyl) (Chemo).   Chemotherapy drug used to treat leukemia. Orphan drug. [TRAWKS-ah-SIT-ah-been].

**Troxatyl** (Chemo).   See *troxacitabine*. [TRAWS-ah-til].

**Trusopt** (Ophth).   See *dorzolamide*. [TROO-sawpt].

**Truvada** (Anti-infec) (generic *emtricitabine, tenofovir*).   Combination nucleoside reverse transcriptase inhibitor and nucleotide analog reverse transcriptase inhibitor antiviral drug used to treat HIV and AIDS. Tablet: 200 mg/300 mg. [troo-VAYdah].

**Trycet** (Analges) (generic *acetaminophen, propoxyphene*).   Combination Schedule IV nonnarcotic and narcotic analgesic drug for pain. Tablet: 325 mg/100 mg. [TRY-set].

**trypan blue** (VisionBlue) (Ophth).   Dye solution used to stain the anterior capsule during eye surgery. Ophthalmic solution: 0.06%. [TRY-pan BLOO].

**trypsin** (Granulderm, Granulex) (Derm).   Enzyme drug used topically on the skin to debride burns and wounds. Aerosol spray. [TRIP-sin].

**T/Scalp** (Derm).   See *hydrocortisone*. [T-skalp].

**tuberculin purified protein derivative** (Aplisol, Tubersol) (Pulm).   Diagnostic test that uses the drug tuberculin purified protein derivative (PPD) derived from *Mycobacterium tuberculosis;* the solution is injected under the skin to test for exposure to tuberculosis (the Mantoux test). Intradermal injection: 5 TU/0.1 mL. [too-BER-kyoo-lin].

**Tubersol** (Pulm).   See *tuberculin purified protein derivative*. [TOO-ber-sawl].

**Tucks** (Anes, GI).   See *pramoxine*. [TUKS].

**Tucks Ointment** (Derm).   See *hydrocortisone*. [TUKS].

**tumor necrosis factor-binding protein** (Anti-infec).   Used to treat HIV and AIDS. Orphan drug. [TOO-mer neh-KROH-sis].

**Tums Ultra** (GI).   See *calcium carbonate*. [TUMS UL-trah].

**Tussionex** (ENT) (generic *chlorpheniramine, hydrocodone*).   Combination Schedule III antihistamine and narcotic antitussive drug used to treat severe coughs. Oral liquid: 8 mg/10 mg. [TUS-ee-oh-neks].

**Tussi-Organidin NR, Tussi-Organidin-S NR** (ENT) (generic *codeine, guaifenesin*).   Combination Schedule V narcotic antitussive and expectorant drug used to treat severe, productive coughs. Liquid: 10 mg/300 mg. [TUS-ee-or-GAN-ih-din].

**Tussirex** (ENT) (generic *codeine, pheniramine, phenylephrine, sodium citrate*).   Combination Schedule V narcotic antitussive, antihistamine, decongestant, and expectorant drug used to treat severe, productive coughs. Syrup: 10 mg/13.33 mg/4.17 mg/83 mg. [TUS-ee-reks].

**Tusstat** (ENT).   See *diphenhydramine*. [TUS-stat].

**Twin-K** (Uro).   See *potassium*. [TWIN-K].

**Twinrix** (GI) (generic *inactivated hepatitis A virus, recombinant hepatitis B virus*).   Combination vaccine used to prevent hepatitis A and hepatitis B. Intramuscular: 720 EL.U./20 mcg per mL. [TWIN-riks].

**TwoCal HN** (GI).   Lactose-free nutritional supplement. Powder (to be reconstituted). [TOO-kal H-N].

**Tycolene P.M.** (Neuro) (generic *acetaminophen, diphenhydramine*).   Combination over-the-counter analgesic and antihistamine drug used to relieve pain and induce sleep. Tablet: 500 mg/25 mg. [TY-koh-leen P-M].

**Tykerb** (Chemo).   See *lapatinib*. [TY-kerb].

**Tylenol, Tylenol Arthritis, Tylenol Caplets, Tylenol Children's Meltaways, Tylenol Children's Soft Chews, Tylenol 8 Hour, Tylenol Extended Relief, Tylenol Extra Strength, Tylenol Infants' Drops, Tylenol Junior Strength, Tylenol Regular Strength, Tylenol Sore Throat** (Analges).   See *acetaminophen*. [TY-leh-nawl].

**Tylenol Allergy Complete NightTime, Tylenol Flu NightTime Maximum Strength** (ENT) (generic *acetaminophen, diphenhydramine, pseudo-ephedrine*).   Combination over-the-counter analgesic, antihistamine, and decongestant drug. Gelcap/tablet: 500 mg/25 mg/30 mg. [TY-leh-nawl].

**Tylenol Allergy Multi-Symptom** (ENT) (generic *acetaminophen, chlorpheniramine, phenylephrine*).   Combination over-the-counter analgesic, antihistamine, and decongestant drug. Tablet: 325 mg/2 mg/5 mg. [TY-leh-nawl].

**Tylenol Children's Cold, Tylenol Children's Cold Plus Nighttime** (ENT) (generic *acetaminophen, chlorpheniramine, pseudoephedrine*).   Combination over-the-counter analgesic, antihistamine, and decongestant drug. Tablet: 325 mg/2 mg/15 mg/30 mg. [TY-leh-nawl].

**Tylenol Cold Complete** (ENT) (generic *acetaminophen, chlorpheniramine, dextromethorphan, pseudoephedrine*). Combination over-the-counter analgesic, antihistamine, nonnarcotic antitussive, and decongestant drug. Liquid: 160 mg/1 mg/5 mg/15 mg.

**Tylenol Cold Non-Drowsy, Tylenol Flu Maximum Strength Non-Drowsy,** (ENT) (generic *acetaminophen, dextro-methorphan, pseudoephedrine*).   Combination over-the-counter analgesic, nonnarcotic antitussive, and decongestant drug. Tablet: 500 mg/15 mg/30 mg. Tablet: 325 mg/15 mg/30 mg. Gelcap: 500 mg/15 mg/30 mg. [TY-leh-nawl].

**Tylenol Cough & Sore Throat Daytime** (ENT) (generic *acetaminophen, dextromethorphan*).   Combination over-the-counter analgesic and antitussive drug. Liquid: 166.7 mg/5 mg. [TY-leh-nawl].

**Tylenol Flu Nighttime Maximum Strength** (ENT) (generic *acetaminophen, dextromethorphan, doxylamine, pseudoephedrine*).   Combination over-the-counter analgesic, nonnarcotic antitussive, antihistamine, and decongestant drug. Liquid: 167 mg/5 mg/2.1 mg/10 mg. [TY-leh-nawl].

**Tylenol Infants' Plus Cold and Cough** (ENT) (generic *acetaminophen, dextromethorphan, phenylephrine*). Combination over-the-counter analgesic, nonnarcotic antitussive and decongestant drug. Drops: 80 mg/ 2.5 mg/1.25 mg. [TY-leh-nawl].

**Tylenol PM, Extra Strength; Tylenol PM Gelcaps, Extra Strength** (Neuro) (generic *acetaminophen, diphenhydramine*).   Over-the-counter combination analgesic and antihistamine drug used to relieve pain and induce sleep. Capsule: 500 mg/25 mg. Tablet: 500 mg/ 25 mg. [TY-leh-nawl].

**Tylenol Severe Allergy** (ENT) (generic *acetaminophen, diphenhydramine*).   Combination over-the-counter analgesic and antihistamine drug to treat allergies. Gelcap/tablet: 500 mg/12.5 mg, 500 mg/25mg. [TY-leh-nawl].

**Tylenol Severe Sinus Congestion** (ENT) (generic *guaifenesin, pseudoephedrine*).   Combination over-the-counter expectorant and decongestant drug. Tablet: 200 mg/30 mg. [TY-leh-nawl].

**Tylenol Sinus NightTime** (ENT) (generic *acetaminophen, doxylamine, pseudoephedrine*).   Combination over-the-counter analgesic, antihistamine, and decongestant drug. Tablet: 500 mg/6.25 mg/30 mg. [TY-leh-nawl].

**Tylenol w/ Codeine** (Analges) (generic *acetaminophen, codeine*).   Schedule V combination nonnarcotic and narcotic analgesic drug for pain. Liquid: 120 mg/12 mg. [TY-leh-naw with KOH-deenl].

**Tylenol w/ Codeine No. 2** (Analges) (generic *acetaminophen, codeine*).   Schedule III combination nonnarcotic and narcotic analgesic drug for pain. Tablet: 300 mg/15 mg. [TY-leh-nawl with KOH-deen].

**Tylenol w/ Codeine No. 3** (Analges) (generic *acetaminophen, codeine*).   Schedule III combination nonnarcotic and narcotic analgesic drug for pain. Tablet: 300 mg/30 mg. [TY-leh-nawl with KOH-deen].

**Tylenol w/ Codeine No. 4** (Analges) (generic *acetaminophen, codeine*).   Schedule III combination nonnarcotic and narcotic analgesic drug for pain. Tablet: 300 mg/60 mg. [TY-leh-nawl with KOH-deen].

**Tylox** (Analges) (generic *acetaminophen, oxycodone*). Combination Schedule II nonnarcotic and narcotic analgesic drug for pain. Capsule: 500 mg/5 mg. [TY-lawks].

**tyloxapol** (Enuclene, Supervent) (Ophth, Pulm).   Used to clean and lubricate an artificial eye (Enuclene); orphan drug used to treat cystic fibrosis (Supervent). Ophthalmic solution: 0.25%. [ty-LAWKs-ah-pohl].

**Tysabri** (GI, Neuro).   See *natalizumab*. [tih-SAB-ree].

**Tyzeka** (Anti-infec, GI).   See *telbivudine*. [ty-ZEK-ah].

**Tyzine, Tyzine Pediatric** (ENT).   See *tetrahydrolzoline*. [TY-zeen].

**UAA** (Uro) (generic *atropine, hyoscyamine, methenamine, methylene blue, phenyl salicylate*).    Combination urinary tract antispasmodic, anti-infective, antiseptic, and analgesic drug used to treat urinary tract infections with pain and spasms. Tablet: 0.03 mg/0.03 mg/40.8 mg/5.4 mg/18.1 mg. [U-A-A].

**ubiquinol** (Cardio, Neuro).    Used to treat Huntington's chorea; used to treat congestive heart failure in children. Orphan drug. [yoo-BIH-kwih-nawl].

**Ucephan** (Hem) (generic *benzoate, phenylacetate*).    Combination drug used to prevent and treat increased levels of ammonia in the blood in patients with abnormalities of the enzymes that produce urea. Orphan drug. [yoo-SEF-an].

**U-cort** (Derm).    See *hydrocortisone*. [YOO-kort].

**Uendex** (Pulm).    See *dextran sulfate*. [yoo-EN-deks].

**Ultane** (Anes).    See *sevoflurane*. [UL-tayn].

**Ultiva** (Anes).    See *remifentanil*. [ul-TEE-vah].

**Ultracal** (GI).    Lactose-free nutritional supplement. Liquid. [UL-trah-kal].

**Ultrace, Ultrase MT 12, Ultrase MT 18, Ultrase MT 20** (GI) (generic *amylase, lipase, protease*).    Combination digestive enzyme drug used as replacement therapy. Capsule: 20,000 units/4500 units/25,000 units; 39,000 units/ 12,000 units/39,000 units; 58,500 units/18,000 units/ 58,500 units; 65,000 units/20,000 units/65,000 units. [UL-trays].

**Ultracet** (Analges) (generic *acetaminophen, tramadol*).    Combination nonnarcotic analgesic drug. Tablet: 325 mg/ 37.5 mg. [UL-trah-set].

**ultralente insulin** (Endo).    Long-acting insulin. Subcutaneous: 100 units/mL. [UL-trah-LEN-tay IN-soo-lin].

**Ultram** (Analges).    See *tramadol*. [UL-tram].

**Ultra Tears** (Ophth).    Over-the-counter artificial tears for dry eyes. Ophthalmic solution. [UL-trah TEERZ].

**Ultratrace** (Chemo).    See *iobenguane*. [UL-trah-trays].

**Ultravate** (Derm).    See *halobetasol*. [UL-trah-vayt].

**ultraviolet light** (Derm).    See *PUVA*. [UL-trah-VY-oh-let LITE].

**Umecta** (Derm).    See *urea*. [yoo-MEK-tah].

**Unasyn** (Anti-infec) (generic *ampicillin, sulbactam*).    Combination penicillin-type antibiotoic and penicillinase inhibitor drug used to treat penicillin-resistant bacterial infections. Intramuscular or intravenous (powder to be reconstituted): 1 g/0.5 g, 2 g/1 g. [YOO-nah-sin].

**undecylenic acid** (Cruex Aerosol, Cruex Powder, Desenex Powder, Desenex Soap, Fungoid AF) (Derm).    Over-the-counter antifungal drug used topically to treat tinea (ringworm) fungal skin infection. Cream: 8%, 20%. Liquid: 25%. Powder: 10%, 19%, 12%, 25%. Soap. [UN-deh-sy-LEN-ik AS-id].

**Unguentine** (Derm) (generic *phenol, zinc oxide*).    Combination over-the-counter anesthestic and astringent drug used topically on the skin. [UN-gwen-teen].

**Unguentine Maximum Strength** (Anes, Derm).    See *benzocaine*. [UN-gwen-teen].

**Unguentine Plus** (Anes, Derm) See *lidocaine*. [UN-gwen-teen].

**Uniphyl** (Pulm).    See *theophylline*. [YOO-nih-fil].

**Uniretic** (Cardio) (generic *moexipril, hydrochlorothiazide*).    Combination ACE inhibitor and diuretic drug used to treat hypertension. Tablet: 7.5 mg/12.5 mg, 15 mg/12.5 mg, 15 mg/25 mg. [YOO-nih-REH-tik].

**Unisom Maximum Strength SleepGels** (Neuro).    See *diphenydramine*. [YOO-nih-sawm].

**Unisom Nighttime Sleep-Aid** (Neuro).    See *doxylamine*. [YOO-nih-sawm].

**Unisom with Pain Relief** (Neuro) (generic *acetaminophen, diphenhydramine*).    Combination analgesic and antihistamine drug used to relieve pain and induce sleep. Tablet: 650 mg/50 mg. [YOO-nih-sawm].

**Unithroid** (Endo).    See *levothyroxine*. [YOO-nih-throyd].

**Univasc** (Cardio).    See *moexipril*. [YOO-nih-vask].

**Uracid** (Derm, Uro).    See *methionine*. [YOOR-ah-sid].

**urea** (Carmol 40, Kerafoam, Keralac, Keralac Nailstik, Neurosolve, Umecta, Ureaphil, Vanamide) (Derm, Neuro, OB/GYN, Ophth).    Osmotic diuretic drug used to treat cerebral edema and increased intracranial pressure; used to treat increased intraocular pressure and glaucoma; injected into the amniotic fluid to induce abortion; used topically to debride and treat eczema, diaper rash, skin irritation, and itching; orphan drug used to treat retinitis pigmentosa (Neurosolve). Cream: 10%, 20%, 40%, 50%. Topical emulsion: 40%. Gel: 40%, 50%. Lotion: 10%, 25%, 35%, 40%. Ointment: 50%. Topical suspension: 40%, 50%. Intravenous or intra-amniotic injection: 40 g/150 mL. [yoo-REE-ah]

**Ureaphil** (Neuro, Ophth).    See *urea*. [yoo-REE-ah-fil].

**Urecholine** (Uro).    See *bethanechol*. [YOOR-eh-KOH-leen].

**Urelle** (Uro) (generic *hyoscyamine, methenamine, methylene blue, phenyl salicylate*).    Combination drug with a urinary tract antispasmodic, anti-infective, antiseptic, and analgesic drug; used to treat urinary tract infections with pain and spasms. Tablet: 0.12 mg/81 mg/10.8 mg/32.4 mg. [yoo-REL].

**Uretron D/S** (Uro) (generic *hyoscyamine, methenamine, methylene blue, phenyl salicylate*).    Combination urinary tract antispasmodic, anti-infective, antiseptic, and analgesic drug; used to treat urinary tract infections with pain and spasms. Tablet: 0.12 mg/120 mg/10.8 mg/36.2 mg. [YOOR-eh-trawn D-S].

**Urex** (Anti-infec, Uro).    See *methenamine*. [YOOR-eks].

**Urimar T** (Uro) (generic *hyoscyamine, methenamine, methylene blue, phenyl salicylate*).    Combination urinary tract antispasmodic, anti-infective, antiseptic, and analgesic drug; used to treat urinary tract infections with pain and spasms. Tablet: 0.12 mg, 120 mg/10.8 mg/36.2 mg. [YOOR-ih-mar T].

**Urimax** (Uro) (generic *hyoscyamine, methenamine, methylene blue, phenyl salicylate*).   Combination urinary tract antispasmodic, anti-infective, antiseptic, and analgesic drug; used to treat urinary tract infections with pain and spasms. Tablet: 0.12 mg/81.6 mg/10.8 mg/36.2 mg/. [YOOR-ih-maks].

**Urised** (Uro) (generic *atropine, hyoscyamine, methenamine, methylene blue, phenyl salicylate*).   Combination urinary tract antispasmodic, anti-infective, antiseptic, and analgesic drug; used to treat urinary tract infections with pain and spasms. Tablet: 0.03 mg/0.03 mg/40.8 mg/5.4 mg/18.1 mg. [YOOR-ih-sed].

**Urisedamine** (Uro) (generic *hyoscyamine, methenamine*).   Combination urinary tract antispasmodic and urinary anti-infective drug; used to treat urinary tract infections with pain and spasms. Tablet: 0.15 mg/500 mg. [YOOR-ih-SED-ah-meen].

**Uriseptic** (Uro) (generic *atropine, hyoscyamine, methenamine, methylene blue, phenyl salicylate*).   Combination urinary tract antispasmodic, anti-infective, antiseptic, and analgesic drug; used to treat urinary tract infections with pain and spasms. Tablet: 0.03 mg/0.03 mg/40.8 mg/5.4 mg/18.1 mg. [YOOR-ih-SEP-tik].

**Urispas** (Uro).   See *flavoxate.* [YOOR-ih-spaz].

**UriSym** (Uro) (generic *hyoscyamine, methenamine, methylene blue, phenyl salicylate*).   Combination urinary tract antispasmodic, anti-infective, antiseptic, and analgesic drug; used to urinary tract infections with pain and spasms. Capsule: 0.12 mg/100 mg/10.8 mg/40 mg. [YOOR-ih-sim].

**Uritin** (Uro) (generic *atropine, hyoscyamine, methenamine, methylene blue, phenyl salicylate*).   Combination urinary tract antispasmodic, anti-infective, antiseptic, and analgesic drug; used to treat urinary tract infections with pain and spasms. Tablet: 0.03 mg/0.03 mg/40.8 mg/5.4 mg/18.1 mg. [YOOR-ih-tin]

**Uritact DS** (Uro) (generic *atropine, hyoscyamine, methenamine, methylene blue, phenyl salicylate*).   Combination urinary tract antispasmodic, anti-infective, antiseptic, and analgesic drug; used to treat urinary tract infections with pain and spasms. Tablet: 0.06 mg/ 0.06 mg/81.6 mg/10.8 mg/36.2 mg. [YOOR-ih-takt D-S].

**Uro Blue** (Uro) (generic *hyoscyamine, methenamine, methylene blue, phenyl salicylate*).   Combination urinary tract antispasmodic, anti-infective, antiseptic, and analgesic drug; used to treat urinary tract infections with pain and spasms. Tablet: 0.12 mg/120 mg/10.8 mg/36.2 mg. [YOOR-oh BLOO].

**Urocit-K** (Ortho, Uro).   See *potassium citrate.* [YOOR-oh-sit-K].

**urofollitropin** (Bravelle, Fertinex, Metrodin) (Endo, OB/GYN).   Follicle-stimulating hormone drug used to stimulate ovulation and treat infertility in women; used with assisted reproductive technology; orphan drug used to stimulate ovulation in women with polycystic ovaries;

orphan drug used to treat low sperm count and infertility in men with pituitary gland malfunction. Subcutaneous (powder to be reconstituted): 75 units/2 mL. [YOOR-oh-FOH-lih-TROH-pin].

**urogastrone** (Ophth).   Used to promote healing after corneal transplant surgery. Orphan drug. [YOOR-oh-GAS-trohn].

**Urogesic** (Uro).   See *phenazopyridine.* [YOOR-oh-JEE-sik].

**Urogesic Blue** (Uro) (generic *hyoscyamine, methenamine, methylene blue, phenyl salicylate*).   Combination urinary tract antispasmodic, anti-infective, antiseptic, and analgesic drug; used to treat urinary tract infections with pain and spasms. Tablet: 0.12 mg/81.6 mg/10.8 mg/36.2 mg. [YOOR-oh-JEE-sik BLOO].

**Urolene Blue** (Emerg, Uro).   See *methylene blue.* [YOOR-oh-leen BLOO].

**Uroquid-Acid No. 2** (Uro) (generic *methenamine, sodium acid phosphate*).   Combination urinary tract anti-infective and urinary acidifier drug; used to treat urinary tract infections. Tablet: 500 mg/500 mg. [YOOR-oh-kwid AS-id].

**URSO 250, URSO Forte** (GI).   See *ursodiol.* [UR-soh].

**ursodiol** (Actigall, URSO 250, URSO Forte) (GI).   Used to dissolve gallstones in patients who cannot undergo gallbladder surgery. Capsule: 300 mg. Tablet: 250 mg, 500 mg. [UR-soh-DY-ol].

**Uroxatral** (Uro).   See *alfuzosin.* [YOOR-oh-ZAY-trawl].

**UTI Relief** (Uro).   See *phenazopyridine.* [U-T-I ree-LEEF].

**Uvadex** (Derm).   See *methoxsalen.* [YOO-vah-deks].

**Vagifem** (OB/GYN).   See *estradiol.* [VAJ-ih-fem].

**Vagisil** (Anes, OB/GYN).   See *benzocaine.* [VAJ-ih-sil].

**Vagistat-1** (OB/GYN).   See *tioconazole.* [VAJ-ih-stat-1].

**Vagistat 3 Combination Pack** (OB/GYN).   See *miconazole.* [VAJ-ih-stat 3].

**valacyclovir** (Valtrex) (Anti-infec, Derm, OB/GYN).   Antiviral drug used to treat herpes zoster (shingles); used to treat herpes simplex type 1 virus (cold sores); used to treat herpes simplex type 2 virus (genital herpes) in immunocompromised patients. Tablet: 500 mg, 1 g. [VAL-ah-SY-kloh-veer].

**Valcyte** (Anti-infec).   See *valganciclovir.* [VAL-site].

**valganciclovir** (Valcyte) (Anti-infec).   Antiviral drug used to treat cytomegalovirus infection of the retina in patients with AIDS and in kidney or heart transplant patients. Tablet: 450 mg. [VAL-gan-SY-kloh-veer].

**Valium** (GI, Neuro, Ortho, Psych).   See *diazepam.* [VAL-ee-um].

**Valortim** (Emerg).   Used to treat anthrax from bioterrorism. Orphan drug. [vah-LOR-tim].

**valproic acid** (Depacon, Depakene, Depakote, Depakote ER, Stavzor) (GI, Neuro, Psych).   Anticonvulsant drug used to treat tonic-clonic, absence, simple partial, and complex partial seizures; used to treat the mania of manic-depressive disorder; used to prevent migraine headaches; orphan drug used to treat adenomatous polyps in the colon. Capsule:

125 mg, 250 mg, 500 mg. Sprinkle capsule: 125 mg. Delayed-release tablet: 125 mg, 250 mg, 500 mg. Liquid: 250 mg/5 mL. Intravenous: 100 mg/mL. [val-PROH-ik AS-id].

**valrubicin** (Valstar) (Chemo). Chemotherapy antibiotic drug used to treat bladder cancer. Intravesical (within the bladder) injection: 40 mg/mL. Orphan drug. [val-ROO-bih-sin]

**valsartan** (Diovan) (Cardio). Angiotensin II receptor blocker drug used to treat hypertension and congestive heart failure; used to decrease the risk of death after a myocardial infarction. Tablet: 40 mg, 80 mg, 160 mg, 320 mg. [val-SAR-tan],

**Valstar** (Chemo). See *valrubicin*. [VAL-star].

**Valtrex** (Anti-infec, Derm, OB/GYN). See *valacyclovir*. [VAL-treks].

**Vanamide** (Derm). See *urea*. [VAN-ah-mide].

**Vancocin** (Anti-infec). See *vancomycin*. [VAN-koh-sin].

**Vancoled** (Anti-infec). See *vancomycin*. [VAN-koh-led].

**vancomycin** (Vancocin, Vancoled) (Anti-infec). Antibiotic drug used to treat severe bacterial infections; used to treat methicillin-resistant staphylococcus (MRSA) infections; used to treat endocarditis; used orally to treat enterocolitis due to *S. aureus*. Pulvule: 125 mg, 250 mg. Liquid (powder to be reconstituted): 1 g. Intravenous (powder to be reconstituted): 500 mg, 1 g. [van-koh-MY-sin].

**Vandazole** (OB/GYN). See *metronidazole*. [VAN-dah-zohl].

**vandetanib** (Zactima) (Chemo). Chemotherapy drug used to treat thyroid cancer. Orphan drug. [van-DET-ah-nib].

**Vaniqa** (Derm). See *eflornithine*. [VAN-ih-kah].

**Vanocin** (Derm) (generic *sodium sulfacetamide, sulfur*). Combination anti-infective and keratolytic drug used topically on the skin to treat acne vulgaris. Lotion: 10%/5% [VAN-oh-sin].

**Vanos** (Derm). See *fluocinonide*. [VAN-ohs].

**Vanquish** (Analges) (generic *acetaminophen, aspirin, caffeine*). Combination over-the-counter nonsalicylate and salicylate analgesic and caffeine drug. Caplet: 194 mg/227 mg/33 mg. [VAN-kwish].

**Vantas** (Chemo). See *histrelin*. [VAN-tas].

**Vantin** (Anti-infec). See *cefpodoxime*. [VAN-tin].

**vapreotide** (Octastatin, Sanvar) (Endo, GI). Used to treat acromegaly; used to treat carcinoid tumor; used to treat gastric, intestinal, and pancreatic fistulas; used to treat bleeding esophageal varices. Orphan drug. [vah-PREE-oh-tide].

**Vaprisol** (Endo). See *conivaptan*. [VAP-rih-sawl].

**Vaqta** (GI). See *hepatitis A vaccine*. [VAK-tah].

**vardenafil** (Levitra) (Uro). PDE5 inhibitor drug used to treat male impotence due to erectile dysfunction. Tablet: 2.5 mg, 5 mg, 10 mg, 20 mg. [var-DEN-ah-fil].

**varenicline** (Chantix) (Pulm). Nicotine antagonist drug that binds to nicotine receptors and blocks the effect of nicotine; used to help stop smoking. Tablet: 0.5 mg, 1 mg. [vah-REN-ih-kleen].

**Varivax** (Misc). Used to prevent varicella in children. Subcutaneous: Vaccine. [VAIR-ih-vaks].

**Vaseretic** (Cardio) (generic *enalapril, hydrochlorothiazide*). Combination ACE inhibitor and diuretic drug used to treat hypertension. Tablet: 5 mg/ 12.5 mg, 10 mg/25 mg. [VAY-seh-REH-tik].

**Vasocidin** (Ophth) (generic *prednisolone, sulfacetamide*). Combination corticosteroid and sulfonamide anti-infective drug used topically in the eyes to treat inflammation and bacterial infections. Ophthalmic solution: 0.25%/10%. [VAY-soh-SY-din].

**Vasodilan** (Cardio). See *isoxsuprine*. [VAY-soh-DY-lan].

**vasopressin** (Pitressin) (Endo, GI). Antidiuretic hormone drug used as replacement therapy to treat diabetes insipidus; used to treat bleeding esophageal varices; used to prevent postoperative abdominal distention. Intramuscular or subcutaneous: 20 pressor units/mL. [VAY-soh-PRES-in].

**Vasotec** (Cardio). See *enalapril*. [VAY-soh-tek].

**VaxSyn HIV-1** (Anti-infec). Antigen drug used to treat HIV and AIDS. Orphan drug. [VAKS-sin H-I-V-1].

**VaZol** (Derm, ENT). See *brompheniramine*. [VAY-zawl].

**VCF** (OB/GYN). See *nonoxynol-9*. [V-C-F].

**Vectibix** (Chemo). See *panitumumab*. [VEK-tih-biks].

**vecuronium** (Norcuron) (Anes, Pulm). Neuromuscular blocker drug used during surgery; used to treat patients who are intubated and on the ventilator. Intravenous (powder to be reconstituted): 10 mg, 20 mg. [veh-kyoor-OH-nee-um].

**Veetids** (Anti-infec). See *penicillin V*. [VEE-tids].

**Velban** (Chemo). See *vinblastine*. [VEL-ban].

**Velcade** (Chemo). See *bortezomib*. [VEL-kayd].

**Velivet** (OB/GYN) (generic *desogestrel, ethinyl estradiol*). Combination triphasic oral contraceptive drug. Pill pack, 28-day: (7 hormone tablets) 0.1 mg/25 mcg; (7 hormone tablets) 0.125 mg/25 mcg; (7 hormone tablets) 0.15 mg/ 25 mcg; (7 inert tablets). [VEL-ih-vet].

**venlafaxine** (Effexor, Effexor XR) (OB/GYN, Psych). Serotonin and norepinephrine reuptake inhibitor (SNRI) drug used to treat depression, anxiety disorder, social anxiety, and premenstrual dysphoric disorder; used to treat the hot flashes of menopause. Extended-release capsule: 37.5 mg, 75 mg, 150 mg. Tablet: 25 mg, 37.5 mg, 50 mg, 75 mg, 100 mg. [VEN-lah-FAK-seen].

**Venofer** (Hem, Uro). See *iron sucrose*. [VEN-oh-fer].

**Ventavis** (Cardio). See *iloprost*. [ven-TAV-is].

**Venticute** (Pulm). Used to treat adult respiratory distress syndrome. Orphan drug. [VEN-tih-kyoot].

**Ventolin HFA** (Pulm). See *albuterol*. [VEN-toh-lin H-F-A].

**VePesid** (Chemo). See *etoposide*. [veh-PEH-sid].

**Veramyst** (ENT). See *fluticasone*. [VAIR-ah-mist].

**verapamil** (Calan, Calan SR, Covera-HS, Isoptin SR, Verelan, Verelan PM) (Analges, Cardio).   Calcium channel blocker drug used to prevent and treat angina pectoris; used to treat hypertension; used to treat atrial flutter, atrial fibrillation, and ventricular tachycardia; used to treat hypertrophic cardiomyopathy; used to prevent migraine headaches. Extended-release capsule: 100 mg, 120 mg, 180 mg, 200 mg, 240 mg, 300 mg, 360 mg. Tablet: 40 mg, 80 mg, 120 mg. Extended-release tablet: 120 mg, 180 mg, 240 mg. Intravenous: 2.5 mg/mL. [veh-RAP-ah-mil].

**Verdeso** (Derm).   See *desonide.* [ver-DES-oh].

**Veregen** (Anti-infec, OB/GYN).   See *kunecatechins.* [VAIR-eh-jen].

**Verelan, Verelan PM** (Analges, Cardio).   See *verapamil.* [VEER-eh-lan].

**Vermox** (Misc).   See *mebendazole.* [VER-mawks].

**Veronate** (Anti-infec).   Used to prevent bacterial septicemia in premature infants. Orphan drug. [VAIR-oh-nayt].

**Vesanoid** (Chemo).   See *tretinoin.* [VES-ah-noyd].

**Vesicare** (Uro).   See *solifenacin.* [VES-ih-kair].

**Versiclear** (Derm) (generic *sodium thiosulfate, salicylic acid*).   Combination antifungal and keratolytic drug used topically on the skin to treat tinea (ringworm) fungal infection. Lotion: 25%/1%. [VER-sih-kleer].

**verteporfin** (Visudyne) (Ophth).   Phototherapy drug used to treat age-related macular degeneration; used to treat ocular histoplasmosis. Intravenous (followed by exposure to red laser light to activate the drug): 2 mg/mL. [VER-teh-POR-fin].

**Vexol** (Ophth).   See *rimexolone.* [VEK-sawl].

**Vfend** (Anti-infec).   See *voriconazole.* [V-fend].

**Viagra** (Uro).   See *sildenafil.* [vy-AG-rah].

**Vianain** (Derm) (generic *anasain, comosain*).   Combination enzyme drug used topically to debride severe burns. Orphan drug. [VY-ah-nayn].

**Vibramycin** (Anti-infec).   See *doxycycline.* [VY-brah-MY-sin].

**Vibra-Tabs** (Anti-infec).   See *doxycycline.* [VY-brah-tabs].

**Vibrilase** (Derm).   See *vibriolysin.* [VIB-rih-lays].

**vibriolysin** (Vibrilase) (Derm).   Used to debride severe burns. Orphan drug. [VIB-ree-oh-LY-sin].

**Vicks 44 Cough Relief** (ENT). See *dextromethorphan.* [VIKS 44].

**Vicks 44M Cough, Cold & Flu** (ENT) (generic *acetaminophen, chlorpheniramine, dextromethorphan, pseudoephedrine*).   Combination over-the-counter analgesic, antihistamine, nonnarcotic antitussive, and decongestant drug. Liquid: 160 mg/1 mg/5 mg/15 mg. Liquid: 162.5 mg/1 mg/7.5 mg/15 mg. [VIKS].

**Vicks 44D Cough & Head Congestion** (ENT) (generic *dextromethorphan, pseudoephedrine*).   Combination over-the-counter antitussive and decongestant drug. Liquid: 10 mg/20 mg. [VIKS].

**Vicks NyQuil Multi-Symptom Cold/Flu** (ENT) (generic *acetaminophen, dextromethorphan, doxylamine, pseudoephedrine*).   Combination over-the-counter analgesic, nonnarcotic antitussive, antihistamine, and decongestant drug. Liquid: 167 mg/5 mg/2.1 mg/10 mg. LiquiCap: 325 mg/15 mg/6.25 mg/30 mg. [VIKS].

**Vicks NyQuil Cough** (ENT) (generic *dextromethorphan, doxylamine*).   Combination over-the-counter nonnarcotic antitussive and antihistamine drug. Syrup: 5 mg/2.1 mg. [VIKS].

**Vicks Sinex Ultra Fine Mist** (ENT).   See *phenylephrine.* [VIKS SY-neks].

**Vicks Sinex 12-Hour** (ENT).   See *oxymetazoline.* [VIKS-SY-neks].

**Vicodin, Vicodin ES, Vicodin HP** (Analges) (generic *acetaminophen, hydrocodone*).   Combination Schedule III nonnarcotic and narcotic analgesic drug for pain. Tablet: 500 mg/5 mg, 750 mg/7.5 mg, 660 mg/10 mg. [VY-koh-din].

**Vicoprofen** (Analges) (generic *hydrocodone, ibuprofen*).   Combination Schedule III narcotic and NSAID analgesic drug for pain. Tablet: 7.5 mg/200 mg. [VY-koh-PROH-fen].

**Vidaza** (Chemo, Hem).   See *azacitidine.* [vy-DAY-zah].

**Videx, Videx EC** (Anti-infec).   See *didanosine.* [VY-deks].

**Vigamox** (Anti-infec, Ophth).   See *moxifloxacin.* [VIG-ah-mawks].

**viloxazine** (Catatrol) (Neuro).   Used to treat narcolepsy. Orphan drug. [vih-LAWK-sah-zeen].

**vinblastine** (Velban) (Chemo).   Mitosis inhibitor chemotherapy drug used to treat cancer of the breast and testicle; used to treat Hodgkin's lymphoma, mycosis fungoides, and Kaposi's sarcoma. Intravenous: 1 mg/mL. [vin-BLAS-teen].

**Vincasar PFS** (Chemo, Hem).   See *vincristine.* [VIN-kah-sar P-F-S].

**vincristine** (Vincasar PFS) (Chemo, Hem).   Mitosis inhibitor chemotherapy drug used to treat cancer of the brain, breast, lung, muscle, and bladder; used to treat leukemia, Hodgkin's lymphoma, non-Hodgkin's lymphoma, multiple myeloma, Wilms' tumor, and Kaposi's sarcoma; used to treat thrombocytopenia purpura. Intravenous: 1 mg/mL. [vin-KRIS-teen].

**vinorelbine** (Navelbine) (Chemo).   Mitosis inhibitor chemotherapy drug used to treat cancer of the lung, breast, uterus, ovary, and cervix; used to treat Hodgkin's lymphoma, non-Hodgkin's lymphoma, and Kaposi's sarcoma. Intravenous: 10 mg/mL. [vih-NOH-rel-been].

**Viokase 8, Viokase 16** (GI) (generic *amylase, lipase, protease*).   Combination digestive enzyme drug used as replacement therapy. Tablet: 30,000 units/8000 units/30,000 units; 60,000 units/16,000 units/60,000 units. Powder (to be reconstituted): 70,000 units/16,800 units/70,000 units. [VY-oh-kays].

**Viprinex** (Hem).   See *ancrod.* [VIH-prih-neks].

**Viracept** (Anti-infec).   See *nelfinavir.* [VEER-ah-sept].

**Viramune** (Anti-infec).   See *nevirapine.* [VEER-ah-myoon].

**Virazole** (Anti-infec, Pulm).   See *ribivarin.* [VY-rah-zohl].

**Viread** (Anti-infec).   See *tenofovir.* [VY-reed].

**Virilon** (Chemo, Endo).    See *methyltestosterone.* [VEER-eh-lawn].

**Viroptic** (Ophth).    See *trifluridine.* [veer-AWP-tik].

**virulizin** (Chemo).    Used to treat pancreatic cancer. Orphan drug. [vih-ROO-lih-zin].

**Viscoat** (Ophth) (generic *chondroitin, sodium hyaluronate*).    Combination aqueous humor replacement drug injected into the anterior chamber during eye surgery. Intraocular injection: 40 mg/30 mg per mL. [VIS-koht].

**Visicol** (GI).    See *sodium phosphate.* [VIS-ih-kawl].

**Visine, Visine Advanced Relief** (Ophth).    See *tetrahydrozoline.* [VY-zeen].

**Visine LR** (Ophth).    See *oxymetazoline.* [VY-zeen L-R].

**VisionBlue** (Ophth).    See *trypan blue.* [VIH-zhun-BLOO].

**Visken** (Cardio).    See *pindolol.* [VIS-ken].

**Vistaril** (Anes, Derm, Psych).    See *hydroxyzine.* [VIS-tah-ril].

**Vistide** (Anti-infec, Ophth).    See *cidofovir.* [VIS-tide].

**Visudyne** (Ophth).    See *verteporfin.* [VIZ-yoo-dine].

**Vital High Nitrogen** (GI).    Lactose-free nutritional supplement. Powder (to be reconstituted). [VY-tal HY NY-troh-jen].

**vitamin B$_{12}$** (Misc).    See *cyanocobalamin.* [VY-tah-min B-12].

**vitamin C** (Misc).    See *ascorbic acid.* [VY-tah-min C].

**vitamin K** (Hem).    See *phytonadione.* [VY-tah-min K].

**Vitaxin** (Chemo).    Used to treat malignant melanoma. Orphan drug. [vy-TAK-sin].

**Vitelle Nestrex** (OB/GYN, Pulm).    See *pyridoxine.* [vih-TEL NES-treks].

**Vitrase** (Misc).    See *hyaluronidase.* [VIH-trays].

**Vitrasert** (Anti-infec, Ophth).    See *ganciclovir.* [VIH-trah-sert].

**Vivactil** (Analges, Neuro, OB/GYN, Psych).    See *protriptyline.* [vy-VAK-til].

**Vivaglobin, Vivaglobin P** (Anti-infec, Misc).    See *human immune globulin.* [VY-vah-GLOH-bin].

**Vivelle, Vivelle-Dot** (OB/GYN, Ortho).    See *estradiol.* [vy-VEL].

**Vivitrol** (Psych).    See *naltrexone.* [VIV-ih-trawl].

**Vivonex T.E.N.** (GI).    Lactose-free nutritional supplement. Powder (to be reconstituted). [VIH-voh-neks T-E-N].

**Voltaren, Voltaren Gel, Voltaren-XR** (Analges).    See *diclofenac.* [vol-TAIR-en].

**Voluven** (I.V.).    See *hydroethyl starch.* [VAWL-yoo-ven].

**Vopac** (Analges) (generic *acetaminophen, codeine*).    Combination Schedule III nonnarcotic and narcotic analgesic drug for pain.    Tablet: 650 mg/30 mg. [VOH-pak].

**Voraxaze** (Chemo).    See *glucarpidase.* [voh-RAWK-says].

**voriconazole** (Vfend) (Anti-infec).    Antifungal drug used to treat severe systemic fungal and yeast infections such as aspergillosis and candidiasis. Tablet: 50 mg, 200 mg. Intravenous: 40 mg/mL. [VOR-ih-KAWN-ah-zohl].

**vorinostat** (Zolinza) (Chemo).    Chemotherapy drug used to treat mycosis fungoides. Capsule: 100 mg. [voh-RIN-oh-stat].

**VoSpire ER** (Pulm).    See *albuterol.* [voh-SPYR].

**Vumon** (Chemo).    See *teniposide.* [VYOO-mawn].

**Vusion** (Derm) (generic *miconazole, zinc oxide*).    Combination antiyeast and astringent drug used topically to treat diaper rash associated with a yeast infection. Ointment: 0.25%/15%. [VYOO-shun].

**Vytorin** (Cardio) (generic *ezetimibe, simvastatin*).    Combination drug to lower the serum cholesterol level. Tablet: 10 mg/10 mg, 10 mg/20 mg, 10 mg/40 mg, 10 mg/80 mg. [VY-tohr-in].

**Vyvanse** (Psych).    See *lisdexamfetamine.* [VY-vans].

**warfarin** (Coumadin, Jantoven) (Cardio, Hem, Neuro, Pulm).    Anticoagulant drug used to prevent deep venous thrombosis, pulmonary embolism, and a second myocardial infarction or stroke; used in patients with atrial fibrillation and artificial heart valves to prevent clots from forming. Tablet: 1 mg, 2 mg, 2.5 mg, 3 mg, 4 mg, 5 mg, 6 mg, 7.5 mg, 10 mg. Intravenous: 2 mg/mL. [WAR-fah-rin].

**Wart-Off** (Derm).    See *salicylic acid.* [WART-off].

**WelChol** (Cardio, Endo).    See *colesevelam.* [WEL-kawl]

**Wellbutrin, Wellbutrin SR, Wellbutrin XL** (GI, Psych).    See *bupropion.* [wel-BYOO-trin].

**Wellcovorin** (Chemo).    See *leucovorin.* [WEL-koh-VOR-in].

**Wellferon** (Anti-infec).    See *interferon alfa-n1.* [wel-FAIR-awn].

**Westcort** (Derm).    See *hydrocortisone.* [WEST-kort].

**Westhroid** (Endo).    See *desiccated thyroid.* [WEST-throid].

**Whitfield's Ointment** (Derm) (generic *benzoic acid, salicylic acid*).    Combination over-the-counter antifungal and keratolytic drug used topically to treat tinea (ringworm) on the skin. Ointment: 6%/3%. [WHIT-feeld].

**WinRho SDF** (Hem, OB/GYN).    Immunoglobulin drug used to treat immune thrombocytopenia purpura; used after abortion, amniocentesis, or chorionic villus sampling to treat an Rh-negative mother with an Rh-positive baby to prevent hemorrhagic disease of the newborn in a subsequent pregnancy. Intramuscular or intravenous (powder to be reconstituted): 600 units (120 mcg), 1500 units (300 mcg), 2500 units (500 mcg), 5000 units (1000 mcg), 15,000 units (3000 mcg). [WIN-roh S-D-F].

**Women's Tylenol Multi-Symptom Menstrual Relief** (OB/GYN) (generic *acetaminophen, pamabrom*).    Combination over-the-counter analgesic and diuretic drug used to treat dysmenorrhea. Caplet: 500 mg/25 mg. [TY-leh-nawl].

**Wyanoids Relief Factor** (GI) (generic *cocoa butter, shark liver oil*).    Emollient drug used topically to treat hemorrhoids. Suppository. [WHY-ah-noyds].

**Wytensin** (Cardio).    See *guanabenz.* [why-TEN-sin].

**Xalatan** (Ophth).    See *lantanoprost.* [ZAL-ah-tan].

**Xanax** (GI, OB/GYN, Psych). See *alprazolam*. [ZAN-aks].

**Xcytrin** (Chemo) (generic *gadolinium, motexafin*). Combination radioactive drug and chemotherapy drug used to treat brain cancer. Orphan drug. [ek-SY-trin].

**Xeloda** (Chemo). See *capecitabine*. [zeh-LOH-dah].

**Xenazine** (Neuro, Psych). See *tetrabenazine*. [ZEN-ah-zeen].

**Xenical** (GI). See *orlistat*. [ZEN-ih-kal].

**Xerac AC** (Derm). See *aluminum chloride*. [ZEER-ak A-C].

**Xerecept** (Neuro). See *corticotropin-releasing factor*. [ZEER-ah-sept].

**Xibrom** (Ophth). See *bromfenac*. [ZY-brawm].

**Xifaxan** (Anti-infec). See *rifaximin*. [zy-FAK-san].

**Xigris** (Hem). See *drotrecogin alfa*. [ZY-gris].

**Xodol** (Analges) (generic *acetaminophen, hydrocodone*). Combination Schedule III nonnarcotic and narcotic analgesic drug for pain. Capsule: 300 mg/5 mg, 300 mg/7.5 mg, 300 mg/10 mg. [ZOH-dawl].

**Xolair** (Pulm). See *omalizumab*. [ZOH-lair].

**Xolegel** (Derm). See *ketoconazole*. [ZOH-leh-jel].

**Xolegel Duo** (Derm) (generic *ketoconazole, pyrithione zinc*). Combination antifungal and antiseborrheic drug used topically to treat seborrheic dermatitis. Gel/shampoo: 2%/1%. [ZOH-leh-jel DOO-oh].

**Xomazyme-H65** (Chemo). Immunosuppressant drug used to treat graft-versus-host disease after organ transplantation or bone marrow transplantation. Orphan drug. [ZOH-mah-zime H-65].

**Xomazyme-791** (Chemo). Immunosuppressant drug used to treat colon and rectal cancer. Orphan drug. [ZOH-mah-zime-791].

**Xopenex, Xopenex HFA** (Pulm). See *levalbuterol*. [ZOH-peh-neks].

**X-Prep Bowel Evacuant Kit-1** (GI) (generic *bisacodyl, docusate, senna*). Combination over-the-counter irritant/stimulant and stool softener bowel evacuant drug. Oral liquid, oral tablets, suppository. [X-prep].

**X-Prep Liquid** (GI). See *sennosides*. [X-prep].

**Xylocaine, Xylocaine MPF, Xylocaine Viscous** (Anes, Derm, ENT, GI). See *lidocaine*. [ZY-loh-kayn].

**xylometazoline** (Otrivin, Otrivin Pediatric Nasal) (ENT). Over-the-counter decongestant drug used to treat nasal stuffiness due to colds and allergies. Nasal drops/spray: 0.05%, 0.1%. [ZY-loh-MET-ah-ZOH-leen].

**Xyntha** (Hem). See *factor VIII*. [ZIN-thah].

**Xyralid** (Derm, GI) (generic *hydrocortisone, lidocaine*). Combination corticosteroid and anesthetic drug used topically on the skin to treat inflammation and itching; used to treat hemorrhoids. Cream 1%/3%. [ZY-rah-lid].

**Xyrem** (Neuro). See *oxybate*. [ZY-rem].

**Xyzal** (Derm, ENT). See *levocetirizine*. [ZY-zawl].

**Yasmin** (OB/GYN) (generic *drospirenone, ethinyl estradiol*). Combination monophasic oral contraceptive drug. Pill pack, 28-day: (21 hormone tablets) 3 mg/30 mcg; (7 inert tablets). [YAZ-min].

**YAZ** (OB/GYN, Psych) (generic *drospirenone, ethinyl estradiol*). Combination monophasic oral contraceptive drug; used to treat premenstrual dysphoric disorder. Pill pack, 28-day: (24 hormone tablets) 3 mg/20 mcg; (4 inert tablets). [YAZ].

**Yocon** (Uro). See *yohimbine*. [YOH kawn].

**Yodoxin** (Anti-Infec). See *iodoquinol*. [yoh-DAWK-sin].

**yohimbine** (Aphrodyne, Yocon) (Uro). Used to treat male impotence. Tablet: 5.4 mg. [yoh-HIM-been].

**Yondelis** (Chemo). See *trabectedin*. [yawn-DEL-is].

**Zactima** (Chemo). See *vandetanib*. [ZAK-tih-mah].

**Zadaxin** (Chemo, GI). See *thymalfasin*. [zah-DAK-sin].

**Zaditor** (Ophth). See *ketotifen*. [ZAD-ih-tor].

**zafirlukast** (Accolate) (Pulm). Leukotriene receptor blocker drug used to prevent and treat asthma. Tablet: 10 mg, 20 mg. [zah-FIR-loo-kast].

**zalcitabine** (Hivid) (Anti-infec). Nucleoside reverse transcriptase inhibitor antiviral drug used to treat HIV and AIDS. Tablet: 0.375 mg, 0.75 mg. [zal-SY-tah-been].

**zaleplon** (Sonata) (Neuro). Schedule IV nonbarbiturate sedative drug used to treat insomnia. Capsule: 5 mg, 10 mg. [ZAL-eh-plawn].

**Zamyl** (Chemo). See *lintuzumab*. [ZAH-mil].

**Zanaflex** (Neuro, Ortho). See *tizanidine*. [ZAN-ah-fleks].

**zanamivir** (Relenza) (Anti-infec, Pulm). Antiviral drug used to treat influenza A or influenza B virus infection. Blister pak (powder for inhalation): 5 mg. [zan-AM-ih-veer].

**Zanosar** (Chemo). See *streptozocin*. [ZAN-oh-sar].

**Zantac, Zantac 75, Zantac 150 Maximum Strength, Zantac EFFERdose** (GI). See *ranitidine*. [ZAN-tak].

**Zarnestra** (Chemo). See *tipifarnib*. [zar-NES-trah].

**Zarontin** (Neuro). See *ethosuximide*. [zah-RAWN-tin].

**Zaroxolyn** (Cardio, Uro). See *metolazone*. [zah-RAWK-soh-lin].

**Zavesca** (Misc). See *miglustat*. [zah-VES-kah].

**Zazole** (OB/GYN). See *terconazole*. [ZAY-zohl].

**Zeasorb-AF** (Derm). See *miconazole*. [ZEE-ah-sorb-A-F].

**Zebeta** (Cardio). See *bisoprolol*. [zeh-BAY-tah].

**Zecnil** (GI). See *somatostatin*. [ZEK-nil].

**Zegerid** (GI) (generic *omeprazole, sodium bicarbonate*). Combination proton pump inhibitor and antacid drug used to treat esophagitis and GERD. Capsule: 20 mg/1100 mg. Powder (to be reconstituted to an oral liquid): 20 mg/1680 mg, 40 mg/1680 mg. [ZEH-geh-rid].

**Zelapar** (Neuro). See *selegiline*. [ZEL-ah-par].

**Zemaira** (Pulm). See *alpha$_1$-proteinase inhibitor*. [zeh-MAIR-ah].

**Zemplar** (Endo). See *paricalcitol*. [ZEM-plar].

**Zemuron** (Anes, Pulm). See *rocuronium*. [ZEM-yoor-awn].

**Zenapax** (Chemo, Uro). See *daclizumab*. [ZEE-nah-paks].

**Zephiran** (Derm).   See *benzalkonium*. [ZEF-ih-ran].

**Zerit** (Anti-infec).   See *stavudine*. [ZAIR-it].

**Zestoretic** (Cardio) (generic *lisinopril, hydrochlorothiazide*). Combination ACE inhibitor and diuretic drug used to treat hypertension. Tablet: 10 mg/12.5 mg, 20 mg/12.5 mg, 20 mg/25 mg. [ZES-toh-REH-tik].

**Zestril** (Cardio).   See *lisinopril*. [ZES-tril].

**Zetuvet** (Derm) (generic *sodium sulfacetamide, sulfur*) Combination keratolytic drug used topically on the skin to treat acne vulgaris. Suspension or wash: 10%/5%. [ZEE-tah-set].

**Zetar** (Derm).   See *coal tar*. [ZEE-tar].

**Zetia** (Cardio).   See *ezetimibe*. [ZET-ee-ah].

**Zevalin** (Chemo) (generic *ibritumomab, indium-111, yttrium-90*).   Combination monoclonal antibody and radioactive monoclonal antibody drug used to treat non-Hodgkin's lymphoma. Intravenous: 3.2 mg/2 mL. [ZEV-AH-LIN].

**Ziac** (Cardio) (generic *bisoprolol, hydrochlorothiazide*). Combination beta-blocker and diuretic drug used to treat hypertension. Tablet: 2.5 mg/6.25 mg, 5 mg/6.25 mg, 10 mg/6.25 mg. [ZY-ak].

**Ziagen** (Anti-infec).   See *abacavir*. [ZY-ah-jen].

**Ziana** (Derm) (generic *clindamycin, tretinoin*).   Combination antibiotic and vitamin-A type drug used topically on the skin to treat acne vulgaris. Gel: 1.2%/0.025%. [zy-AN-ah].

**ziconotide** (Prialt) (Analges).   Used to treat severe, chronic pain in patients who cannot take other analgesic drugs. Intrathecal solution: 25 mcg/mL, 100 mcg/mL. [zih-KAWN-oh-tide].

**zidovudine** (Retrovir) (Anti-infec).   Nucleoside reverse transcriptase inhibitor antiviral drug used to treat HIV and AIDS; used to prevent transmission of HIV from mother to fetus before birth. Capsule: 100 mg. Tablet: 300 mg. Syrup: 50 mg/5 mL.Oral liquid: 50 mg/5 mL. Intravenous: 10 mg/mL. [zy-DOH-vyoo-deen].

**Zilactin-B Medicated** (Anes, ENT).   See *benzocaine*. [ZY-lak-tin].

**Zilactin-L** (Anes, Derm).   See *lidocaine*. [ZY-lak-tin].

**zileuton** (Zyflo CR) (Pulm).   Leukotriene receptor blocker drug used to prevent and treat asthma. Controlled-release tablet: 600 mg. [zy-LOO-ton].

**Zinacef** (Anti-infec).   See *cefuroxime*. [ZIN-ah-sef].

**zinc acetate** (Galzin) (Misc).   Used to treat Wilson's disease. Orphan drug. [ZINK AS-eh-tayt].

**Zincon** (Derm).   See *pyrithione zinc*. [ZIN-con].

**zinc oxide** (Dr. Smith's Adult Care, Dr. Smith's Diaper Ointment, Tronolane Suppository) (Derm, GI). Over-the-counter astringent and protectant drug used topically to treat skin irritation, diaper rash, and dry, oozing skin; used to treat the swelling and pain of hemorrhoids (Tronolane). Lotion: 1%. Ointment: 10%, 20%. Suppository. [ZINK AWK-side].

**Zinecard** (Cardio, Chemo).   See *dexrazoxane*. [ZIN-eh-kard].

**Zingo** (Anes).   See *lidocaine*. [ZING-goh].

**ziprasidone** (Geodon) (Neuro, Psych).   Antipsychotic drug used to treat schizophrenia; used to treat mania in patients with manic-depressive disorder; used to treat psychosis and agitation in patients with Alzheimer's disease and Parkinson's disease. Capsule: 20 mg, 40 mg, 60 mg, 80 mg. Intramuscular: 20 mg. [zih-PRAS-ih-dohn].

**Ziradryl** (Derm) (generic *diphenhydramine, zinc oxide*). Combination over-the-counter antihistamine and astringent drug used topically on the skin to treat itching and oozing. Lotion: 1%. [ZEER-ah-dril].

**Zixoryn** (Hem).   See *flumicinol*. [zik-SOR-rin].

**Zithromax** (Anti-infec).   See *azithromycin*. [ZIH-throh-maks].

**Zmax** (Anti-infec).   See *azithromycin*. [Z-maks].

**ZNP Bar** (Derm).   See *pyrithione zinc*. [Z-N-P].

**Zocor** (Cardio).   See *simvastatin*. [ZOH-kor].

**Zoderm** (Derm).   See *benzoyl peroxide*. [ZOH-derm].

**Zofran, Zofran ODT** (Chemo, GI).   See *ondansetron*. [ZOH-fran].

**Zoladex** (Chemo, OB/GYN).   See *goserelin*. [ZOL-ah-deks].

**zoledronic acid** (Reclast, Zometa) (Chemo, Ortho).   Bone resorption inhibitor drug used to treat osteoporosis in postmenopausal women; used to treat hypercalcemia caused by malignancy; used to treat bony metastases of tumors; used to treat Paget's disease; used to treat multiple myeloma. Intravenous: 4 mg/5 mL, 4 mg/100 mL. [zoh-leh-DROH-nik AS-id].

**Zolinza** (Chemo).   See *vorinostat*. [zoh-LIN-zah].

**zolmitriptan** (Zomig, Zomig ZMT) (Analges).   Serotonin receptor agonist drug used to treat migraine headaches. Nasal spray: 5 mg/spray. Tablet: 2.5 mg, 5 mg, Orally disintegrating tablet: 2.5 mg. [ZOL-mih-TRIP-tan].

**Zoloft** (Psych).   See *sertraline*. [ZOH-lawft].

**zolpidem** (Ambien, Ambien CR) (Neuro).   Schedule IV sedative drug used to treat insomnia. Tablet: 5 mg, 10 mg. Extended-release tablet: 6.25 mg, 12.5 mg. [ZOL-pih-dem].

**Zometa** (Chemo, Ortho).   See *zoledronic acid*. [zoh-MEE-tah].

**Zomig, Zomig ZMT** (Analges).   See *zolmitriptan*. [ZOH-mig].

**Zonalon** (Derm).   See *doxepin*. [ZOH-nah-lawn].

**Zonegran** (Neuro).   See *zonisamide*. [ZOH-neh-gran].

**zonisamide** (Zonegran) (Neuro).   Anticonvulsant drug used to treat complex partial and simple partial seizures. Capsule: 25 mg, 50 mg, 100 mg. [zoh-NIS-ah-mide].

**Zorbtive** (Endo, GI).   See *somatropin*. [ZORB-tiv].

**ZORprin** (Analges).   See *aspirin*. [ZOR-prin].

**Zostavax** (Derm).   Used to prevent shingles (herpes zoster) from occurring in older adults. Subcutaneous: Vaccine. [ZAWS-tah-vaks].

**Zostrix, Zostrix-HP, Zostrix Neuropathy Cream** (Derm, Ortho, Neuro).   See *capsaicin*. [ZAW-striks].

**zosuquidar** (Chemo).   Chemotherapy drug used to treat leukemia. Orphan drug. [zoh-SOO-kwih-dar].

**Zosyn** (Anti-infec) (generic *piperacillin, tazobactam*). Combination penicillin-type antibiotic and penicillinase inhibitor drug used to treat penicillin-resistant bacteria. Intravenous (powder to be reconstituted): 2 g/0.25 g, 3 g/375 g, 4 g/0.5 g. [ZOH-sin].

**Zovia 1/35E, Zovia 1/50** (OB/GYN) (generic *ethynodiol, ethinyl estradiol*).   Combination monophasic oral contraceptive drug. Pill pack (Compack), 21-day: (21 hormone tablets) 1 mg/35 mcg. Pill pack (Compack), 28-day: (21 hormone tablets) 1 mg/35 mcg; (7 inert tablets). Pill pack (Compack), 21-day: (21 hormone tablets) 1 mg/50 mcg. Pill pack (Compack), 28-day: (21 hormone tablets) 1 mg/50 mcg; (7 inert tablets). [ZOH-vee-ah].

**Zovirax** (Anti-infec, Derm, OB/GYN).   See *acyclovir.* [zoh-VY-raks].

**Zucapsaicin** (ENT).   See *civamide.* [ZOO-kap-SAY-ih-sin].

**Zurase** (Chemo).   Used to prevent hyperuricemia and tumor lysis syndrome in patients receiving chemotherapy. Orphan drug. [ZOOR-ays].

**Z-Xtra** (Derm) (generic *benzocaine, zinc oxide*). Combination over-the-counter anesthetic and astringent drug used topically to numb the skin and decrease oozing. [z-EK-strah].

**Zyban** (Psych, Pulm).   See *bupropion.* [ZY-ban].

**Zydone** (Analges) (generic *acetaminophen, hydrocodone*). Combination Schedule III nonsalicylate and narcotic analgesic drug for pain. Tablet: 400 mg/5 mg, 400 mg/7.5 mg, 400 mg/10 mg. [ZY-dohn].

**Zyflo CR** (Pulm).   See *zileuton.* [ZY-floh C-R].

**Zylet** (Ophth) (generic *ioteprednol, tobramycin*). Combination corticosteroid and antibiotic drug used topically in the eyes to treat inflammation and bacterial infections. Ophthalmic suspension: 0.5%/0.3%. [ZY-let].

**Zyloprim** (Chemo, Ortho, Uro).   See *allopurinol.* [ZY-loh-prim].

**Zymar** (Ophth).   See *gatafloxacin.* [ZY-mar].

**Zymine** (Derm, ENT, Ophth).   See *triprolidine.* [ZY-meen].

**Zyprexa, Zyprexa Zydis** (Neuro, Psych).   See *olanzapine.* [zy-PREK-sah].

**Zyrtec, Children's Zyrtec Allergy, Children's Zyrtec Hives Relief** (Derm, ENT).   See *cetirizine.* [ZIR-tek].

**Zyrtec-D 12 Hour** (Derm, ENT) (generic *cetirizine, pseudoephedrine*).   Combination antihistamine and decongestant drug used to treat seasonal and perennial allergies and allergic rhinitis; used to treat allergic skin reactions with itching. Tablet: 5 mg/120 mg. [ZIR-tek].

**Zytopic** (Ophth).   See *triamcinolone.* [zy-TAW-pik].

**Zyvox** (Anti-infec).   See *linezolid.* [ZY-vawks].

# *Photo Credits*

**Page XXI:** David W. Harbaugh.

## Chapter 1

**Page 4:** (top) Steve Bartholomew © Dorling Kindersley. **Page 5:** Elena Dorfman © Pearson Education/PH College. **Page 6:** © Phil Schermeister/CORBIS. **Page 8:** Getty Images, Inc. **Page 9:** Copyright Eli Lilly and Company. Used with permission. **Page 12:** National Library of Medicine. **Page 17:** Getty Images, Inc. **Page 20:** (bottom) Copyright Novartis Pharmaceuticals Corporation. Reprinted with permission.

## Chapter 2

**Page 23:** Jacob Halaska © Photolibrary.com. **Page 28:** David W. Harbaugh. **Page 34:** (bottom) Copyright Eli Lilly and Company. Used with permission.

## Chapter 3

**Page 36:** Boehringer Ingelheim Pharmaceuticals, Inc. **Page 37:** (bottom) David W. Harbaugh. **Page 40:** (top) Nathan Eldridge © Pearson Education/PH College, (bottom) Michal Heron © Pearson Education/PH College. **Page 41:** Used with permission of Roxane Laboratories, Inc. **Page 42:** (top) David W. Harbaugh, (bottom) Registered Trademark of Pfizer Inc. Reproduced with Permission. **Page 43:** Corbis © Pearson Education/PH College. **Page 45:** (bottom) © Pearson Education/PH College.

## Chapter 4

**Page 47:** Jenny Thomas Photography. **Page 49:** (top) David Young-Wolff © PhotoEdit Inc. **Page 50:** John Greim/Science Photo Library © Photo Researchers, Inc. **Page 52:** Photo reprinted courtesy of BD (Becton, Dickinson and Company). **Page 53:** Elena Dorfman © Pearson Education/PH College. **Page 55:** Nathan Eldridge © Pearson Education/PH College.

## Chapter 5

**Page 67:** © ScienceCartoonsPlus.com. **Page 69:** David W. Harbaugh. **Page 70:** Corbis—Brand X Pictures. **Page 75:** David W. Harbaugh. **Page 77:** Photo reprinted courtesy of BD (Becton, Dickinson and Company).

## Chapter 6

**Page 83:** © Frozen Images/The Image Works. **Page 85:** © Pearson Education/PH College. **Page 91:** © Pearson Education/PH College. **Page 92:** (bottom) Getty Images. **Page 93:** (top) Corbis—Brand X Pictures. **Page 95:** © Pearson Education/PH College.

## Chapter 7

**Page 103:** Copyright Abbott Labs. Reprinted with permission. **Page 107:** (top) Reproduced with Permission of Pfizer Inc. All rights reserved, (bottom) Merck & Co., Inc. **Page 108:** Reproduced with permission of GlaxoSmithKline. **Page 112:** (top, bottom) © Pearson Education/PH College.

## Chapter 8

**Page 117:** (top) Michael Newman © PhotoEdit Inc. **Page 120:** AstraZeneca Pharmaceuticals LP. **Page 121:** AstraZeneca Pharmaceuticals LP. **Page 128:** (bottom) Reproduced with Permission of Pfizer Inc. All rights reserved. **Page 134:** Copyright GlaxoSmithKline. Used with permission.

## Chapter 9

**Page 138:** (bottom) Copyright Novartis Pharmaceuticals Corporation. Reprinted with permission. **Page 142:** Yoav Levy © Phototake NYC. **Page 144:** Jane Burton © Dorling Kindersley. **Page 150:** (top, bottom) © Pearson Education/PH College.

## Chapter 10

**Page 154:** Reproduced with the permission of Schering Corporation and Key Pharmaceuticals, Inc. All rights reserved. PROVENTIL is a registered trademark of Schering Corporation. **Page 155:** (top) Copyright GlaxoSmithKline. Used with permission. **Page 158:** The label for the product Singulair 10mg is reproduced with permission of Merck & Co., Inc., copyright owner. **Page 166:** (bottom, left and right) Copyright GlaxoSmithKline. Used with permission.

## Chapter 11

**Page 171:** Copyright Novartis Pharmaceuticals Corporation. Reprinted with permission. **Page 173:** Reproduced with Permission of Pfizer Inc. All rights reserved. **Page 174:** The label for the product Cozaar 25 mg is reproduced with permission of Merck & Co., Inc., copyright owner. **Page 177:** Registered Trademark of Pfizer Inc. Reproduced with Permission. **Page 178:** The label for the product Zocor 40 mg is reproduced with permission of Merck & Co., Inc., copyright owner. **Page 180:** (top) Used with permission of Roxane Laboratories, Inc. **Page 182:** www.imageafter.com. **Page 188:** Nathan Eldridge © Pearson Education/PH College. **Page 191:** © Pearson Education/PH College. **Page 192:** (bottom) Registered Trademark of Pfizer Inc. Reproduced with Permission. **Page 193:** (top) Registered Trademark of Pfizer Inc. Reproduced with Permission.

## Chapter 12

**Page 202:** Skatz © Amgen Inc. **Page 203:** Getty Images. **Page 204:** © Pearson Education/PH College.

## Chapter 13

**Page 208:** B. Daemmrich © The Image Works. **Page 210:** Custom Medical Stock Photo, Inc. **Page 212:** Reuters NewMedia Inc © Reuters Limited. **Page 213:** Saturn Stills © Photo Researchers, Inc. **Page 214:** Custom Medical Stock Photo, Inc. **Page 217:** David W. Harbaugh. **Page 221:** Reproduced with Permission of Pfizer Inc. All rights reserved. **Page 228:** Custom Medical Stock Photo, Inc.

## Chapter 14

**Page 233:** (top) Copyright Eli Lilly and Company. Used with permission, (bottom) SIU BioMed © Custom Medical Stock Photo, Inc.

# Index